FUNDAMENTAL
IMMUNOLOGY

SECOND EDITION

FUNDAMENTAL IMMUNOLOGY

SECOND EDITION

Robert M. Coleman
University of Massachusetts
at Lowell

Mary F. Lombard
Regis College

Raymond E. Sicard
University of Minnesota

 Wm. C. Brown Publishers

Book Team

Editor *Colin H. Wheatley*
Developmental Editor *Elizabeth M. Sievers*
Production Editor *Marlys Nekola*
Designer *Christopher E. Reese*
Art Editor *Mary E. Swift*
Photo Editor *Carrie Burger*
Visuals Processor *Mary E. Swift*

Wm. C. Brown Publishers

President *G. Franklin Lewis*
Vice President, Publisher *George Wm. Bergquist*
Vice President, Operations and Production *Beverly Kolz*
National Sales Manager *Virginia S. Moffat*
Group Sales Manager *Vincent R. Di Blasi*
Vice President, Editor in Chief *Edward G. Jaffe*
Marketing Manager *John W. Calhoun*
Advertising Manager *Amy Schmitz*
Managing Editor, Production *Colleen A. Yonda*
Manager of Visuals and Design *Faye M. Schilling*
Production Editorial Manager *Julie A. Kennedy*
Production Editorial Manager *Ann Fuerste*
Publishing Services Manager *Karen J. Slaght*

WCB Group

President and Chief Executive Officer *Mark C. Falb*
Chairman of the Board *Wm. C. Brown*

Copyeditor Beatrice Sussman

Library of Congress Catalog Card Number: 91-71607

ISBN 0-697-11310-8

Printed in the United States of America by Wm. C. Brown Publishers, 2460 Kerper Boulevard, Dubuque, IA 52001

10 9 8 7 6 5 4 3 2 1

CONTENTS

P R E F A C E

Numerous advances continue to be made in immunology. Although some do not substantively alter our perception of the essential functioning of the immune system, they extend our understanding of how this is accomplished. *Fundamental Immunology* was revised for two reasons. First, periodic revision is required to maintain current perspectives on the topics presented. This is especially important in a field like immunology. Second, we wished to incorporate suggestions for reorganization intended to make immunology more accessible to beginning students.

The first edition of *Fundamental Immunology* was written to make immunology more accessible to students at an early stage in their academic careers. The positive responses to the first edition encouraged us to continue in this endeavor. As in the first edition, the second edition of *Fundamental Immunology* introduces the reader to various aspects of immunology through discussions incorporating both traditional topics in immunology and background information intended for the relatively uninitiated. In particular, section 1, Introduction, provides a general orientation to immunology. Certain concepts and the major effectors of immune responses are introduced and later, more detailed, discussions anticipated. Section 2, Essentials of Immunological Expression, then presents the central aspects of humoral and cellular immune responses, both nonspecific and specific. Finally, section 3, Immunity and Disease, and section 4, Ontogeny and Phylogeny of Immunity, explore special topics in immunology. Advances occurring since the first edition have been incorporated into the text, and relevant citations added to the list of additional readings following each chapter.

Numerous suggestions from users of the first edition have guided us in revising the text. The second edition of *Fundamental Immunology* incorporates three major changes. First, background information has been consolidated and abbreviated, reducing the total number of chapters in the second edition. For example, the introductory section has been reduced from four chapters in the first edition to two chapters in the second. In addition, discussion of agents of infectious disease has been reduced from two chapters to one (chapter 11). Second, discussion of certain aspects of immune responses has been reorganized, modifying section 2. For example, chapter 3, Effectors of Humoral Immunity, and chapter 5, Antibody Production, Regulation, and Diversity, reflect inclusion of information about B cell differentiation that had formerly appeared in other chapters. In addition, discussion of cellular immunity has been reorganized to emphasize the nature and roles of effectors of nonspecific (chapter 8) and specific (chapter 9) cellular immunity. Third, certain topics have been expanded to reflect major attention that has been focused on them in the last few years. In particular, this has led to inclusion of chapters on immune tolerance and suppression (chapter 10) and on acquired immune deficiency syndrome (chapter 15). Both topics had formerly comprised sections of chapters in the first edition.

The central pedagogy of the second edition of *Fundamental Immunology* retains the major features of the first edition. Each section and unit is preceded by a brief statement, orienting the reader to the focus of that chapter or unit. This is reinforced by chapter overviews and a short list of concepts central to each chapter. These devices anticipate the thrust of each chapter and provide a perspective for the reader in the discussions that follow. Chapter summaries then recapitulate the essential points presented. Numerous tables and figures are provided throughout to assist the reader in grasping the topics discussed. These are supplemented by a glossary, four appendices, and two review tables (located inside the front and back covers).

The information within these pedagogical devices has been revised to reflect new material. In addition, the list of terms within the glossary has been expanded. Furthermore, the usefulness of the chapter summaries to the reader has been enhanced by adding references to page numbers where discussion for each point can be found.

We are grateful to users of the first edition and reviewers of the second edition for sharing their thoughts and reactions with us. For improvements to the second edition of *Fundamental Immunology* we gratefully acknowledge the assistance of Thomas Wolf, Washburn University; Doris L. Lefkowitz, Texas Tech University; Robert I. Krasner, Providence College; Yvonne Boyd-Bartlett, V.A. Medical Center, New York, N.Y.; Linda C. Twining, Northeast Missouri State University; Kent R. Thomas, Kansas

Newman College; Dean A. Hoganson, Drake University; Linda D. Caren, California State University, Northridge; Fred M. McCorkle, Central Michigan University; and Kay Doyle, University of Massachusetts at Lowell. We also wish to thank the editorial and production staff at Wm. C. Brown for their efforts in guiding this project through its several stages.

For those instances in which we fall short of our goal, we assume responsibility. Nevertheless, in our continued endeavor to bring the central concepts and excitement of the field of immunology to others, we invite comments, suggestions, and corrections from our readers and colleagues.

R. M. C.
M. F. L.
R. E. S.

Introduction

UNIT *1* Overview of Immunology

Mastery of any subject requires an understanding of the language used, familiarity with the nature and operation of the components or tools, and an appreciation of the broader context into which the subject fits. Accordingly, unit 1 provides the essential background and framework for an exploration of the immune system and its role in disease. Chapter 1, Introduction to the Study of Immunology, provides an orientation to health and disease as contrasting states in our endeavor to maintain homeostasis and introduces you to some of the language of immunology. This chapter acquaints you with several general mechanisms of disease. In addition, certain of the central concepts and terminology encountered throughout this book are introduced. Moreover, chapter 1 provides a historical context by tracing some of the major developments that have occurred in the field of immunology. The tools through which immunity is expressed are defined in chapter 2, Cells and Tissues of the Immune System. Here the composition of the immune system is presented and the major players are identified. Consequently, this unit provides a general foundation for exploring the functional expression of the immune system that is presented in section 2.

CHAPTER 1

Introduction to the Study of Immunology

OVERVIEW

The role of homeostasis in health and disease is outlined. Major components of the internal environment and certain classes of cells that play significant roles in preserving the organism's steady state are described. A general description of types and causes of disease states is provided. In addition, a brief survey of developments in our understanding of immunity is presented. Moreover, the central elements involved in immune responses are identified and introduced.

CONCEPTS

1. Cells live in an internal environment whose nature is actively maintained in a dynamic steady state.

2. Disease represents a disturbance of this steady state.

3. Disease can arise from a variety of sources, which include infection by foreign agents, cellular transformation, or failure of regulatory organs to function properly.

4. Protection against infective agents, known as immunity, may be innate or can be acquired. Expressions of this protection can make use of circulating factors, specific cell types, or a combination of both.

5. Immune responses are usually triggered by exposure to foreign substances, called antigens, and often evoke the production of specific antagonists, called antibodies. Alternatively, the immune response can be expressed by the direct participation of specific effector cells.

6. Several cell types, each with its own assigned role, constitute the immune system and are responsible for host defense and immunity.

Each of us is a self-contained world. We exist within a larger environment that we recognize outside ourselves. Yet we contain, within ourselves, another environment, an internal environment, in which our individual cells live. If we reflect momentarily over the past weeks or months, we can recall that we felt healthy most of the time, but on occasion we felt sick or out of sorts. We contrast these two states by our own perception of how we feel. But what do these conditions of healthy and sick actually reflect?

■   ■   ■   ■   ■   ■   ■   ■   ■   ■

CONCEPTS OF HEALTH AND DISEASE

In this section, we examine what it means physiologically to be healthy. In addition, we consider, in similar terms, what has occurred to make us feel sick. Last, a number of categories of disease conditions are defined, and a general sense of how these might be caused is provided.

Health and Homeostasis

When we feel healthy we experience a sense of physical and mental well-being. The body appears to be in harmony with the external environment, and there is order in bodily functions. In contrast, when we are ill, our bodies are not in harmony with the external environment, and disorder appears to exist in bodily functions. In short, physically and mentally we do not feel comfortable; there is a functional sense of *dis*-ease. Good health, then, reflects a harmonious balance among the various bodily organ systems. This order and harmony is achieved through a complex interaction of these systems to ensure the maintenance of steady-state conditions within our internal environment.

Homeostasis

The internal environment consists of the body fluids that bathe and nourish every cell of our bodies. The term **homeostasis,** from the Greek *homeos* (the same) and *stasis* (standing), is used to describe the actively maintained steady-state conditions existing in healthy individuals. This notion has existed for some time. The renowned French physiologist **Claude Bernard** (1813–1878), is responsible for introducing, in the 1850s, the notion of an **internal environment,** *le milieu intérieur,* as an integral factor in health and disease. However, it was not until the 1930s that the term homeostasis was introduced by Harvard physiologist **Walter Bradford Cannon** (1875–1945), to describe the steady-state conditions and the processes involved in their maintenance.

It is important to discriminate between homeostasis and equilibrium. **Equilibrium,** which occurs in any chemical reaction, is achieved through essentially *passive* activities of the components involved as a balance is created within the system. If a change is brought about in part of the system, a *new* "final state," or *equilibrium point,* is reached (fig. 1.1*a*). In contrast, through homeostasis, the steady state is *actively* maintained by means of regulatory adjustments that compensate for efforts to impose change on the internal environment. In this case, a temporary change occurs within the system, but the self-regulatory processes of homeostasis eventually restore the *original* steady-state conditions (fig. 1.1*b*).

For example, if additional substance is added to one side of a two-compartment system in chemical equilibrium, the balance is disturbed. As a result of the law of mass action, particles eventually redistribute themselves between both compartments to achieve a *new balance* within the system. This is shown in figure 1.1*a*. In the biological system governed by homeostasis, the situation is different. If the state of the internal environment is altered, it is reestablished. For instance, after eating a meal our blood glucose level rises. This causes glucose to be removed from the blood and stored, thereby reducing the blood glucose level. On the other hand, if we miss a meal, our blood glucose level drops; glucose is then returned to the blood, thus raising the level to the desired steady state. This is diagrammatically portrayed in figure 1.1*b*. In effect, the equilibrium state is affected by and is dependent upon existing conditions, whereas the steady state of homeostasis is essentially *independent* of external conditions.

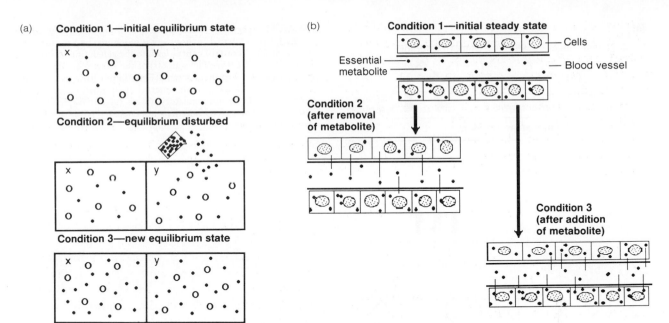

FIGURE 1.1 Equilibrium and homeostasis. (*a*) At equilibrium, there is a balance between the contents of compartment X and compartment Y (*condition 1*). If additional substance is added to one compartment (*condition 2*), redistribution between both compartments will occur in order to establish a **new** equilibrium state (*condition 3*). Both equilibrium states (*conditions 1 and 3*) are different. (*b*) In the case of homeostasis, steady-state conditions exist (*condition 1*) that are ac-

tively maintained. If an essential component is removed, adjustments are made that lead to their replacement to reestablish the **original** steady state (*condition 2*). If, on the other hand, the level of an essential component is increased, activities are initiated to remove the excess, thereby restoring the **original** steady state (*condition 3*). All three steady-state conditions are the same.

The efficient operation of our bodies in homeostasis depends upon three factors. First, there must be a **sensor** to monitor the internal environment and detect when a change occurs. Second, there must be an **effector** to produce an appropriate response to the change sensed. The communication between sensor and effector is called *input*. The action of the effector is called *output*. In addition, there must be **feedback** to the effector, providing information about the consequences of its activity. Feedback is considered **positive** if it causes the output of the effector to be *increased*. **Negative** feedback, on the other hand, *decreases* the output of the effector. The relationship among these factors can be schematically represented as in figure 1.2.

Body Fluids

We are air-breathing organisms; however, the individual cells that make up the tissues and organs of our bodies are actually bathed in fluid. This fluid environment provided for each cell is the means through which

essential substances (e.g., nutrients and oxygen) are delivered to them and wastes (e.g., metabolic byproducts and carbon dioxide) are eliminated. Moreover, it is through this medium that many facets of communication between cells occur.

The body fluids are found in three compartments. These are (1) the **cardiovascular system,** which is comprised of the heart, veins, arteries, and capillaries; (2) the **lymphatic system,** which consists of lymph nodes and a system of veinlike channels; and (3) the **interstitial fluid,** which includes all extracellular fluids not found within the other two enclosed networks. Figure 1.3 depicts the interrelationship among these enclosed compartments, the interstitial fluid, and the cells that they bathe and nourish.

The interstitial fluid is the immediate environment for most cells. Its composition is greatly affected by interactions with the cardiovascular system. The cardiovascular system plays a very significant role as the conduit for delivery of oxygen and nutrients to,

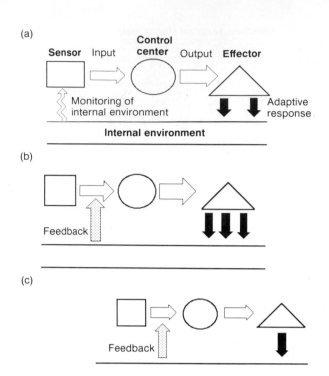

(a)

Sensor   Input   **Control center**   Output   **Effector**

Monitoring of internal environment

Adaptive response

Internal environment

(b)

Feedback

(c)

Feedback

FIGURE 1.2 Schematic representation of homeostatic regulatory systems. (*a*) The internal environment is monitored by a **sensor.** The sensor's *input* to a **control center** leads to the generation of an *output* "signal" to an **effector.** The action(s) of the effector are directed at countering the change in the internal environment that was detected by the sensor. *Feedback* from the internal environment modifies the continued activity of this regulatory system. (*b*) *Positive* feedback *increases* the level of activity initially stimulated. (*c*) *Negative* feedback *decreases* the activity caused by the change.

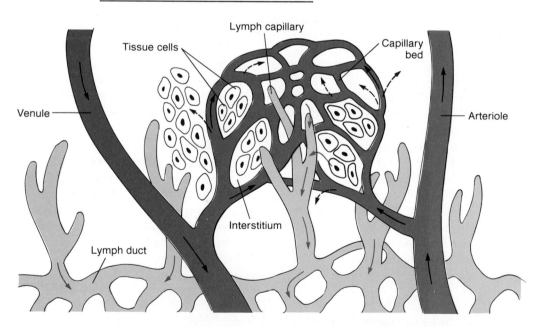

Lymph capillary

Tissue cells

Capillary bed

Venule

Arteriole

Interstitium

Lymph duct

FIGURE 1.3 Interrelationship among compartments of the internal environment. The cells of the body are bathed directly by the **interstitial fluid.** This compartment communicates with **capillaries** of the *lymphatic* and *cardiovascular* systems. Through this association, essential materials (nutrients, oxygen, etc.) and wastes (carbon dioxide, metabolic byproducts, etc.) can be exchanged. *Solid arrows* depict the general direction of circulatory flow (*black arrows* depict cardiovascular flow, arterial to venous; *colored arrows* depict lymphatic flow). *Broken arrows* represent exchange between compartments. (From Kent M. Van De Graaff, *Human Anatomy.* Copyright © 1984 Wm. C. Brown Publishers, Dubuque, Iowa. All rights reserved. Reprinted by permission.)

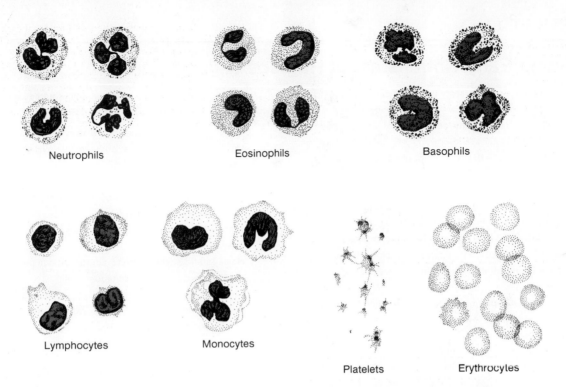

Neutrophils   **Eosinophils**   **Basophils**

Lymphocytes   **Monocytes**   **Platelets**   **Erythrocytes**

FIGURE 1.4 Cells found in human blood. Human blood contains erythrocytes, platelets, and a variety of leukocytes. The leukocytes are classified according to physical attributes readily distinguished in stained blood smears. These cells are *monocytes, lymphocytes, eosino-* *phils* (containing large pinkish-orange granules), *basophils* (containing large purplish-black granules), and *neutrophils* (containing only small cytoplasmic granules).

and the means through which wastes are removed from, the interstitial fluid. These functions are accomplished by the fluid contained within this system, the blood. Blood, which accounts for approximately 8% of body weight, is composed of a fluid phase, plasma, and a particulate phase, the blood cells.

Plasma is responsible for *transporting nutrients, wastes, and informational molecules* which pass as signals between cells. This function is accomplished when nutrients are absorbed through the walls of the intestines, when oxygen dissolves into the blood after crossing the alveoli of the lungs, and following secretion of hormones by endocrine glands. Final elimination of waste is ultimately achieved only by filtration of the plasma by the kidneys. In addition to serving as a solvent, plasma contains a number of molecules that enable it to gel, or *clot*. This transformation from a liquid to colloidal state provides one means of defense

against excessive blood loss after injury. Other molecules, like those in the complement system, participate in *defense* of the organism (discussed in chapter 6).

Blood Cells

The particulate phase of blood contains three major types of cells. These are **erythrocytes** (red blood cells), **leukocytes** (white blood cells), and **platelets.** The appearance of these cells, based on their features in stained blood smears, can be seen in figure 1.4.

Erythrocytes   The small (7 μm diameter), round, enucleate (no nucleus) erythrocytes are the most abundant of the formed elements of blood. There are typically between 2 and 5 $\times$ 10^{12} erythrocytes in every liter of blood. This mass of cells accounts for 40% to 48% of blood volume. (The *hematocrit* refers to the volume of blood due to packed red blood cells. Thus,

Some Early Notions about Homeostasis

Throughout history efforts have been made to understand how the human body works. Although many individuals have contributed to generating this knowledge, two in particular stand out for their contributions to the concept of homeostasis.

The first is Claude Bernard, whose failure to succeed as a playwright led to a career in medicine and research. His many contributions to the field of physiology include the notion that there is an internal environment (*milieu intérieur*) that is important to health and survival. Bernard's concept of the internal environment and the role it played was rather different than the notion that we have today.

To Bernard, all life could be placed into one of three categories: (1) latent life, (2) oscillating life, and (3) constant life. *Latent life* did not actively manifest the features of life. Seeds, spores, and the cysts of some invertebrate species fell into this group. *Oscillating life,* whose manifestations of life were strongly influenced by the external environment, included all cold-blooded animals. *Constant life,* for which manifestations of life appeared to be free of influence from the external environment, contained all complex higher organisms.

From the language used, it would appear that Bernard might well have considered an internal environment for all three forms of life (definitely for oscillating and constant life). However, it is probable that he expected constancy of that environment only among the more complex organisms.

Nevertheless, Bernard's seminal thinking provided an important framework in which physiological studies were to be conducted. A further major step was provided nearly 50 years later by Walter Bradford Cannon. He introduced the term homeostasis to describe the steady-state conditions existing within the internal environment and provided the essential ground rules for homeostatic control.

The central points of this notion of homeostatic control, first published in 1926, are as follows:

1. In open systems, like our bodies, that are subjected to continued disturbances, constancy is evidence that adaptive mechanisms exist.
2. Homeostatic conditions persist because tendencies toward change are resisted by increased effectiveness of adapting factors.
3. A homeostatic agent acts in only one way at any given point.
4. Homeostatic agents that are antagonistic in one region may cooperate in another.
5. Regulating systems that determine a homeostatic state may be composed of cooperating factors acting simultaneously or successively.
6. When a factor is known that shifts the homeostatic state in one direction, it is reasonable to seek an automatic control of the factor(s) having an opposite effect.

Although several of these postulates seem rather obvious, their formulation into a coherent scheme provided a significant advancement in our understanding of physiological control. It is a credit to Cannon's insightful genius that these general rules have held fast since they were proposed. Advances over the past several decades have been guided by them and have confirmed and refined them.

Bernard, C. Lessons on the phenomenon of life common to animals and vegetables.

Cannon, W. B. Physiological regulation of normal states: some tentative postulates concerning biological homeostatics. In *Homeostasis: Origin of the Concept.* L. L. Langley (ed.). Dowden, Hutchinson, & Ross, Stroudsburg, Penna. 1973.

a hematocrit of 42 means that 42% of a person's blood volume is due to red blood cell mass.) Each erythrocyte carries within it an abundant store of *hemoglobin.* This protein is responsible for the majority of the blood's oxygen-carrying capacity. On average, there are approximately 130 to 170 grams of hemoglobin in every liter of blood. It is the oxygenated hemoglobin of the erythrocytes that imparts the reddish color to blood.

Since oxygen delivery and carbon dioxide elimination are essential for cell survival, an adequate supply of erythrocytes is an important factor in homeostasis. Individual erythrocytes have a lifespan of approximately 120 days. Under normal circumstances, 1% to 2% of the erythrocyte population must be replaced every day. Erythrocyte precursors, nucleated *pronormoblasts,* in the bone marrow ensure this replacement through the process of **erythropoiesis** (from the Greek *erythro* [red (blood cells)] and *poiesis* [producing]).

When the oxygen-carrying capacity of the blood falls substantially, a condition of **anemia** exists. This condition reflects *a diminished ability to deliver oxygen to the cells,* at least by normal standards. Any condition that decreases the number of erythrocytes, the hematocrit, or more importantly, the hemoglobin level causes a state of anemia. This triggers the release of the hormone **erythropoietin** from the kidneys and leads to stimulated erythropoiesis in the bone marrow (fig. 1.5). If the hemoglobin level can be restored, the former steady state is regained; if not, a disease state exists.

Leukocytes   The largest cells of the blood are leukocytes. Although they are the least numerous blood cells (approximately 6 to $10 \times 10^9/L$), several distinct types can be identified: *lymphocytes, monocytes,* and *granulocytes* (neutrophils, basophils, and eosinophils), which are shown in figure 1.4. Leukocytes can be classified either *morphologically* (by physical appearance) or *functionally* (table 1.1). For example, we can distinguish **mononuclear cells** from **granulocytes** in that the former have a single nucleus, while the latter contain cytoplasmic granules and might have a multilobed nucleus. Alternatively, we can identify these cells as

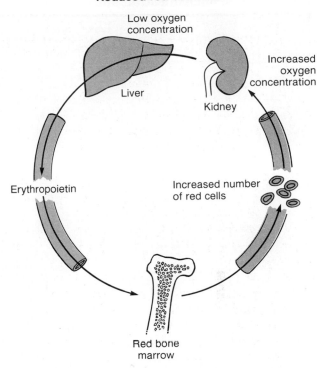

Reduced red cell mass

FIGURE 1.5   Regulation of adequate erythrocyte mass. Reduction in erythrocyte (red blood cell) mass leads to a *low oxygen concentration* in the blood. This causes **erythropoietin** to be released. This hormone acts on the red bone marrow, which increases erythropoiesis. The result is an increased number of red blood cells and *increased oxygen concentration.*

phagocytes, based on their ability to perform phagocytosis, or as **immunocytes,** because of their roles in immune responses. Leukocytes participate in maintaining homeostasis by (1) removing undesirable materials from the internal environment and (2) destroying noncontributing (defective or transformed) cells. Further discussions about the particular roles played by the various leukocyte types are provided in later chapters.

Platelets   In reality, platelets are *fragments of the cytoplasm* of a parent cell found within the bone marrow. This cell, the **megakaryocyte,** buds off pieces of its cytoplasm that emigrate to the bloodstream.

TABLE 1.1 Classification and Characteristics of Blood Leukocytes

Cell Type	Classification		Characteristics
	Morphological	**Functional**	
Lymphocyte	Mononuclear	Immunocyte	Small leukocyte (4–12 μm) with round nucleus that occupies most of cell; can play one of several roles in immune response, depending upon its specific type
Monocyte	Mononuclear	Phagocyte/immunocyte	Large leukocyte (15–30 μm) with prominent nucleus; has readily visible cytoplasmic area; can interact with lymphocytes in immune responses; is active phagocyte among tissues
Neutrophil	Granulocyte	Phagocyte	Leukocyte whose size (12–15 μm) is intermediate between that of monocytes and lymphocytes; has characteristic multilobed nucleus and several nonspecific granules in its cytoplasm; acts as major phagocyte in acute inflammation
Basophil	Granulocyte	Phagocyte/immunocyte	Is similar in size to neutrophils but distinguished by presence of abundant basophilic (darkly staining) specific granules in cytoplasm that often obscure nucleus; contains and releases bioactive substances such as histamine; functions in inflammation and immune responses
Eosinophil	Granulocyte	Phagocyte/immunocyte	Is similar in size to neutrophils with bilobed nucleus and prominent eosinophilic (orange-red) specific granules; is active in parasitic infection.

There these minute particles (approximately 150 to 300 $\times$ 10^9/L) circulate with their stores of bioactive substances until needed. The principal homeostatic role associated with these cellular fragments is in the process of **hemostasis,** or stopping blood flow (from the Greek *hemo* [blood] and *stasis* [standing]). Once activated, platelets participate with the plasma proteins involved in clotting to seal off damage to blood vessels. Platelets accomplish this by releasing their bioactive products which promote vasoconstriction, thereby reducing the size of the blood vessel and decreasing blood flow through that area. In addition, they adhere to the blood vessel wall and aggregate in clumps, forming a plug over the damage in the vessel. Furthermore, platelets release factors that interact with plasma clotting proteins to achieve production of a fibrin clot.

Disease

On a continuing basis, our internal environment is assaulted by elements from the external environment. In most instances, our self-regulatory mechanisms are adequate to meet the challenge. For example, when it gets cold, we shiver, thereby generating more heat; but we sweat if it gets too hot. If we bump against a hard object, we might sustain a bruise. This reflects slight blood loss but effective repair. When we catch a cold, we experience greater discomfort and for a longer period. This suggests a more serious challenge to our steady-state balance, but again one that we eventually overcome. However, this condition contrasts somewhat from the previous examples in that the body was pushed beyond the normal steady-state conditions, and substantially greater effort was required to restore homeostasis. With this illustration, we begin to enter the realm of disease.

TABLE 1.2 Some Categories and Causes of Diseases

Category	Cause	Examples
Infectious Diseases	Viruses	Measles, infectious hepatitis
	Bacteria	Pneumonia, tuberculosis
	Fungi	Yeast infections, histoplasmosis
	Parasitic protozoa	Malaria, amebic dysentery
	Parasitic worms	Trichinosis, tapeworm, schistosomiasis
Cancer	Radiation, chemical carcinogens, tumor viruses	Leukemia, osteosarcoma, neuroblastoma, lung or breast cancers
Immune Disorders	Variable	
Excessive response		Allergies
Inadequate response		AIDS
Inappropriate response		Lupus erythematosus
Genetic Disorders	Defective or missing genes	Diabetes
Degenerative Diseases	"Breakdown" due to aging	Alzheimer's disease

Disease can be considered *a state in which homeostatic balance is severely challenged and disturbed.* In the disease state, homeostasis is not achieved, although considerable effort might be expended in attempting to do so. It is only when the adaptive responses of our regulatory systems are successful in restoring homeostasis that a cure occurs. Failure of these responses to improve the situation is associated with continuation of the disease, whereas a diminishing ability to respond adaptively ultimately leads to death.

In the following sections we outline some categories of disease and briefly examine some of their causes.

Categories of Disease

There are many diseases and afflictions that affect the human organism. Attempting to understand each one individually would present an enormous task, were we not able to group them in some fashion. One convenient way to approach the study of diseases is to focus on the means by which they come about. Since similar disease-causing agents are likely to produce disturbances in homeostatic balance through similar mechanisms, we can more easily uncover principles of **pathogenesis** (the process by which disease comes about; from the Greek *patho* [pain or disease] and *genesis*

[birth or origin]). In addition, this strategy also enables us to see common modes of defense and adaptation to disease.

Some causes of disease states are *infectious biological agents* (e.g., bacteria, viruses, and parasites), *chemical or physical modification of cellular expression* (cancer), *genetic defects,* and *nutritional imbalances* (table 1.2).

Infectious Diseases

Each year thousands of children in tropical Africa are bitten by mosquitoes, become seriously ill, and many die. They become afflicted with the infectious disease, malaria. While taking a blood meal, the mosquitoes release small, single-celled parasites into the children. These parasites become established within the erythrocytes and eventually cause the destruction of erythrocytes, liver and kidney cells, and possibly even brain cells. In doing so, these parasites disturb the normal steady-state conditions of the individual. The body attempts to reestablish homeostatic balance but unfortunately does not always succeed.

This is a common pattern with infectious diseases. A foreign organism gains entry into a human host. Within its human host, this parasite steals nutrients intended for the host's cells. If the organism thrives and multiplies, it presents a threat to homeostasis as it usurps nutrients and damages the host's cells. The body responds in self-defense with one of three results possible: (1) removing the invader, *cure;* (2) failing to destroy the intruder, *death to the host;* or (3) holding the parasite in check, a precarious *stalemate* that can lead to a new challenge at any time.

Biological Agents of Disease   The vast majority of human diseases are caused by biological agents—*viruses, bacteria, fungi, protozoa,* and *worms.* Infectious diseases caused by these agents have often influenced the course of history. For example, smallpox contributed to the downfall of the Aztec and Inca civilizations in Central and South America. In addition, the bubonic plague (the "Black Death") of the Middle Ages took its toll worldwide.

Microscopic biological agents are responsible for a broad range of infectious and communicable diseases. *Viruses,* which cannot reproduce outside of host cells, are responsible for the common cold, influenza, measles, mumps, polio, warts, rabies, infectious hepatitis, genital herpes, and acquired immune deficiency syndrome (AIDS). *Bacteria* cause strep throat, staph infections, pneumonia, tuberculosis, leprosy, syphilis, and gonorrhea. *Parasitic protozoa* can be blamed for diseases like amebic dysentery, sleeping sickness, toxoplasmosis, and malaria.

Multicellular parasites exist as well. The most prevalent of these parasites are the worms (also referred to clinically as helminths). *Worms,* which can range from a fraction of an inch to over 50 feet in length, produce a wide variety of afflictions. Parasitic worms invade various host tissues and organs. Among the sites commonly affected by worms are blood, intestines, lung, liver, urinary system, heart, skin, muscle, brain, and eye.

The involvement of microorganisms (viruses and bacteria) and parasites (protozoa and helminths [worms]) in disease, and the role of the immune system in meeting the challenge of infectious diseases is explored further in unit 4 (chapters 11 and 12).

Cancer

Diseases also are caused by other than infectious agents. Some, like cancer, are believed to be caused by physical or chemical insult to the body (although there is evidence that some cancers are caused by viruses). We constantly encounter warnings to avoid cigarettes, watch what we eat and drink, and avoid too much exposure to the sun and x-rays. These warnings are intended to alert us to dangers associated with **radiation** (physical insults) and **carcinogens** (literally, ulcer producing, from the Greek *carcino* [ulcer] and *gene* [birth or origin]) (chemical insults) as potential means through which cancer arises.

Ideally, the 100 trillion or more cells that comprise our adult bodies are in dynamic equilibrium with each other and with the external environment. Old and worn-out cells are replaced. The disparate healthy cell types exhibit integrated and coordinated behavior. In contrast, a **tumor,** or *neoplasm* (from the Greek *neo* [new] and *plas* [form]), is a mass of cells that is abnormal and discordant. *These cells do not respond to regulatory signals* and thus display uncoordinated behavior. A tumor can exist either as a solid mass, or nodule, or be dispersed. Nevertheless, the individual tumor cells are derived from a single cell that was converted, or *transformed,* into a tumor "stem cell" following interaction with an inducing agent. This interaction caused the cell's genetic machinery to be changed. The result is a cell that no longer responds to normal homeostatic controls. When this rogue, or outlaw, cell reproduces it creates more like itself, creating a tumor.

The tumors that are eventually produced can be either benign or malignant. **Benign tumors** tend to have a more mature appearance; that is, the cells that make up the tumor tend to *resemble normal cells.* **Malignant tumors,** on the other hand, contain cells that *appear less differentiated* and contrast more strikingly with normal cells. Malignant tumors grow more rapidly than benign tumors because their cells divide more frequently. Furthermore, malignant cells are more invasive and more destructive. They can **metastasize** (from the Greek *meta* [to change or between] and *stasis* [stand], thus to relocate or to stand between); that is, they can *break free of the parent tumor and spread to a distant site to seed a new tumor.* As a result, malignant tumors invade tissues where they displace normal cells and interrupt vital functions. These tumors are cancers.

The Causes of Disease: Malevolent Spirits to Microbes

Today we realize that there is an identifiable cause for every disease. We do not always know the nature of the causative agent nor the manner in which it brings about the disease state. Nonetheless, we are certain of a specific cause that we can eventually understand and counteract. However, this way of thinking has not always existed.

What prehistoric humans believed caused disease is a matter for conjecture. But by the time of **Hippocrates** (460–377 B.C.), fairly definite notions had been established, systematized, and used as a basis for diagnosis and even treatment. Central to the ancient Greek school was the belief that good health and its converse, disease, resulted from changes in the balance of the **four principal humors:** *blood, phlegm, yellow bile,* and *black bile.* When these were in balance, health prevailed. If an imbalance occurred, disease resulted. The humor that predominated dictated the nature of the manifestations. Even today we encounter vestiges of that scheme in our speech. The designations of *sanguine, phlegmatic, choleric,* and *melancholic* personalities owe their origins to the concept of the four humors.

The prevalent thinking from the ancient Greeks through the Middle Ages seemed to be that disease was caused by black magic, evil spirits, the will of God, or other supernatural agencies. A major step away from this nonproductive view of disease occurred in 1546. In that year, **Girolamo Francastoro** (1483–1553) published his work, *Contagion, Contagious Diseases and their Treatment.* For the first time, disease was attributed to natural causes. **Contagion** was defined as *an infection that can be passed from one thing to another.* Curiously, Fracastoro used a term for "germ" to describe the infectious or contagious principle. Although his notions of germs and contagious disease were different from our own, his approach paved the way for others.

Substantial progress in further detailing the origins of infectious disease was hampered by the **theory of spontaneous generation.** If organisms, in particular infectious organisms, can arise spontaneously, when and where disease might manifest itself was unpredictable. Moreover, attempting to trace the progression of an infectious disease presented nearly insurmountable obstacles. The invention of the microscope made it possible to see plant and animal cells and the "minuscule beings" that we refer to as bacteria and protozoa. But this alone was not sufficient to significantly advance the understanding of the causes of diseases, the ways in which they progressed, and how infectious diseases were transmitted.

Through the efforts of **Louis Pasteur** (1822–1895) and others, the theory of spontaneous generation was eventually overthrown. This notion that *life could arise only from life* was refined by **Rudolf Virchow** (1821–1902), who added the corollary that *cells were derived from preexisting cells.* (This idea had profound implications for noninfectious diseases. For example, this postulates that cancer cells must have arisen from previously normal cells of the body.) But to **Robert Koch** (1843–1910) goes the distinction of having formulated the *credo for identifying the causative agents of infectious diseases,* known as Koch's **four postulates**: 1. The causative agent (e.g., bacteria) must be isolated from an infected individual. 2. The agent must be propagated in isolated culture. 3. Products (e.g., bacteria) of this culturing must be capable of infecting a noninfected host. 4. The same agent must be recovered from this second host.

This framework is still used today in attempting to discover the causative agent of any new disease. Two recent epidemics illustrate the point: (1) legionnaires' disease (named for an outbreak among persons attending an American Legion convention in Philadelphia in 1976), caused by a bacterium, *Legionella pneumophila,* and (2) acquired immuno deficiency syndrome (AIDS) (named for its consequences on the immune system). AIDS is transmitted by infected body fluids and secretions and is caused by a virus (human immunodeficiency virus [HIV], formerly human T lymphotrophic virus-III / lymphadenopathy virus [HTLV-III / LAV]).

Brock, T. *Milestones in Microbiology.* Prentice-Hall, Englewood Cliffs, New Jersey, 1961.

Bullock, W. *The History of Bacteriology.* Dover Publications, Inc., New York, 1979.

Lechevalier, H. A., and Solotorovsky, M. *Three Centuries of Microbiology.* Dover Publications, Inc., New York, 1974.

Tumor, or cancer, cells are derived from normal cells. Cancer cells have *altered genetic expression* resulting either from mutation and/or activation of cancer-causing genes or **oncogenes** (from the Greek *onco* [mass or tumor]) or from mutation or inactivation of **repressor genes,** following exposure to physical or chemical insult (e.g., radiation or carcinogens). Fortunately, even after prolonged (chronic) exposure, most normal cells do not mutate, express pronounced oncogene activity, or display impaired repressor gene expression. Moreover, cells that mutate usually die. Furthermore, in order to survive and produce a tumor, the transformed cell must escape elimination by the body's defense mechanisms.

Despite these obstacles, one in four humans will probably produce cancerous cells in response to environmental factors during their lives. The likelihood that cancer will manifest itself seems greater in some individuals than in others. This is a result of differences in individual ability to respond and adapt to the environment that are determined by genetic constitution. In other words, there is apparent *inherited susceptibility* to cancer. For example, the frequency of occurrence of specific forms of cancer in individuals inheriting particular genetic disorders (e.g., albinism and immune deficiencies) is greater than that observed in the general population. In addition, studies of identical twins and close relations suggest increased incidence of certain cancers. Although the evidence for this is not overwhelming, the frequency of occurrence of cancer appears much greater than can be expected from chance alone.

Several hypotheses have been offered to account for the transformation of a normal cell to a tumor cell. These hypotheses suggest that tumors arise alternatively from *physical* or *chemical injury, viral infection,* or a breakdown in normal cellular expression resulting from an *accumulation of errors* in function. The nature of tumors and the several mechanisms through which they arise are discussed in greater detail in chapter 17, Cancer.

Normal healthy individuals usually possess an **immune surveillance** system that is potentially capable of recognizing and destroying cancer cells. Some researchers have suggested that most of us probably develop, and temporarily have, transformed cells from time to time throughout life. These cells are recognized as foreign and readily destroyed by immune surveillance mechanisms. However, this defense system is not always effective. Chapter 18, Tumor Immunology, examines the interactions that occur between tumor (cancer) cells and the immune system.

Immunological Diseases

Our immune systems probably evolved primarily to *recognize, regulate,* and *remove foreign agents* and *abnormal or worn-out cells.* These strategies operate to ensure our protection, good health, and survival. Under certain circumstances, however, this system might bring harm, rather than good, to the body. Immune response to an infective organism, for example, might also cause significant, albeit unintended, damage to normal cells in the target area. On the other hand, the immune system, at times, might *react inappropriately* (excessively, insufficiently, or in a misdirected manner) to substances encountered in our environment.

Hypersensitivity   When an immune response seems to be *exaggerated,* we are dealing with **hypersensitivity** reactions. Two well-known forms of hypersensitivity reactions are atopic disease (e.g., allergies) and anaphylaxis (exaggerated reactions to foreign substances to which an individual has become sensitized). Allergic reactions can be *localized,* producing wheals (e.g., blisters), or *generalized* with accompanying intestinal cramps, nausea, respiratory obstruction, lowered blood pressure, and shock. Reactions to poison ivy and poison oak produce localized allergic reactions that can be quite irritating. On the other hand, allergic reactions occasionally can lead to life-threatening responses such as anaphylactic shock. Penicillin and insect venoms are two substances associated with anaphylactic responses. Hypersensitivity is explored in chapter 13.

Autoimmunity   The immune system functions to protect the integrity of the individual. Nevertheless, occasionally this function goes awry and the immune system *attacks normal cells of the body.* This is known as an **autoimmune** response. The disorders that result can be caused either by *autosensitized lymphocytes* (lymphocytes that become activated by an individual's own cells or their products) or *autoantibodies* (antibodies against an individual's own cells or their products). Autoimmune responses can be *organ specific* or *systemic*. Examples of autoimmune diseases that are organ specific are acquired hemolytic anemia (erythrocytes are the target cells destroyed with anemia resulting) and myasthenia gravis (where antibodies attack acetylcholine receptors on skeletal muscle fibers, impairing neuromuscular interaction leading to muscle weakness and motor disorders). Lupus erythematosus is an example of a systemic autoimmune disorder in which antinuclear (anti-DNA) antibodies are produced. In lupus, damage to skin, joints, lymph nodes, spleen, liver, lungs, gastrointestinal tract, and kidneys is not uncommon. Further discussion of autoimmune phenomena can be found in chapter 16.

Immune Deficiency   In contrast to an overreactive or misdirected immune system causing bodily injury, an underreactive immune system can be harmful by enabling other agents to cause damage. Our environment constantly exposes us to viruses, bacteria, and other disease-causing agents. These are more likely to be effective in producing a disease in an individual who is **immunodeficient,** since the *mechanisms intended to combat these agents are in a weakened state.*

Immune deficiency can be *congenital* (present at birth) or *acquired* (appearing later in life). Congenital immune deficiencies involve a failure of one or more components of the immune system to develop properly. This might be the result of some genetic defect or a consequence of damage (chemical or physical) occurring during a critical stage of fetal development. Acquired immune deficiencies arise later in life, after immune competence has already been expressed. These deficiencies are the consequence of damage to components of the immune system. Damage to the immune system can arise through direct insult to cells of the immune system (e.g., as in AIDS) or in conjunction with other disorders such as diabetes, alcoholic cirrhosis, malnutrition, and sickle cell disease. In other instances, the immune system becomes damaged as a result of efforts to treat other disorders. Immunosuppressant drugs used on organ transplant recipients and chemotherapy or radiotherapy used to treat cancer patients provide two examples of therapeutic regimens

that can impair the performance of the immune system. Mechanisms through which immune deficiencies arise, and their consequences to the organism, provide the focus for chapter 14.

Other Causes of Disease

In addition to the factors discussed earlier, disease can be brought about by a variety of other means. In an oversimplified manner, we can classify these into (1) genetic, (2) degenerative, (3) environmental, (4) psychogenic, and (5) iatrogenic.

Genetic defects express themselves early. Many lead to spontaneous abortion or stillbirth. If the child is born, however, problems invariably arise since deficiencies or alterations of the gene pool can easily impair an individual's ability to maintain homeostasis. Having a gene that produces a defective hemoglobin molecule leads to an impaired ability to properly satisfy oxygen demands of the body's cells. Sickle cell anemia is an example of this type of genetic disorder. In contrast, *degenerative* causes of disease are typically associated with the elderly. These seem to be a consequence of the aging process and most often affect the cardiovascular system, the kidneys, the lungs, and the brain.

Environmental causes of disease can manifest themselves at any time. This category encompasses mechanical, physical, and chemical agents. For example, consuming alcohol or smoking during pregnancy can lead to congenital defects in the newborn child. Alternatively, these same agents can produce cirrhosis of the liver and lung cancer in an adult. *Nutritional imbalance* represents yet another example. However, in this instance, cells are being deprived of essential materials, rather than being subjected to damaging insult. A common factor of all these agents is that they exert their harmful effects by damaging cells and tissues, thereby impairing their abilities to participate effectively in maintaining homeostasis.

An individual's emotional state can also lead to the expression of disease. This *psychogenic* means of influencing disease expression is probably related to alterations in the functioning of the body's regulatory systems, in particular the nervous and endocrine systems.

On occasion, the efforts of modern medicine might themselves contribute to the expression of disease. Such conditions are referred to as *iatrogenic*. The examples of immune deficiency induced by treatments of cancer patients or transplant recipients are cases where efforts to control one set of problems might give rise to another.

The classifications provided earlier represent tools of convenience. They do not provide rigid compartments into which we might place one disease or another. They enable us more readily to see relationships in how diseases come about, manifest themselves, and can be treated. Several of the causative agents of disease can give rise to the same disease, although by different means. Moreover, two or more of these agents might interact in giving rise to a disease. Nevertheless, all share a *common denominator—they create an imbalance within our internal environments and challenge our regulatory systems.* They cause disease by destroying, even temporarily, the harmonious balance of homeostasis.

IMMUNITY AND IMMUNOLOGICAL EFFECTORS

A host of notable ideas and significant concepts about the immune system and its function have evolved over the last few decades (see appendix B, Milestones in the History of Immunology, for a summary chronological survey). It is now clear that the immune system is an extremely complex *surveillance system* providing a remarkably adaptable set of responses, *geared to maintaining homeostasis and health.* Recent evidence indicates that this system is intimately influenced by and interacts with the nervous and endocrine systems.

Immune responses constitute the principal means of defense against pathogenic microorganisms and cells that are transformed into cancer cells. Defense is based on a unique surveillance system that recognizes, responds, and remembers. In addition, the immune system is intimately involved in the expression, or lack of expression, of *allergies, autoimmune disease, immune deficiency states,* and *transplantation reactions* to healthy tissues or organs used to replace diseased ones. In any of these immune responses, genes,

macromolecules, and cells of the immune system are responsible for an intricate communicating system that generates *specific effector proteins* (**antibodies**) and *cells* (**lymphocytes**).

Before exploring the immune system in detail (in later chapters), let us become acquainted with this intricate system in a general way.

The Scope of Immunology

Immunology is the *study of the immune system.* This system has evolved primarily as a surveillance system for the body's defense against cells or substances that are nonself or altered self. Immunology deals basically with questions of how and why the body reacts to almost anything alien, foreign, or nonself entering its domain. It also explores responsiveness to self-components that have become recognizably abnormal or transformed. Immunology involves the study of processes and events, by which the body *attempts to defend and maintain constancy of its internal environment* against disease-causing agents, toxic substances, and abnormal cells.

Many studies of the immune system are directed at the nature of the response, or lack of response, to a variety of factors. These include disease agents, cancer cells, vaccines, tolerogens (agents that induce immune tolerance), blood transfusions, tissue and organ transplants, and allergens (agents that induce allergic reactions). In addition, studies of the immune system endeavor to understand reactions to self-components that have or have not been altered. Moreover, a substantial part of immunology today is *non-disease oriented* and used as a *tool* to solve problems in cellular and molecular biology and biochemistry.

This section provides an introduction to certain important terms and concepts in the field of immunology. In addition, the development of some of these concepts is explored briefly.

Immunity

Our understanding of immunity, and the role played by the immune system, has changed dramatically over the years. Early interest in immunity developed in ignorance of both the existence of an immune system

TABLE 1.3 Major Categories of Immune Protection and Mechanisms of Their Expression

Type of Immunity or Means of Expression	Characteristic Features
Type of Immunity	
Innate	Protection against infective agents that is present at birth; this includes a variety of defenses that are not antigen specific
Acquired	Protection against infective agents that is not present at birth but rather comes about later in life
Active	Protection acquired through generation of immune products by immunized individual, e.g., following vaccination; it is antigen specific
Passive	Protection acquired as a result of receiving immune products that have been generated from another source; it is antigen specific
Mechanism of Expression	
Humoral immunity	Defense that is accomplished through activity of circulating immune products
Cellular immunity	Defense provided by direct involvement of specific cell types, rather than by circulating immune products

and of the nature of causative agents of disease. Nevertheless, as a result of advances made in several areas of the biological and medical sciences, a coherent picture of the nature and function of the immune system has emerged. This picture contains knowledge of three major categories of immune protection that are provided through two primary mechanisms (table 1.3). Since a historical examination of changes in concepts of immunity provides valuable insights into the operation of the immune system, certain of these trends and their contributions are briefly reviewed.

Innate, Nonspecific Immunity

Immunological defenses can be either generalized and nonspecific (i.e., not directed against particular agents) or focused and specific (provoked in response to particular agents). For example, *at birth,* humans must normally depend on nonspecific, or innate, defense measures. These innate defenses (immunity) contrast with acquired immunity, which is specific (discussed later). Innate immunity is ordinarily provided along with the specific passive immunity derived from the mother. **Nonspecific immunity** includes critical *physical* (e.g., body temperature) and *anatomic* (e.g., the skin) barriers to microbial invasion. It also includes *biochemical substances* (e.g., complement) in body fluids, which may be detrimental to infectious agents. Potentially infectious microorganisms might be discharged by our ability to salivate, express tears, cough, and sneeze. *Normal flora* also can be antagonistic to infectious agents. Above all, perhaps, is the protection derived from baseline *cellular effectors.* This includes cytolysis by nonspecific killer lymphocytes and phagocytosis on the part of macrophages, monocytes, and neutrophils of the body. Killer cells and phagocytes in the immune individual can become even more effective in their ability to kill, engulf, and digest infectious microorganisms. Acquired immunity not only adds specific resistance to the body's defensive posture, it enhances innate mechanisms of resistance as well.

Active Immunity

Although ancient civilizations might not have been aware of the causative agents of infectious disease, writings of prominent observers like Hippocrates and Thucydides reveal their awareness of resistance to second attacks of certain diseases, such as smallpox. In fact, efforts by Chinese and Arab physicians to "immunize" against smallpox date back to the eleventh century. Since smallpox killed one in four afflicted individuals, these pioneering physicians sought to protect healthy persons from smallpox by giving them a mild case of the disease. However, it was not until the early eighteenth century that similar efforts were introduced into Europe. At that time, Lady Mary Montagu (the wife of the British ambassador to the Ottoman Empire) introduced a procedure known as *variolation* to

England, after having had her own son variolated. This rather dangerous procedure involved taking fluid from the vesicles of individuals with mild cases of variola (as smallpox was called) and inoculating it into the bloodstream of the person to be "variolated." The variolated person usually became ill and was contagious. Despite an average mortality of 1% to 2%, the fact that survivors acquired protection against natural smallpox provided substantial appeal. As a result, variolation spread rapidly throughout England and Western Europe.

Toward the end of the eighteenth century, a dairy maid noticed that her friends who developed cowpox (*vaccinia*) from her herd never became ill with the dreaded smallpox (variola). She communicated this observation to **Edward Jenner,** an English general practitioner, who tested this hypothesis by inoculating human "volunteers" with fluid from a cowpox pustule (sore). The *vaccinated* individuals subsequently developed mild reactions. After recovery, these individuals did not contract smallpox when exposed. Jenner's vaccination was a safer treatment than variolation since the vaccinia (cowpox) fluid produced only mild, noncontagious reactions rather than the more violent, contagious reactions often seen using variola (smallpox) fluid. This represented the first induction of active immunity, or resistance, to infection in humans using a safe vaccine. Jenner reported the results of this study in 1796. The terms vaccine and vaccination are still used today, although vaccinia virus is rarely used to immunize against smallpox today. Nevertheless, vaccinia virus is frequently used in the production of many modern vaccines (discussed in chapter 12). Modern vaccines contain various foreign substances (often proteins) capable of stimulating an immune response.

Nearly 100 years later, **Louis Pasteur** and his colleagues experimentally extended the concept of vaccination. They discovered that certain bacteria lost their **virulence** (their ability to cause disease) after extensive culturing in the laboratory. Pasteur suggested that microorganisms that had lost their virulence might still be capable of providing immunity. In essence, he postulated that the properties of a disease-causing organism that were responsible for immunity were not changed when that organism became avirulent. If this

was true, then such materials might be "ideal" vaccines, providing effective and safe means of immunization.

Jenner's original vaccine contained cowpox (vaccinia) virus. This virus was later shown to be very similar to smallpox virus (variola). Vaccinia virus was sufficiently different from smallpox virus in that it produced only mild responses in infected humans; nevertheless, it resembled the smallpox virus immunogenically enough to provoke an immune response that protected against smallpox. Thus, Jenner's vaccine represented the first "live" vaccine. In contrast, Pasteur's idea was to use the *same* organism that caused the disease in question to produce a live vaccine. In order to do this, he had to weaken, or attenuate, the organism so that it could not cause the disease.

In 1881 Pasteur performed a now classic experiment. He vaccinated sheep with attenuated anthrax bacilli and dramatically demonstrated protection against anthrax, a disease that is rapidly fatal in humans (fig. 1.6). Since that time, numerous attenuated vaccines have been developed and used to immunize humans against disease. In addition to smallpox, diseases that have been controlled in this manner include tuberculosis, yellow fever, rubella, measles, and polio. However, despite their benefits, live vaccines can be dangerous when used in immunologically incompetent individuals, in pregnant women (at least to the fetus), and occasionally in normal recipients.

Jenner's and Pasteur's use of vaccination illustrate attempts at active immunization. In these instances, experimental or clinical (and subclinical) exposure to disease agents was used to *stimulate an active immune response* resulting in varying degrees of humoral (mediated by antibodies and serum complement) and cell-mediated (requiring active participation of lymphocytes) immunity, or resistance, to disease. The *acquired* adaptive immunity is active since the response was initiated and developed in the individual. Moreover, these can be considered an *artificial means* of producing active immunity. A modified form of the pathogen was used to stimulate an immune response, without producing the disease. This can be contrasted with **natural active immunity** that occurs in recovering from infection by the native disease-causing

Prior to 1881 the rule pertaining to anthrax was as follows:

Sheep   +   Live anthrax bacilli   =   Death

To prove that he could immunize sheep against the ravages of anthrax, Pasteur performed the following public experiment at Pouilly-le-Fort in 1881.

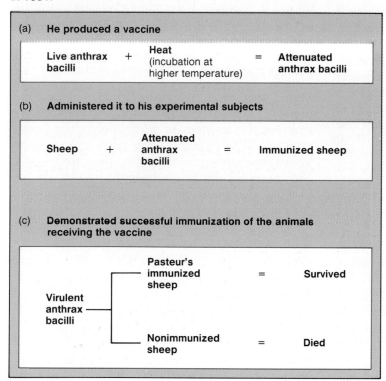

(a)   **He produced a vaccine**

Live anthrax bacilli   +   Heat (incubation at higher temperature)   =   Attenuated anthrax bacilli

(b)   **Administered it to his experimental subjects**

Sheep   +   Attenuated anthrax bacilli   =   Immunized sheep

(c)   **Demonstrated successful immunization of the animals receiving the vaccine**

Virulent anthrax bacilli —
- Pasteur's immunized sheep = Survived
- Nonimmunized sheep = Died

FIGURE 1.6 Pasteur's experiment demonstrating immunization against anthrax.

agent. In this case, the pathogenic organism not only stimulates an immune response, it can also produce the disease.

Passive Immunity

By the late nineteenth century, the medical and scientific communities realized that immunity could theoretically be acquired against a broad range of diseases. Such immunity could be actively acquired by vaccination with the disease-causing microorganisms, preferably in an attenuated state. In addition, they knew that this specific protection against the disease agent was not present from birth. However, they did not know how immunity was conferred or from where in the body it originated. An initial glimpse into answers to these questions was acquired in 1888, when **Richet** and **Hericourt** showed that the blood of an immunized animal possessed protective properties. They were able to confer partial protection against infection with staphylococci by inoculating blood from an immunized animal. A year later, serum from immunized animals was shown to clump, or agglutinate, bacteria used as the vaccine. Agglutination did not occur if normal (nonimmune) serum was used or if a different strain of bacteria was used. The reaction was, therefore, specifically between the immune serum and the inoculating bacteria.

The acquisition of immunity demonstrated by Richet and Hericourt did not require an active immune response by the recipient. Rather, the recipient acquired its immunity, ready-made, from another animal that had actively developed its own immunity following vaccination. *Passive* immunization refers to the *transfer of antibodies* or, in some cases, products of effector cells *from an immune individual to a nonimmune individual.* **Natural passive humoral immunity** is transferred from mother to child across the placenta or in the mother's milk (colostrum) in the form of low molecular weight antibodies.

Humoral Immunity

Although blood had been shown to be involved in immunity, the mechanism, or mechanisms, through which protection against infective agents was expressed had yet to be defined. Several investigators provided evidence for the existence of **circulating,** or **humoral, factors.** As Richet and Hericourt had shown, these humoral factors could provide protection against an infective organism or cause their *agglutination.* By 1890 **von Behring** and **Kitasato** had shown that serum from animals immunized with diphtheria or tetanus toxoid could neutralize the harmful effects of the toxins. The factor in blood or serum of immunized animals responsible for immunity became known as an *antibody* in the late 1890s.

Antibodies were not the only agents of humoral immunity, however. In the early 1890s, **Bordet** showed that *immune sera could dissolve, or lyse, certain bacteria.* He also discovered serum from one individual could lyse erythrocytes from another individual, in certain instances. He suggested that two factors, both present in serum, were responsible for this phenomenon. These two factors were later defined as antibody and **complement.** Of these two, antibody provided specific recognition of the target cells (bacteria or erythrocytes), while complement was the component actually responsible for lysing the cells.

Humoral immunity, then, provided protection against infectious agents, or their toxic products, through the activities of circulating factors in the blood. Two factors were recognized as agents of humoral immunity by the end of the nineteenth century, antibodies and complement. By that time, the following activities were associated with antibodies: (1) agglutination of bacteria, (2) precipitation of immunogenic substances and toxins, (3) lysis of target bacteria and red blood cells in the presence of complement, and (4) enhancement of the activity of certain cells.

Cellular Immunity

While others were considering aspects of humoral immunity, a Russian biologist, **Elie Metchnikoff,** was studying the activities of white blood cells (leukocytes). In 1883 he showed that some leukocytes engulfed microorganisms. Formerly, most investigators had concluded that microorganisms invaded the leukocytes. However, following repeated observations, Metchnikoff became convinced that the *leukocytes were the aggressors.* He named these engulfing cells "phagocytes," meaning devouring cells. He also noted that this *phagocytic activity was greatly enhanced in immunized animals* and in animals recovering from infections. In addition, he was the first to observe the ability of phagocytes to leave the bloodstream by active penetration of the blood vessel wall. He subsequently suggested that *phagocytic leukocytes also played a role in inflammation.*

Metchnikoff challenged the notion that humoral immunity provided the primary means of defense for an organism. He staunchly believed that this was provided by phagocytes. Thus, a concept of **cellular immunity** emerged. According to this concept, *cells constitute the primary line of defense* against infective agents. When a microorganism gains entry into its host, whether through a wound or through infective transmission, phagocytes become activated. They then mount an aggressive assault on the intruders and, if successful, rid the host's body of the insulting organisms. In this scheme, humoral agents are not required. Metchnikoff's original conception of cellular immunity relied heavily upon the aggressive nature of phagocytes. However, our present notion of cellular immunity integrates phagocytes with other effector cells and places primary emphasis on certain classes of lymphocytes (described later) for specific cellular immunity.

Integration of Humoral and Cellular Immunity

For a time, an intense conflict existed between advocates of the two theories. However, around the turn of the century, it became increasingly obvious that both cellular and humoral factors were involved in acquired immunity. For example, Metchnikoff had observed that microorganisms were more effectively engulfed in immunized than in nonimmunized animals. In addition, Wright and Douglas, in 1903, demonstrated that immune serum contained a factor that adhered to microorganisms (similar to those used to immunize the animal), making them more easily engulfed by phagocytes. Cells and humoral factors thus appeared capable of cooperation in defending the body.

Later, it became apparent that nonspecific immunity, present at birth, might be mediated, in part, by humoral factors in body secretions and, in part, by phagocytes. On the other hand, specific immunity, acquired after birth by exposure to disease or through immunization, might be mediated by specific antibodies and by specific cells. Today, it is known that immune responses involve interactions of both humoral and cellular immunity.

Antigens

Invasive viruses, bacteria, fungi, protozoa, worms, cancer cells, foreign tissues, and worn out cells can exhibit, produce, or release nonself substances known as antigens. **Antigens** are *substances that can stimulate an immune response* and, given the opportunity, *react specifically by binding with the effector molecules* (**antibodies**) and *effector cells* (**lymphocytes**) produced. (For further discussion of antigens see chapter 3, Effectors of Humoral Immunity.) This definition of an antigen focuses on two important properties that were formally identified by Obermayer and Pick in 1903, namely, **immunogenicity** (the capacity to stimulate the formation of antibodies) and **specificity** (the ability to react specifically with these antibodies). This latter property means that in a humoral immune response an antigen reacts selectively with its corresponding antibody and not with any of the variety of antibodies formed in response to other antigens. Similarly, in a cell-mediated immune response, an antigen induces selective activation of some, but not all, effector cells.

Nature of Antigens

Most antigens are proteins, but some contain carbohydrates, lipids, or nucleic acids. Some antigens are more **immunogenic,** or *capable of eliciting an immune response,* than others. An antigen, such as a protein, can possess a number of small chemical groupings that are called **antigenic-determinant groups.** Any one determinant group, under appropriate conditions, *can stimulate the formation of a particular kind of antibody molecule or effector cell.* Thus, a pure protein antigen might give rise to many distinct antibodies and effector cells.

Immunogenicity and specificity of antigens can be altered by chemical treatment. For example, attaching various chemical groups to protein antigens can cause different antibodies to be formed. In 1921 Landsteiner coined the term **hapten** to describe these specific chemical groups that are, by themselves, incapable of stimulating antibody formation but, when associated with proteins, are capable of doing so.

Tolerogens

Antigens do not always exhibit immunogenicity or evoke antibody formation, however. In some instances, an antigen presented at one concentration might induce *specific immunological unresponsiveness,* or **tolerance,** while at another concentration it might promote immunity. An antigen that induces tolerance is referred to as a *tolerogen.*

The notion of immunological tolerance was proposed in 1944 by **Medawar** and **Burnet** and earned them the 1960 Nobel Prize. One important manifestation of tolerance occurs during fetal development. Since an individual's immune system does not normally react against self-components, Burnet suggested that fetal immunocytes were deleted by contact with their specific autoantigens. This process, called *clonal deletion,* supposedly led to removal of immunocytes that would react against self-antigens. In this manner, an individual became tolerant to self-antigens. It has since become clear, however, that mammals possess all the genetic information necessary to react immunologically against self-constituents, although this rarely occurs. Nevertheless, autoimmune responses do occur under certain circumstances. (See chapter 10, Immune Tolerance and Suppression, and chapter 16, Autoimmunity, for further discussions.)

Histocompatibility Antigens

Immunological tolerance has become an exciting and active area of research that is especially relevant to the problems of tissue and organ transplantation. Unless the tissue proposed for transplantation is antigenically identical to that of the intended recipient, the recipient's immune system attempts to reject it. The antigens of tissues that are responsible for evoking immunological responses against grafts are called histocompatibility antigens. They are encoded by genes known as histocompatibility genes, which collectively constitute a **major histocompatibility complex (MHC)**. Thus, MHC products present markers of individual identity. MHC products on human leukocyte surfaces, known as human leukocyte-associated (HLA) antigens have been used extensively in identifying potential donors for transplants. In addition to serving as surface markers for tissue typing, HLA antigens are involved in critical regulatory interactions. Chapter 7, Histocompatibility Systems, explores this topic in greater depth.

Antibodies
Nature of Antibodies

The term **antibody** refers to a spectrum of *proteins that are formed in response to an antigen and that react specifically with that antigen.* Antibodies belong to a group of proteins known as **immunoglobulins (Igs)**. There are five major classes of immunoglobulins (*IgG, IgM, IgA, IgD,* and *IgE*), each with specialized properties (see chapter 3, Effectors of Humoral Immunity). These are easily distinguished on the basis of their characteristic heavy polypeptide chains.

 IgG is the most common class and plays a critical role in most humoral responses. All antibody molecules, regardless of class, have a basic four-chain structure consisting of *two identical* **light (L)** and *two*

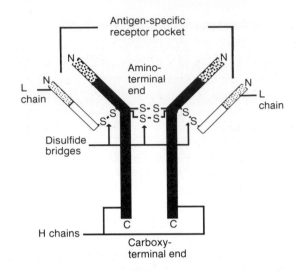

FIGURE 1.7 General structure of an antibody molecule. The basic structure of an antibody molecule is represented by IgG. This molecule has two heavy (H) and two light (L) polypeptide chains that are linked to each other as depicted. Constant regions of these chains are shown in *solid color* (white or black), while the variable regions are *stippled.* The variable regions are responsible for the specificity shown for a particular antigen. In addition, carbohydrate moieties (not depicted) are attached to the H chains at several sites (see chapter 3 for additional details).

identical **heavy (H) polypeptide chains** (fig. 1.7). Portions of both L and H chains vary uniquely in different antibody molecules. *Variable regions* in each L and H chain *form a specific receptor or "pocket,"* which is genetically programmed and *complementary to a specific antigenic determinant.* Thus, two identical receptor sites for binding specific antigenic determinants are present on each four-chain structure. The *variable sequence* of amino acids at amino-terminal ends of the randomly paired L and H chains is essentially *responsible for the antibody specificity* expressed. The specificity of an antibody molecule is, therefore, a product of gene expression. Antibody specificity refers to the *ability of an antibody to discriminate between two antigenic determinants.* The structure of antibody molecules was elucidated in the late 1950s by **Porter, Edelman,** and others. The value of these studies, which provided the basis for a more thorough understanding of the chemistry of antibody specificity and the mechanism of antigen-antibody binding, was recognized by the award of the 1972 Nobel Prize in Physiology to Porter and Edelman.

Antibody Formation

The existence of antibodies was known, or suspected, during the last decades of the nineteenth century. It was clear, almost from the start, that many kinds of antibodies must either exist or be capable of being formed. However, it was unclear how a cell made a specific antibody when stimulated by a particular antigen. Moreover, it was not known whether a cell could produce more than one kind of antibody molecule. For example, did a cell have a program for each specific antibody that required antigen *selection,* or did it have a program for producing a molecule that could be influenced by any antigen, thereby giving the antibody its specificity by *instruction?*

In 1896 Paul Ehrlich suggested that cells already knew how to make specific antibodies. He proposed that antibody-forming cells had specific side chains that acted as receptors for antigens. When a complementary antigen bound to this receptor, it triggered the new synthesis of side chains, which were subsequently released into the blood as antibodies specific for that antigen. This "key (antigen) in a lock (antibody)" hypothesis was not generally accepted at that time, however.

Since that time, numerous hypotheses to account for antibody production have arisen. One of the more popular hypotheses appeared in 1955. In that year, **Jerne** and **Burnet** postulated that each of us has a large heterogeneous population of lymphocytes, each of which is capable of binding antigens of a single specificity (fig. 1.8). If the proper antigen binds to that specific receptor, the cell can become activated, undergo division, and produce a clone of antibody-forming plasma cells. This model is known as the **clonal selection theory.** It is so called because the antigen "selects," or binds, to a particular cell that then produces a clone of itself. It should be noted that this cell already "knows" how to make a *specific* antibody, which is expressed on its surface as a receptor for the antigen.

Cellular Components

The *major cellular components* of the immune system are **lymphocytes, antigen-presenting cells (APCs)**, and **phagocytes** (table 1.4). These cells are responsible for

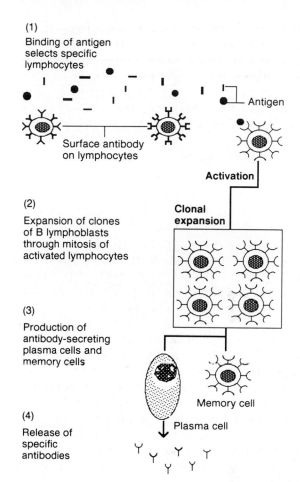

(1)
Binding of antigen selects specific lymphocytes

Antigen

Surface antibody on lymphocytes

Activation

(2)
Expansion of clones of B lymphoblasts through mitosis of activated lymphocytes

Clonal expansion

(3)
Production of antibody-secreting plasma cells and memory cells

Memory cell

(4)
Release of specific antibodies

Plasma cell

FIGURE 1.8 Antigen-specific clonal selection in an immune response. Lymphocytes possess surface antibodies of a single specificity. If the complementary antigen binds to that receptor, activation occurs leading to the formation, by clonal expansion, of a population of cells that either produce antibodies against that antigen (plasma cells) or remember that antigen upon subsequent exposure (memory cells). Note that differences in appearances of the antibodies depicted represent distinctive identities of the antibodies, not the nature of antigen recognition or binding.

bringing about defensive responses that are generalized (nonspecific) or triggered by and focused on particular antigens (antigen specific).

Lymphocytes

Lymphocytes have the remarkable ability to *recognize, bind, and interact with antigens by means of unique antibody receptors* on their membrane surfaces. A single

TABLE 1.4 Major Cell Types of the Immune System

Cell Type	Characteristics and Functions
Lymphocytes	
B cells	Differentiate in bursa of Fabricius (birds) or bone marrow (mammals); respond to specific antigens by production of antibody-producing plasma cells or memory cells; are responsible for expression of humoral immunity
T cells	Differentiate in thymus gland; are responsible for expression of cellular immunity; include subclasses responsible for immune regulation
Null cells	Do not express B or T cell antigens; are responsible for responses that are not antigen specific
Antigen-Presenting Cells	Are diverse group of cell types (e.g., macrophages and dendritic cells); are first cells to encounter and interact with antigen; present antigen in conjunction with self-markers
Phagocytes	Are diverse group of cell types (e.g., macrophages and neutrophils); physically remove immunologically marked antigens by engulfment

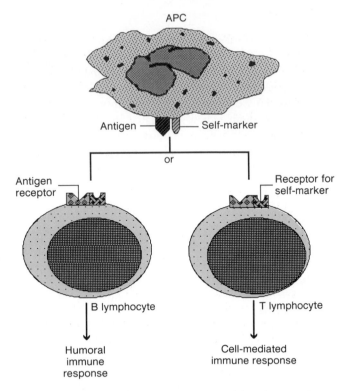

FIGURE 1.9 Interaction between an APC and lymphocytes. Antigen, in association with self-markers, can be processed for presentation to lymphocytes to initiate a specific immune response. Since APCs can interact with either B or T cells, the nature of the response depends upon the type of lymphocyte activated, not the APC. Activation and expression of B cells, in these circumstances, might require the assistance of T cells.

lymphocyte, or a clone of identical lymphocytes, possesses *monospecific receptors* that essentially *bind a* **single type** of antigenic determinant. There are two major classes of **antigen-reactive lymphocytes: B and T cells.**

 B lymphocytes are primarily responsible for *humoral, or antibody, responses,* while **T lymphocytes** are responsible for *specific cell-mediated responses.* The several subclasses of B and T lymphocytes cooperate to provide a dual defensive system against numerous insults. Further discussions of these cells and their central roles in immune responses are presented in chapter 2 and in units 2 and 3, respectively.

Antigen-Presenting Cells

Antigen-presenting cells, such as **macrophages** and **dendritic cells,** make a triad with T and B cells during most humoral and cell-mediated responses (fig. 1.9). They may be the first cells to encounter antigen that has entered the body. They subsequently appear to *process the antigen and then present it, in association with a self-marker,* to the major lymphocyte participants. An immune response subsequently follows. Details of the interactions between antigen-presenting cells and lymphocytes can be found in chapter 3, Effectors of Humoral Immunity and chapter 9, Effectors of Specific Cellular Immunity.

Phagocytes

Completion of an immune response includes *physical removal of the antigen.* This might be expressed in the form of phagocytic ingestion of antigen-antibody complexes or of antibody-tagged infective cells and their debris. Cells that are responsible for this aspect of immunological defense are **macrophages** and **phagocytic leukocytes** (granulocytes).

S U M M A R Y

1. Health represents the state of harmonious balance between the internal and external environments. [p. 4]
2. The tendency to actively preserve the normal steady-state conditions of the internal environment is called homeostasis. [p. 4]
3. The internal environment, which provides the fluid environment for all cells, consists of the cardiovascular and lymphatic systems and the interstitial fluid. This internal environment makes available to the cells all substances essential for life and communication and ensures the elimination of waste materials. [pp. 5–7]
4. The cardiovascular compartment contains a complex medium called blood. The plasma, or fluid, portion of blood functions to transport a variety of dissolved nutrients and waste products. The particulate phase of blood contains cells responsible for gas exchange (erythrocytes) and defense (phagocytic leukocytes and immunocytes and platelets). [pp. 7–10]
5. Disease represents the state when normal homeostatic balance is disturbed, when the organism is no longer in harmony with its environment. [pp. 10–11]
6. Causes of disease include infectious biological agents, modification of cellular expression (cancer), alterations in the status of immune function, genetic change, environmental factors, and degeneration. [p. 11]
7. Infectious diseases are caused by biological agents: (a) viruses (infectious hepatitis), (b) bacteria (tuberculosis), (c) fungi (histoplasmosis), (d) protozoa (malaria), and (e) worms (trichinosis). [pp. 11–12]

8. Cancer is characterized by a population of cells that function atypically and do not respond to normal regulatory control. Tumors can be either benign or malignant. Several theories exist to explain how transformation of a normal cell to a tumor (cancer) cell can be accomplished. [pp. 12–14]
9. Immunological diseases can cause harm to the individual directly or by default. Hypersensitivity (overreactive) and autoimmune (directed against oneself) reactions cause direct harm to the organism. Immune deficiency states cause damage by default by failing to effectively counteract foreign substances or invading organisms. [pp. 14–15]
10. Disease can also arise from a variety of other sources. These include genetic, degenerative, environmental, psychogenic, and iatrogenic causes. [pp. 15–16]
11. The immune system plays an important role in maintaining homeostasis and health. A significant aspect of this role is involved in defense against foreign substances and infective agents. [p. 16]
12. Immunology is the field of study that is concerned with understanding the immune system and processes through which it works. [p. 16]
13. Protection against the effects of infective agents is known as immunity. It can be innate or acquired actively or passively. [pp. 16–17]
14. Innate immunity is not acquired, but rather is present from birth. In contrast to acquired immunity that is antigen specific, innate immunity is not antigen specific. [p. 17]
15. Active acquired immunity is the result of the generation of immune products by an individual following exposure to an inducing agent. The inducing agent can be artificially introduced in the form of a vaccine. [pp. 17–19]
16. Passively acquired immunity comes about through the presentation to an individual of immune products developed by some other source. [pp. 19–20]
17. Immunological responses can be defined as humoral when they are mediated primarily by

antibodies and complement or cellular when they are mediated by cellular effector cells. Integration between these two pathways is common in the expression of immunity. [pp. 20–21]

18. Antigens are substances that can elicit an immune response. The ability of an antigen to provoke an immune response depends upon its chemical and physical properties. [p. 21]

19. Two important classes of antigens are tolerogens and major histocompatibility antigens. Tolerogens are antigens that can produce a state of immunological nonresponsiveness, or tolerance. Major histocompatibility antigens are antigens that play a central role in self-recognition and graft rejection. [pp. 21–22]

20. Antibodies are molecules produced in response to particular antigens for which they are specific. Antibodies are plasma proteins known as immunoglobulins. Five major classes of immunoglobulins exist in mammals. [pp. 22–23]

21. The major cells of the immune system are lymphocytes, antigen-presenting cells, and phagocytes. Collectively, these cells are responsible for recognizing "offending" antigens, mounting specific reactions against them, and eliminating them from the host. [pp. 23–25]

READINGS

Boyd, W., and Sheldon, H. *Introduction to the Study of Disease.* Lea & Febiger, Philadelphia, 1984.

Brock, T. D. (ed.). *Milestones in Microbiology.* Prentice-Hall, Englewood Cliffs, New Jersey, 1961.

Cannon, W. B. *The Wisdom of the Body.* W. W. Norton & Co., Inc., New York, 1963.

Caplan, A. L., Engelhardt, H. T., Jr., and McCartney, J. J. (eds.). *Concepts of Health and Disease: Interdisciplinary Perspectives.* Addison-Wesley Publishing Co., Reading, Mass., 1981.

de Kruif, P. *Microbe Hunters.* Pocket Books, New York, 1953.

Ehrlich, P. *Studies in Immunity.* Wiley Publishing Co., New York, 1910.

Glasser, R. J. *The Body is the Hero.* Random House, New York, 1976.

Guyton, A. C. *Human Physiology and Mechanisms of Disease.* 3d ed. W. B. Saunders Co., Philadelphia, 1982.

Hill, R. B., and LaVia, M. F. (eds.) *Principles of Pathobiology.* 3d ed. Oxford University Press, Inc., New York, 1980.

Kent, T. H., Hart, M. N., and Shires, T. K. *Introduction to Human Disease.* Appleton-Century-Crofts, New York, 1979.

Langley, L. L. (ed.). *Homeostasis: Origins of the Concept.* Dowden, Hutchinson, & Ross, Stroudsburg, Penna., 1973.

Metchnikoff, E. *Lectures on the Comparative Pathology of Inflammation.* Dover Publications, Inc., New York, 1968. (Reprint of the English edition published by Kegan Paul, Trench, Tübner & Co., Ltd., in 1893.)

Metchnikoff, E. *L'immunité dans les Maladies Infectieuses.* Masson, New York, 1901.

Parish, H. J. *A History of Immunization.* Livingston Press, Wynnewood, Penna., 1965.

Price, S. A., and Wilson, L. M. *Pathophysiology: Clinical Concepts of Disease Processes.* 2d ed. McGraw-Hill Book Co., New York, 1982.

Schmidt, J. E. *Medical Discoveries: Who and When.* Thomas Publishers, Caldwell, Texas, 1959.

Silverstein, A. M. *A History of Immunology.* Academic Press, San Diego, Calif., 1989.

CHAPTER 2

Cells and Tissues of the Immune System

OVERVIEW

The principal organs of the immune system are identified and their structures and functions are outlined. A general description is provided of the cells of the immune system. Distinguishing features and functions of the disparate cell types are stressed.

CONCEPTS

1. The organs of the immune system provide appropriate microenvironments for the proliferation, maturation, and differentiation of the cells that execute immunological functions.

2. The various cells of the immune system have surface markers and receptors that serve to identify them and relate to the roles that they perform.

In any country, order may be threatened by the "unlawful" or disorderly, often violent, conduct of some members of society. Consequently, a variety of defensive and regulatory postures are established to protect the society. Just as society has evolved mechanisms for preserving itself (an external environment), it is not surprising to find that nature has devised a defensive system that can actively combat threats to the order of the internal environment. This defensive system contains *special surveillance units,* cells *capable of specific recognition and subsequent response* to these identifiable dangers, which effect a number of unique protective measures.

This chapter examines the structural organization of the immune system. In addition, the several classes of cells that are responsible for the functions of the immune system are introduced and characterized. This provides the cornerstone for the exploration of immunological activities and the role of the immune system in disease that follows.

■　■　■　■　■　■　■　■　■

ARCHITECTURE OF THE IMMUNE SYSTEM

The immune system consists of a network of lymphoid organs, tissues, and cells (fig. 2.1 and table 2.1) and the products of these cells (e.g., cytokines [growth factors and regulatory agents], cytotoxic substances, and antibodies). The primary lymphatic organs are the bone marrow and thymus, where immature lymphocytes differentiate into antigen-sensitive, mature B (for bursa-equivalent) and T (for thymus-processed) cells, respectively. (The significance of these designations is explained later.) The principal secondary lymphatic organs are the spleen and lymph nodes. Other secondary lymphoid organs include the adenoids, tonsils, lymphoid (Peyer's) patches of the small intestine, and the appendix. All secondary lymphoid organs serve as areas where lymphocytes may encounter and bind antigen, whereupon they proliferate and differentiate into fully mature, antigen-specific effector cells.

These hemopoietic and lymphoid organs undergo change in organization throughout development. Many of these changes reflect structural and ar-

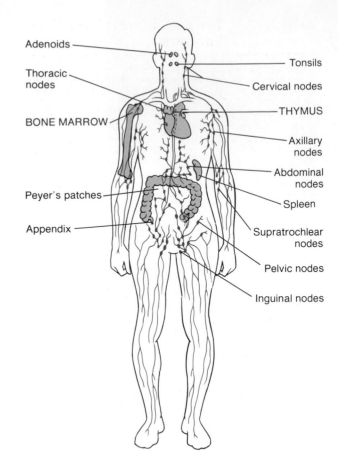

FIGURE 2.1　Organs of the immune system. Primary (*uppercase*) and secondary (*upper- and lowercase*) organs of the immune system are represented. In addition, several of the lymph node regions are designated.

chitectural reorganization. However, certain of these changes are functional and have profound influence on the development of our immune responses. Discussion of acquisition of immune competence during development is deferred until chapter 20, Development of Immunity. In this chapter, our attention is focused on lymphoid organs and effector cells of the immune system found in adults, since our objective here is to introduce you to the major participants in immune responses. Units 2 and 3 elaborate on factors involved in the maturation and function of major effectors of humoral and cellular immune responses.

TABLE 2.1 Lymphoid Organs and Their Functions

Lymphoid Organs	Functions
Primary Lymphoid Organs	
Bone marrow	Is major site of hemopoiesis (production of all major blood cell types); provides microenvironment for antigen-independent differentiation of B cells; provides antigen-processing environment; is possible equivalent of bursa of Fabricius
Thymus	Provides environment for antigen-independent differentiation of T cells; produces hormonal factors important for T cell maturation
Bursa of Fabricius	Provides environment responsible for B cell maturation (found only in birds)
Secondary Lymphoid Organs	
Spleen	Acts as temporary reserve site for lymphocytes; provides antigen-processing environment; is auxiliary site of hemopoiesis (in extraordinary circumstances)
Regional lymph nodes; adenoids, tonsils, Peyer's patches, appendix	Are temporary holding sites for recirculating lymphocytes; provide antigen-processing environment

Primary Lymphoid Organs

Bone Marrow

In adults, **red bone marrow** serves as the *major source of all blood cells,* including lymphocytes. It is found in the cavities of most bones in the body including the skull, ribs, sternum, femur, and spine. However, the distribution of red marrow diminishes with age. Red bone marrow is compartmentalized into hemopoietic and vascular areas. The principal architecture of hemopoietic (blood-forming) marrow consists of sinusoids arranged peripherally around a central vein (fig. 2.2). Within these sinusoids are found the precursors

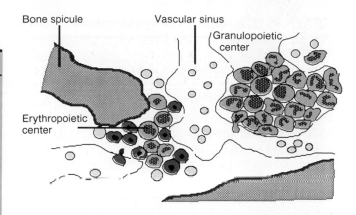

FIGURE 2.2 Sinusoid of red bone marrow. The major architectural subunit of hemopoiesis in the bone marrow is the sinusoid. Through this organization, hemopoiesis occurs in intimate association with veins into which the newly formed blood cells can readily migrate.

(*blast cells*) of the different blood cell lines and their more mature descendants. For example, a particular sinusoid might contain several myeloblasts (granulocyte progenitor cells) surrounded by larger numbers of more mature granulocytes. This pocket reflects proliferation and maturation of granulocytes from the precursor pool. Bone marrow, thus, contains various intermediate and mature forms of erythrocytes, monocytes, granulocytes, lymphocytes, and megakaryocytes.

In addition to definitive progenitor cells for each blood cell type, there seems to be a generalized progenitor cell capable of yielding any of the blood cell lines. This ultimate progenitor is called a **stem cell.** This remarkably renewable pluripotent stem cell is believed to have a lymphoid morphology (appearance), and its existence is inferred from its ability to repopulate all of the blood cells in a lethally irradiated animal. The various stem cells and hemopoietic precursors are summarized in table 2.2.

Bone marrow is not only the source of all blood cell classes, but it also provides the *microenvironment for the antigen-independent differentiation of B cells.* (As shown in later chapters, lymphocytes undergo two major stages of differentiation. One is independent of antigen [antigen independent] and leads to the production of B and T classes of lymphocytes. The other is dependent upon exposure to antigen [antigen dependent] and leads to the production of clones of lymphocytes that are reactive to the provoking antigen.)

TABLE 2.2 Classes of Hemopoietic Stem Cells

Stem Cell	Mature Progeny
Pluripotent Stem Cells (broad potential)	
Colony-forming unit–lymphoid-myeloid (CFU-LM)	All blood cell types
Colony-forming unit–spleen (CFU-S)	All nonlymphocytic blood cells
Pluripotent Stem Cells (limited potential)	
Colony-forming unit–culture (CFU-C)	Granulocytes and monocytes
Unipotential Stem Cells	
Burst-forming unit–erythroid (BFU-E)	Erythrocytes
Cluster-forming unit–erythroid (CFU-E)	Erythrocytes
Colony-forming unit–thromboid (CFU-T)	Platelets
Differentiated Progenitor Cells	
Lymphoblasts	B and T lymphocytes
Megakaryoblasts	Megakaryocytes/platelets
Monoblasts	Monocytes
Myeloblasts	Any granulocyte type
Pronormoblasts (proerythroblast, prorubriblast)	Erythrocytes

Relationships among these precursors are depicted in figure 2.7.

These cells display an immense repertoire of antigen receptors at maturity. Moreover, bone marrow serves as a secondary lymphoid organ where mature, virgin, antigen-reactive lymphocytes (T and B cell) may respond to antigen trapped by antigen-presenting cells, such as macrophages. Thus, bone marrow may provide an antigen-processing environment, as does the spleen.

Thymus

The **thymus** is considered a critical organ of the immune system. It is responsible for the *antigen-independent maturation and development of T lymphocytes* that effect cell-mediated immunity and regulate most humoral and cell-mediated responses.

The thymus is a bilobed, grayish, lympho-epithelial organ, located just above the heart and beneath the breastbone. It consists of a reticular network filled with a mass of lymphocytes, and a small number of epithelial cells (fig. 2.3). In adults, the thymus consists of many lobules, each containing a cortex, or outer region, and a medulla, or central region. The medulla contains mature, virgin T cells that have emigrated from the cortex, and layers of comparatively large epithelial cells. Polypeptide hormones produced by the epithelial cells appear to provide (or at least significantly contribute to) the microenvironment that promotes antigen-independent differentiation of primitive thymocytes. (See chapter 20, Development of Immunity, for a discussion of the thymic hormones and their influence on the differentiation of T cells.)

Progenitor lymphocytes migrate through the bloodstream from the bone marrow to the thymus for the maturation process. Maturation involves many divisional steps, and only the emergent progeny are capable of carrying out T cell–related functions. The thymus is one of the most active sites of lymphocyte proliferation. However, most cells die in the process. Only 5% of the cells produced actually leave the thymus as viable cells. Some believe this apparent waste may represent the elimination of lymphocyte clones that react against self, along with cells that sustained lethal mutations or genetic abnormalities during faulty divisions. Those that do survive, however, are functional antigen-reactive T cells.

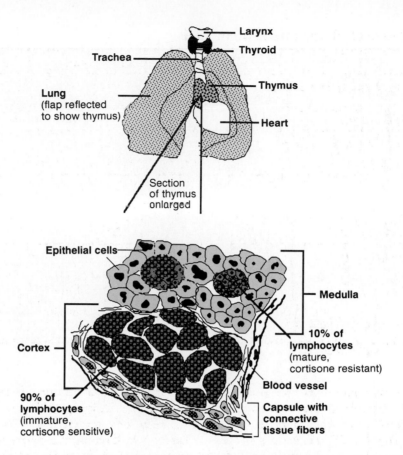

FIGURE 2.3 Thymus. The thymus gland contains cortical and medullary regions that differ in their cellular organization. The major features of these differences are illustrated in this sketch of a section (lobule) of the thymus.

The thymus reaches peak activity in childhood and attains its largest size at puberty. Thereafter, it gradually becomes smaller and is extremely small in old age. Early in life the thymus is critical for T cell maturation and if the thymus is removed shortly after birth (referred to as neonatal thymectomy), normal cell-mediated immune responses fail to develop. Accordingly, the individual does not reject histoincompatible tissue transplants (see chapter 7, Histocompatibility Systems); blood lymphocyte levels are drastically reduced, and the response to most antigens is poor or absent. Impaired thymic development may be associated with immune deficiency disorders, cancer, and autoimmune disease (see unit 5, Damaging and Defective Immune Responses).

Bursa of Fabricius

While the thymus serves as a central lymphoid organ to control maturation of T lymphocytes concerned largely with cell-mediated immunity, the **bursa of Fabricius,** in birds, is responsible for the *antigen-independent maturation of B cells* involved in humoral immunity. The bursa is a lymphoepithelial organ seen as an intestinal pouch in birds, but not in mammals. It is lined with epithelial cells which cover outer cortical and inner medullary areas that are packed with B cells and plasma cells. If the bursa is surgically removed, a procedure known as bursectomy, birds may have normal cell-mediated immune responses, but they express little, if any, antibody-producing capability. Like

The Nude Mouse

Ordinarily, an individual is born with a full complement of organs and tissues. Assuming that there are no associated organic, or other, disorders this individual can be expected to display all normal physiological functions. Nevertheless, from time to time, individuals are born displaying one defect or another in function. These are sometimes traced to genetic alterations or deficiencies.

One instance of a genetic defect with far-reaching consequences for immunological function has emerged. This is the genetically defective *nude, or hairless, mouse*. Nude mice are **homozygous** for the recessive allele, Nu (Nu/Nu). Having the **Nu/Nu genotype** leads to a condition characterized by (1) absence of a thymus, (2) failure of hair growth, and (3) endocrine abnormalities. Since these mice are also sterile, they are produced by breeding mice that are carriers of the recessive trait.

The nude mouse provides a natural experiment that *mimics* conditions seen by neonatal thymectomy. Since full immunological competence does not exist at birth (at least not in mice), neonatal thymectomy leads to impairment of immune function because of a failure of the T cell component of the immune system to function. A similar situation is expected in nude mice. Nonetheless, nude mice have a T cell population (between 2% and 20% of splenocytes carry the Thy-1 antigen, an indicator of T cell differentiation), yet these cells fail to differentiate into functionally active, mature T cells. Moreover, these mice possess a B cell component and display effective humoral immunity. Accordingly, nude mice provide an excellent *model for studying T cell function*. Studies have found that some of the functions of the thymus can be restored to nude, or thymectomized, mice by the administration of extracts of thymus tissue, which consist of hormones and thymic factors. This enables investigators to explore factors that are involved in the regulation of T cell commitment and differentiation. In addition, nude mice can be used to propagate certain human cancer cells that otherwise would be destroyed readily in normal mice.

Thus, the unique deficiencies displayed by athymic (nude) mice provide a convenient natural laboratory in which to explore several aspects of immunological function. Of particular significance are questions of B/T cell dichotomy and environmental influences on the maturation and differentiation of T cells.

Pantelouris, E. M. Absence of thymus in a mouse mutant. *Nature* (London) 217:370. 1968

Bevan, M. J. Thymic education. Hünig T. T-cell function and specificity in athymic mice. Scollay, R. Intrathymic events in the differentiation of T lymphocytes: A continuing enigma. Robinson, J. H., and Jordan, R. K. Thymus in vitro. In *T Lymphocytes Today*. J. R. Inglis (ed). Elsevier Science Publishers, Amsterdam, 1983.

the thymus, the bursa starts to shrink or atrophy at puberty. The organ serves as the hemopoietic-inducing microenvironment for progenitor B cells in birds.

The mammalian equivalent of the bursa of Fabricius appears to be the **red bone marrow.** Thus, the two functional compartments of immune maturation in humans, and all mammals, are the thymus and the bursa equivalent (quite possibly the bone marrow), which process T and B lymphocytes, respectively.

Secondary Lymphoid Organs

The lymph nodes, spleen, adenoids, tonsils, lymphoid patches of the gut, and the appendix are all areas where **mature T** and **B lymphocytes** may have an opportunity to bind antigen and **undergo further antigen-dependent differentiation.** It is here that the active immune response begins. All of these lymphoid organs are capable of *trapping antigen,* which normally involves large tissue phagocytes, known as macrophages. These peripheral lymphatic organs *concentrate antigens from all parts of the body.* Since the system contains recirculating lymphocytes, which pass from the blood through the lymphoid tissues and back to the blood, it virtually ensures that circulating antigen-reactive lymphocytes with the proper receptors will encounter these antigens. Furthermore, the size of the lymphocyte pool suggests that there are lymphocytes available to "fit"

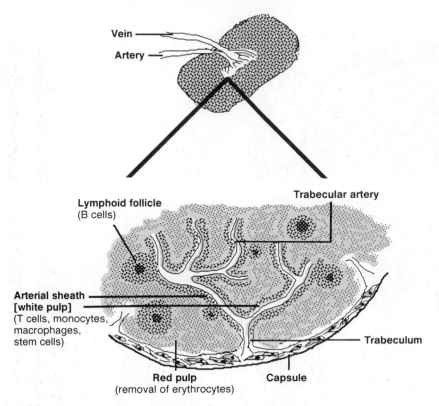

FIGURE 2.4 Spleen. The basic organization of the spleen, showing regions of red pulp and white pulp, is represented. Note the intimate apposition of white pulp to the trabecular artery.

any type of antigen. Thus, the traffic of lymphocytes between the blood, lymphoid tissues, and lymph enables antigen-reactive cells to bind antigen and, in turn, be recruited to sites where the action is occurring.

During the course of normal lymphocyte circulation, lymphocytes leave the blood and accumulate in lymphatic tissues, as if by a homing instinct, to set up B and T cell areas. Here they reside temporarily before returning to the circulation. The normal steady input and output of cells among lymphoid organs is disrupted during a primary immune response, and dramatically so following a secondary immune response, as seen by a sharp fall in cell output. Within 24 hours of the time an antigen becomes localized in the lymph nodes (or spleen), there is a depletion of antigen-reactive cells from the circulating pool of lymphocytes. This temporary cessation of lymphocyte recirculation is called lymph node shutdown. Approximately three days later, activated cells are released into circulation.

In this regard, the system further serves to transport products and cells of the immune response (in large part antibodies and antigen-specific effector T cells) to the tissues through the bloodstream.

The Spleen

The spleen is a large, encapsulated, lymphoid organ. By means of the evident macrophages, it filters out antigens that enter the bloodstream. The cortex of the spleen contains packed lymphocytes with germinal centers and a medulla containing a variety of cell types. Basically there are two types of tissues in the spleen, referred to as the lymphoid, or white pulp, of the cortex, and the erythroid, or red pulp, of the medulla (fig. 2.4). T cells are diffusely packed in the white pulp, with the follicles primarily composed of B cells.

Most lymphocytes enter and leave the spleen by way of the bloodstream. The white pulp forms a sheath around entering blood vessels, thereby permit-

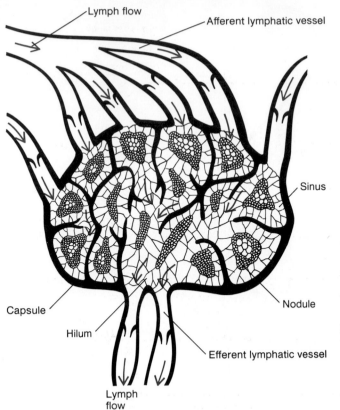

FIGURE 2.5 Lymph node. The organization of a representative lymph node is depicted. Its position relative to lymphatic flow is shown by the arrows. The nodules present are analogous to the germinal centers seen in the spleen (see fig. 2.4).

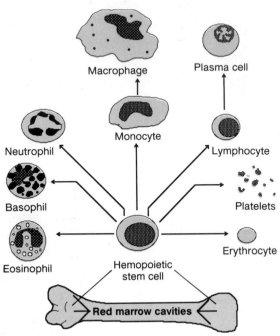

FIGURE 2.6 Cell types derived from bone marrow stem cells. Through differentiation of the stem cell into specific precursors, and their subsequent proliferation and maturation, each of the blood cell types depicted can be produced by the bone marrow. (See also plate 1.)

ting circulating B and T cells to enter and leave the spleen by traversing the walls of small incoming arterioles and outgoing veins (fig. 2.4). The red pulp is involved in removing old red blood cells and is a reserve site for hemopoiesis during pathological states.

Lymph Nodes

Lymph nodes are small, bean-shaped organs that act as filters. They are located at major junctions of the network of lymphatic channels (fig. 2.5). They consist of an outer cortex and an inner medulla. If antigens enter the body via the respiratory or gastrointestinal tracts, they must pass through the regional lymph nodes, as well as the adenoids, tonsils, Peyer's patches, and the appendix. The antigens might pass, via lymphatic channels, through several lymph nodes with increasing likelihood of being trapped by macrophages. Particulate matter, such as bacteria, might be phago-

cytized. These antigens have the opportunity to react with immigrant B and T cells entering, or already localized in, different areas of the lymph node.

B cells and plasma cells are accumulated in subcapsular follicles, while T cells occupy spaces between them in the diffuse cortex. If an animal has been primed or stimulated by antigen, rapidly dividing B lymphocytes can be seen in the germinal center of each follicle. The size of the germinal center is proportional to the intensity of antigenic stimulation and can be greatly enlarged during a secondary immune response.

CELLS OF THE IMMUNE SYSTEM
Hemopoiesis

Cells that participate in the immune response originate in the bone marrow (fig. 2.6) through **hemopoiesis,** the *process of blood cell formation.* Most blood cells have

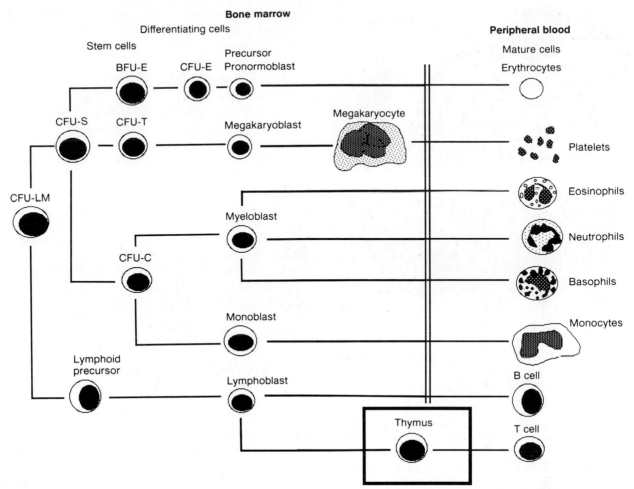

FIGURE 2.7 Classes of stem cells and their lineages. The various stem cells and their relationships to each other are outlined. The progression from left to right is achieved through differentiation. Each successive movement toward the right further limits the potential of the stem cell.

relatively short and unique lifespans according to cell type. Moreover, their numbers remain relatively constant through a homeostatic process of programmed replenishment. This means that there is a set rate at which new cells of a particular type (e.g., granulocytes) are formed. Should the number of cells be reduced, as for example might occur following infection, then the rate of production is increased in order to keep the circulating level constant. Similarly, if the number of those cells were increased, then the rate of production would be temporarily reduced. Maintaining a relatively constant number of erythrocytes in the circulation (a stable hematocrit), with a corresponding increase in erythropoiesis after acute blood loss (see fig. 1.5), also illustrates this point.

Whether each type of blood cell has a separate renewal system, or is derived from a common precursor cell, was a formidable question for many years. (Review table 2.2 for a summary of stem and precursor cells.) It is now clear that both theories are partly correct (fig. 2.7). Experimental evidence supports the existence of both pluripotent and several classes of unipotent hemopoietic stem cells. These **pluripotential stem cells** display two important features: (1) they are able to *maintain a population of pluripotent stem cells* and (2) they are able to *differentiate into the various cell types*. However, there appears to be a hierarchy of such cells, represented as a continuum with different potentials for proliferation and differentiation.

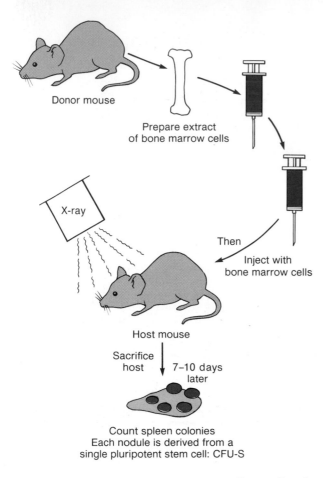

Donor mouse

Prepare extract
of bone marrow cells

X-ray

Then

Inject with
bone marrow cells

Host mouse

Sacrifice
host   7–10 days
            later

Count spleen colonies
Each nodule is derived from a
single pluripotent stem cell: CFU-S

FIGURE 2.8 Spleen colony assay. Bone marrow cells are collected from a healthy donor mouse. These are injected into a previously irradiated recipient mouse. After 7 to 10 days, the spleen of the host is removed and the nodular colonies present are counted. Each colony formed was derived from a single precursor stem cell designated as CFU-S.

The first pluripotent stem cell to be defined was the *spleen colony-forming unit.* Till and McCulloch showed that colonies of hemopoietic cells could form within, and on the surface of, spleens of lethally irradiated mice following injection with appropriate dilutions of murine (mouse) bone marrow cells (fig. 2.8). The nodules of colonies were comprised of pure or mixed populations of erythroid, granulocytic, or megakaryocytic cell lines, as well as undifferentiated cells. The cell giving rise to these clones is termed the *colony-forming unit–spleen (CFU-S),* which is now believed to represent a restricted pluripotent stem cell that can be

found in bone marrow, spleen, and blood. The CFU-S normally displays a low degree of proliferation, although it possesses extensive self-renewal and differentiation capacity or potential.

The relationship of lymphocyte differentiation to the CFU-S is unclear. Most investigators indicate that the CFU-S does not give rise to the lymphoid series. Based on recent studies by Abramson and his colleagues, it now appears that both CFU-S and lymphoid progenitors arise from a more primitive and less restricted pluripotent stem cell, which they term *colony-forming unit– lymphoid-myeloid (CFU-LM).*

Two basic models attempt to describe the mechanisms governing transformation of pluripotent stem cells into one or another specific line of hemopoietic differentiation. The first model of stem cell regulation considers commitment to be a random process, possibly related to mutational occurrences. The second model is deterministic, suggesting that local environmental factors direct the differentiation pathway taken by pluripotent stem cells. Curry and Trentin have coined the phrase **hematopoietic inductive microenvironment** to describe this influence on stem cell differentiation. Accordingly, if a pluripotent stem cell migrates, or "homes," into an *erythroid inductive microenvironment,* it can be acted upon and influenced by factors, including erythropoietin. Consequently, it will be induced to differentiate into the erythroid cell line and eventually form mature erythrocytes. Similarly, if a lymphocyte progenitor migrates to *lymphocyte-inducing microenvironments,* it can be acted on by local hormones or inducing factors to undergo antigen-independent differentiation into a mature antigen-reactive lymphocyte. (See chapters 5, 9, and 20 for further discussions.)

At least *two* **lymphocyte-inducing microenvironments** exist. The microenvironment for *induction of thymic (T) lymphocytes* is the **thymus;** while the microenvironment for *induction of bursal (B) lymphocytes* is the **bursa of Fabricius** (in birds) or its equivalent (presumably the **red bone marrow,** in mammals). Within the thymus gland, a CFU-LM can be induced by thymic hormones, such as a thymopoietin, to differentiate into a T lymphocyte. Within the bursa (or bone marrow) on the other hand, a CFU-LM can be induced by other factors to differentiate into

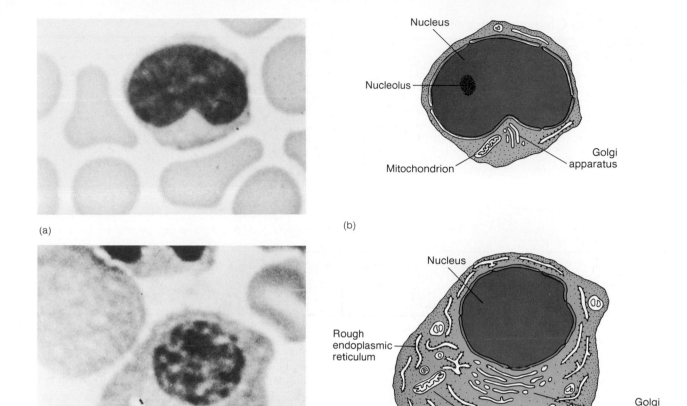

Nucleus

Nucleolus

Mitochondrion

Golgi apparatus

(b)

Nucleus

Rough endoplasmic reticulum

Golgi apparatus

Mitochondria

(a)

(c)

(d)

FIGURE 2.9 Lymphoid cells. Photomicrographs (*a, c*) and sketches of the likely ultrastructure (*b, d*), depicting the organelles of the same cell, are presented for a circulating **lymphocyte** (*a, b*) and a **plasma** cell (*c, d*). (See also plates 2*e* and 2*f*.) (Parts *a* and *c* From Hyun, B. H., Ashton, J. K., and Dolan, K. *Practical Hematology.* 1975. W. B. Saunders Co., Philadelphia.)

a B lymphocyte. These cells subsequently can undergo antigen-dependent differentiation to become the specific effectors of cell-mediated and humoral immune responses, respectively.

Since the discovery of the CFU-S, evidence has accumulated for the existence of intermediate compartments of stem cells, which are committed to specific lines of hemopoiesis. For example, stem cells committed to erythropoiesis are represented by a primitive burst-forming unit–erythroid, a late burst-forming unit–erythroid, and the recently discovered cluster-forming unit–erythroid. In terms of parent to progeny relationships, the primitive burst-forming unit is believed to reside close to CFU-S, while the cluster-forming cell is perhaps the immediate precursor to the pronormoblast, the first morphologically recognizable

cell of the erythroid series. Committed stem cells, likewise, have been elucidated for the granulocyte-monocyte-macrophage series, the megakaryocytic lineage for platelets, and they presumably exist for the lymphoid cell lines as well.

Lymphoid Cells

Lymphocytes are ovoid cells, about 8 to 12 μm in diameter, that are mobile and circulate throughout the body. Lymphocytes possess the unique structural and functional ability to recognize and respond to antigens. Two major classes of lymphocytes are recognized which are designated *T cells and B cells*. T and B cells are indistinguishable by conventional light microscopy (fig. 2.9*a*). Each cell is almost entirely filled

TABLE 2.3 Characteristics of Various Lymphocyte Classes

| Lymphocyte | Surface Markers or Features of T and B Cells | |
	Human	Mouse
T Cells		
Immature	CD5; CD1; CD2	Thy-1; Ly-1,2,3; and TL
Mature subsets		
T_H cells and T_D cells	CD4; CD3; TCR	Thy-1; Ly-1; L3T4; Qa1
T_S cells and T_C cells	CD8; CD3; TCR	Thy-1; Ly-2,3
Activated T cells	HLA-DR; CD25 (Tac)	Ia
B Cells		
B lymphocytes	CD19–22; C1R; mIg	Lyb-2,3,5; mIg
Plasma cells	?	PC.1
Null Cells		
K, NK, NC, LAK	Display neither T nor B cell markers NK1; CD11b; CD16	

NC, natural cytotoxic cell; LAK, lymphokine-activated killer cell.

K, killer cell; NK, natural killer cell; TCR, T cell receptor.

by the nucleus. Nevertheless, T and B lymphocytes can be distinguished from one another and from other leukocytes on the basis of surface markers.

Classification of lymphocytes on the basis of surface markers makes use of two important classes of characteristics. One of these is known as the **cluster designation (CD)**. CDs represent families of surface antigens that can be recognized by specific antibodies produced against them. Thus, a cell displaying CD1 is identified by the binding of antibodies against CD1. Each class of leukocyte displays a diagnostic pattern of CDs. For example, CD3 is expressed only by T cells, CD19 only by B cells, CD64 only by monocytes, CD66 only by granulocytes, and CD68 only by macrophages. In contrast, CD18 and CD45 are expressed by a variety of leukocyte types. Moreover, the pattern of CDs expressed by leukocytes also changes as a function of cell differentiation and maturation. For example, CD9 is expressed by pre-B cells, while CD76 is expressed by mature B cells and CD77 is expressed by resting B cells, whereas CD69 is expressed by activated B cells. (In 1989 the Fourth International Workshop on Human Leukocyte Differentiation Antigens recognized and codified more than 78 distinct CDs. See appendix D.)

The other diagnostic feature used to classify lymphocytes is the nature of **antigen recognition receptors** expressed. Antigen recognition is accomplished by means of *membrane-bound (surface) immunoglobulins (mIgs)* by B cells or by an equivalent molecule called the *T cell receptor (TCR)* by T cells. Unlike CDs, which can serve as diagnostic features for all leukocytes, antigen recognition receptors are limited to B and T lymphocytes. These receptors are required for B and T cells to be antigen reactive. Moreover, mIgs and TCRs confer specificity to antigen recognition by these cells. (The nature of these receptors and their roles in activation of immune responses is explored in chapters 3, 5, and 9.)

Examples of some of the characteristics of various human and murine (mice) lymphocyte classes are presented in table 2.3. Note that the markers identified illustrate only some distinctions among these cells; a complete list of all markers expressed by any cell type is not provided.

Among circulating lymphocytes, approximately 20% to 30% are antigen-reactive B cells, 65% to 75% are T cells, and less than 5% are null cells (i.e., not identifiable as either B or T cells on the basis of surface markers). The number of lymphocytes in the body is enormous, perhaps over a trillion cells, constituting approximately 1% of the body's total weight.

Specific binding of antigen by membrane-bound receptors can stimulate the transformation of small lymphocytes into larger forms, with more abundant cytoplasm, and larger numbers of mitochondria and ribosomes. Some large B lymphocytes can undergo antigen-dependent differentiation into **plasma cells,** which are filled with endoplasmic reticulum (fig. 2.9c), indicative of active antibody synthesis. Other large lymphocytes may revert back to small cells following antigen stimulation, and function as **memory lymphocytes.** (See unit 2 for further discussion of B cell differentiation during immune responses.) T cells can undergo analogous activation by exposure to antigen; however, changes in physical appearance are not as dramatic. (See unit 3 for further discussion of T cell differentiation during immune responses.)

Identification of specific populations and subpopulations of cells that participate in the immune response has become critical in immunology. We simply cannot understand when, how, and where such cells originate; what they do under a variety of conditions; or how they may be manipulated for our best interest, unless they can be identified, isolated, and functionally evaluated. Further understanding of their pivotal roles in normal immune protection, immune deficiency, and immune pathology or disease depends upon continual expansion of our knowledge of these cells.

T Lymphocytes

T lymphocytes are *critically involved in both humoral and cell-mediated immune responses.* They are, therefore, intimately related to our well-being. Indeed, the very quality and quantity of life may be dependent on proper numbers of healthy T cells. If T cell formation or T cell populations, once formed, are adversely affected as a result of, for example, genetic defects, disease, drugs, radiation, or the aging process, individuals may become especially susceptible to certain viral, intracellular parasitic, malignant, and autoimmune diseases.

T cells may be detected, isolated, and assessed largely due to the *surface markers* expressed (as self-antigens), which permit identification (see table 2.3 and plate 3a–c). Pluripotent stem cells in the bone marrow give rise to progenitor T cells, which migrate to the thymus. Once they enter the cortex, or outer portion of the thymus, they are called thymocytes. As a T cell matures, the nature and distribution of surface markers (including CDs and TCRs) change. In particular, the characteristics of TCRs on individual T cells change during antigen-independent differentiation and ultimately contribute to the antigen specificity displayed by mature T lymphocytes. These surface markers and receptors provide a powerful tool for studying the differentiation process, since through them T cells can be identified at various stages of development. (Changes in the expression of differentiation antigens and TCRs during T cell maturation are examined more closely in chapters 9 and 20.)

All members of the class of cells known as T cells, whether immature or mature, including subpopulations in or out of the thymus, share antigen(s) that are not present on B lymphocytes. In mice, this antigen is known as **theta (θ)** or **Thy-1.** The human counterpart markers are CD5, CD3, and CD2. Within T cell populations there are subpopulations distinguished by specific subset antigens, for example Ly-2,3 (murine) and CD4 or CD8 (human). Furthermore, T cells express histocompatibility antigens that are distinct for each individual and that can vary on T cell subsets.

Major histocompatibility antigens are products of a cluster of linked genes known as the **major histocompatibility complex** (**MHC**) (discussed in chapter 7). Genes of the I region of the murine MHC exert dramatic control over immune responses. *Immune response (Ir) gene products* (Ia antigens) may be displayed on lymphocytes as well as macrophages and influence or restrict T and B cell activities. The D region of the human MHC appears to be analogous to the mouse I region.

Several **subclasses of T cells** have been identified that can be discriminated on the basis of their roles in immune responses. For example, some T cells regulate humoral and cell-mediated responses by providing help, whereas other T cells may suppress a response, if necessary (see table 2.4). *T helper cells* (T_H) and *T suppressor cells* (T_S) possess distinct antigens, which identify them (see table 2.3). Other T cells are neither helpers nor suppressors, but serve as *cytotoxic effector cells* (T_C); while still other T cells (T_D) *mediate*

TABLE 2.4 Classes of Lymphocytes

Lymphocyte	Role
T Cells	
T_H cells	Provide "assistance," or potentiate expression of immune function by other lymphocytes
T_S cells	Suppress or impair expression of immune function by other lymphocytes
T_C cells	Bring about cytolysis and cell death of "targets"
T_D cells	Recruit and regulate a variety of nonspecific blood cells and macrophages in expression of delayed (Type IV) hypersensitivity reactions
B Cells	
B lymphocytes	Proliferate/mature into antibody-producing cells
Plasma cells	Are mature, active antibody-producing cells
Null Cells	
Various killer cell types: K, NK, NC, LAK	Bring about cytolysis and death of target cells

delayed-type hypersensitivity reactions by recruiting and regulating a variety of nonspecific blood cells and macrophages. Both T_C and T_D cells may be directly involved in the rejection of tissue transplants that are incompatible to the host.

Thus, T cells share a common class antigen (Thy-1 [mouse]; or CD5, CD3, CD2 [human]) and express TCRs that distinguish them from B cells. In addition, they display MHC antigens representing self. Moreover, they express different antigens during the maturation process (differentiation antigens). Furthermore, the different types of T cells exhibit subset antigens reflecting their specific functions.

B Lymphocytes

Lymphocytes with readily demonstrable **mIg** are termed **B cells.** These cells are derived from pluripotent stem cells in the bone marrow. Progenitor B lymphocytes (pre-B cells) may migrate to several bursa equivalent sites to mature, but it is perhaps more likely that they mature in the bone marrow itself, and then emigrate to the secondary lymphoid organs. Pre-B cells are large lymphoid cells that are recognized by the presence of diffuse heavy chains of immunoglobulins (Igs) belonging to the IgM class (see chapter 3, Effectors of Humoral Immunity). As B cells differentiate and develop into mature antigen-reactive cells, they begin to express membrane-bound monomeric IgM at the cell surface. Later, Igs of other classes might also reside on B lymphocyte membranes. *Most circulating B lymphocytes express both IgM and IgD,* while very few express IgG, IgA, or IgE. Other receptors and antigens serve to mark or distinguish immature and mature B cells and their subpopulations from other cells of the immune system (see table 2.3).

Immature and mature B cells are readily identified by the presence of prominent mIg receptors. These Ig molecules in the membrane serve as *specific receptors for antigen* and, thus, are analogous to TCRs. They can be detected by staining cell suspensions with fluorescent antibodies to the appropriate Ig. In addition, a number of B cell differentiation antigens and markers have been described to distinguish immature and mature B cells. The primary markers are Ly-5 (and possibly 3, 4, and 7) on mature mouse B cells and Ly-1 (primarily a T cell antigen) on immature mouse B cells (analogous to CD5 antigen on human B cell subpopulations). (Further discussions of changes in surface markers occurring during B cell development are presented in chapters 4 and 20.) Moreover, most B cells *express class II MHC gene products,* or Ia antigens, in the mouse and HLA-DR antigens in humans. (These will be discussed in greater detail in chapter 7, Histocompatibility Systems.)

Plasma Cells

Plasma cells are *fully differentiated antibody-synthesizing cells.* They are derived from large transitional B lymphocytes following activation of small B lymphocytes and populate the lymphoid organs in the immunized host. A plasma cell can be distinguished by its eccentric nucleus, numerous ovoid mitochondria, abundant rough endoplasmic reticulum, and prominent Golgi

Assays for Lymphocyte Surface Antigens

Most of the information that we have concerning the nature of B and T cell surface antigens has been derived from studies of inbred, congenic, and mutant strains of mice. A **congenic strain** refers to a line of mice that is *identical to a particular inbred strain, except for one or a few genes.* Using a variety of these animals, antibodies have been produced against a number of different surface antigens.

To produce an antiserum, cells from one strain of mouse are injected into another strain of mouse. Cells from the first strain might possess an antigen not present in the cells from the other strain. Such an antigen is called an alloantigen, and the antiserum that is produced is called an alloantiserum. Thus, an **alloantigen** is an antigen that is *produced by some individuals* (or animal strains) but *not by others of the same species.* The presence of at least one different antigen is necessary in order to produce alloantibodies.

Such specific alloantibodies are often used to identify cell surface antigens by **cytotoxicity assays.** If antibodies bind to specific surface antigenic determinants on lymphocytes, the addition of serum complement (a family of serum proteins) can cause *lysis of the cell membrane* and cell death. To help distinguish dead cells

from live cells, a selective dye is used (e.g., trypan blue), which is excluded by living cells but passively enters and stains dead cells. Thus, *complement-dependent antibody lysis* can be used as a cytotoxicity assay to detect a particular alloantigen. This is useful for identification and discrimination of cell types.

Immunofluorescence and immunoenzymology afford other practical methods for identifying surface markers or antigens. In **immunofluorescence,** the identifying antibodies are labeled with a fluorescent dye, so that the particular lymphocytes possessing complementary-binding antigens can be distinguished when viewed with a fluorescence microscope (see plates 3a and 3e). With **immunoenzymology**, an enzyme (e.g., peroxidase) is attached to the antibody. The complex is then visualized by the formation of reaction products generated by the enzyme in the presence of a suitable substrate.

Cantor, H., and Boyse, E. A. Regulation of cellular and humoral immune responses by T-cell subclasses. *Cold Spring Harbor Symposium on Quantitative Biology* **41**:23, 1976.

Mishell, B. B., and Shiigi, S. M. (eds). *Selected Methods in Cellular Immunology.* W. H. Freeman & Co. Publishers, San Francisco, 1980.

Raff, M. C. Two distinct populations of peripheral lymphocytes in mice distinguished by immunofluorescence. *Immunology* **19**:637, 1970.

apparatus (see fig. 2.9d and plate 2f). It is, thus, well adapted for efficient production and packaging of antibodies.

Plasma cells possess a *unique PC (plasma cell) antigen* not found on their B cell precursors, but they *do not express Ia antigens or surface Ig receptors.* The antibody secreted by a single plasma cell (or specific clone) may be of any class (e.g., IgM, IgG, IgA, or IgE) but the antigen-binding specificity will be identical to that of the receptor expressed by the original B cell precursor. Plasma cells are relatively short-lived (days), compared with small circulating B lymphocytes, which may live for years. Plasma cells are probably capable of dividing only a few times.

Non-T and Non-B Lymphocytes

A small population of lymphocytes, called **null cells,** *do not express characteristics of either T cells or B cells.* They do not possess normal levels of Thy-1 (or CD5) antigen nor do they express TCRs or mIg. The majority of these cells are large granular lymphocytes that are derived from pluripotent stem cells in the bone marrow. From their point of origin they appear to migrate particularly to the spleen and lymph nodes, although there is a significant population in the blood (up to 5% of the lymphocytes present). In addition, a few null cells in circulation might be stem cells or immature T or B cells.

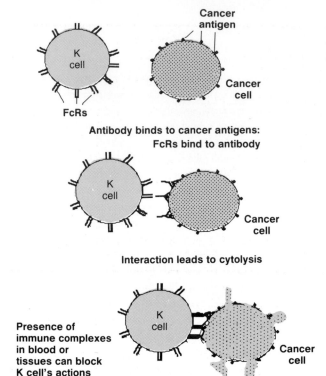

Antibody binds to cancer antigens:
FcRs bind to antibody

Interaction leads to cytolysis

Presence of immune complexes in blood or tissues can block K cell's actions

FIGURE 2.10 Antibody-dependent cellular cytotoxicity reaction. The mechanism in antibody-dependent cellular cytotoxicity is represented for an interaction between a K cell (effector) and a cancer cell (target). (See also plate 2e.)

Null cells appear quite heterogeneous with respect to surface markers expressed. Most null cells *possess receptors for IgG.* By binding to antibodies that are complexed with surface antigens on target cells, they are able to kill or cytolyze the cell through a mechanism known as *antibody-dependent cellular cytotoxicity (ADCC)* (depicted in fig. 2.10). In this capacity, null cells can be referred to as **killer (K), natural killer (NK),** and **natural cytotoxic (NC) cells.** NK cells are neither adherent nor phagocytic, as macrophages, nor do they display antigen-specific cytotoxicity, as T$_C$ cells. Nevertheless, they are spontaneously cytotoxic to a variety of targets, including certain cancer cells, although the means by which NK cells can recognize their pathological target cells is unknown and remains an active area of interest to investigators.

In addition to antibody receptors, some null cells display *receptors for lymphokines* (bioactive products of antigen-specific T cells that can modulate target cell responses) such as interferon (IFN) and interleukin 2 (IL-2). Nonspecific cytotoxic lymphocytes that have become activated in this way are known as **lymphokine-activated killer (LAK) cells.** (Further discussion of null cells and their contributions to nonspecific cellular immune responses is presented in chapter 8.) Moreover, null cells also can display Ly-3 antigens and certain unique antigens such as NK1 detected by monoclonal antibodies.

Surface Receptors

Lymphocytes possess a variety of surface receptors capable of binding a broad range of substances. These include receptors for *foreign antigens* and *self-determinants* of the MHC; *immune complexes* (complexes of antibodies and antigens); *complement; lymphokines; mitogens* (substances that stimulate mitosis); *hormones; viruses;* and *erythrocytes* (table 2.5). Following binding of one or another of these substances to its receptor, T cells may be stimulated into an active state and B cells may initiate a particular activity that reflects the nature of the **ligand** (any molecule that forms a complex with another molecule, such as an antigen complexing with an antibody receptor).

The first class of receptor that we consider are **antigen receptors.** Membrane-bound Ig, or mIg, clearly distinguishes B from T cells by its very presence. Any single B cell, or clone of B cells, possesses mIg receptors *specific for only one* (monospecific) *antigenic determinant.* Thus, the billions of B cells in our bodies display a diversity of receptors capable of reacting with any antigenic determinant that might be encountered. *Receptor Ig and secreted Ig,* relative to a single cell or clone of cells, *are identical in the* **variable** regions of the antibody molecules, and thus show the same specificity for antigen. (See unit 2 for further discussions of immunogenetics and Ig structure.) The nature of TCRs for antigens is somewhat similar to B cell receptors in that antigen recognition depends on variable domains within the protein molecules. In contrast to B cells, however, the *TCR is not an Ig* (see chapter 9 for a more detailed discussion of the TCR).

TABLE 2.5 Lymphocyte Surface Receptors

Receptor	Features	Distribution
Antigen receptors	Are mIg that react against specific foreign antigens	B cells
	Are non-Ig protein heterodimers that bind specific foreign antigens	T cells
MHC receptors	Recognize particular "self"-antigens	B and T cells
Fc receptors	Recognize Fc fragment of Igs	B and T cells; null cells; phagocytes
Complement receptors	Bind active fragments of C3 of complement system	Mature B cells; phagocytes
Lymphokine/monokine receptors	Bind lymphocyte or monocyte factors such as interleukins	B and T cells (different specificities)
Mitogen receptors	Recognize lipopolysaccharide or plant lectin (nonspecific) mitogenic factors	B cells and T cells

A second important class of receptors are antibody receptors known as **Fc receptors (FcRs)**. All cell types of the immune system contain populations or subpopulations with FcRs for IgG, and some express receptors for other Ig classes as well. These receptors recognize a portion of an antibody molecule that is not concerned with antigen binding and is composed of two constant portions of the heavy chains. This domain of the Ig molecule is called the *Fc fragment* (fragment crystallizable).

FcRs are also found on other cells involved in immune function. Their presence on macrophages permits binding, followed by enhanced engulfment and destruction of otherwise host-damaging immune complexes. FcRs on macrophages, granulocytes, NK, and K cells may also allow such cells to become specifically cytotoxic to certain target cells through ADCC reactions. Eosinophils, for example, possess low-affinity FcRs for IgE (see chapter 12). Basophils and mast cells, on the other hand, possess high-affinity receptors for IgE, which might be involved in hypersensitivity reactions (see chapter 13). FcRs can be detected by observing rosette formation when FcR-bearing cells are allowed to react with red cells coated with antibodies (of the IgG class) to red cell antigens.

Complement receptors represent a third class of surface receptors. Complement consists of a family of blood proteins that are identified by a number—for example, complement component 3 (C3) or complement component 5 (C5). In immune responses, proteins of the complement system can become associated with antigen-antibody complexes (see chapter 6). Receptors for components of the complement system are referred to as complement receptors (CRs). Immature B cells lack CRs, whereas mature B cells possess receptors for products of C3 identified as C3b (CR1) and C3d (CR2). Selective receptors for products of C3 (C3a, C3b, C3d) or of C5 (C5a) can also be expressed on macrophages, monocytes, and granulocytes, where their importance in adherence, enhanced phagocytosis, and chemotactic activity is well known. Such receptors might permit B cells to interact with other cells but a clear role has not been determined. CRs are also detected by rosetting techniques (see highlight 2.3).

Another important class of receptors are the **cytokine receptors.** Cytokines (the general classification) are secretory products of particular cells that act on other cells. Lymphokines refer to products of lymphocytes, while monokines are produced and released by monocytes or macrophages. These secretions, in turn, act on other cell populations. For example, the monokine, interleukin 1 (IL-1), acts on lymphocytes, NK cells, and fibroblasts. B cells possess receptors for

Assays for Lymphocyte Surface Receptors

ntigenic determinants displayed in the plasma membrane can be detected by specific reagent antibodies (engendered against alloantigens) and are used to identify cell types or subpopulations. Membrane receptors are also macromolecules that can be characteristic of specific cell types. Receptors have known binding affinities for specific ligands.

Specific lymphocyte receptors can be treated as antigens, for identification purposes, and can be detected by cytotoxic and antibody-labeling techniques (see highlight 2.2). They can also be detected by **rosetting assays.**

An *erythrocyte rosette* (e-rosette) consists of a *lymphocyte surrounded by red cells* attached to its surface CD2 receptors. For example, human T cells bind sheep red blood cells to form a rosette, while B cells do not. The rosetting assay, which might appear trivial at first glance, has become a widely accepted means of identifying human T cells.

Since the first report of this finding, a number of modified rosette assays have been employed for the detection of other receptors. In these cases, red cells are coated with appropriate reagent ligand. By observing for rosettes, we can determine whether or not members of a particular lymphocyte population possess the receptor in question.

The general format of any rosetting assay is as follows:

1. Erythrocytes (e.g., sheep, pig, or human) are coated with the ligand of interest.
2. Coated red cells and the lymphocytes to be tested are then mixed and allowed to react over a period of time.
3. The preparation is next observed for rosette formation.

The presence of rosettes provides evidence for the presence of receptor-positive lymphocytes. In addition, the number of rosetting centers provides an index of how many lymphocytes with a receptor for the ligand are in the population tested.

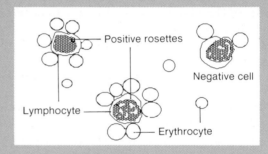

FIGURE 2.A Rosette formation.

IL-1 and B cell growth factors (lymphokines produced by activated T cells, which include IL-2). B cells also possess receptors for factors produced by activated T cells, which contribute to B cell differentiation. T cells have receptors for IL-1 and IL-2. (The roles of several important lymphokines and monokines in immune responses are discussed in context throughout units 2 and 3.)

Yet another class of receptors are the **mitogen receptors.** Substances that promote cell division, or mitosis, are called mitogens. Thus, the ligands that bind to these receptors promote the proliferation of B or T cells. T cell mitogens differ from B cell mitogens. One class of mitogen consists of lipopolysaccharides (LPS) derived from the cell walls of gram-negative bacteria. These substances can act as specific antigens in mice at one concentration and as a mitogen at higher concentrations. Thus, in the B cell repertoire of antigen-reactive clones, monoclonal and polyclonal activation can be identified. Monoclonal activation, which is activation of one or a few clones, represents an antigen-specific response to low LPS concentrations. In contrast, polyclonal activation, which is activation of many clones, represents an apparently indiscriminate response to higher concentrations of LPS as a mitogen. Human B cells do not exhibit LPS receptors, but they can be stimulated by pokeweed (*Phytolacca americana*) mitogens.

A second class of mitogens are the lectins. These are glycoproteins produced by some plants that bind specifically to certain sugar residues present in glycoprotein receptors exhibited on certain cell surfaces. Phytohemagglutinin (PHA) is a lectin from the red kidney bean (*Phaseolus vulgaris*) that binds to both T and B lymphocytes, but only stimulates T cells to divide. Concanavalin A (Con A), a lectin extracted from the black bean (*Conavalia ensiformis*), binds to T cells and acts as a T cell mitogen for both immature and mature cells. Selective T cell mitogens have served to distinguish T cells from B cells and act as polyclonal T cell activators. An antigen stimulates a specific antigen-reactive clone of T or B cell. T cell mitogens, on the other hand, stimulate any clone of T cells, regardless of their binding specificity for antigen. In this regard, mitogens have been very useful in the study of T cell function.

Receptors also are present *for other signal molecules,* for example, hormones and neurotransmitters. Receptors for endorphins and acetylcholine have been identified on lymphocytes. Although their precise role is not yet clear, they undoubtedly mediate communications from the other regulatory systems. In addition, T cells express *receptors for nonspecific binding to erythrocytes.* This reaction is energy dependent, since it can be blocked by metabolic poisons; moreover, it is a nonantigenic interaction.

Most membrane antigenic determinants and receptors will undergo surface redistribution when they combine with complementary molecules at body temperature. After several minutes the material aggregates into patches over the entire cell surface. Dispersed patches then coalesce and localize at one pole of the cell, forming a polar cap (fig. 2.11). The process may be easily visualized by staining cells with fluorescent antibodies directed to the Ig receptors. If monovalent labeled antibodies are used (rather than divalent or multivalent) redistribution doesn't occur, suggesting that crosslinking of receptors is necessary for patching

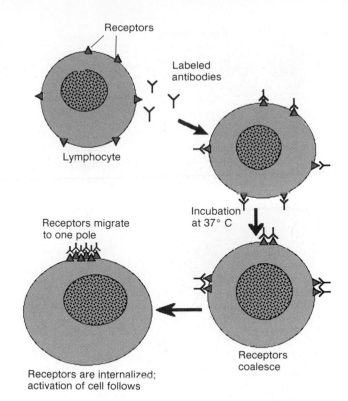

FIGURE 2.11 Polar cap formation. The events in the relocation of surface receptors to create a cap (capping) are outlined. This process was originally described using labeled antibodies to follow redistribution of antibody-receptor complexes over the lymphocyte surface.

and capping. This capping event, which is usually followed by internalization of the components by pinocytosis, requires metabolic activity. Therefore, conditions that depress mobility of the fluid membrane inhibit or block capping (e.g., low temperatures). Cells normally lose surface determinants and/or receptors. Accordingly, after B cells lose mIg, they can reexpress these receptors within eight hours, suggesting dynamic turnover in surface markers. The capping and internalization events suggest that this process might be a key step in cell activation, not only for B and T lymphocytes, but for other cells of the immune system as well. The intracellular events that follow are now the focus of research interest.

Antigen-Presenting Cells

A number of different cell types have been described as **antigen-presenting cells (APCs)**. In addition to

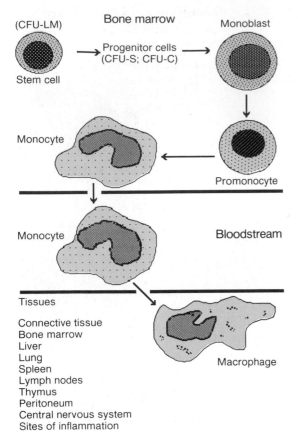

FIGURE 2.12 Derivation of macrophages. The developmental history leading to the formation of a macrophage is schematically represented.

presenting antigen to effector lymphocytes, many of these cells perform nonspecific immunological functions (e.g., phagocytosis and cytotoxicity). Moreover, each shares in the key ability to *present foreign antigen, in association with self-MHC antigen, to antigen-reactive lymphocytes.* Induction of humoral and cell-mediated immunity cannot occur efficiently in the absence of APCs; that is, with lymphocytes alone. Two types of APCs—dendritic cells and macrophages—are discussed as illustrations.

Dendritic Cells

Dendritic cells are APCs that are found in the skin (Langerhans' cells), thymus (medulla), lymph nodes (cortex and paracortex), and spleen and other secondary lymphoid organs. They are large, adherent,

motile cells, possessing numerous and prominent pseudopodia that represent approximately 1% of the cells in the tissues in which they reside. Langerhans' cells, with characteristic Birbeck granules (clubbed shaped) can migrate to the lymph nodes following binding of antigen and present the antigen to T cells in the paracortex. These follicular cells are also seen forming cellular interconnections in the cortical B cell areas.

Macrophages

Macrophages are seen in association with dendritic cells and, until recently, were considered to be the primary APCs. Mononuclear phagocytes originate from precursor cells in the bone marrow, circulate for a short time in the blood as monocytes, and then emigrate into tissues where they develop into macrophages (fig. 2.12). Circulating monocytes are larger than lymphocytes (15 to 30 μm) providing space for large numbers of lysosomes (fig. 2.13 and plate 2*d*). They can secrete enzymes and soluble products that act on other cells in a number of ways. Only after leaving the bloodstream do monocytes acquire full functional competence as phagocytes and APCs through metamorphosing into macrophages. Although most tissue macrophages, whether they are fixed or wandering, are derived from blood monocytes, they may be formed by local proliferation in tissues as well. Macrophages are found in the connective tissues, liver, lungs, lymph nodes, spleen, bone marrow, serous cavities, nervous tissues, skin, and synovia (joint fluids) where they may be identified by a variety of names.

Macrophages play at least three **major roles**: (1) *antigen processing and presentation,* (2) *production and release of immune response modifiers,* and (3) *phagocytosis.* Macrophages, or other APCs, are required for the induction of both humoral and cell-mediated responses. They can bind, process, and present antigens to lymphocytes. This is an integral step in initiating antigen-dependent differentiation of lymphocytes (discussed further in chapters 3 and 9). In addition, macrophages produce some of the major components of complement, IFNs, prostaglandins, and monokines such as IL-1. These substances help promote expression of both nonspecific and specific cell-mediated immune responses (see chapters 8 and 9 for further discussion). Furthermore, macrophages adhere readily to glass and

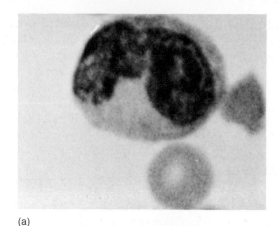

(a)

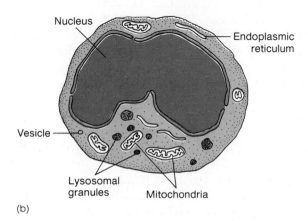

(b)

FIGURE 2.13 Monocyte. (*a*) Photomicrograph and (*b*) ultrastructure. (See also plate 2*d*.) (Part *a* from Hyun, B. H., Ashton, J. K., and Dolan, K. *Practical Hematology.* 1975. W. B. Saunders Co., Philadelphia.)

plastic (even attempting to engulf them), are actively motile, and are intensely phagocytic. Although macrophages do not possess specific antigen receptors, they apparently can bind, ingest, and degrade virtually any type of antigen. Moreover, they can bind immune complexes (free or attached to cells) by means of FcRs or CRs, then engulf and digest them. This role may be significant during bouts of immune complex disease, when immune complexes can be damaging to critical tissues of the body. Macrophages also can exhibit ADCC reactions and can be made to express tumoricidal activity by products of lymphocytes.

TABLE 2.6 Nonlymphoid Cells Involved in Immune Responses

Cells	Actions
Dendritic cells	Process antigens for presentation to lymphocytes
Monocytes/macrophages	Process antigens for presentation to lymphocytes; produce and release monokines (e.g., IL-1) to modulate lymphocyte function; are phagocytic and release chemotactic factors in immune-mediated inflammation
Neutrophils	Engage in phagocytosis and antibody-dependent cytotoxicity
Eosinophils	Modulate hypersensitivity reactions; participate in parasite destruction and removal
Basophils/mast cells	Mediate Type I (immediate) hypersensitivity reactions; release chemotactic factors in inflammation
Platelets	Potentiate vascular responses in immune-mediated inflammatory reactions

Other Cells Involved in Immunological Responses

In addition to APCs, the lymphoid cells are assisted in their surveillance and defensive functions by granulocytes and platelets (table 2.6). Although these cells might have alternative primary functions, each is suited to play a role in immune surveillance and defense.

Neutrophils

Approximately 60% of the circulating leukocytes in humans are neutrophils. Mature neutrophils have five-lobed nuclei, and are therefore designated as polymorphonuclear neutrophils (PMNs) (fig. 2.14*a* and plate 2*a*). PMNs are derived from the pluripotent stem cells, as are all cells of the blood. Their primary function is that of *phagocytosis* of foreign, aberrant, or dead cells

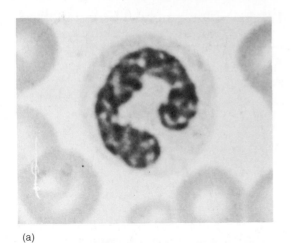

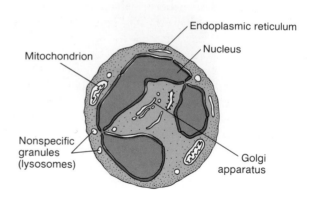

(a)

Mitochondrion

Endoplasmic reticulum

Nucleus

Nonspecific granules (lysosomes)

Golgi apparatus

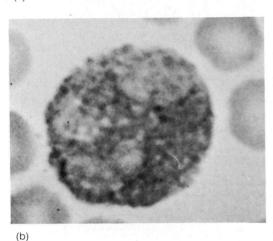

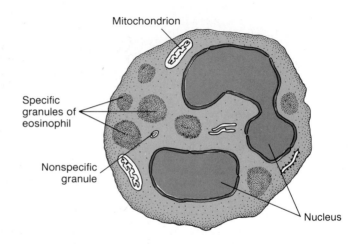

(b)

Mitochondrion

Specific granules of eosinophil

Nonspecific granule

Nucleus

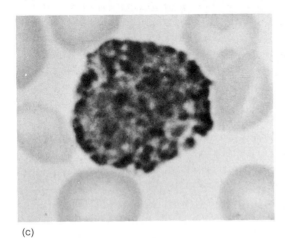

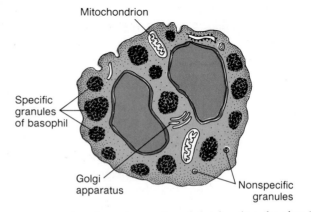

(c)

Mitochondrion

Specific granules of basophil

Golgi apparatus

Nonspecific granules

FIGURE 2.14 Granulocytes. The three types of granulocytes (neutrophil [*a*], eosinophil [*b*], and basophil [*c*]), and the probable appearance of their major cytoplasmic organelles, are shown in the accompanying photomicrographs and sketches. (See also plate 2*a*–*c*.) (Parts *a, b,* and *c* from Hyun, B. H., Ashton, J. K., and Dolan, K. *Practical Hematology.* 1975. W. B. Saunders Co., Philadelphia.)

and pinocytosis of pathological immune complexes. They can also exhibit *ADCC*. These cells are especially capable of rapid activation and mobilization in response to chemotactic stimuli, such as bacterial products or activated components of complement (C5a). A variety of receptors (e.g., FcR, CR1, and CR2) are increasingly displayed following activation. During the early stages of inflammation, arising from infectious and/or immune complex disease, PMNs are the most prominent cell type. At an inflammatory site, PMNs bind, ingest, or lyse (and in essence remove) the foreign or aberrant target.

Eosinophils

Granulocytes containing prominent acidophilic (because of their affinity for the acidic dye, eosin) granules are called eosinophils (fig. 2.14*b* and plate 2*b*). These cells have bilobed nuclei and abundant ribosomes and mitochondria. They account for 3% to 5% of the white blood cells. During certain allergic conditions, and during certain parasitic infections, the numbers of eosinophils can increase dramatically. Through their phagocytic/pinocytic potentials, eosinophils can engulf and remove immune complexes and can inactivate certain allergic mediators. Eosinophils *possess FcRs and can mediate ADCC*. They respond to chemotactic factors released by T cells that have been activated by helminthic (worm) antigens. They can bind to worm larvae (such as schistosomulae) coated with IgG, degranulate, and release toxic proteins which are damaging to the parasites. They can also respond to chemotactic products released by basophils and mast cells. For example, eosinophils can release enzymes (e.g., histaminase), which inactivate pharmacologically active mediators of Type I hypersensitivity reactions (e.g., histamine), that have been secreted by basophils and mast cells.

Basophils and Mast Cells

Basophils of the blood comprise less than 1% of white blood cells. Both blood basophils and their tissue counterparts, mast cells, possess prominent, randomly distributed basophilic (because of their affinity for the aniline dyes) granules (fig. 2.14*c* and plate 2*c*). These granules contain eosinophil chemotactic factors and *pharmacological mediators of Type I hypersensitivities* (see chapter 13, Hypersensitivity). These granules release their contents when stimulated with allergens that specifically bind to IgE (and crosslink these molecules) that has become attached to the basophil through high-affinity FcRs. Basophils also possess FcRs for IgG and receptors for C3a, C3b, and C5a, suggesting a *capability to exhibit ADCC, phagocytosis, and chemotaxis.*

Mast cells are generally quite similar to basophils in terms of morphology, receptors expressed, and function. They are not, however, homogeneous, and there appear to be at least two subpopulations that exhibit some critical physiological and morphological differences. One population is found in the mucosa of the lungs and intestine and the other in the connective tissues near blood vessels. Differences in these cells, the number and size of granules, density of receptors expressed, pharmacological properties, lifespan, and response to drugs can bear significantly on potential control and treatment of allergies.

Platelets

Platelets are small, cytoplasmic fragments having a diameter less than half that of erythrocytes. They are derived from large megakaryocytes in the bone marrow. They possess small granules, class I MHC antigens, and FcRs for IgG and IgE. Platelets are not only important in *blood clotting* (as a producer of thromboplastin), but they are also critically involved in *hypersensitivity reactions and the inflammatory process.* They are capable of releasing permeability-increasing substances, such as histamine, following aggregation and degranulation. Platelets can be induced to aggregate and degranulate by platelet-activating factor, immune complexes, and C3a, and C5a. Platelet-activating factor is produced by a variety of cells, for example, basophils and mast cells, following interaction with allergens or immune complexes and complement factors.

...system consists of a network of
..., and cells. The primary lymphatic
...e bone marrow and thymus, while
...mphatic organs include the spleen,
lymph nodes, adenoids, tonsils, Peyer's patches
(intestines), and appendix. [p. 28]

2. The bone marrow is where all blood cell types
arise from stem cell precursors. It also provides
the microenvironment for the antigen-
independent differentiation of B cells. [pp. 28–30]

3. The thymus provides the environment for
antigen-independent differentiation of T
lymphocytes. [pp. 30–31]

4. The bursa of Fabricius is an organ found in birds
where differentiation of B cells occurs. It does
not exist in mammals, but its role is believed to
be assumed by the bone marrow. [pp. 31–32]

5. The secondary lymphatic organs trap antigens
and provide sites for interaction between
antigens and the cells of the immune system.
[pp. 32–34]

6. Through the process of hemopoiesis, the various
classes of blood cells are derived in the bone
marrow. This is accomplished by the progressive
differentiation of stem cells. There appear to be
populations of both pluripotential and
unipotential stem cells. The unipotential
precursors are called blast cells and give rise to
one cell type only. [pp. 34–37]

7. The lymphoid cells include T and B
lymphocytes, plasma cells, and null cells. These
can be distinguished by the surface antigens they
express. [pp. 37–39]

8. T cells, which are involved in cell-mediated
immune reactions, can be characterized by the
presence of Thy-1 (mouse) or CD5 (human).
[p. 39]

9. Several T cell subsets can be distinguished
functionally. These are designated as: T_H
(helper) and T_S (suppressor) cells, which assist or
suppress humoral and cell-mediated response; T_C
cells (cytotoxic effector), which mediate direct
cytotoxicity; and T_D cells, which mediate
delayed-type hypersensitivity reactions. [pp. 39–40]

10. B cells are responsible for humoral immunity.
They can be identified by the presence of
membrane-bound (surface) immunoglobulin.
Most circulating B cells express IgM and IgD on
their surfaces. Plasma cells are the fully
differentiated antibody-producing cells derived
from B cells. [pp. 40–41]

11. Null cells do not display markers identifying
them as either T or B cells. Included among null
cells are K and NK cells. These cells are capable
of antibody-dependent cellular cytotoxicity.
[pp. 41–42]

12. Lymphoid cells also carry a variety of surface
receptors. The most significant of these are
receptors for foreign antigens, self-determinants
of the major histocompatibility system, immune
complex (Fc), complement, lymphokines, and
mitogens. Receptors can redistribute over the
membrane surface and display a phenomenon
called capping. [pp. 42–45]

13. Antigen-presenting cells enhance the efficiency
of immune responses by presenting antigen, in
association with self-MHC antigen, to antigen-
reactive lymphocytes. Dendritic cells and
macrophages represent the principal antigen-
presenting cells. [pp. 45–47]

14. Granulocytes and platelets provide support for
immunological reactions. Neutrophils contribute
chiefly as phagocytes. Eosinophils play a role in
helminthic infections and in certain
hypersensitivity reactions. Basophils and mast
cells appear to be active in and augment allergic
reactions. Platelets play a significant role in
blood coagulation, but are also activated
following reactions with allergens, immune
complexes, and complement. [pp. 47–49]

READINGS

Butterworth, A. E., and David, J. R. Eosinophil function. *New England Journal of Medicine.* **304**:154, 1981.

Erslev, A. J., and Gabuzda, T. G. *The Pathophysiology of Blood.* 2d ed. W. B. Saunders Co., Philadelphia, 1979.

Groopman, J. E., Molina, J. M., and Scadden, D. T. Hematopoietic growth factors: biology and clinical applications. *New England Journal of Medicine.* **321**:1449, 1989.

Haberman, R., and Holden, H. Natural cell-mediated immunity. *Advances in Cancer Research* **27**:305, 1978.

Inglis, J. R. (ed.). *T Lymphocytes Today.* Elsevier Science Publishers, Amsterdam, 1983.

Jensen, P. E. Protein synthesis in antigen processing. *Journal of Immunology* **141**:2545, 1988.

Knapp, W., Rieber, P., Dörkin, B., et al. Towards a better definition of human leucocyte surface molecules. *Immunology Today* **10**:253, 1989.

Mahmoud, A. A. F., and Austen, K. F. *The Eosinophil in Health and Disease.* Grune & Stratton, Inc., New York, 1980.

Murphy, P. *The Neutrophil.* Plenum Publishing Co., New York, 1976.

Nakayama, N., Hatake, K., Miyajima, A., et al. Colony-stimulating factors, cytokines and hematopoiesis. *Current Opinion in Immunology* **2**:68, 1989.

Nathan, D. G. Regulation of hematopoiesis. *Pediatric Research* **27**:423, 1990.

Otten, G. Antigen processing and presentation. *Current Opinion in Immunology* **2**:204, 1989.

Reinherz, E. L., and Schlossman, S. F. Regulation of the immune response: Inducer and suppressor T lymphocyte subsets in human beings. *New England Journal of Medicine* **303**:370, 1980.

Ritter, M. A., and Larché, M. T and B cell ontogeny and phylogeny. *Current Opinion in Immunology* **1**:203, 1988.

Steinmann, R. M. The dendiritic cell system and its role in immunogenicity. *Annual Review of Immunology* **9**:271, 1991.

Vernon-Roberts, B. *The Macrophage.* Cambridge University Press, Cambridge, 1972.

Weiss, L. *The Blood Cells and Hematopoietic Tissues.* McGraw-Hill Book Co., New York, 1977.

Weller, P. F. The immunobiology of eosinophils. *New England Journal of Medicine* **324:** 1110, 1991.

Essentials of Immunological Expression

This section explores central elements responsible for the expression of humoral and cell-mediated immune responses. Unit 2 provides discussion of humoral immunity. This includes exploration of the cells responsible for the production of antibodies (chapter 3), interactions between antibodies and antigens (chapter 4), the nature and diversity of antibody types (chapter 5), and an adjunct system of circulating nonantibody molecules (the complement system) used in immunological defense (chapter 6). Unit 3 examines cellular immunity. This includes discussion of histocompatibility systems (chapter 7) which provide the basis for specific cellular immune responses, the major cell types responsible for cell-mediated immune responses (chapters 8 and 9), and mechanisms underlying natural immunological tolerance and immune suppression (chapter 10). Accordingly, this unit provides a basic understanding of how the immune system functions and provides a foundation for appreciating immunological expression under diverse conditions, as examined in section 3.

2 Humoral Immunity

Humoral immunity represents one of the major arms of the immune system. In humoral immunity, the immune response is mediated by specific antibodies that are directed against the stimulating antigen(s). This unit explores the bases for humoral immunity. Chapter 3, Effectors of Humoral Immunity, characterizes the nature of humoral immune responses. In particular, the nature of antigens and their relationship to immunogenicity are described. In addition, the nature and properties of humoral effectors, antibodies, are presented. Moreover, models to account for how the humoral arm of the immune system is able to respond specifically to almost any antigen presented are discussed. Interactions between antigens and antibodies are outlined in chapter 4, Antigen-Antibody Reactions. In addition, this chapter explains how several of these reactions can be used to quantify antigen or antibody concentrations. The genetic background and mechanisms through which diverse antibodies can be produced are explored in chapter 5, Antibody Production, Regulation, and Diversity. Unit 2 concludes with chapter 6, Complement and its Role in Immune Responses, which discusses humoral defenses provided by an intricate system of nonimmunoglobulin cytolytic agents that can play an active role in immune responses.

3 Effectors of Humoral Immunity

OVERVIEW

This chapter explores the nature of the molecules (antigens) that provoke immune responses and the effector molecules (antibodies) formed during humoral immune responses. Theories of antibody formation are presented and the technology used to produce pure, structurally identical antibodies in animal cell and bacterial cultures is examined. In addition, the structural basis for antigen and antibody diversity is described. Moreover, the functional and structural differences exhibited by the five major classes of immunoglobulins are discussed.

CONCEPTS

1. Antigens are molecules that can interact with the combining sites of antibodies. The distinct chemical groups of antigens that interact with antibody molecules are known as antigenic determinants or epitopes. An antibody's selective discrimination among different epitopes is called specificity.

2. The ability to stimulate immune responses is termed immunogenicity. Immunogenicity depends upon the nature of the antigen, the mode of its presentation, and the nature and condition of the host.

3. Through the mechanism of clonal selection, a foreign antigen selectively binds to specific lymphocyte(s) displaying complementary receptors. In humoral immune responses, these cells, once activated, give rise to progeny that make antibodies against particular epitopes (plasma cells) or retain memory of exposure to those epitopes (memory cells).

4. Individual plasma cells normally produce only one structurally distinct kind of antibody. Since there are many different plasma cells, serum (and extravascular fluid) contains a heterogeneous population of antibodies referred to as immmunoglobulins.

5. Methods have been devised to produce homogeneous populations of monoclonal antibodies using isolated antibody-producing cells in culture or bacteria to which antibody genes have been transferred.

6. All immunoglobulins share a basic monomeric structure consisting of heavy and light chains that can be subdivided into specific regions or domains. Proteolytic treatment of immunoglobulins yields antigen-binding fragments and a crystallizable fragment, which does not bind antigen, indicating that immunoglobulin molecules are multifunctional.

7. Several classes and subclasses of immunoglobulins exist that are functionally and structurally distinct.

This chapter considers the molecules that stimulate humoral immune responses, called **antigens (Ags)**, and the effector molecules produced during the humoral immune response, known as **antibodies (Abs)**. The first portion of the chapter focuses on the nature of Ags and factors influencing their ability to elicit an effective immune response. For example, why are some Ags more provocative than others? Why do some hosts respond more than others? Why might several different classes of Ab molecules be formed in response to a single Ag?

The remainder of the chapter examines the structure and function of Abs, which are proteins known as **immunoglobulins (Igs)**. There are five distinct classes, and several subclasses, of Ig molecules. The major classes are designated IgG, IgM, IgA, IgD, and IgE. Each class (and subclass) exhibits certain unique functions and differs from the others in amino acid composition, carbohydrate content, charge, and size. The structural diversity of Ab molecules within any class or subclass appears almost boundless. Each human being may naturally possess over a billion structurally distinct Abs. The structural configuration of each particular Ab, in areas where Ag is bound, has a different specificity or "face," as individually distinct and identifiable as each of our own faces. The basis for Ab specificity, namely, a molecule's ability to discriminate between one antigenic determinant and another, is examined. The nature of the design capability that permits mammals to construct a remarkable repertoire of structurally distinct Ab molecules is discussed in the following chapter.

Early investigators thought that Ab specificity might be due to folding of the molecule to fit the Ag (acting as a template). With technical advances, later researchers suggested that Ab specificity might be based on the primary structure of molecules and, therefore, be genetically determined. Models of Ab formation relating to structurally adaptive, versus structurally preformed, Abs were subsequently proposed. These hypotheses demonstrated an urgent need for pure, or homogeneous, antigenically distinct Abs for structural analysis. This need was ingeniously satisfied by 1975.

Since that time, interest in Ab structure and its relationship to function has intensified and attracted an increasing number of investigators.

■   ■   ■   ■   ■   ■   ■   ■   ■   ■

ANTIGENS AND IMMUNOGENICITY

The adaptive immune system recognizes foreign molecules and subsequently produces specific new products. These new products appear in the form of Abs and effector cells that are capable of binding specifically with the foreign molecules that triggered their formation. An **Ag** is *any substance that can bind to specific Ab molecules or specific Ag receptors on lymphocytes.* Soluble and cell-bound proteins constitute the largest group of naturally occurring Ags. In addition, polysaccharides, lipids, and nucleic acids (often associated with proteins) also can be antigenic.

A complete Ag can induce specific immune responses and react with the products of those responses. The *distinct chemical groups within Ag molecules that can bind specifically to the Ag-binding site* (paratope) of Ab molecules (fig. 3.1), or T cell receptors (discussed in chapter 9), are called antigenic determinants or **epitopes.** A *complete Ag is multideterminant* (i.e., it possesses several epitopes). A single Ag with several distinct epitopes could induce and specifically bind to the paratopes of several different Ab molecules. There can be as many different species of Abs (and effector T cell clones) produced as there are functional epitopes within the Ag.

An *incomplete Ag,* or **hapten,** is a chemically defined substance of low molecular weight that *cannot* induce an adaptive immune response by itself. Nevertheless, haptens can induce a response if combined with larger macromolecules (normally proteins), which serve as carriers (see the following section). This response, however, requires assistance from T helper (T_H) lymphocytes. In contrast to complete Ags, haptens contain a *single epitope*.

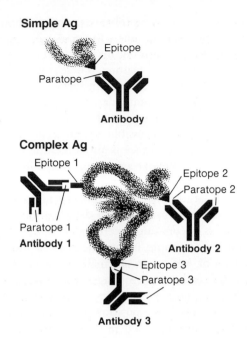

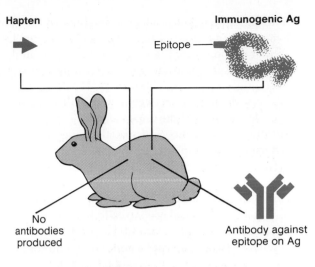

FIGURE 3.1 Physical relationship between epitope and paratope. The antigenic determinant, or epitope, is complementary to the antibody-combining site, or paratope. The result is a "matched fit" between these two domains. In response to a simple Ag (which might express but a single epitope), specific antibody complementary to that single epitope will appear. On the other hand, a complex Ag (expressing several unique epitopes) can induce the production of several types of antibodies, each with specificity against a single epitope.

Epitopes as Antigenic Determinants

Our understanding of epitopes as antigenic determinants is due, in large part, to the early studies of **Karl Landsteiner.** A significant portion of his work focused on the role of haptens in immune responses. A hapten, which does not by itself provoke an immune response, can stimulate an immune response if covalently coupled to a suitable carrier (fig. 3.2). The hapten is too small to engage T and B cells simultaneously. However, if the hapten is conjugated to an appropriate carrier, a T cell recognizes an epitope of this protein and a B cell the haptenic determinant. Antihapten Ab is produced (and anticarrier Ab as well, since other B cells may recognize epitopes of the carrier molecule).

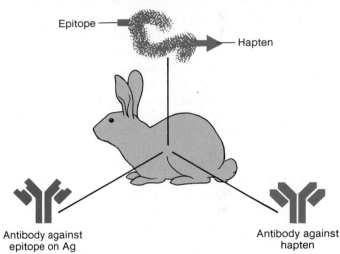

FIGURE 3.2 Effect of carrier on immunogenicity of hapten. Haptens, as small molecules, are incapable of inducing an immune response when presented alone. This is markedly different from what occurs when a more complex, immunogenic Ag is presented. In this instance, antibody directed against the specific epitope(s) of that Ag can be produced. However, if hapten is linked to a large molecule (which is used as a carrier), the hapten might then appear immunogenic. Under these conditions, antibody is produced, not only against the epitope of the immunogenic carrier molecule but against the epitope of the hapten as well.

The antihapten Abs produced then bind to the hapten even when it is not linked to the carrier protein. Landsteiner demonstrated that virtually any chemical substance can serve as an antigenic determinant or epitope, if conjugated to a suitable carrier. He discovered that Abs can distinguish between structurally similar haptens. He also noted the importance of acid radicals, position of substituents, and spatial arrangements in the determinant groups (see chapter 4, Antigen-Antibody Reactions, for further discussion). In addition he showed that Abs may recognize overall three-dimensional shape of an antigenic determinant, rather than any specific chemical property. This led to the concept of structural complementarity between the convex antigenic determinants and a concave Ab-binding site.

Epitope Characteristics

An Ab that is specific for an Ag binds noncovalently to a region of the molecule's surface known as an epitope. Naturally occurring epitopes are relatively small, for example, four to six amino acid or sugar residues. The convex epitope area might be only 2×3 nm across. At these dimensions, an epitope can fit into the Ab-binding site. Thus, large proteins and oligosaccharides can express many different and/or identical (repeating) epitopes.

The Ab-combining site, or paratope, is a concave pocket shaped to match the convexity of the epitope. Linus Pauling showed that an epitope and its binding site must become closely related, for most of the forces responsible for binding are short-range (less than 4 Å). These include hydrophobic and van der Waals forces, which are spherically symmetrical, and hydrogen bridges, which are directional and require matching of the reactants. Electrostatic forces might also contribute; however, they act at a distance. Accordingly, formation of stable immune complexes normally occur only when the epitope and the paratope fit "jigsaw fashion."

The more hydrophilic regions of a protein surface are most likely to be antigenic. However, the entire exposed surface of a protein can be antigenic, although only a few of these epitopes may actually evoke an immune response in any given individual. The epitope, of course, must be readily accessible to an Ag receptor. Consequently, the convex, protruding parts

of the protein surface are probably the most prominent normally functional epitopes. Molecular cartography has been used to plot contour maps of proteins, in order to quantify their surface features. These studies showed that the highest peaks on protein surfaces usually coincided with experimentally determined antigenic epitopes. These protruding parts of the molecular surface are generally most accessible to Ab molecules. Although most of the surface is antigenic, the potential of different areas to evoke an immune response appears to vary greatly. In addition, critical epitopes can be isolated inside large molecules, exposed only when the molecule unfolds during partial denaturation or processing. This occurs under certain, often perturbing, conditions, for example, in catabolism of the molecule. Catabolism of Ags occurs normally in Ag-presenting cells (APCs) such as macrophages. However, if Ag is completely catabolized, epitopes are destroyed.

Not only is the position of an epitope within a large molecule important in determining its ability to induce an immune response, but the position of each subunit within the epitope may also be important. For example, each of the amino acid residues comprising a given accessible epitope might contribute unequally to binding with an Ab paratope. Thus, some components of an epitope are more *immunodominant* than others. When the epitope is a terminal sequence, the terminal residue of that sequence is almost invariably the immunodominant subunit.

Any amino acid can contribute to a protein epitope; however, some are more common than others. Since epitopes bind to Abs through multiple noncovalent bonds—which can include interactions between charged groups and hydropohbic bonds—residues whose side chains carry a charge (e.g., lysine and glutamic acid) or which enter into hydrophobic interactions (e.g., alanine, leucine, tyrosine, and valine) are common in epitopes. Residues that are not part of the epitope might not bind to Ab, but might influence Ag conformation and affect epitope binding. Substitution of even a single amino acid in an epitope can affect binding to Ab. Flexibility between adjacent residues in the epitope might also be significant. Local mobile adjustments can permit a better fit between epitope and Ab-binding site, with improved binding efficiency (see chapter 4 for discussion of Ag-Ab interactions).

Sequential and Conformational Epitopes

Antigenicity of protein molecules resides either in short peptide segments serving as sequence epitopes, discrete conformational epitopes, or in combinations of both. Specific Ab populations can be formed in response to either type of epitope. Epitopes whose specificity is determined by the sequence of subunits (e.g., amino acids or monosaccharide units) are designated *sequential determinants*. Sequential determinants can be composed of terminal or internal sequences of the Ag. Sequential epitopes are located in hydrophilic regions of the molecule. *Conformational determinants,* on the other hand, are epitopes whose specificity depends on the spatial folding or configuration of the Ag molecule. For example, Abs generated to isolated chains of a complex protein molecule (such as lysozyme or insulin) might not react with intact molecules. Conformational epitopes are normally associated with globular proteins and helical structures.

Epitopes can be continuous or discontinuous. If Abs bind to a contiguous sequence of amino acids, the determinant is continuous. A discontinuous determinant, in contrast, is comprised of residues that are separated from one another in the sequence of the protein, but are brought together by folding. Conformational determinants can be sequential or discontinuous, but sequential determinants are always continuous.

Immunogenicity

Immunogenicity refers to the *relative ability of an Ag to stimulate immune responses.* In order for a molecule to be considered an Ag, it need only be capable of binding to a specific Ab molecule (or T cell receptor). However, only Ags that provoke immune responses are immunogenic and can be called **immunogens.** The immunogenicity of an Ag depends upon its general molecular characteristics, the manner in which it is presented, and the nature of the individual being immunized or exposed to the Ag. Selected characteristics of Ags and immunogens are compared in table 3.1.

Immunogens

The most potent immunogens are proteins with molecular weights (MW) greater than 100 kD. Extremely small molecules, such as amino acids or

TABLE 3.1 Comparison between Antigen and Immunogen

Characteristic	Antigen	Immunogen
Relation to immune system	Can bind to antibody-combining site	Can bind to antibody-combining site; can stimulate immune responses
Nature of molecule	Can be any molecule (protein, lipid polysaccharide, nucleic acid)	Are molecules differing from those present in host
Size of molecule	Can be any size; however, epitope generally consists of 4–6 subunits (2–3 nm across)	Size affects efficiency: >100 kD (most effective); 10–100 kD (variable immunogenicity); <10 kD (not usually independently immunogenic; haptens)

monosaccharides, are not immunogenic. Molecules with MWs of less than 1 kD can bind to Ab, but they are not immunogenic unless coupled with a large carrier protein. Molecules between 1 and 10 kD might be only weakly immunogenic by themselves, and these Ags also might require conjugation to carriers to generate suitable responses.

Foreignness of a conventional Ag is critical for immunogenicity, for the host distinguishes self from nonself and "normally" does not respond to self. Generally, the more a protein Ag differs from host proteins, the more potent it is as an immunogen. The healthy body is immunologically tolerant of nearly all self-Ags that would be immunogenic in a foreign host. (Tolerance is explored in greater detail in chapter 10.) However, during certain diseases, tolerance can be broken and pathological autoimmune reactions might occur. These appear as humoral and/or cell-mediated responses to some self-Ags. However, physiological autoimmune reactions also might occur. For example, the immune system might recognize and respond to specific self-Abs (auto-Abs) and effector cells generated during an immune response. This mechanism, proposed by Jerne, is believed to represent one means of immune regulation (see Idiotypic Regulation in chapter 5).

Molecular *complexity* is another important aspect of immunogenicity. Polymers of identical repeating units, even though they are massive, are generally very poorly immunogenic. The synthetic substances nylon and Teflon, which are chemically simplistic (repeats of a single core subunit), do not stimulate immune responses.

Antigen Administration

Every Ag has an optimal immunogenic dose range. Thus, the amount of Ag used in immunization procedures can be quite critical. Too much, or too little, Ag might not elicit a response. An Ag, in fact, could establish a state of tolerance in which the animal fails to form Abs or effector cells (see chapter 10, Immune Tolerance and Suppression). Any substance that can induce Ab formation can establish tolerance that is specific and directed to particular determinants. Furthermore, effectiveness varies with the route of administration and the presence or absence of potentiators.

Response to an immunogen can be enhanced by the use of adjuvants. *Adjuvants* are compounds that potentiate the immune response when mixed and administered with Ags. Adjuvants contribute to greater and more prolonged Ab production and increased effector cell counts. Adjuvants can act in several ways: (1) to alter the distribution and persistence of Ags within the host, (2) to stimulate lymphocytes nonspecifically, (3) to activate macrophages, or (4) to perhaps alter traffic of circulating lymphocytes. In some instances, combinations of these processes might occur. A commonly used adjuvant was developed originally by Freund. It is a stable water-in-oil emulsion, which may (complete) or may not (incomplete) contain killed *Mycobacterium tuberculosis*. A concentration of immunogen, which might be ineffective when injected intravenously, might be effective if given intraperitoneally with Freund's complete adjuvant. However, this adjuvant cannot be used in humans and must be replaced by other adjuvants such as alum or killed *Bordetella pertussis*.

Routes commonly used for immunization include inoculations of Ag (1) into skeletal muscle (intramuscular), (2) under the skin (subcutaneous), (3) into a vein (intravenous), (4) into the abdominal cavity (intraperitoneal), and (5) into the skin (intradermal [usually multiple injections]). On the other hand, some Ags might be inhaled, ingested, or applied to the skin. In addition, foreign Ags might be presented to a host by tissue or organ transplants (see chapter 19, Transplantation Immunology). Regardless of the route of administration, most Ags eventually become distributed throughout the body by means of the lymphatic and blood vessels. Although a combination of humoral and cell-mediated immune responses might follow Ag administration, the route of administration can influence the type of response that occurs. For example, cell-mediated responses can be enhanced by intradermal injection of Ag. In addition, the route of administration can influence the dominant class of Abs that are formed. Accordingly, preferential synthesis of IgA occurs when immunogens are inhaled or introduced into the intestine. In this instance, B cells in the area are committed to produce IgA.

Protein Ags are more immunogenic when administered in aggregated rather than soluble form. For example, Ag-Ab complexes, in slight Ag excess, and chemically cross-linked protein molecules are highly immunogenic. In addition, a high degree of chemical complexity appears to be important for immunogenicity. Synthetic homopolymers, for example, are nonimmunogenic, regardless of their molecular weight. This is quite different from the immunogenicity of native proteins (which are heteropolymers of amino acids), which is influenced by molecular weight (see table 3.1). In essence, the immunogenicity of an Ag increases as the structural diversity of the Ag increases.

Antigen Presentation and Epitope Recognition

Expression of an immune response requires that Ag interact with the lymphocytes that are ultimately activated. Ags can be classified according to how they are presented to lymphocytes and how immunogenic epitopes are recognized by B and T cells specific for these epitopes. Most protein Ags are thymus dependent. This means that Ab production by activated B lymphocytes (plasma cells) cannot occur without assistance from T_H cells. **T-dependent Ags** contain specific epitopes that activate B cells and other specific epitopes that activate T_H cells. On the other hand, **T-independent Ags** elicit Ab formation without assistance from T_H cells. These latter Ags often are polysaccharides, lipids, and nucleic acids with repeating epitopes.

B lymphocytes can recognize both protein and nonprotein Ags. T lymphocytes, however, recognize only protein Ags. B cell responses to nonprotein Ags, therefore, might not require assistance from T cells. B cells appear to bind epitopes on the surface of intact, native protein but fail to recognize epitopes of denatured or processed proteins. Structural conformation of the Ag appears to be critical for B cell activation. T cells, on the other hand, can bind epitopes that have been separated from the native molecule. Thus, T cells can respond to small, cleaved peptides (epitopes) that were "buried" inside native protein. This seems reasonable since T cells require that protein Ag be processed by accessory cells before presentation. Furthermore, recognition of the small (processed) epitopes requires that they be presented in conjunction with self-proteins on the surface of APCs (see chapters 5 and 9 for further discussions).

The Immunized Host

The intrinsic ability of an individual to respond to a particular Ag (including specific epitopes) is controlled by immune response (Ir) genes of the histocompatibility complex. Ir genes encode self-protein molecules that form critical associations with processed Ags displayed by APCs (discussed in chapter 5). These genes determine whether a response occurs and influence the nature of the response itself (see chapter 7, Histocompatibility Systems, for discussion of these genes). In addition, the health, age, and sex of the immunized host bears on the response to foreign Ags. In general, the very young and the very old respond less effectively than adults. Disease, poor nutrition, and stress also can affect the expression of immune responses; usually their impact is negative. Moreover, adult males do not respond immunologically as well as young adult females.

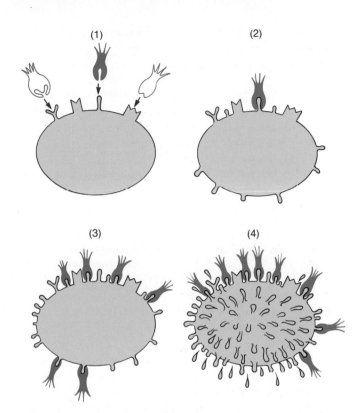

FIGURE 3.3 Ehrlich's elective theory of antibody formation. Ehrlich proposed that one of a variety of preformed receptors (antibodies) on cell surfaces (*panel 1*) might bind to a specific Ag, depicted in black (*panel 2*). Formation of the immune complex would then lead to a selective increase in the number of receptors for that particular Ag (*panel 3*), with subsequent secretion of antibodies (*panel 4*). (From Ehrlich, P. On immunity with special reference to cell life. *Proceedings of the Royal Society* [London], Series B **66:**424, 1900, by permission of the Royal Society, London.)

THEORIES OF ANTIBODY FORMATION

Instructive Versus Elective Theories of Antibody Formation

Resolution of the question of how specific Abs are produced to diverse Ags resulted from the collective efforts of several investigators. During the last century, **Paul Ehrlich** suggested that the human body possessed a full range of *preformed Abs* (fig. 3.3) and proposed an elective theory of Ab formation. Ehrlich's proposal, based on the *selection* of preformed receptors

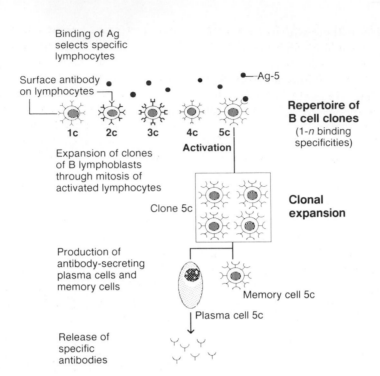

FIGURE 3.4 Clonal selection theory. Foreign Ag, designated in this example as Ag-5, enters the body, where it encounters circulating lymphocytes, each with a different Ag-binding specificity. Ag-5 will combine with only one, or a small number, of the lymphocyte pool that possess complementary receptors (5c). The B lymphocyte "selected" by Ag-5 becomes activated. This causes it to proliferate and differentiate, producing a clone of antibody-secreting plasma cells and memory cells.

(Abs), became less acceptable when it was learned that Abs can be produced against Ags that are not normally encountered in nature. Furthermore, even though Abs exhibited a variety of specificities, studies during the 1940s suggested that they might be chemically similar, since methods then available did not detect chemical differences.

Within this setting, **Linus Pauling** suggested that Ab specificity might be due to "molding" or *folding of the molecule to fit an Ag "template."* Advocates of this model suggested that, after dissociation from the Ag template, appropriate bonds and electrostatic forces would form to maintain and stabilize the three-dimensional structure of the Ab. This, and many other **instructive theories of Ab formation,** became quite popular. However, subsequent studies showed that the instructional theory was not valid for many reasons. For example, once protein molecules could be sequenced, it became clear that tertiary structure depended on primary structure (the amino acid sequence) of the molecule, not on reaction with a template.

Clonal Selection Theory

In 1955 **Niels Jerne** introduced the concept of preformed Ab molecules with a wide range of specificities, which he referred to as *natural Ab.* A **clonal selection theory** of Ab formation was proposed in 1957 by **F. M. Burnet** that resembled and reaffirmed aspects of Ehrlich's earlier selective model. Ehrlich had proposed that, before exposure to Ag, an individual possessed immune cells displaying receptors of many different specificities. When one of these cells bound an Ag, more receptors of that specificity were produced and shed as specific Abs. Thus, an *Ag selected a specific receptor* (Ab), from the many available, *for expanded production.* One way of depicting the operation of the clonal selection model is presented in figure 3.4.

The clonal selection model proposed that each of us possesses heterogeneous clones of lymphocytes, each displaying monospecific receptors capable of binding a specific antigenic determinant. When a foreign Ag (e.g., the substance designated Ag-5 in fig. 3.4) enters the body, it might subsequently encounter circulating lymphocytes, each with different specificities. The foreign Ag is able to combine with cells in the lymphocyte pool that possess complementary receptors. The B cell "selected" becomes activated, then proliferates and differentiates, giving rise to a clone of Ab-secreting plasma cells and memory cells.

In this model, the specificity of the Ag-binding lymphocytes resides in the structure of the receptor molecules, which are Igs (Abs) located in B lymphocyte membranes. The heterogeneous clones of B cells originally developed from pluripotent stem cells in the bone marrow by *Ag-independent differentiation.* Interaction of a particular foreign antigenic determinant with the monospecific receptors on a B lymphocyte stimulates cell division and differentiation. The result is a clone of identical daughter cells. Derived from this clone, through *Ag-dependent differentiation,* are plasma cells, which make only Ab of the same specificity as the Ab receptor, and memory cells, which will be capable of more rapid response to a second exposure to this same Ag.

"Selection" and activation of a lymphocyte by Ag is determined by complementarity between the Ag and the surface Abs (receptors) of the lymphocyte. Thus, an Ag with x number of antigenic determinants could stimulate x number of clones.

Burnet proposed that cells that developed autoimmune receptors (forbidden clones) were eliminated (or suppressed) by early encounter with self-Ags. Although not originally hypothesized, clonal selection implies that Ag selection and activation of T cells also occurs, and is similarly based on monospecific receptor-binding activity. Although the T cell receptor is not an Ig, but a disulfide-linked glycoprotein dimer, it can exhibit structural diversity by somatic gene rearrangements much like Ig genes (see chapter 5 for further discussion).

NATURE OF ANTIBODIES
Access to Pure Antibodies

Abs are protein molecules called **immunoglobulins,** which are formed, for the most part, in response to the entry of foreign Ag(s) into the body, via injection or infection (detailed in chapter 5). Several kinds of Abs may be formed against a single Ag possessing several determinants. Following release from plasma cells, Abs are present in highest concentration in the plasma. They can be found, however, in many body fluids including milk, tears, urine, and in secretions of the respiratory, digestive, and genitourinary tracts. Abs are most easily obtained from plasma or serum.

Abs or Igs are not, of course, the only proteins in serum as revealed by an electrophoretic scan (fig. 3.5). They may be separated from other serum proteins according to the particular biochemical characteristics they possess. For example, if we add increasing concentrations of a salt such as ammonium sulfate to serum, Igs become insoluble and "come out" of solution at one concentration, while other proteins become insoluble at a higher or lower salt concentration. Thus, we can "salt out" Igs from serum, pour off the other proteins still in solution, and resolubilize our isolated Igs in dilute salt solution.

With time, workers found that the Igs isolated were heterogeneous. Isolates were found to contain five classes of Igs designated as IgG, IgM, IgA, IgE, and IgD, along with a number of subclasses. Some classes were larger in size than others, and these proteins settled or sedimented more rapidly when centrifuged at high speeds. The overall electrostatic charge was found to differ among classes and subclasses. Normal serum concentrations of Ig classes varied, ranging from the most common (IgG) to the least common (IgE). Moreover, Igs within any respective class or subclass exhibited diverse specificities for Ags, as well as diverse antigenic markers of their own. Thus, a preparation of serum IgG, for example, would contain Abs of different specificities (against known and unknown Ags). In addition, these Abs were also antigenically different from each other. Consequently, any attempt to analyze the structure of an Ab exhibiting specificity for a particular Ag (determinant) was nearly impossible in view of the heterogeneity of Abs present.

As early as 1935, however, it was known that specific Abs could be removed from serum by allowing the serum to react with complementary Ag. In a short time, the insoluble Ag-Ab complexes formed (under certain conditions) would "fall," or precipitate, out of solution. The immune complexes then could be removed, dissociated in high salt concentrations, and free

Hemolytic Plaque Assay

Progress in our understanding of biological principles has been marked by increased refinement of our knowledge of the component systems. For example, our understanding of the immune system has become progressively more sophisticated as we have become more fully aware of the nature and mechanisms of immune response. Often this advancement in our understanding has depended upon technical developments. This has been the case with respect to our current understanding of the mechanism of humoral immunity.

The **clonal selection theory**, published in 1959, implied that a *single plasma cell,* or a clone of plasma cells, *produced only one kind of Ab,* that is, specific for one Ag (determinant). Providing conclusive evidence bearing on this postulate (either in support or challenging it) presented a considerable challenge. **Jerne and Nordin** in 1963 introduced a technique that permitted study of Ig secretion by *individual* cells, the hemolytic plaque assay.

The hemolytic plaque assay is based on the ability of Abs, secreted by a single plasma cell (mature B lymphocyte), to bind to an antigenic determinant on an erythrocyte. This can be either a red blood cell Ag or an Ag that has been covalently attached to a red blood cell.

In Figure 3.A, the basic direct technique (using sheep red blood cells [SRBC]) was used to immunize a mouse. B lymphocytes were then collected,

mixed with SRBC, and suspended in melted agarose gel. The agarose was spread thinly on a microscope slide, allowed to solidify, and incubated in a moist chamber. During incubation, some B cells secreted Abs. These Abs bound to Ag on the SRBC. Fresh serum complement then was added. This lysed any red blood cells that had absorbed Ab, producing a clear zone of lysis (a plaque) around the B cell. The number of plaques is proportional to the number of Ab-secreting B cells present.

The direct technique detects only Abs of the IgM class since they are very efficient in fixing complement. An additional step is required to detect IgG. This entails using anti-IgG Abs, which enhance complement fixation. In addition, the basic technique can be modified, so that cells secreting hormones or lymphokines can be detected, known as *reverse plaque assays.*

Studies using this technique provided evidence that supported the one-cell-one-Ab corollary of the clonal selection theory. For this contribution and his numerous other remarkable accomplishments in the field of immunology, Jerne was awarded the Nobel Prize for Physiology or Medicine in 1984.

Jerne, N. K., and Nordin, A. A. Plaque formation in agar by single antibody-producing cells. *Science* **140**:405, 1963.

Jerne, N. K., Henry, C., Nordin, A. A., et al. Plaque forming cells: methodology and theory. *Transplantation Reviews* **18**:130 1, 1974.

Abs recovered, yielding a "purified" preparation of Abs containing only molecules reactive to the Ag in question. Problems remained, however, since only small quantities of Abs could be obtained in this way. More importantly, such "purified" Abs contained a mixture of molecules specific to the different determinants of the Ag, since they were derived from several clones of plasma cells. It became clear that until homogeneous Abs became available, investigation of primary Ab structure, and its relationship to Ab specificity and other functional activities, was not feasible.

Monoclonal Antibodies

Myeloma Proteins

One answer to the seemingly unsolvable problem of obtaining pure Ab molecules was derived from the study of myeloma proteins in the 1960s. Plasma cells normally form only one specific kind of Ab in relatively small quantities. It was observed that sometimes plasma cells in humans (and in mice) become transformed, or cancerous, giving rise to plasma cell tumors, called myelomas or plasmacytomas. Cells in any particular tumor may presumably be derived from a single

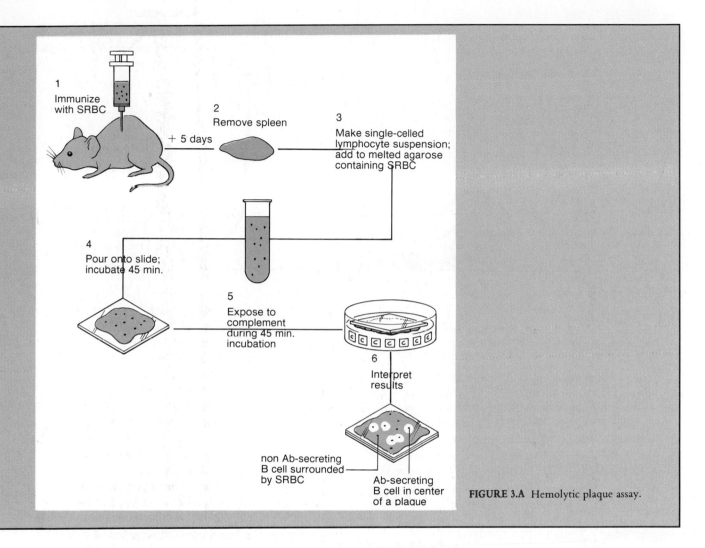

1
Immunize
with SRBC

+ 5 days

2
Remove spleen

3
Make single-celled
lymphocyte suspension;
add to melted agarose
containing SRBC

4
Pour onto slide;
incubate 45 min.

5
Expose to
complement
during 45 min.
incubation

6
Interpret
results

non Ab-secreting
B cell surrounded
by SRBC

Ab-secreting
B cell in center
of a plaque

FIGURE 3.A Hemolytic plaque assay.

transformed plasma cell yielding a monoclonal plasma cell neoplasm. Thus, each monoclonal tumor is composed of identical cells, which produce homogeneous Igs or myeloma proteins, often in large quantities. The globulins may be intact Abs, or parts of an Ab molecule consisting only of either light (L) polypeptide chains (known as Bence-Jones proteins) or heavy (H) polypeptide chains.

In any event, these proteins are derived from a *single clone of plasma cells,* in contrast to normal Igs in serum, which are derived from many clones of plasma cells. Myeloma tumor cells may be transferred from one mouse to another, or maintained in culture, thereby providing large quantities of pure monoclonal antibody (MAb) for analysis. In many, perhaps most instances, the Ag specific to a particular myeloma protein is unknown. This is, of course, a serious limitation. Nevertheless, myeloma proteins provided the first pure Igs, in quantity, for amino acid sequence studies.

Hybridomas

In 1960 a spontaneous cell fusion was observed and, in 1973, Cotton and Milstein fused mouse and rat myeloma cells, forming hybrids capable of secreting both

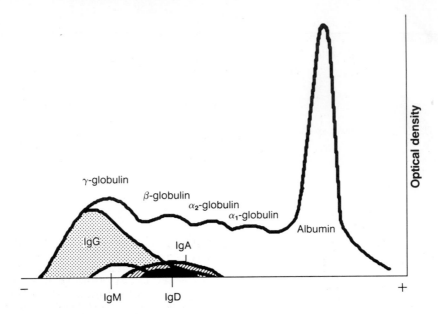

FIGURE 3.5 Separation of serum proteins by electrophoresis. This figure shows zone electrophoresis patterns of separated major serum proteins. A small volume of human serum was applied to a cellulose acetate strip. Electrophoresis was conducted in an alkaline buffer, over a period of 90 minutes, with proteins migrating to the anode (+), on the basis of their surface charge. Densitometric scanning of the stained cellulose acetate shows the relative concentrations (optical density) of the separated protein peaks. The five major electrophoretic bands distinguished include albumin, α_1-globulin, α_2-globulin, β-globulin, and γ-globulin. Four classes of Igs fall within the γ-, β-, and α_1-globulin peaks.

Igs. During this time, cell culture and cell fusion techniques were being developed. The stage was set and, in 1975, **Kohler** and **Milstein** provided an ingenious method for the production of MAbs against any Ag of choice. They produced an "immortal" Ab-secreting clone of cells by fusing the nucleus of a myeloma cell with that of a normal Ab-producing cell (fig. 3.6). They were awarded the Nobel Prize for Physiology or Medicine in 1984 for this striking achievement.

As outlined in figure 3.6, MAbs can be produced as follows. Splenocytes or lymphocytes, from immunized mice, are mixed in the presence of a fusing agent (e.g., Sendai virus or polyethylene glycol) with myeloma cells that have been mutated so that they do not secrete their own Igs. The myeloma cells used lack a critical enzyme, necessary for purine metabolism by an alternate pathway, that splenocytes and hybrids possess.

After fusion, the mixture of cells is cultured in a selection medium (hypoxanthine-aminopterin-thymidine [HAT]). The aminopterin in the medium blocks purine synthesis, thereby requiring that cells use the alternative purine pathway for growth. Nonfused myeloma cells die because they do not possess the enzyme (hypoxanthine phosphoribosyl transferase [HPRT]) required by this pathway. Nonfused splenocytes die naturally within a few days. The hybridomas (fused myeloma and spleen cells), however, reproduce (doubling every 24 to 48 hours). Cultures producing Ab are identified, and single cells from these cultures are isolated and allowed to reproduce clones of cells, making a single type of Ab.

Clones derived from fused cells permitted the mass production of homogeneous Abs by the hybrid cells (*hybridomas*), either in culture or as ascites in mice. If, for example, hybridomas were injected into mice, serous fluid in the abdominal cavity (ascites fluid) would contain very high concentrations of MAb. With the availability of large quantities of homogeneous Abs or MAbs (to known antigenic determinants), structural studies were intensified. It had become clear that access to an understanding of the biologic activities of Abs is through structure.

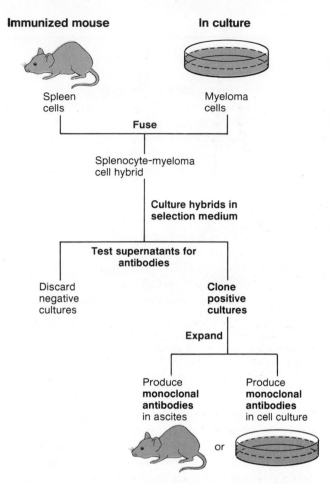

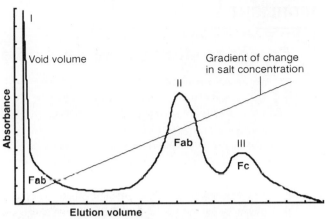

FIGURE 3.7 Profile of γ-globulin following papain digestion. Rabbit γ-globulin (IgG) was digested and cleaved into fragments with papain. It was then dialyzed and chromatographed on a column of carboxymethylcellulose, which separates molecules on the basis of net electric charge. Fractions were eluted in buffers of increasing salt concentration and the protein concentrations monitored. Two identical Fab (antigen binding) fragments and an Fc (crystallizable) fragment were isolated.

FIGURE 3.6 Production of monoclonal antibodies. Spleen cells or lymphocytes, from an immunized mouse, are fused with myeloma cells. The cells are suspended in a selection medium, distributed into multiwell plates, and cultured. The selection medium supports growth of hybridomas (lymphocytes fused with myeloma cells) but not myeloma cells. Unfused spleen cells or lymphocytes die naturally, within a few days. Culture supernatants are screened for antibody when cell growth is observed. Single hybridoma cells, from any well containing antibody, are cloned so that monoclonal antibodies can be produced, in culture or as ascites in mice. (Fusing agents used are Sendai virus or, more commonly, polyethylene glycol, selection medium used is HAT.) Myeloma cells are killed in HAT since (1) aminopterin blocks synthesis of purine and pyrimidines and (2) myeloma cells do not possess an enzyme, HPRT, which would permit them to use an alternative metabolic pathway, using hypoxanthine. Splenocytes and, therefore, hybridomas possess HPRT.

Immunoglobulins from Cloned Antibody Genes

In 1989 two research teams (Lerner and associates in the United States and Winter and associates in England) presented a new method for producing MAbs using re-

combinant DNA technology. In brief, Ig genes can be isolated from the B lymphocytes; these genes can be cloned and expressed in bacteria (see highlight 3.2). With this method, large quantities of unique MAbs can be generated, detected, and recovered in a short period of time. In addition, more recombinant MAb clones can be screened than hybridoma clones within the same time. This facilitates identification and selection of clones producing desired MAbs for study or therapeutic application. Moreover, applications of recombinant technology promise to make possible the production of tailor-made MAbs for therapeutic use.

ANTIBODY STRUCTURE
Subunits of Immunoglobulins

Even before purified preparations of Abs were readily available, early workers deduced considerable information about the structure of Igs. In the mid-1950s **Rodney Porter** treated IgG from rabbit serum with the proteolytic enzyme papain, which cleaved the molecule into three fragments. The digested material was separated on carboxymethylcellulose columns, which segregate molecules on the basis of net electric charge (fig. 3.7). Each fraction sedimentated at 3.5S in

Designer Monoclonal Antibodies

Recent advances in molecular biology have provided tools for rapidly producing large quantities of selected cell products that ordinarily are available in limited quantity. Recombinant DNA technology (sometimes referred to as genetic engineering) has enabled investigators to produce hormones, growth factors, and other biological response modifiers in quantities that have facilitated characterizing their physiological roles or have made them more readily available for therapeutic application. More recently, specific applications of this technology have advanced efforts at producing highly purified monospecific Igs in quantity. On the one hand, specific Igs now can be mass produced using applications of this technology. On the other hand, this same technology can be exploited to produce Igs of desired specificity—in a sense, made-to-order (or designer) Abs.

A schematic outline of this procedure is presented in figure 3.B. Total mRNA is isolated from B lymphocytes obtained from the blood of humans or the blood, spleen, or lymph nodes of mice and used to produce complementary DNA (cDNA). The cDNA sequences for the Ig H and L chain is amplified by the polymerase chain reaction (PCR) using appropriate primers. The H and L chain gene products are then digested with restriction enzymes into small DNA fragments. These are then inserted (ligated) into a viral vector (bacteriophage-λ) and used to infect bacteria (e.g., *Escherichia coli*). The virus grows lytically, and the expressed Ab can be readily detected with labeled Ag in the phage plaques that form.

Using the PCR, cDNA sequences can be greatly amplified. Subsequently, an Ab cDNA library (with possibly 10^{12} members) can be generated. A bacteriophage "library" of Ab genes is a depository of cloned genes from which an individual clone can be picked to obtain a desired Ab, much as we select a book from a conventional library. In only about two days a million clones (single viral plaques containing Ab molecules) can be screened with Ag. Since Ab molecules are composed of L and H chains, separate variable H and L chain gene libraries must be constructed. These two libraries are then "fused" randomly to form a combinatorial library capable of coexpressing the variable H and L chains of Ab molecules. The Abs present in bacteriophage plaques are then screened with labeled Ag.

Detection of Ab in the plaques is accomplished following adsorption to a carefully oriented nitrocellulose filter that is then incubated with Ag. The oriented nitrocellulose filter creates a map of the original virus plaque positions. Specific Ab can be detected at particular locations on the nitrocellulose membrane through reaction with the Ag. These positions on the nitrocellulose filter identify the locations of the original phage plaques expressing Ab with affinity for the Ag. These plaques can then be used to identify clones for subsequent expansion. Since tens of thousands of phage plaques can be screened with a single membrane, it is possible to screen millions of clones in less than a week.

With this technology an expanded variety of pure MAbs can be produced in quantity by bacteria rather than by animals or their cells. In this way, more structurally

---

the ultracentrifuge, and each had a MW of approximately 50 kD. Peaks I and II retained the Ag-binding capacity of intact molecules and were referred to as **Fab fragments,** for *fragment Ag binding.* Subsequent analysis showed that these fragments were identical in accord with the bivalency of Ab monomers (discussed below). The other fragment did not combine with Ag, but was readily converted into protein crystals, indi-

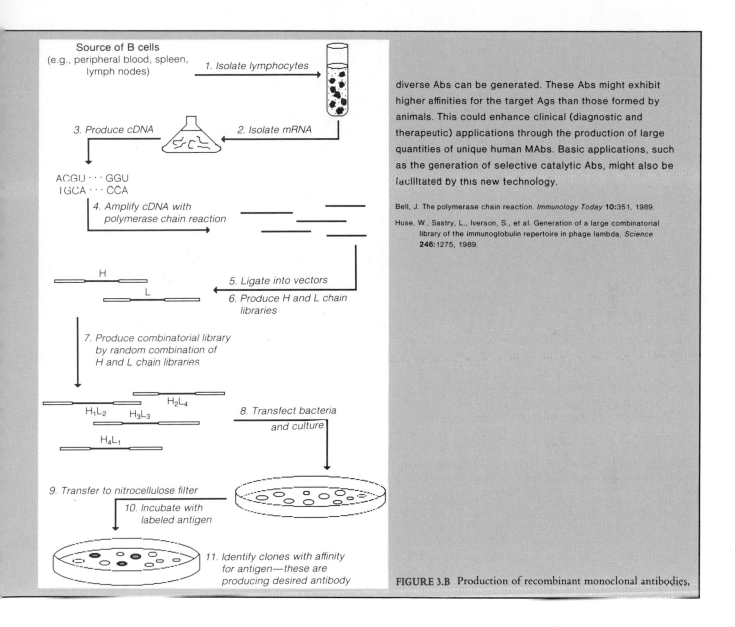

Source of B cells
(e.g., peripheral blood, spleen,
lymph nodes)

1. Isolate lymphocytes

3. Produce cDNA   *2. Isolate mRNA*

ACGU ··· GGU
TGCA ··· CCA

*4. Amplify cDNA with
polymerase chain reaction*

5. Ligate into vectors

H

L

*6. Produce H and L chain
libraries*

*7. Produce combinatorial library
by random combination of
H and L chain libraries*

H_1L_2 H_3L_3 H_2L_4

H_4L_1

*8. Transfect bacteria
and culture*

9. Transfer to nitrocellulose filter

*10. Incubate with
labeled antigen*

*11. Identify clones with affinity
for antigen—these are
producing desired antibody*

FIGURE 3.B Production of recombinant monoclonal antibodies.

diverse Abs can be generated. These Abs might exhibit higher affinities for the target Ags than those formed by animals. This could enhance clinical (diagnostic and therapeutic) applications through the production of large quantities of unique human MAbs. Basic applications, such as the generation of selective catalytic Abs, might also be facilitated by this new technology.

Bell, J. The polymerase chain reaction. *Immunology Today* **10:**351, 1989.

Huse, W., Sastry, L., Iverson, S., et al. Generation of a large combinatorial library of the immunoglobulin repertoire in phage lambda. *Science* **246:**1275, 1989.

cating "purity," and hence called **Fc,** for *fragment crystallizable.* The Fc fragment was found to contain carbohydrate and to mediate a number of effector functions expressed by intact Ab molecules. These include binding of complement, which is a very important effector mechanism (see chapter 6, Complement and its Role in Immune Responses) and binding to cell receptors (Fc receptors [FcRs]). The Fc region of Ig

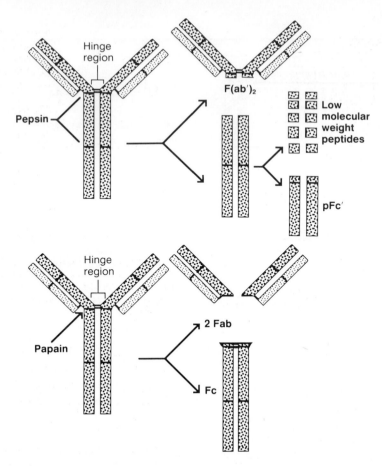

FIGURE 3.8 Comparison of pepsin and papain digestion of IgG. Pepsin cleaves the H chains of IgG on the carboxy-terminal side of the interchain disulfide bonds of the hinge region. A large fragment designated F(ab')₂, with two Ag-binding sites, is formed. Pepsin also degrades part of the Fc portion to small peptides and leaves a dimer of the C-terminal quarter of the chain, termed pFc'. Papain cleaves the H chains on the amino-terminal side of the interchain disulfide bonds of the hinge region. Disulfide bonds may, however, be broken since papain is used in the presence of reducing agents. Papain digestion yields two identical Fab (Ag-binding) fragments and a readily crystallizable Fc fragment.

molecules is also related to the secretory capability of Ig molecules following synthesis and to the passage of IgG molecules across the placenta. Porter also showed that antigenic determinants that distinguish one class of Ab from another were located on the Fc fragment.

Pepsin was found by Nisonoff to be another useful enzyme that generates two major fragments: (1) a large fragment, designated **F(ab')₂,** which encompasses two Fab regions that are linked by the hinge region and (2) a **pFc** fragment similar to the Fc fragment cleaved by papain (fig. 3.8). F(ab')₂ fragments bind two identical antigenic determinants similar to intact Ab. Preparations of F(ab')₂ are particularly useful for cell-binding studies requiring discrimination of Ag and Fc receptors.

By 1960 **Gerald Edelman** and colleagues had treated IgG with reducing agents, such as mercaptoethanol, in the presence of urea, and split the molecule (disulfide bonds reduced) into four peptide chains. Reassociation was prevented with an alkylating agent such as iodoacetate. The chains were then separated on the basis of size by Sephadex chromatography or gel filtration, a recently evolved technique at that time (fig. 3.9). Edelman's group obtained *two L chains,* each

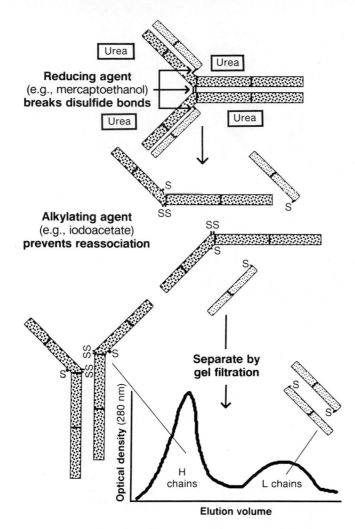

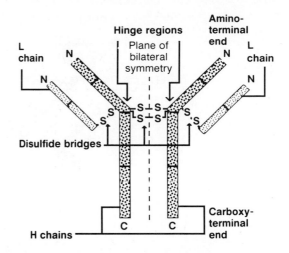

FIGURE 3.10 Basic Ig structure. The basic Ig unit is common to all classes of Ig. It consists of two identical L polypeptide chains linked by interchain disulfide bonds to two identical H polypeptide chains. The N (H₂N) and C (COOH) terminals of the polypeptide chains are designated.

FIGURE 3.9 Separation of Ig H and L chains. γ₂-Globulin (IgG) was treated with a reducing agent (mercaptoethanol), breaking disulfide (—S—S—) bonds. The reduced bonds were prevented from reforming by addition of an alkylating agent (iodoacetic acid). Fragments were then separated, on the basis of molecular size, by gel filtration. H chains were eluted first, followed by L chains. H chains were found to have a molecular weight of 50 kD and L chains 25 kD, suggesting that an intact Ig molecule (150 kD) contained two H and two L chains.

having a MW of about 25 kD, and *two H chains,* about twice as heavy as the L chains. The number of L chains formed equaled the number of H chains formed, suggesting that the intact IgG molecule (150 kD) contained two H and two L chains.

In 1962 Porter proposed a basic structure for Igs, a four-chain bilaterally symmetrical form, on the basis of proteolytic cleavage data (fig. 3.10). Two L chains were each linked to an H chain by a disulfide bond, and two H chains were linked together by one or more disulfide bonds. Later it became clear that one or more of these **basic monomeric structures (H₂L₂)** is found in *all classes of Igs.* Elucidation of Ig structure beyond this model was almost entirely dependent on the availability of "pure" Igs.

Structural Basis for Antibody Diversity

With the availability of homogeneous Igs (with defined specificities), it soon became evident that the two H chains were always identical in a given molecule, as were the L chains (fig. 3.11). H chains of homogeneous IgG contained about 440 residues, whereas L chains possessed about 220 amino acids. Data derived from sequencing of L chains showed that the N-terminal half of the chain differed substantially between different molecules and was referred to as the **variable (V) region.** The other half of the L chain, near the C terminal, showed little sequence variability from one chain to another and was called the **constant (C) region.** A similar pattern was found in the H chain.

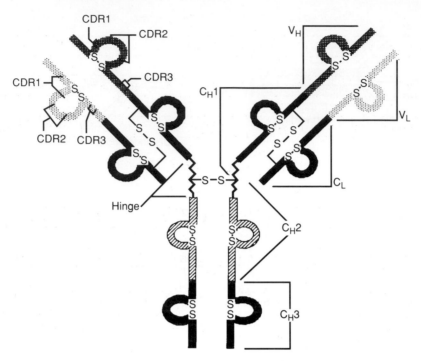

FIGURE 3.11 Monomeric Ig: V and C domains. L and H chains possess globular domains of about 110 amino acids containing approximately 60 residues linked by intradisulfide bridges. The first domain is the variable (V) region, and the remaining domains (three or four depending upon the Ig class) occur in the constant (C) regions of both types of chains. Each C domain has distinct functions, other than Ag binding, and displays degrees of homology with the other C domains. The relative locations of the regions of high variability (CDRs) are noted for both H and L chains.

The V region of the H chain, however, was only 25% as long as the C region. Each L and H chain was composed of linearly arranged domains of approximately 110 amino acids. Each domain contained an intrachain disulfide bridge of about 60 residues. The first domain made up the V region, and the remaining domains were assigned to the C region of the chain.

There are five classes of **H chains,** each designated by a Greek letter reflecting the major Ig class in which it appears: *gamma* (γ) in IgG, *mu* (μ) in IgM, *alpha* (α) in IgA, *epsilon* (ϵ) in IgE, and *delta* (δ) in IgD. H chains are distinguishable on the basis of amino acid sequences in their C regions and even by the number of C segments present. Two classes of **L chains,** known as *kappa* (κ) and *lambda* (λ), were distinguished by the amino acid sequences in their C regions (fig. 3.12). An Ab of any Ig class or subclass was found to contain *either* κ *or* λ L chains, *never both*. Ratios of λ and κ chains varied considerably within mammalian species. Only 5% of mouse Abs, for example, carried λ chains in contrast to human Abs, where over 40% may possess λ chains.

Analysis of L chains has shown that they may be further divided into subgroups. Human κ chains, for example, exhibit four such subgroups, while six subgroups have been defined for λ chains. Each subgroup contains certain amino acids in defined positions that are never changed, while other amino acids that localize nearby may display pronounced variability.

Light Chain Variable Regions

Sequence studies of N-terminal domains of L chains showed them to be highly variable, but interestingly the heterogeneity observed was not uniform. *Hypervariable subregions* were observed in three sites within κ and λ V regions. Each hypervariable region consisted of approximately 10 amino acids, which serve as **con-**

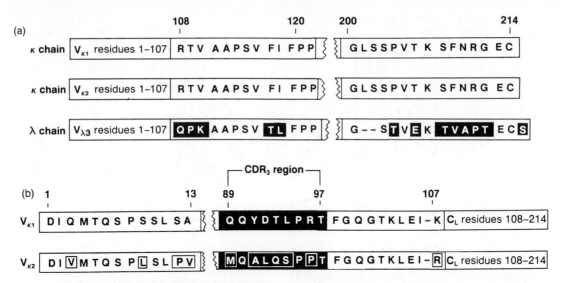

FIGURE 3.12 κ and λ L chains. Two classes (isotypes) of L chains, present in every individual, differ significantly in their C regions and are designated κ or λ. The marked sequence differences between the C regions of κ and λ chains are depicted in *a. Note:* Although the two κ chains, Vκ1 and Vκ2, may differ in the V region (*b*), they do not differ in the C region (*a*). Homologies are always high between C domains, but not necessarily 100%, between κ (or λ) C regions of even a single group. (See table 3.4 on page 000 for a key to single-letter abbreviations for amino acid residues.)

tact residues for Ab binding (see following). They function essentially as *complementarity-determining regions* (CDRs) with respect to the binding of an Ag.

The three *hypervariability subregions* (or CDRs) of an L chain (along with the hypervariability subregions of an H chain) *determine the Ab specificity of a molecule*. Inside a V region, there were subregions of preserved, fairly constant, amino acid sequences in between the CDRs, which were common to all members of a V region family (κ or λ). Such framework sequences may contribute to the conformation of the V region and the shape of the Ab-binding site.

Index of Variability

When sequences of V regions of κ, λ, or H chains are compared, the three hypervariable subregions show the greatest sequence variability. Measurement of variability at any given amino acid position may be derived from the following formula developed by Kabat and colleagues:

Thus, an index of variability may range from 1, for a completely invariant position, to a maximum of 400 for a position in which all 20 amino acids were found with equal frequency. For example, if only one kind of amino acid has been found at a given position in 20 sequenced L chains, the index is 1. If, on the other hand, 20 different kinds of amino acids have been found at a given position in 20 sequenced L chains, then the index is 400. Thus, the degree of variability may be graphically expressed (qualitatively and quantitatively) for L and H chain V regions.

The structure of the V region of human L chains showing the degree of variability at each amino acid position may be seen in figure 3.13. The CDRs of L chains occupy positions 24 to 34 (CDR1), 50 to 56 (CDR2), and 89 to 97 (CDR3). The framework residues (FRs) occupy positions 1 to 23 (FR1), 35 to 49 (FR2), 57 to 88 (FR3) and 98 to 107 (FR4).

$$\text{Variability} = \frac{\text{Number of different amino acids found at a given position}}{\text{Frequency of the most common amino acid at that position}}$$

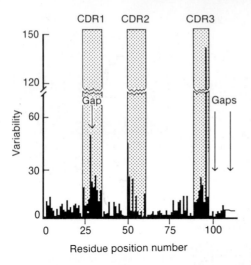

FIGURE 3.13 Degree of variability in V regions of L chains. The degree of variability, at each position, is depicted for the entire V region (110 amino acids) of representative Ig L chains. The degree of variability (or index) is calculated as the number of different amino acids found at a given position, divided by the frequency of the most common amino acid at that position. Note the three areas of hypervariability making up CDR1, CDR2, and CDR3. (Adapted from Kabat, E. A., Wu, T. T., and Bilofsky, H. *Sequence of Immunoglobulin Chains.* U.S. Department of Health, Education, and Welfare, 1977.)

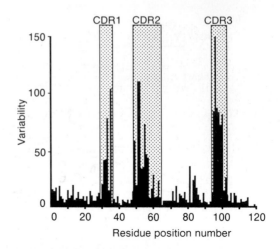

FIGURE 3.14 Degree of variability in V regions of H chains. The degree of variability, at each different position, is graphically represented for the entire V region of Ig H chains. Note the three areas of hypervariability making up CDR1, CDR2, and CDR3. (Adapted from Kabat, E. A., Wu, T. T., and Bilofsky, H. *Sequence of Immunoglobulin Chains.* U.S. Department of Health, Education, and Welfare, 1977.)

Heavy Chain Variable Regions

Here the CDRs may occupy positions 31 to 35 (CDR1); 50 to 65 (CDR2); and 96 to 102 (CDR3), as seen in a variability plot (fig. 3.14). These subregions of hypervariability contribute to the formation of the Ab-binding site, along with the CDRs of the L chain. An Ab-binding site is formed by the pairing of an H chain V region with an L chain V region. Framework subregions at positions 1 to 30 (FR1); 36 to 49 (FR2); 60 to 95 (FR3), and 103 to 113 (FR4) "push" and "pull" CDRs as they do L chains and, therefore, influence the shape of the Ab-binding site.

THE ANTIBODY-BINDING SITE

Ag binding had been shown by Porter to occur in the Fab fragments of Ab molecules, with the H chain portion usually playing a dominant role in the binding efficiency observed. To identify amino acid residues that form the active binding site, Jonathan Singer and colleagues devised a method known as affinity labeling. Using this technique, an antigenic determinant (hapten) can be radiolabeled and modified so that, on contacting and binding to its complementary Ab, it remains bound to the active site. The Ab is digested enzymatically. Fragments can then be sequenced, and the amino acids to which Ag became (and remained) attached identified through the radioactive label.

Using this method, investigators learned that labeled amino acids were derived from both H and L chains and were associated with the hypervariable or CDR subregions. Thus, widely separated **CDRs of both chains** appeared to *participate in the formation of the Ag-combining site* in the amino-terminal region of the Fab fragments. The high degree of sequence variability encountered in these regions is a major contributing factor of the diversity of Ag specificities displayed by Ig molecules.

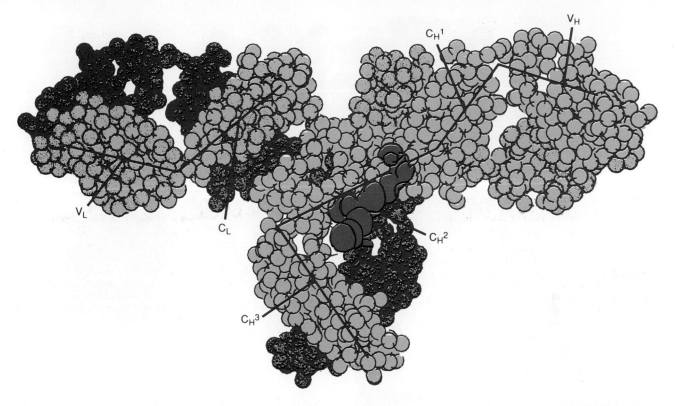

FIGURE 3.15 Model of IgG. This is a three-dimensional, computer-generated model of myeloma IgG. One H chain is white; the other is shaded darkly. The two L chains are shaded lightly. Carbohydrate, bound to the Fc fragment of the H chains, is shown in solid color. Domains of one L chain and one H chain are highlighted. (From Silverton, E. W., Navia, M. A., and Davies, D. R. Three-dimensional structure of an intact human immunoglobulin. *Proceedings of the National Academy of Sciences* [USA] **74**:5140, 1977, by permission.)

Three-Dimensional Models

A three-dimensional model of IgG, based on x-ray crystallographic studies, is seen in figure 3.15. The **Ag-binding region** of the Ab molecule *involves variable portions of both L and H chains,* which fold to form a three-dimensional mold or cavity into which an antigenic determinant "fits" (fig. 3.16). The tertiary structure of the combining site was derived from x-ray diffraction studies of immune complexes. Using this method, it was possible to determine the position and orientation of the Ag.

Figure 3.16 depicts diagrammatically an Ag (hapten) in contact with the binding site of an Ab. The data was obtained by x-ray crystallography of a human IgG myeloma protein that binds a derivative of vitamin K. The size of the cleft of the Ag-binding site, in this case, is about 15 Å $\times$ 6 Å $\times$ 6 Å. The size of the cavity, however, may vary according to the primary structure of the hypervariable subregions.

Igs, as other proteins, spontaneously assumes a particular shape, or tertiary structure, based on a given sequence of amino acids, which is influenced by the carbohydrates present. However, CDR conformation may be influenced more by length than by sequence of the hypervariable subregions. Using techniques from molecular biology, CDRs from one Ab have been shown to switch to another's framework and retain the Ag-binding specificity of the CDR donor. On the other hand, the hybrid Ab expressed an altered idiotype (see following under Idiotypic Determinants).

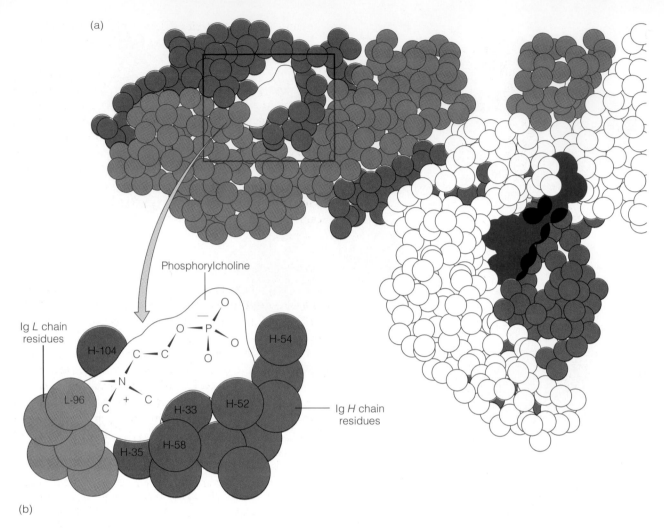

(a)

Phosphorylcholine

Ig L chain
residues

H-104

L-96

H-33

H-35   H-58

H-54

H-52

Ig H chain
residues

(b)

FIGURE 3.16 Antibody-combining site in contact with hapten. (*a*) This figure depicts an IgG antibody-combining site that has bound a hapten (phosphorylcholine). (*b*) An expansion of the inset of (*a*) shows the interaction of hapten with the CDR residues at the site, as determined by x-ray crystallography. Amino acid residues of H chain CDRs (H-33, H-35, H-52, H-54, H-58, H-104) and L chain CDRs (L-96) are shown in contact with hapten. Note that in this instance, the hapten lies closer to the H chain portion of the antibody than to the L chain.

It appears that we possess an unclear understanding, at present, of how particular combinations of CDRs give rise to particular surface topologies. Rees, at Oxford University, predicts that it will eventually be possible to construct binding-site topologies knowing only the structure of the Ag and the sequences of the matching CDRs. He and others are exploiting the methods of protein engineering in examination of computer-derived models of combining sites.

IMMUNOGLOBULINS AS ANTIGENS

Since Igs are high MW glycoproteins, they can serve as very potent Ags (immunogens). Differences in amino acid sequences between Ig classes, subclasses, types, and specific kinds of Abs largely determine the antigenic specificity of Igs. Igs carry three major categories of antigenic determinants: **isotypic, allotypic,** and **idiotypic** (fig. 3.17).

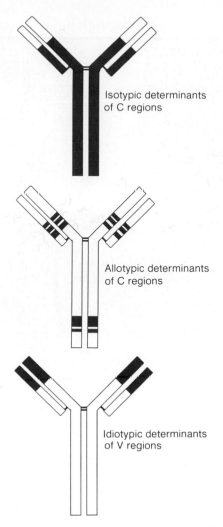

Isotypic determinants
of C regions

Allotypic determinants
of C regions

Idiotypic determinants
of V regions

FIGURE 3.17 Location of isotypic, allotypic, and idiotypic Ig determinants. *Isotypic Ig determinants (dark area)* are amino acid residues that distinguish H chain classes (IgG, IgM, IgA, IgD, IgE) and subclasses (IgG1, IgG2, IgG3, IgG4, and IgA1 and IgA2), as well as L chain types (κ and λ). They are located in the C domains of Ig chains, in all individuals. *Allotypic determinants (dark area)* are distinct amino acid residues located primarily in γ and α H chains and κ L chains. They are possessed by some but not all individuals. *Idiotypic determinants (dark area)* are located in the V regions of L and H chains, at or near the antibody-combining sites.

Isotypic Determinants

These determinants *distinguish the C regions of the H chain classes (and subclasses) and the L chain types.* Each isotype is encoded by a distinct gene that is characteristic for a particular mammalian species and is present in all members of that species. Thus, each human being carries Igs representing all the human isotypes in the serum.

Abs to these determinants may be raised by injecting Ig from one species into another species. Each Ig class (IgG, IgM, IgA, IgD, and IgE) possesses a specific isotypic determinant on its H chain. Similarly, each Ig subclass can be distinguished by a different H chain isotypic determinant. We all possess two types of L chains, which can be identified by their isotypic determinants, either κ or λ, located in the C region. Thus, an antiserum against a γ H chain, for example, can identify IgG, as distinct from other Ig classes, in any human serum.

Allotypic Determinants

The second group of *antigenic determinants are those found on the Igs of some, but not all, members of a particular species.* Allotypic determinants reflect genetic polymorphism of Igs within one species. Thus, individuals of a given species possess a given Ig class that either does or does not carry a certain allotypic determinant. Abs can be formed against an allotypic determinant by injecting Igs into another member of the species that does not possess the alloantigen. In humans, a number of allotypic markers have been discovered on Igs: G_m on γ H chains, K_m on κ L chains, A_m on α H chains, and H_v on variable H chains. The alleles in a heterozygous individual are codominant, although at the level of single cells only one or the other allele is expressed, which is known as allelic exclusion. The same V_H allotype may be associated with several different classes of H chain. There are, for example, about 25 different G_m determinants, designated by two numbers. The first number indicates the Ig subclass on which it appears, and the second number (in parentheses) the allotype, such as $G_{3m(11)}$. Allotypes have been used to identify peoples and show familial relationships.

Possession of certain allotypic determinants has been related, in some instances, to certain disease risks. For example, individuals possessing $G_{1m(3)}$ and $G_{3m(5)}$ appear to have increased risk of developing an autoimmune thyroid disorder. In some abnormal situations, Abs develop against a G_m allotypic determinant in the same person possessing the allotype, seen predominantly in individuals with rheumatoid arthritis.

TABLE 3.2 Physical and Biological Characteristics of Human Immunoglobulin Isotypes

Characteristic	Immunoglobulin Isotype				
	IgA	IgD	IgE	IgG	IgM
Biophysical and Chemical Traits					
Molecular weight (kD)	385*	160–184	160–200	150–170	146–970
Sedimentation coefficient (S_w)	7–9, 11*	7	8	7	7–19
Electrophoretic mobility	β-γ	γ	β-γ	γ	β
Carbohydrate content (%)	7–11	9–14	12	2–3	12
Heavy chain class†	$\alpha_1\alpha_2$	δ	ϵ	$\gamma_1\gamma_2\gamma_3\gamma_4$	μ
Light chain class	κ or λ	κ or λ	κ or λ	κ or λ	κ or λ
Biological Characteristics					
Serum concentration (mg/dL)	50–400	1.5–40	≤0.005	800–1,600	50–200
Half-life (days)	6	3	2	21	5
Complement binding‡	Alt.	None	None	Class.	Class.
Binding to tissue§	None	None	Homol.	Heterol.	None
Secretion from serous membranes	Yes*	No	Yes	No	No
Placental passage	No	No	No	Yes	No

*Secretory IgA.

†Multiple isotypes exist for Iga (IgA1 and IgA2) and IgG(IgG1, IgG2, IgG3, and IgG4).

‡Alt. = alternate pathway; Class. = classical pathway.

§Homol. = homologous tissues; Heterol. = heterologous tissues.

Idiotypic Determinants

The third group of antigenic determinants of Igs exists as a result of unique structures generated by the hypervariable subregions (or CDRs) on L and H chains. These antigenic determinants are called **idiotopes,** analogous to epitopes of classical Ags. Kieber-Emmons and Kohler have classified idiotopes as α-*idiotopes,* those that lie outside the Ag-binding site; β-*idiotopes,* those that are close to the Ag-binding site; and γ-*idiotopes,* those formed by the Ag-binding site. Thus antiidiotopic Abs may (1) not affect the binding site (α); (2) exhibit noncompetitive interference (β) of Ag binding; or (3) specifically block Ag binding (γ). An idiotype refers to the particular collection of antigenic determinants or idiotopes possessed by a specific Ab molecule.

Antiidiotypic Abs may be formed in self naturally or induced artificially in self, as well as in allo-typically identical members of a species under certain conditions. The significance of these molecules relates to their importance for immune regulation (see chapter 5), immunization procedures involving substitution for classical Ags (e.g., using bioengineered Ags), and specific immune suppression against transplantation and autoantigens (see Chapter 19).

PROPERTIES OF IMMUNOGLOBULIN CLASSES

Igs can be divided into classes and subclasses consistent with characteristics that are independent of their ability to bind Ags. They can be divided according to different antigenic properties into *five major isotypes:* IgG, IgA, IgM, IgD, and IgE. As can be seen in table 3.2, the various classes differ with respect to chemical and physical features and function.

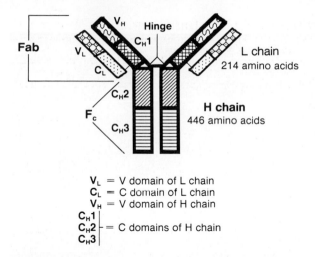

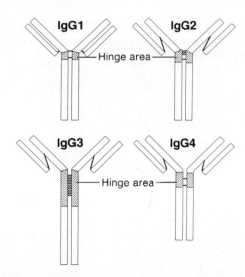

V_L = V domain of L chain
C_L = C domain of L chain
V_H = V domain of H chain
C_H1
C_H2 = C domains of H chain
C_H3

FIGURE 3.18 Structure of IgG. V_L and V_H domains exhibit sequence variability and hypervariability. The remaining sections of the polypeptide chains are relatively constant and are designated as C_L or C_H domains. All domains are stabilized by intrachain disulfide bonds (—S—S—). The C_H region is divided into three homology units (C_H1, C_H2, and C_H3). The molecule has two binding sites at the N-terminal end, composed of the hypervariable regions of both V_L and V_H chains. The distance between the two sites may vary since the hinge region is flexible. Carbohydrate is associated with the C_H2 domain, which may also serve as a site for complement fixation. C_H1 may bind certain complement fragments, and C_H2 and C_H3 may bind to FcRs on certain cells, and they also serve as sites for binding of *Staphylococcus* Protein A.

FIGURE 3.19 Structure of IgG subclasses. Interchain disulfide bridges in different human IgG subclasses are quite diverse, in contrast to the constancy of intrachain disulfide bonds. All disulfide bridges are localized in the hinge regions (*shaded area*). The H chain cysteine residue, forming the H-L chain bond in IgG subclasses 2, 3, and 4, is much closer to the amino terminus than IgG1. Variations in the number and arrangement of the interdisulfide bonds may be related to subclass function.

Immunoglobulin G

IgG is the most abundant class of Ig in the body, constituting approximately 75% of the total Igs and distributed equally within the intravascular and extravascular pools. Very little IgG is produced during the early stages of the primary response to Ag, but it is the major form of Ab produced during the secondary response. IgG is also the most commonly seen myeloma protein.

The basic structure of IgG, illustrating the various domains, is shown in figure 3.18. There are four subclasses of human IgG (1, 2, 3, and 4). Each subclass can be identified by a characteristic determinant localized on the H chain, and each exhibits different numbers and arrangements of the interchain disulfide bonds (fig. 3.19).

Table 3.3 compares some prominent IgG subclass characteristics, including their ability to fix complement and bind protein A. It is known that IgG3 is

most effective in binding complement, followed by IgG1 and IgG2, which bears significantly on many immune activities (see chapter 6, Complement and its Role in Immune Responses). The ability of IgG to bind to Protein A (from *Staphylococcus aureus*) and Protein G (from group G streptococci) has facilitated several applications, including Ig isolation.

IgG is the only class that can pass across the placenta and is responsible, in part, for the protection of the infant during the first few months of life. IgG2 does not cross the placenta as well as the other subclasses, and may not cross at all in some cases. IgG is also found, along with IgA, in the milk during the first few weeks after birth, providing additional protection if the infant is breast fed.

Macrophages and monocytes bear Fc receptors which bind to the Fc portion of IgG1 and IgG3 in the C_H3 domain. Such binding permits these cells to exhibit Ab-dependent cellular cytotoxicity, as

TABLE 3.3 Characteristics of Human IgG Isotypes

Characteristic	IgG Isotype			
	IgG1	IgG2	IgG3	IgG4
H chain type	γ^1	γ^2	γ^3	γ^4
Number of disulfide bridges	2	4	13	2
Allotypes (G_m group)	1, 2, 4, 17, 22	24	3, 5, 6, 13, 14, 15, 16	—
Crosses placenta	Yes	Possibly	Yes	Yes
Binds complement	Yes	Possibly	Yes	No
Binds to macrophages, neutrophils, and eosinophils	Yes	Possibly	Yes	Possibly
Binds to heterologous tissue	Yes	No	Yes	Yes
Binds to Protein A	Yes	Yes	No	Yes
Binds to Protein G	Yes	Yes	Yes	Yes

Source: Modified from Hanson, L. A., and Wigzell, H. *Immunology.* Butterworths, London, 1983.

described for other cell types. As a class, IgG usually exhibits rather high affinity for Ag, which may permit efficient neutralization of poisons or toxins. Most Ab responses probably involve all four subclasses of IgG, but some responses may be restricted, as seen, for example, by the comparative ability of the various subclasses to fix complement, bind to macrophages, or cross the placenta.

Immunoglobulin M

About 10% of normal serum Igs consist of this class. IgM normally exists as a pentamer, consisting of five Ig subunits, with a MW of about 900 kD. In contrast to IgG, the larger IgM remains in the serum almost exclusively and is not usually found extravascularly in body spaces or secretions. Pentameric IgM is apparently too large to cross the placenta.

The H μ chain has four C_H domains rather than three, as seen in the H chains of IgG. The subunits are held together by disulfide bonds between the C_H3 domains (fig. 3.20). There are a number of carbohydrate units associated with the μ chain. Moreover, there is an additional peptide chain called the joining (J) chain. The J chain may be largely responsible for the polymerization process, which occurs shortly before the molecule is secreted by the plasma cell.

IgM Abs are the *first Igs* on the scene following Ag challenge and are, therefore, important as a first *specific* defensive measure against infectious agents of disease. Each of the five subunits has two Ag-binding sites and all ten sites (valence of 10) are identical, with respect to binding specificity. Individually, each binding site may express low affinity for an antigenic determinant, but collectively they can exhibit pronounced avidity. In addition, IgM is more efficient than IgG in activating complement. Complement may bind to several Fc regions of pentameric IgM simultaneously, thereby initiating the complement cascade and target cell lysis with a single molecule. Conceivably, only a few molecules of avid IgM, arriving early in the area following bacterial invasion, could represent a significant defensive measure. IgM is also important as an Ag receptor, where it occurs in monomeric form on early B lymphocytes. In certain disease states, such as lupus erythematosus and rheumatoid arthritis, IgM may occur in monomeric form in rather high concentrations. Monomeric IgM has a lower avidity for Ag than does the pentameric form.

Immunoglobulin A

IgA constitutes about 15% of human serum Igs, where it exists primarily as a monomeric Ig (fig. 3.21). Perhaps the most important form is the dimeric form,

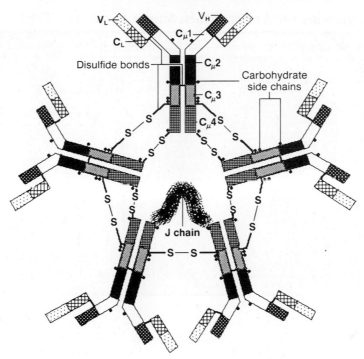

FIGURE 3.20 Structure of IgM. IgM consists of five monomeric subunits, joined by disulfide bridges in both the C_H3 and C_H4 domains, which are linked to a J chain. μ chains lack a hinge region but have four, rather than three, C_H domains. The subunits are, nevertheless, quite flexible. Each of the five monomers has a molecular weight of about 180 kD and the J chain 15 kD. The IgM pentamer possesses 10 identical Ag-binding sites, permitting multivalent binding, if the Ag has repeating determinants.

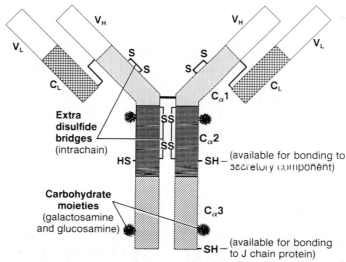

FIGURE 3.21 Structure of monomeric IgA. In this diagram, the approximate location of oligosaccharides at multiple sites are shown. Additional intrachain disulfide bridges are indicated. These bonds are peculiar to IgA and complement the normal intradisulfide bonds, which stabilize each globular domain of all Ig classes (not shown). The penultimate cysteine residue may be linked to a J chain in polymeric forms. Two cysteine residues in the C_H2 domain may be involved in the covalent binding of secretory component (see fig. 3.22).

TABLE 3.4 Abbreviations for Amino Acids: Single-Letter and Triplet Codes

Amino Acid	Single Letter	Triplet	Amino Acid	Single Letter	Triplet
alanine	A	ala	histidine	H	his
arginine	R	arg	isoleucine	I	ile
asparagine	N	asn	leucine	L	leu
aspartic acid	D	asp	lysine	K	lys
asp/arg (not distinguished)	B	asx	methionine	M	met
			phenylalanine	F	phe
cysteine	C	cys	proline	P	pro
glutamic acid	E	glu	serine	S	ser
glutamine	Q	gln	threonine	T	thr
glu/gln; or pyrrolidone carboxylic acid (not distinguished)	Z	glx	tryptophan	W	trp
			tyrosine	Y	tyr
glycine	G	gly	valine	V	val

known as *secretory IgA* (sIgA) (fig. 3.22). IgA is the predominant class of Ig in secretions such as milk, tears, nasal fluids, saliva, perspiration, genitourinary secretions, and seromucous secretions of the lung and intestine. Its function is to protect the various exposed epithelial surfaces from pathogenic microorganisms and animal parasites.

Secretory IgA is quite resistant to proteolytic digestion, which may be due in large part to the secretory component. IgA and a polypeptide known as the J chain are synthesized by plasma cells that are associated with epithelial cells. Two molecules of IgA and one J chain are assembled into dimeric IgA that is secreted. Secretory components of sIgA are synthesized by glandular epithelial cells, especially those of the lungs, intestine, and lacrimal (tear) glands. Secreted IgA dimers become strongly bound to secretory components on the surfaces of epithelial cells, where they are produced. The sIgA complex can then be engulfed and subsequently secreted into body fluids. Following release, sIgA can prevent microorganisms from entering body tissues.

There are two subclasses of IgA in humans. Neither subclass can bind complement and activate the classical complement pathway. Nevertheless, IgA can activate the alternative complement pathway and contribute to the killing of coliform bacteria (see chapter 6).

Immunoglobulin D

Less than 1% of the serum Igs (in humans) fall in this class. IgD does not bind complement. Neither does it cross the placenta nor bind to cells via the Fc region. On the other hand, IgD is found on the surface of B lymphocytes, where it serves as an early **Ag receptor.** With progressive maturation of B cells, IgD is replaced by other Igs (see chapter 20, Development of Immunity, for further discussion).

The Fc region of IgD is apparently quite resistant to proteolysis. The Fab regions, by contrast, are quite labile, compared with other Ig classes, and are prone to proteolysis. Calvert recently suggested that the labile structure conceivably plays a role in Ag processing. Accordingly, once bound Ag is taken into the cell, the receptor (IgD) may undergo proteolysis in the endocytic vesicles releasing Ag for interaction with class II molecules (see chapter 7, Histocompatibility Systems). The role of IgD as a modulator of immune responses is under active investigation. The structure of IgD is depicted in figure 3.23.

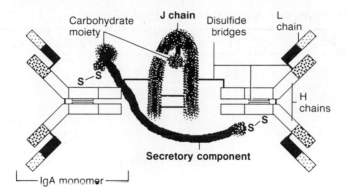

FIGURE 3.22 Structure of secretory IgA. In the dimeric form, two IgA molecules are joined by a J chain, linked to the Fc region (C_H3) by disulfide bridges. The J chain has a molecular weight of about 15 kD. The secretory component is a single polypeptide chain, with a molecular weight of 70 kD, which is covalently linked to the Fc region (C_H2 domain). sIgA has a sedimentation coefficient of about 11S and a molecular weight of approximately 380 kD.

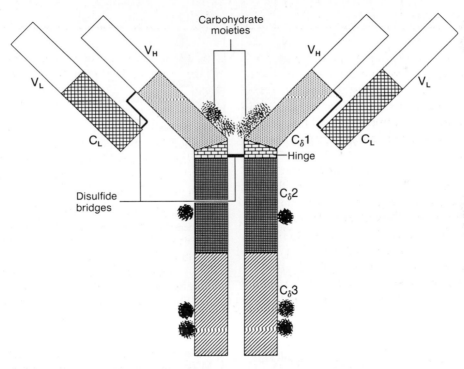

FIGURE 3.23 Structure of IgD. The δ chains are apparently linked to each other by a single disulfide bridge, and each δ chain is linked to an L chain through a cysteine in the C_H1 region, very close to the V domain. Possible sites of glucosamine (carbohydrate) attachment are shown.

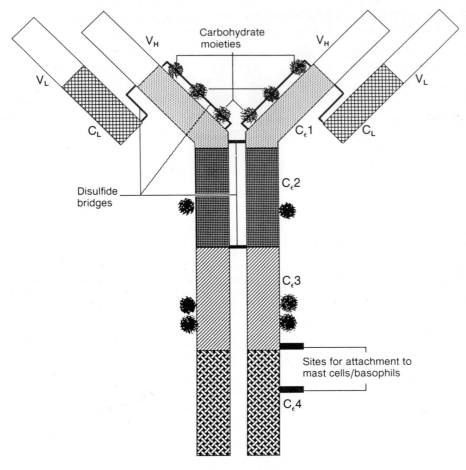

FIGURE 3.24 Structure of IgE. IgE, along with IgM, possesses four C regions in the H chains, in contrast to the other Ig classes. One structural feature of IgE is unique to this class. The molecule has two interchain disulfide bridges separated by a complete domain. Sites for attachment to mast cells or basophils may be located on C_H3 and C_H4 domains.

Immunoglobulin E

IgE is quite important in the body, but it is normally found in extremely low concentrations in the serum. Serum levels increase during allergic responses and certain parasitic diseases. It is associated with allergic, Type I immediate hypersensitivities in which specific IgE molecules may be generated against allergens (see chapter 13, Hypersensitivity). The IgE produced can adhere to, and passively sensitize, basophils and mast cells. This class also plays a role in the active immune response to helminthic disease (see chapter 12, Immunity to Infectious Diseases). The ϵ H chain has four domains in the constant region, similar to μ chains of IgM (fig. 3.24). IgE does not cross the placenta, nor does it fix complement.

S U M M A R Y

1. The adaptive immune system can recognize, and respond to, foreign molecules or antigens, giving rise to increasing quantities of specific antibodies (humoral immunity) and/or effector T cells (cellular immunity). [p. 56]

2. An antigen molecule contains one or more distinct chemical groups, known as antigenic determinants or epitopes, each of which can bind to specific antibody molecules or specific antigen receptors on lymphocytes. [p. 56]

3. An antigenic determinant or epitope cannot, by itself, induce an immune response, but it can bind specifically to the paratope, or antigen-binding site, of a B or T cell receptor. An epitope, or hapten, can be immunogenic if combined with a larger carrier macromolecule. [p. 56]

4. Epitopes whose specificity is determined by the sequence of continuous subunits are called sequence epitopes, whereas conformational epitopes depend on the spatial folding or configuration of the molecule. In the latter instance, subunits of the epitope might not be continuous. [pp. 57–59]

5. The relative ability of an antigen to stimulate immune responses is termed immunogenicity. Although all immunogens are antigenic, not all antigens are immunogenic. The ability of an antigen to be immunogenic depends upon several factors, including the nature of the molecule, mode of presentation, and nature of the host. [p. 59]

6. High molecular weight foreign proteins serve as potent immunogens. Their immunogenicity can be enhanced on administration with an adjuvant, which potentiates an immune response. [pp. 59–60]

7. Most protein antigens require T cell help for the production of antibody and are called T-dependent antigens. These antigens contain specific epitopes that activate B lymphocytes and other epitopes that activate T helper cells. Other antigens do not require T cell help and are called T-independent antigens. These contain repeating epitopes and include polysaccharides, lipids, and nucleic acids. [pp. 60–61]

8. Most T cells recognize antigen only after it has been processed by accessory cells and presented, in association with self-protein, as small epitopes on the accessory cells' surface. Most B cells recognize native, unprocessed antigen with its conformational structure intact. [p. 61]

9. The intrinsic ability of an individual to respond to antigen is influenced by immune response genes, sex, health, nutrition, behavior, and age. [p. 61]

10. In accordance with the clonal selection model, a foreign antigenic determinant "selects" a particular B cell expressing an appropriate surface receptor (an antibody). The antigen becomes bound, thereby stimulating the cell to divide, differentiate, and clonally expand into antibody-secreting and memory cells. [pp. 62–64]

11. Antibodies are protein molecules called immunoglobulins, which are synthesized in plasma cells and found primarily in plasma or serum. They can be found in other body fluids including milk, tears, urine, and secretions of the respiratory, digestive, and genitourinary tracts. [p. 64]

12. Serum immunoglobulins consist of heterogeneous populations of antibodies. These can be identified and separated, according to isotype (class, subclass, group, and subgroup), allotype (genetic markers on Ig chains of some individuals), and idiotype (collection of unique antigenic determinants specific for variable regions). [p. 65]

13. Pure immunoglobulins, required for the study of antibody structure, were first obtained in large quantities from myeloma tumor cells, which could be maintained indefinitely in culture or as ascites in mice. Usually, the complementary antigen to the antibody (myeloma protein) was unknown. [p. 66]

14. Novel techniques for producing monoclonal antibodies have been developed. These include forming hybridomas (fusing spleen cells, from immunized animals, with cancer cells that were nonimmunoglobulin-secreting myeloma cells) and producing recombinant monoclonal antibodies. [pp. 66–67]

15. Treatment of immunoglobulin with the proteolytic enzyme, papain, cleaves the molecule into three fragments. Two of these are identical and antigen binding (Fab fragments), and one does not bind antigen and is crystallizable (Fc fragment). When immunoglobulin is treated with reducing agents, the molecule separates into two light and two heavy chains with molecular weights of 25 and 50 kD, respectively. [pp. 67–70]

16. Two light chains and two heavy chains are linked together by disulfide bonds to yield a basic monomeric structure (H_2L_2) found in all classes of immunoglobulins. [pp. 70–71]

17. Sequencing studies of pure antibodies showed that light and heavy chains contain variable and constant regions with linearly arranged domains of about 110 amino acids. [pp. 71–72]

18. Two classes of light chains, known as kappa (κ) and lambda (λ), are distinguished by the amino acid sequences in the constant regions. Either κ or λ light chains are found in all immunoglobulin classes. [p. 72]

19. Three hypervariable subregions, or complementarity-determining regions, are found within the variable regions of both light and heavy chains. [pp. 72–73]

20. Antibody specificity depends largely on the structure of the complementarity-determining regions, which participate in the formation of the antibody-binding site. The shape of the binding site is influenced, however, by framework residues on either side of the complementarity-determining regions. [p. 73]

21. Variability in the V region may be determined by comparing the number of different amino acids at a given position, with the frequency of the most common amino acid at that position. [pp. 73–74]

22. Amino acids that participate, as contact residues of the binding site, can be detected by affinity labeling. An antigenic determinant is labeled and covalently bound to the binding site for analysis. [p. 74]

23. The tertiary structure of the antibody-binding site was derived from x-ray diffraction studies of immune complexes. With this approach, the position and orientation of the antigenic determinant can be determined. [p. 75]

24. Complementarity-determining regions from one antibody may be switched to another's framework and retain the antigen-binding capacity of the complementarity-determining region donor. [p. 75]

25. Isotypic determinants distinguish constant regions of heavy chain classes and subclasses, as well as light chain types found in all human beings. [p. 77]

26. Allotypic determinants are found on Igs of some, but not all, humans. G_m markers may be found on γ chains, A_m markers on α chains, H_v markers on variable heavy chains, and K_m markers on κ light chains. [p. 77]

27. Idiotypic determinants are unique structures generated conventionally by the hypervariable subregions (or CDRs) on light and heavy chains. These antigenic determinants are called idiotopes. An idiotype refers to a particular collection of idiotopes possessed by a specific antibody molecule. [p. 78]

28. There are five major classes of immunoglobulins: IgG, IgA, IgM, IgD, and IgE. There are also several subclasses (IgG1–4 and IgA1–2). Classes and subclasses differ chemically, physically, and functionally. [p. 78]

29. IgG is the most abundant and the major form of antibody during the secondary response. It can fix complement, cross the placenta, neutralize toxins, enhance phagocytosis, and effect antibody-dependent cellular cytotoxicity. [pp. 79–80]

30. IgM is generally the first immunoglobulin to respond to an antigen and, with 10 antibody-binding sites, exhibits pronounced avidity. IgM

is a very efficient activator of complement. It occurs in monomeric form as an antigen receptor on early B lymphocytes. [p. 80]

31. IgA occurs in several forms, including a dimeric form with secretory component. Secretory IgA is found in exocrine secretions such as milk, tears, saliva, and perspiration, as well as genitourinary secretions and seromucous secretions of the lung and intestine. IgA serves to protect epithelial surfaces from infectious agents. [pp. 80–82]

32. IgD represents less than 1% of the serum immunoglobulins. Perhaps its primary function is that of an antigen receptor on B cells. [p. 82]

33. IgE is found in very low concentrations in the serum of normal individuals. Levels may increase considerably in individuals manifesting allergic reactions and/or parasitic infections. IgE is critically involved in Type I hypersensitivity reactions. It also plays a role in host resistance to helminthic infestations. [p. 84]

R E A D I N G S

Burton, D. R. Immunoglobulin G: functional sites. *Molecular Immunology* **22:**161, 1985.

Calvert, J. E. A function for IgD? *Immunology Today* **7:**136, 1987.

Catty, D. *Antibodies: A Practical Approach.* (Vol. 1). IRL Press, Oxford, 1988.

Davies, D. R., and Metzer, H. Structural basis of antibody function. *Annual Review of Immunology* **1:**87, 1983.

Davis, A., and Shulman, M. IgM—Molecular requirements for its assembly and function. *Immunology Today* **10:**118, 1989.

Goding, J. W. *Monoclonal Antibodies: Principles and Practices.* Academic Press, Inc., New York, 1987.

Grey, H., Sette, A., and Buus, S. How T cells see antigen. *Scientific American* **261:**56, 1989.

Hebert, J., Bernier, D., Boutin, Y., et al. Generation of anti-idiotypic and anti-anti-idiotypic monoclonal antibody in the same fusion. Support of Jerne's Network Theory. *Journal of Immunology* **144:**4256, 1990.

Hilschmann, N., and Craig, L. C. Amino acid sequence studies with Bence-Jones proteins. *Proceedings of the National Academy of Science (USA)* **53:**1403, 1965.

Hoffman, M. Superantigens may shed light on immune puzzle. *Science* **248:**685, 1990.

Koshland, M. E. The coming of age of the immunoglobulin J chain. *Annual Review of Immunology* **3:**425, 1985.

Marx, J. Learning how to bottle the immune system. *Science* **246:**1250, 1989.

Mestecky, J., and McGhee, J. Immunoglobulin A: molecular and cellular interactions involved in IgA biosynthesis and the immune response. *Advances in Immunology* **40:**153, 1987.

Moller, G. (ed.). Immunoglobulin D: structure, synthesis, membrane representation and function. *Immunological Reviews,* Vol. 37, 1977.

Mullis, K. The unusual origin of the polymerase chain reaction. *Scientific American* **262:**56, 1990.

Rees, A. R. The antibody combining site: retrospect and prospect. *Immunology Today* **8**(2):44, 1987.

Saragovi, H. U., Fitzpatrick, D., Raktabutr, A., et al. Design and synthesis of a mimetic from an antibody complimentarity-determining region. *Science* **253:**792, 1991.

Solari, R., and Kraehenbuhl, J. The biosynthesis of secretory component and its role in the transepithelial transport of IgA dimer. *Immunology Today* **6:**17, 1985.

Stevenson, F. K. Idiotypes and diseases. *Immunology Today* **7:**287, 1986.

Winter, G., and Milstein, C. Man-made antibodies. *Nature* **349:**293, 1991.

Wu, T. T., and Kabat, E. A. An analysis of the variable regions of Bence-Jones proteins and myeloma light chains and their implications for antibody complementarity. *Journal of Experimental Medicine* **132:**211, 1970.

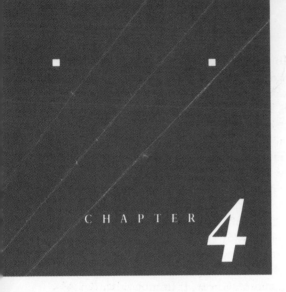

CHAPTER 4

Antigen–Antibody Reactions

OVERVIEW

This chapter discusses immune-complex formation, and the implications and applications of the antigen-antibody interaction. Why an antibody binds to an antigen, where the binding takes place, and under what conditions an antigen-antibody complex might dissociate are considered. A variety of representative techniques for detecting and measuring antigens, antibodies, and their interactions are presented and their importance to biological research or medical diagnostic/therapeutic applications is discussed.

CONCEPTS

1. An antigenic determinant and an antibody bind if they are complementary, spatially close, and if multiple noncovalent bonds form.

2. Antibody affinity reflects the strength of binding between members of an immune complex, while antibody specificity characterizes the ability of the molecule to discriminate one antigenic determinant from another. High-affinity antibody is more specific than low-affinity antibody.

3. Crossreactive antibodies can react with two different antigens that share some identical antigenic determinants or related determinants.

4. A variety of techniques have been developed for detecting and measuring one component of an immune complex when the other is known.

5. Immune-complex formation, which may occur in the body following antigenic insult from microorganisms and animal parasites, can be beneficial or protective. On the other hand, immune complexes formed with self-antigens and allergens can be quite damaging.

Humoral immune responses are mediated by effector molecules known as immunoglobulins (Igs). To be effective, Igs (also known as antibodies [Abs]) must form stable interactions with the antigens (Ags) against which they are directed. These interactions are determined by properties of both the Ab and the Ag. The first part of this chapter explores these properties. Later in this chapter, we examine means of evaluating and quantifying these interactions.

■ ■ ■ ■ ■ ■ ■ ■ ■

ANTIGEN-ANTIBODY BINDING

An Ag-Ab complex forms as a result of the formation of many noncovalent bonds between an antigenic determinant (epitope) and the contact residues (amino acids) of an Ab-binding site. Considerable binding energy develops as a result of the establishment of multiple bonds, which may include hydrogen bridges, charged group attractions, van der Waals forces, and hydrophobic bonds. Nonetheless, the reactants must be close and spatially complementary for binding to occur. The binding pocket must fit the antigenic determinant, and any deviation may cause a decrease in binding energy and attraction. Disruption of the noncovalent bonds can occur if the resulting decrease in binding energy reaches a critical threshold. The reaction is reversible, and neither reactant is changed, in contrast to enzyme-substrate reactions. The reaction follows common laws of mass action and chemical equilibrium.

ANTIBODY AFFINITY

Ab **affinity** refers to the *strength of binding between an Ab-binding site and an antigenic determinant* (monovalent ligand or hapten). Affinity is an expression of attraction that exists, over and above, any steric repulsive or disruptive forces that may exist. The term **avidity,** on the other hand, is used to designate the *strength of binding of a multivalent Ag with an Ab possessing at least two combining sites or an antiserum containing Abs of differing specificities.* For example, an IgM Ab, with ten binding sites, or an IgG molecule, with two binding sites, might become bound to an Ag possessing several identical determinants. The avidity of these Ab-Ag binding reactions is greater than the sum of the intrinsic affinities involved, since all bonds (at all sites) must be broken simultaneously for dissociation to occur. Since natural Ags might possess several epitopes, some identical and some different, the functional affinity or avidity of the combined binding reactions is complex and reflects the various binding equilibria.

Measurement of Antibody Affinity

The intrinsic affinity of an Ab, which can be expressed as an affinity constant, is of interest for several reasons. It can be used to assess Ab specificity (discussed later in chapter) or to examine binding phenomena. It is also of interest since it influences the functional efficiency of Abs. High-affinity Abs, for example, are very desirable for diagnostic, therapeutic, or analytical applications. To determine the affinity of an Ab for a particular ligand, on encounter, we require a means of detecting bound and unbound ligand.

In accordance with the law of mass action, the rate of a reaction is proportional to the concentration of the reactants. Thus,

$$Ag + Ab \leftrightarrow AgAb, \text{ or } k_a[Ag][Ab] = k_d[AgAb]$$

where [Ag] and [Ab] are the concentrations of unbound Ag and Ab, [AgAb] is the concentration of bound Ag and Ab, and k_a and k_d are association and dissociation constants.

At equilibrium, the equilibrium constant $K = k_a/k_d = [AgAb]/[Ag][Ab]$. If all binding sites of an Ab have the same equilibrium constant, then

$$\frac{r}{c} = nK - rK, \text{ or } K = \frac{r}{(n-r)c}$$

where r = moles of ligand bound/mole of Ab, c = concentration of unbound (free) ligand in moles/liter, and n = valence of the Ab (number of ligand-binding sites). K values can vary, for example, from 10^5 liters/mole for low-affinity complexes to 10^{11} liters/mole for high-affinity complexes.

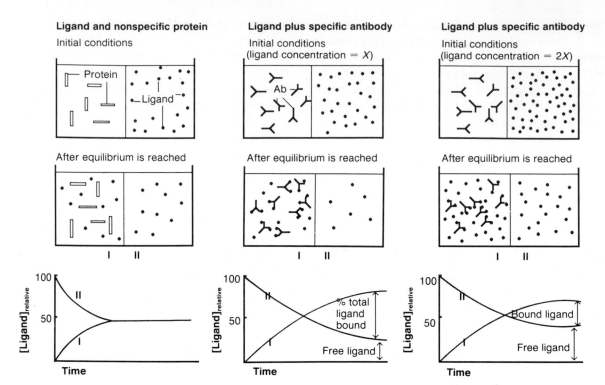

FIGURE 4.1 Equilibrium dialysis for affinity measurements. *Top panel:* A series of dialysis chambers is set up containing constant amounts of Ab (bivalent in this example) and increasing amounts of monovalent ligand. Each chamber contains two compartments (I and II, left and right) separated by a semipermeable membrane. The ligand is labeled and, thus, is readily detectable. The small ligand but not the Ab can freely diffuse across the membrane from one chamber to the other. *Middle panel:* At equilibrium, the following conditions exist. *Left chamber:* Concentration of ligand is equal in both compartments since there was no reaction with the nonspecific protein. *Center and right chambers:* The concentration of ligand in compartment I, in each case, is greater than in compartment II. This occurs because there is binding of ligand to the Abs. Since they are bound, they are not free to diffuse across the membrane. However, the remaining free ligand distributes between both compartments I and II to establish an equilibrium of "free" ligand between these compartments. *Bottom panel:* Plotting relative ligand concentration versus time traces the *net distribution* of ligand between compartments I and II until equilibrium

is reached. The difference between the two curves reflects the percentage of *total* ligand bound to Ab in compartment I. *Left chamber:* No binding occurs. Ligand distributes equally between compartments I and II. *Middle chamber:* Approximately 21% of total ligand (6/28) is free in compartment II. The remaining 79% (22/28) is found in compartment I; however, approximately 58% (16/28) of total ligand occurs bound to Ab [(free ligand + bound ligand in compartment I) − (free ligand in compartment II)]. *Right chamber:* A similar situation exists in this case. Since the concentration of Ab was the same but the concentration of ligand had been increased, the percentage of total ligand bound to Ab is less. Free ligand in compartment II is 36% (20/56); free ligand + bound ligand in compartment I is 64% (36/56); the percentage of total ligand bound to Ab is 28% (16/56) [(free ligand + bound ligand in compartment I) − (free ligand in compartment II)]. Although the same final amount of ligand (16 units) is bound, the percentage of total bound ligand is less because there was a greater initial concentration of ligand.

Monoclonal antibodies (MAbs) are desirable, if available, for affinity determinations since they allow the determination of binding constants for individual Ag-Ab reactions. Several methods are available for measuring the intrinsic affinity of a specific binding reaction. Two simple and useful ways of determining binding constants are equilibrium dialysis and an adaptation of solid-phase radioimmunoassay (RIA).

Equilibrium Dialysis

Determination of binding constants requires that at least one component of the system be univalent (or monovalent). A univalent ligand (or hapten) is most frequently used, but when a multivalent Ag must be employed then univalent Fab fragments of Ab are necessary. In this technique, an equilibrium dialysis chamber containing a membrane permeable to one

TABLE 4.1 Sample Results from a Hypothetical Equilibrium Dialysis Experiment (amount of ligand varies as shown; Ab concentration = 1.5 μM)

Part I—Raw Data

Amount of Ligand Added (μM)	cpm* in Compartment II[†]	cpm in Compartment II	Total cpm [I + II]	Bound cpm [I − II]
0.1	210	1,535	1,745	1,325
0.25	517	3,700	4,217	3,183
0.5	1,051	7,329	8,380	6,278
1.0	1,948	13,322	15,270	11,374
2.5	4,848	31,579	36,427	26,731

Part II—Calculating Results

Bound Ligand[‡] (μM)	c[§] (Free Ligand) (μM)	$\left[\dfrac{\text{Bound ligand}}{\text{Ab concentration}}\right]$	r/c (μM)	K[‖] (μM^{-1})
0.076	0.012	0.051	4.25	2.55
0.189	0.031	0.126	4.06	2.17
0.375	0.063	0.25	3.97	2.27
0.745	0.128	0.497	3.88	2.59
1.330	0.333	0.887	2.66	2.39
				(Average = 2.394)

*cpm = counts per minute of radioactive ligand measured.

[†]For compartment characteristics, refer to figure 4.1, after equilibrium.

[‡]Bound ligand = ([bound cpm]/[total cpm]) × concentration of ligand added.

[§]c (concentration of free ligand) = ([cpm in compartment II]/[Total cpm]) × concentration of ligand added.

[‖]$K = r/[(n - r) \times c]$, where n is valence of binding molecule (for this example, $n = 2$).

component, but not the other, is used. Usually, the ligand used in the assay is the permeable component, while the Ab is the nonpermeable component. Ligands are often labeled with radioisotopes. A series of chambers are set up with constant concentrations of **Ab** and increasing concentrations of ligand. Nonpermeable and permeable components are placed on opposite sides of the membrane. The concentration of freely permeable, labeled ligand is determined on both sides of the membrane, after equilibrium is reached (fig. 4.1). The concentration of bound ligand is obtained by subtracting the concentration of unbound ligand in the Ab-free compartment from the total amount of ligand in the Ab-containing compartment.

Hypothetical results of an equilibrium dialysis experiment in which radiolabeled ligand x is complexed with Ab y are given in table 4.1. In addition to calculating a value for K, the affinity constant can be derived by plotting r/c versus r. This type of representation is called a Scatchard plot (fig. 4.2). K is a constant when MAbs are used, since the Abs are homogeneous with respect to affinity for the ligand. The plot should produce a straight line with a slope designated as $-K$. From this plot we can derive the affinity constant K for the Ab and its valence n.

If the Abs are polyclonal, and heterogeneous with respect to affinity for the ligand, then K is not constant but may range in value. However, using a

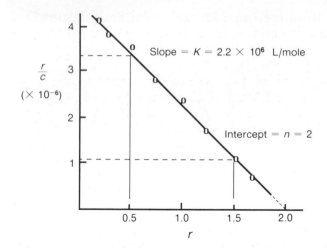

FIGURE 4.2 Scatchard plot of ligand binding by homogeneous Abs. This diagram shows a hypothetical plot, r/c versus r, of monovalent ligand molecules binding with MAbs. The Abs are homogeneous. All of the Ab-combining sites possess the same association constant and, therefore, $r/c = nK - rK$, which is the equation of a straight line. The intercept on the abscissa, $r/c = 0$, is equal to n, and the intercept on the ordinate is equal to nK. The slope, $\Delta y/\Delta x$; $2.2 \times 10^6/L$, provides a measure of K; here $K = 2.2 \times 10^6$ liters/mole. Abbreviations (see also table 4.1 for additional definitions): c is the concentration of free ligand, r is the amount of ligand-bound/Ab concentration, n is the valence (number of binding sites) of Ab, and K is the affinity constant of ligand for Ab.

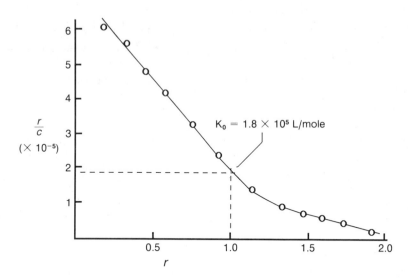

FIGURE 4.3 Scatchard plot of ligand binding of heterogeneous Abs. This is a plot of representative binding results for the reaction of ligand with polyclonal Abs. Departure from linearity is primarily due to heterogeneity of the Ab molecules. Since the Ab-ligand interactions do not give a straight line, an average value for the association constant K_0 may be taken. Thus, K_0 is the reciprocal of the concentration c when $r = 1$ (the point at which an average of one ligand molecule is bound to one Ab molecule [half-saturation]). Here, $K_0 = 1.8 \times 10^5$ liters/mole and may be read directly from the plot, as indicated.

monovalent ligand restricts the heterogeneity observed to subsets of Abs directed against a single determinant, which might nevertheless still exhibit a spectrum of affinities. A Scatchard plot, in this case, is not a straight line (fig. 4.3). In this instance, we can define an average affinity K_0. For divalent Ab, where $n = 2$, the average intrinsic association constant K_0 can be calculated, when half of the Ab-binding sites are occupied (and $r = 1$), from the equation, $K_0 = 1/c$. The average affinity constant can be read directly from the Scatchard plot, since it is the reciprocal of the concentration of free ligand c, when $r = 1$.

Antibody-Binding Constants by Radioimmunoassay

The use of equilibrium dialysis or precipitation techniques require that at least one component of the system be monovalent. RIA can be used to determine affinity constants of MAbs using either monovalent or multivalent ligands. Under certain conditions, cells displaying membrane-bound Ags can also be used. The RIA method has the further advantage that large numbers of samples can be analyzed simultaneously.

The *solid-phase RIA* is a sensitive method that may be used for screening hybridoma cultures for specific Ab activity (fig. 4.4). Soluble Ag, or fixed cells displaying the Ag, are adsorbed to the bottom of multiwelled polyvinyl microtiter plates. Ab activity can then be determined by a two-step incubation. Hybridoma-culture media (which may contain MAbs) is added. If Abs are present, they become bound to the Ag. Following washing procedures, a radiolabeled anti-Ab is added. If the well in question contains the primary Ab (bound to the Ag), it provides a target for the radiolabeled secondary Ab, which now becomes similarly bound. The well is now radioactive and, of course, detectable, whereas a well that did not contain the primary MAb would not be radioactive since no binding of the radioactive secondary Ab could occur.

Frankel and Gerhard developed a method for handling binding data from RIAs, which allows the determination of binding constants. Binding of MAb (mouse) to Ag is determined by incubating different dilutions of Ab in wells containing constant amounts of Ag. Wells are treated, after washing, with radiolabeled antimouse F(ab')$_2$. The amount of bound Ab in each well is then determined by extrapolation of the

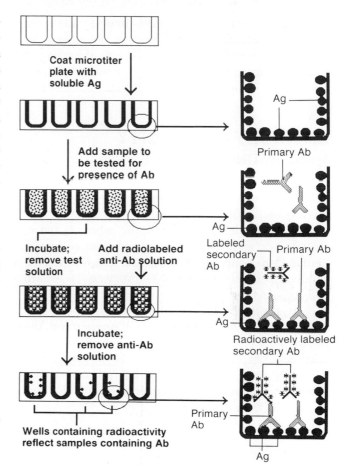

FIGURE 4.4 Solid-phase RIA. A multiwell plate is coated with Ag. Samples being assessed for human Ab are added to each well and incubated. If Ab is present, it becomes bound to the Ag. The plate is washed, and radiolabeled anti-human Ig is added to each well. If the specific primary Ab is present in the well, the radiolabeled secondary Ab (an anti-Ab) will become bound. The solid-phase "hot sandwich" consisting of (1) Ag, (2) specific Ab, and (3) radiolabeled indicator Ab is detected when each well is monitored for radioactivity.

radioactivity bound to a standard curve for Ab of known concentration. The total amount of Ab added to each well for incubation is determined by a binding curve produced at the same time, using increasing Ag concentrations. Ab concentration is then determined as the maximum amount of Ab bound at maximum Ag concentration. A plot of bound Ab/unbound Ab versus bound Ab has a slope of $-nK$, or $-2K$ for divalent Ab.

MAbs can also be ranked simply in the order of their affinities for the same Ag. Van Heyningen and colleagues showed this by measurements of binding of constant, tracer amounts of labeled Ag with increasing dilutions of tissue culture supernatants.

ANTIBODY SPECIFICITY
Specificity Defined

The specificity of an Ab molecule refers to its ability to discriminate between the epitope that stimulated its production and other determinants. Specificity for a set of Abs may be defined as $S = k_h/k_x$, where k_h and k_x are intrinsic affinities for the homologous or immunizing ligand and the heterologous crossreacting ligands, respectively. Thus, Ab specificity can be assessed and compared by affinity measurements.

Generally, *high-affinity Abs are more specific than low-affinity Abs.* An Ab reacts more effectively with the homologous epitope that stimulated its formation than with other heterologous epitopes. However, on rare occasions, an Ab induced by one determinant interacts more strongly with a different determinant. This type of Ab is called a *heteroclitic Ab.*

Crossreactivity

A specific polyclonal antiserum might contain a collection of specific Abs directed against different determinants (and different parts of identical determinants) of an immunizing Ag. Thus, the specificity of the antiserum, reflecting a variety of affinities, refers to the potential binding capability of all the various Abs directed against the Ag. Some Abs engendered against one Ag can **crossreact** with a different Ag, for a number of reasons. For example, they might crossreact if the two different Ags share one or more common epitopes (fig. 4.5) In this regard, immunization with Jenner's smallpox vaccine, containing cowpox (vaccinia virus) Ags, gave protection against smallpox caused by variola virus. The collection of Abs engendered against vaccinia virus contained some Abs capable of reacting with variola Ags, suggesting that two (or more) different viral Ags shared some common determinants.

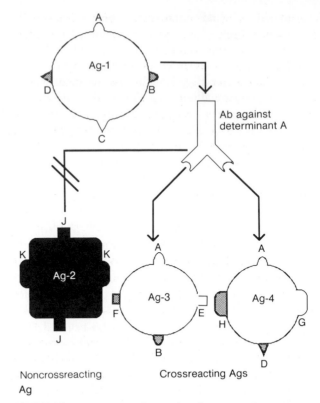

FIGURE 4.5 Crossreactions due to shared antigenic determinants. In this example, Ag-1 stimulates Ab populations versus determinants A, B, C, and D. Some anti-Ag-1 Abs crossreact with Ag-3 and Ag-4 since each possesses determinant A. This population of Abs does not crossreact with Ag-2 since the A determinant is absent.

In 1959 Talmage proposed that polyclonal antiserum generated against a single antigenic determinant would contain a mixture of Abs, with a broad range of specificities. Experimental support for Talmage's hypothesis was obtained in the 1970s. Consequently, the concept of absolute specificity and the strict lock-and-key model for Ag-Ab interaction was modified. Clearly, a particular antigenic determinant might interact with a number of structurally similar binding sites, displayed by different Abs. Moreover, it might react more strongly with some than with others.

Conceivably, some Abs would possess higher intrinsic affinities for the determinant, involving many contact points. On the other hand, weakly crossreacting, or low-affinity Ab, might have only one contact point with the antigenic determinant and be considered essentially nonspecific. Contact points infer hydrogen bonding, hydrophobic bonding, ionic interactions, or combinations of the three between the determinant and the sites within the binding pocket of the Ab. Furthermore, a single Ab-binding pocket might crossreact, with varying degrees of affinity, with a spectrum of related antigenic determinants. In some instances, an Ab-binding site may even crossreact with diverse antigenic determinants (see below).

Are MAbs, serving as Ag receptors on B lymphocyte clones or as secreted products of plasma cell clones, monospecific or multispecific? In the preceding chapter, predetermined Ig receptors were said to be monospecific and, as such, fundamental to the concept of clonal selection. MAbs are, with exceptions, structurally identical and, therefore, possess identical, not merely similar, binding sites and idiotypes. A clone of B lymphocytes produces Ig receptors of one structurally specific kind, and a plasma cell clone produces only one structurally specific kind of Ab. A lymphocyte does not produce diverse or pluripotent Ab molecules. Each MAb molecule exhibits a defined and reproducible intrinsic affinity or singular level of specificity for a homologous ligand. In this sense, MAb might be considered monospecific. On the other hand, MAb may crossreact with several antigenic determinants, albeit with lower affinity. Although specificity for the homologous ligand may be singularly expressed (as $S = k_h/k_x$) the binding site does exhibit limited multispecificity.

Types of Specificity

Specific Ab can distinguish small differences in structure, charge, optical configuration, and conformation of an epitope (see chapter 3, Effectors of Humoral Immunity). By attaching known chemicals to protein carrier molecules, it became possible to stimulate immune responses to well-defined chemical groups, known as haptens. A hapten is a "shelf" chemical that serves as a well-defined antigenic determinant. A comparison of the binding of structurally related haptens appears in figure 4.6.

Other early studies by Landsteiner compared the effect of the chemical nature and configuration of the ligand on the reaction with Ab (fig. 4.7). The importance of the three-dimensional shape of the determinant group appears more significant for Ab recognition than the chemical structure of the ligand in this instance. In 1975 Richards showed that two structurally diverse haptens, 2,4-dinitrophenyl-L-lysine and methylnaphthoquinone, could bind to a myeloma Ig, but with very low affinity. *A single Ab-combining site may possess two separate complementarity locations within the binding pocket,* permitting binding to two different haptens, but to only one at a time. The reacting Ab, in this case, offers only one contact point for either of the haptens, accounting for the low affinity. Another epitope might make three contact points with the Ab (and would have a high affinity).

Antigenicity of protein Ags is strongly dependent on protein conformation. Protein folding brings some amino acids closer together, permitting unique surface exposure, while masking others that might otherwise serve as antigenic determinants. Many proteins consist of several equal or unequal polypeptide chains. Hemoglobin, for example, consists of two pairs of similar polypeptide chains (α and β). Abs against isolated chains are specific for the corresponding polypeptide chains. However, the native tetrameric molecule contains conformational determinants, which are not found on isolated chains. Amino acids, which may be far apart in an isolated chain, may become close together, providing a new antigenic determinant, in a folded molecule. Furthermore, both the Ab and a flexible Ag may be able to induce conformational alterations, optimal for binding. The tertiary conformation is a very stable form of the molecule. For example, if strong acids or bases, or heat, destroy secondary and tertiary structures, unfolding of polypeptide chains occurs and conformational determinants are lost.

DETECTION AND MEASUREMENT OF ANTIGEN-ANTIBODY INTERACTIONS

Ags, or Abs, can be specifically detected and quantified using whichever component is known to identify the other component. Thus, if we wished to detect an Ag

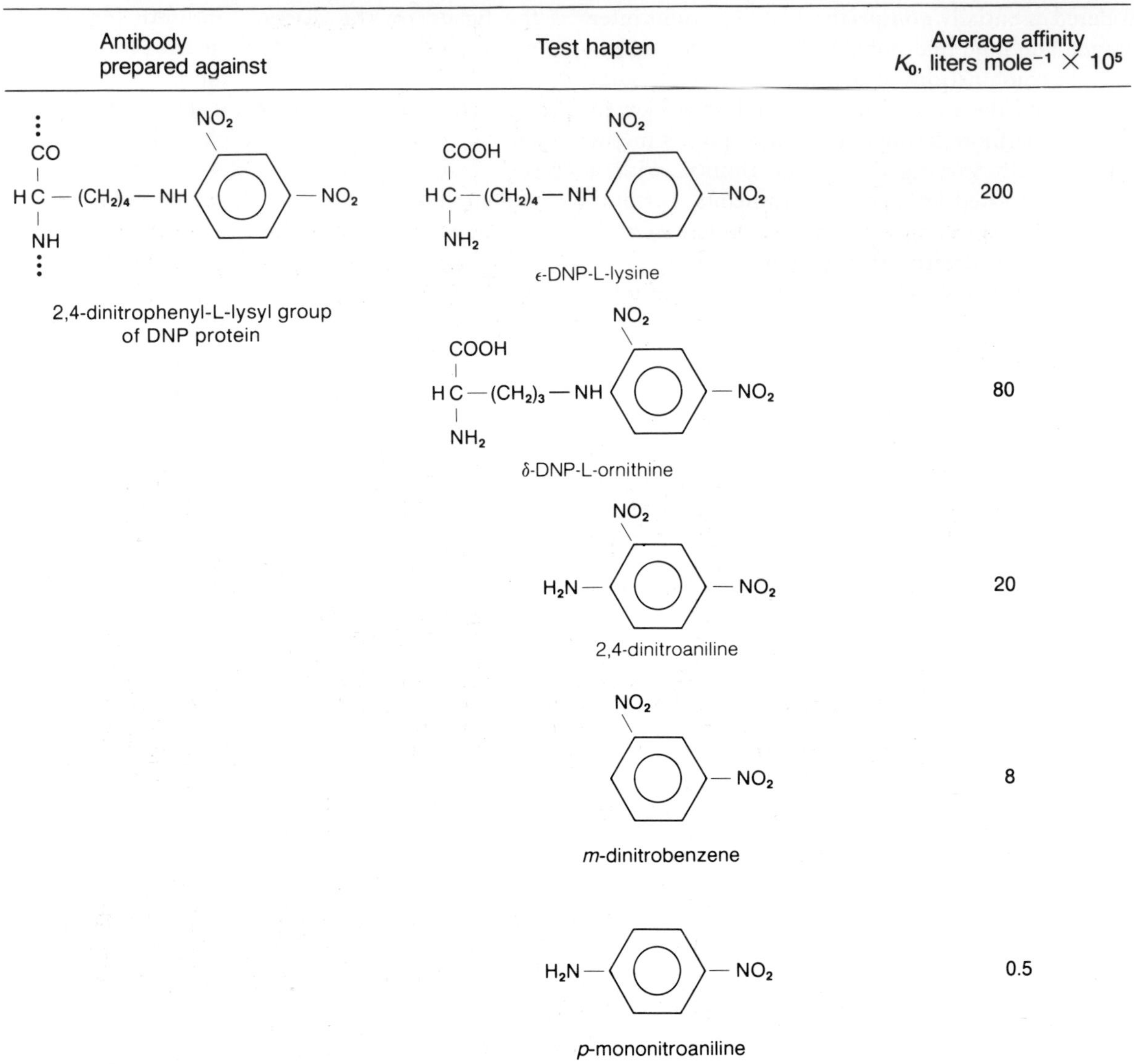

Antibody prepared against	Test hapten	Average affinity K_0, liters mole^{-1} $\times$ 10^5
2,4-dinitrophenyl-L-lysyl group of DNP protein	ε-DNP-L-lysine	200
	δ-DNP-L-ornithine	80
	2,4-dinitroaniline	20
	m-dinitrobenzene	8
	p-mononitroaniline	0.5

FIGURE 4.6 Binding of structurally related haptens. Abs generated against an immunizing hapten bind more strongly to haptenic groups that most resemble the immunogen DNP, dinitrophenyl. (From Eisen, H. N. *Immunology*. Harper & Row Publishers, Inc., Hagerstown, Md., 1980. Original data from Eisen, H. N., and Siskind, G. W. Variation in affinity of antibodies during the immune response. *Biochemistry* **3**:996, 1964.)

(e.g., bacterial, viral, protozoan, helminthic, and cancer Ags, or hormones, drugs, and allergens) an Ab must be known; whereas; if we wished to detect Abs (against any of the Ag examples cited) the Ag must be known. Based on the ability of Abs and Ags to form specific immune complexes, a known Ab or Ag can be used to detect the unknown component. In addition, the composition, quantity, and rate of formation of Ag-Ab complexes can be evaluated. In this section, we examine some methods for detecting and quantifying Ags or Abs.

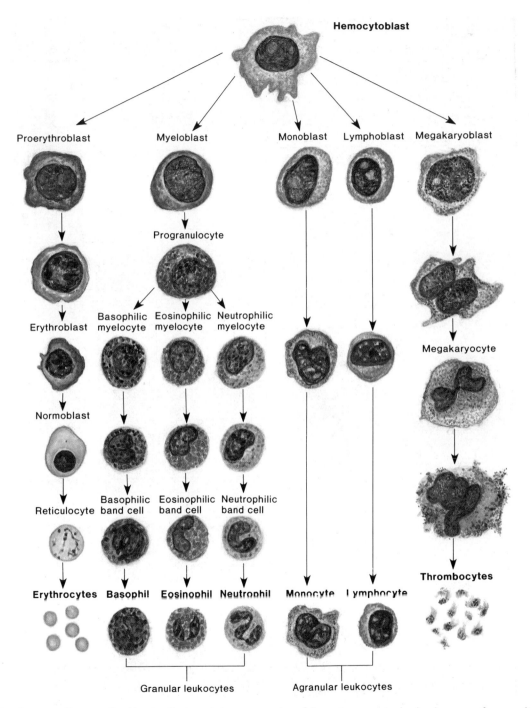

PLATE 1 Development of mammalian blood cells. An artist's representation of the major stages in the development of mammalian erthy-rocytes, leukocytes, and platelets from a hemocytoblast, or stem cell. Refer to Chapter 2 for a discussion of hemopoiesis. (From John W. Hole, Jr., *Human Anatomy and Physiology,* 4th ed. Copyright © 1987 Wm. C. Brown Publishers, Dubuque, Iowa. All Rights Reserved. Reprinted by permission.)

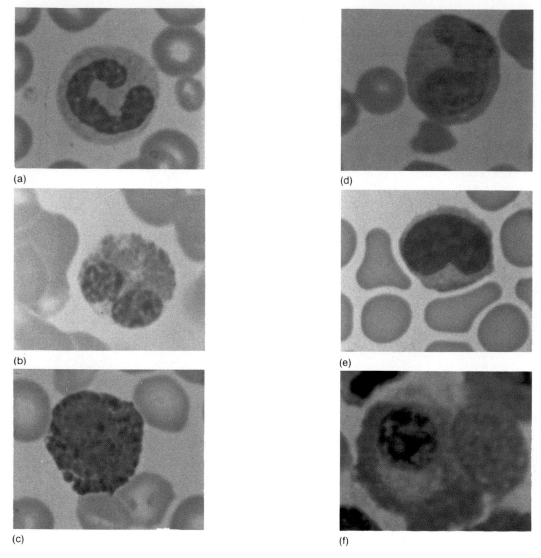

(a)

(b)

(c)

(d)

(e)

(f)

PLATE 2 (*a*) Neutrophil. Note the lightly staining cytoplasm and the narrow, constricted nucleus. Contrast the absence of specific granules in the cytoplasm with *b* and *c*. Contrast the cytoplasmic and nuclear characteristics with those of the monocyte in figure *d*. (*b*) Eosinophil. Note the presence of prominent acidophilic (eosinophilic) specific granules in the cytoplasm. Contrast this with *a* and *c*. (*c*) Basophil. Note the presence of prominent basophilic granules in the cytoplasm. Contrast this with *a* and *b*. (*d*) Monocyte. This large leukocyte can resemble the neutrophil to the untrained observer. Note the grayish-blue cytoplasm and the broad nucleus. Contrast these with the light cytoplasm and narrow nucleus of *a*. (*e*) Lymphocyte. This cell is characterized by a high nuclear to cytoplasmic ratio. This example reveals a substantial amount of cytoplasm and an indented nucleus. However, a full round nucleus with a thin halo of cytoplasm is not an uncommon feature for this cell. (*f*) Plasma cell. This antibody-producing cell is characterized by three distinctive features: (1) a nucleus with substantial heterochromatin (denoted by *darkly stained areas*), (2) a deeply basophilic (bluish) cytoplasm reflecting active protein synthesis; and (3) a distinctive perinuclear "clear zone," which is created by the Golgi complex actively engaged in preparing immunoglobulin (Ig) for secretion. Contrast this appearance with that of the more quiescent circulating lymphocyte in *e*. (Plates *a–f*: Photomicrographs of cells stained with Wright's stain. Plates *a–e* are of cells in peripheral blood; plate *f* is of cells in bone marrow.) (From Hyun, B. H., Ashton, J. K., and Dolan, K. *Practical Hematology.* 1975. W. B. Saunders Co., Philadelphia.)

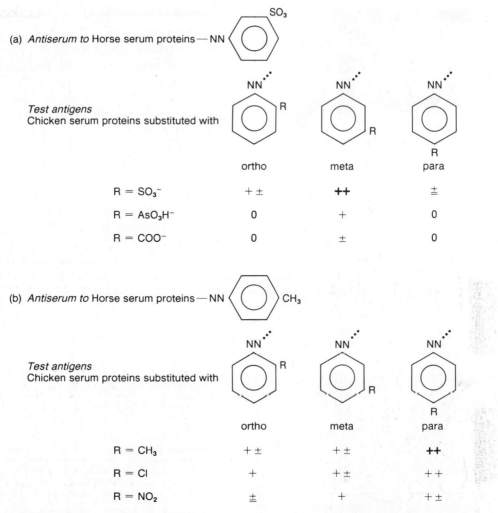

FIGURE 4.7 Effect of position and nature of chemical substituents of haptenic groups on the reaction with Abs. (*a*) Prominent effect of position and nature of acidic substituents of haptenic groups on the reaction between Abs to *m*-azobenzenesulfonate and test Ags. *R* in the test Ag refers to the acidic substituents SO_3^-, AsO_3H^-, and COO^-. The homologous reaction is most intense and shown in bold type. (From Eisen, H. N. *Immunology.* Harper & Row Publishers, Inc., Hagerstown, Md., 1980. Original data from Landsteiner, K., and van der Scheer, J. On cross reactions of immune sera to azoproteins.

Journal of Experimental Medicine **63**:325, 1936.) (*b*) Effect of nature and position of uncharged substituents of haptenic groups on the reactions of Abs generated against the *p*-azotoluidine group and test Ags. *R* in the test Ag refers to uncharged substituents CH_3, Cl, and NO_2. The homologous reaction is shown in bold type. (From Eisen, H. N. *Immunology.* Harper & Row Publishers, Inc., Hagerstown, Md., 1980. Original data from Landsteiner, K., and van der Scheer, J. On the influence of acid groups on the serological specificity of azoproteins. *Journal of Experimental Medicine* **45**:1045, 1927.)

Precipitin Reaction

Interaction between soluble Ag and Ab molecules can produce an insoluble precipitate. For this to occur, the Ag must possess more than one determinant and the Ab must be, at least, divalent (i.e., possess two combining sites). Ags and Abs are able to link together and form a "lattice" (fig. 4.8). If the Abs are monoclonal, rather than polyclonal, *Ag must possess more than one identical determinant* for precipitation to occur. Precipitation reactions are evaluated either qualitatively or quantitatively and are carried out in solution or in semisolid media (gels).

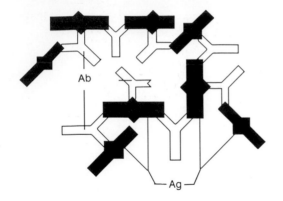

FIGURE 4.8 Ab-Ag crosslinking in a lattice.

Precipitation in Liquids

A rather simple way of detecting and measuring specific polyclonal Abs was described as a quantitative precipitin reaction over 50 years ago by Michael Heidelberger. In this assay, a small volume of soluble Ag, of known concentration, is mixed with homologous antiserum. If Abs are present, a precipitate may form at the interface. This is first seen as a ring. Within a short period of time, a precipitate may settle to the bottom of the tube. If increasing amounts of Ag are allowed to react with a constant amount of antiserum, varying amounts of precipitate form and can be measured. The Ab concentration and molar ratios of the Ab/Ag in the precipitates can be determined (table 4.2; fig. 4.9).

TABLE 4.2 Sample Results from a Hypothetical Precipitin Assay

Part I—Raw Data

Tube Number	Amount of Antiserum Added (ml)	Amount of Ag Added (mg)	Total Quantity of Protein Precipitated (mg)	Amount of Ab Precipitated* (mg)	Results of Assay of Supernatant
1	1.0	0.050	1.975	1.925	Excess Ab
2	1.0	0.100	2.925	2.825	Excess Ab
3	1.0	0.500	3.950	3.450	No Ab; no Ag
4	1.0	0.600	4.125	3.525	No Ab; trace Ag
5	1.0	1.000	3.900	2.900	Excess Ag
6	1.0	2.000	1.800	Cannot be determined	Excess Ag

Part II—Ratio of Ab to Ag in Precipitate

Tube Number	Weight Ratio[†]	Molar Ratio[‡]
1	38.5	7.7
2	28.25	5.65
3	6.9	2.38
4	(5.87)[§]	(1.18)[§]
5	(2.9)[§]	(0.58)[§]
6	Cannot be determined	Cannot be determined

*Amount of Ab precipitated = (total protein precipitated) − (amount of Ag added).

[†]Weight ratio = (amount of Ab precipitated)/(amount of Ag added).

[‡]Molar ratio = (weight ratio)/(MW of Ab/MW of Ag); for this example: MW of Ab = 150 kD, MW of Ag = 30 kD.

[§]Ratio is estimated only, since there is excess Ag in supernatant.

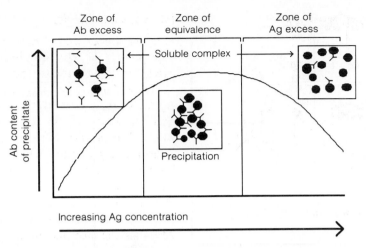

FIGURE 4.9 Precipitin curve. On the ascending curve, or Ab excess zone, the supernatants contain decreasing amounts of free Ab as the equivalence zone is approached. At equivalence (ideally) the supernatants are free of Ab and Ag molecules. Thus, the amount of Ab in the precipitate represents the amount of Ab in the sample being tested. In Ag excess, increasing amounts of free Ag become detectable in the supernatants. Soluble complexes occur in the supernatants in both Ab and Ag excess zones.

In the *equivalence zone,* precipitate is maximum, since the ratio of Ag to Ab is optimal. In tubes where excess Ab is present, there is less precipitate. Moreover, free Ab is still present in the supernatant fluid. When Ag is added in excess, little precipitate forms, although soluble immune complexes and free Ag are present in the supernatant fluid. Obviously, in reactions where there is either Ab or Ag excess, crosslinking is impaired and the formation of heavy complexes is reduced. Thus, it is important to note that critical concentrations of Ag must be added for maximum precipitation of serum Ab.

If immune complexes form in serum, monocytes, neutrophils, and eosinophils attempt to remove them. Complexes formed at equivalence (or in Ab excess) are easily removed. However, small, soluble complexes formed in Ag excess (often with low-affinity Abs) are more difficult to remove. These might gain entrance to tissues, such as the glomeruli of the kidney, or become deposited within vessel walls, causing varying degrees of damage.

Precipitation in Gels

A qualitative (or semiquantitative), double-immunodiffusion assay was developed and introduced by **Ouchterlony** of Sweden. It is based on the diffusion of Ag and Ab molecules through a semisolid gel (e.g., agar) to form precipitates that can be analyzed. A gel-coated petri plate or slide is normally used with wells cut out for Ag and Ab reactants. A large number of geometric arrangements are possible. Some of the simpler forms are depicted in figure 4.10.

Once deposited in wells, Ag and Abs diffuse in all directions, at their own rates, in accordance with their size and shape. When equivalent, or optimal, proportions of Ag and Ab molecules meet, complexes link and form a visible precipitin band. If the concentration of introduced Ab or Ag is in relative excess, the band forms closer to the other well, where the reactants reach equivalence. This technique is very useful for detecting and comparing Ags that may be identical, crossreactive, or nonidentical. Since specific proteins are encoded by specific genes, a comparative study of protein Ags may be used to study genetic relationships.

Single radial immunodiffusion is a simple, quantitative procedure that was developed by Mancini and introduced in 1965. It has been widely adopted for measurement of many Ags present in diverse biologic fluids, including serum Igs. The moderate sensitivity of the method falls in the range of 1 to 3 μg/mL of a protein Ag. In this technique, an Ag is deposited in a well and allowed to diffuse into a gel containing uniformly dispersed specific Abs. As a zone of equivalence

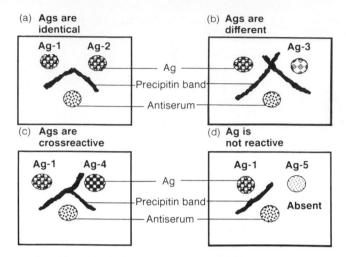

FIGURE 4.10 Ouchterlony technique: double diffusion in gels. In (*a*) the antiserum engendered versus Ag-1 also reacts with test Ag-2 to form a visible precipitin band, at equivalence. This forms a **chevron of identity.** In (*b*) Ag-1 and Ag-3 are compared versus homologous antiserum and a **pattern of nonidentity,** in the form of crossing precipitin bands, indicates that the Ags are different. In (*c*) the antiserum engendered versus Ag-1 is compared with test Ag-4, yielding a pattern of partial identity. This suggests that Ag-4 shares some common antigenic determinants with Ag-1. In (*d*) antiserum versus Ag-1 does not react with Ag-5.

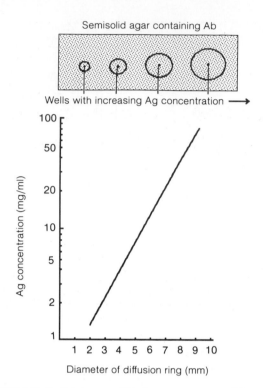

FIGURE 4.11 Radial immunodiffusion measurement of Ag. Standard preparations of increasing concentrations of Ag are placed in wells that have been cut in agar containing dispersed specific Ab (*top panel*). The Ag molecules diffuse into the gel and form a visible precipitin ring, at equivalence. The more concentrated the Ag, the greater the distance the molecules must travel to reach equivalence. The diameter of the diffusion ring is plotted versus the Ag concentration to establish a standard curve. Samples being tested for Ag are then compared.

is established, a ring of precipitate forms around the well. The area, or the diameter, of the ring is proportional to the initial concentration of the Ag placed in the well. From results obtained with known concentrations of Ag, a calibration curve is constructed, permitting quantitation of an unknown Ag (fig. 4.11).

By combining electrophoresis and immune precipitation in gels, Grabar and Williams developed *immunoelectrophoresis,* an ingenious method for analyzing complex Ags in biological fluids. In this powerful technique, a glass slide is covered with molten agar or agarose. Two Ag wells with an Ab trough in between can be cut (other patterns are often employed) with a template. Ag (protein) mixtures for comparison (e.g., serum samples) are then placed in the wells and separated in an electric field over a period of time (perhaps an hour). The electric gradient is discontinued and antiserum is placed in the trough, which parallels the axis of electrophoretic migration. The Abs and Ags diffuse toward each other, and distinct precipitin bands are completely formed where they intersect (at equivalence), within 18 to 24 hours. The middle of each

precipitin band or arc lies nearer the trough than either end, since a greater concentration of protein occurs at the center of each separated antigen "spot." With more Ag available centrally, more Ab is required and precipitation occurs proximal to the trough. The front and tail of the band curves where the Ag concentration is lower, since Ab must diffuse further into the gel to reach equivalence. Separation of serum proteins (Ags) and their reaction with antiserum is represented in figure 4.12. This technique has been useful in comparing proteins in biological fluids from normal and diseased individuals.

In *electroimmunodiffusion* techniques, Ag and Ab reactants are electrically driven together in a gel, rather than simply allowed to come in contact by diffusion.

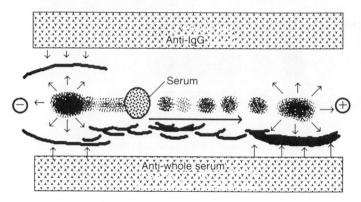

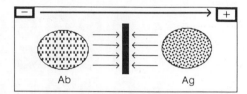

FIGURE 4.13 Double electroimmunodiffusion. Ag and Ab are electrophoresed from separate wells into a gel, under conditions that permit migration in opposite directions (countercurrent immunoelectrophoresis). Precipitin bands may form within minutes.

FIGURE 4.12 Immunoelectrophoresis. A thin layer of agar gel is applied to a slide and a small well cut near the center. Serum is added to the well and electrophoresed to separate serum proteins. (Direction of migration in the electric field is designated by the *bold arrow.*) Antiserum is added to the lower trough and anti-IgG (H chain–specific) Abs to the upper trough. Abs in the troughs diffuse into the agar and encounter diffusing Ags (serum proteins), forming precipitin arcs. (Diffusion is indicated by the *thin arrows.*) Note that IgG migrates more slowly, and albumin more rapidly, than the other serum proteins.

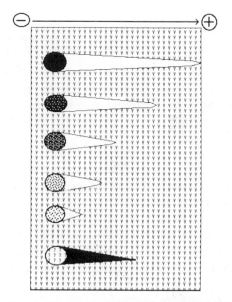

FIGURE 4.14 Rocket immunoelectrophoresis. Ag is placed in a well and electrophoresed into a gel containing Ab. Precipitin patterns resemble rockets since precipitation occurs along the moving boundary of the Ag. The concentration of Ag is proportional to rocket length, or the area under the curve. A standard curve can be made (*white rockets*) for determining concentration of sample Ag (*black rocket*).

Double electroimmunodiffusion involves electrophoresis of both Ab and Ag in a semisolid medium, so that they migrate toward each other. Precipitation occurs at a point intermediate between their origins (fig. 4.13). Results can be obtained in minutes, not hours, and the technique is much more sensitive than simple immunodiffusion. This method is also known as countercurrent immunoelectrophoresis.

Single electroimmunodiffusion, or rocket immunoelectrophoresis, involves electrophoresis of Ag into an agarose gel containing dispersed Ab that does not migrate. The pattern of immunoprecipitation resembles a rocket, since precipitation occurs along the moving boundary of Ag, as it migrates into the agarose (fig. 4.14). The height of the rocket (or the area under the curve), for a given antiserum concentration, is linearly proportionate to the Ag concentration. Thus, the total distance of unknown Ag migration may be evaluated by comparison with known standards.

Immunobeads: Solid-Phase Interactions

A system in which Ab is bound to a solid matrix (solid-phase) can be used as an alternative to presenting Ab in soluble form. One popular solid-phase method makes use of purified Ab (or MAb) covalently bound to polyacrylamide beads, which are often referred to as immunobeads. The polyacrylamide beads provide an inert matrix to which Abs are attached. Thus, the beads provide increased reaction surface area. In addition, the outward orientation of Ab ensures that reactions with Ag occur on the surface of the beads. Two applications of this method are (1) as a reagent in precipitation reactions and (2) as a means of cell identification.

When used as a reagent in precipitation reactions, immunobeads are added as a secondary Ab. Following interaction between Ag and the primary Ab,

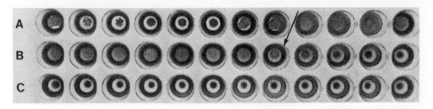

FIGURE 4.15 Indirect (passive) hemagglutination. Soluble Ag is passively adsorbed to red blood cells. Ab is serially diluted and allowed to react with a defined number of Ag-coated erythrocytes that have been placed in each microwell. The reciprocal of the highest Ab dilution to give a visible agglutination reaction is known as the titer. Agglutination may not occur, or occur minimally (as in the precipitin reaction), if Ab is in excess. This is known as the prozone effect. Wells in which agglutination has occurred contain a mat, or sheet, of cells over much of the bottom of the well. Negative reactions are seen as discrete, solid discs of red cells in the bottom of the wells. In row *A*, wells 7 to 12 (*right half*) are positive. Similarly, row *B* is positive to well eight (*designated by arrow*), while wells 9 to 12 are negative. All of the control wells (*row C*) are also negative. The first six wells in row *A* (*left half*) show the prozone effect. (From Virella, G., et al. *Introduction to Medical Immunology*. Marcel Dekker, Inc., New York, 1986.)

immunobeads (with Abs against the primary Ab) couple to the existing Ab-Ag complex, generating a precipitin reaction. Products of this reaction can be recovered by centrifugation.

Cell identification can be achieved using immunobeads carrying Ab against specific markers on the cell type of interest. Reaction between Ab on the immunobeads and surface Ag on the cells leads to rosette formation. These rosettes enable cells expressing markers for which the Ab has specificity to be identified. For example, immunobeads carrying Ab against surface Ig facilitate identification of mature B cells.

Agglutination Reactions
Direct Agglutination

Cells displaying surface Ags can clump or agglutinate when mixed with their antisera. Direct agglutination provides a simple and rapid method for identifying cells if known Abs are available, or of detecting and measuring Abs if known cells are available. The agglutination reaction can be used as a semiquantitative assay. A given number of cells are added to a series of tubes, each containing the same volume of antiserum, at different dilutions. Over time, clumping is observed and the relative strength of an antiserum is expressed as the reciprocal of the highest dilution that causes agglutination. This is known as the agglutination titer of the antiserum. It is indicative of the relative Ab concentration. False-negative agglutination reactions can occur with some antisera in Ab excess (first few dilutions). This is known as the prozone phenomenon. Unagglutinated cells in the prozone actually have Ab molecules

adsorbed on their surfaces, with both sites of bivalent Ab attached to the same cell. At high concentrations of Ab, there may be poor lattice formation and steric hindrance, as observed in the precipitin reaction.

Indirect Agglutination

In direct agglutination, the functional Ags are natural components of the cell wall (bacteria) or cell suface membrane. The same reaction can be extended to a wide variety of soluble Ags by attaching them to the surface of a cell or particle. Red blood cells, and synthetic polymers, are widely used for indirect, or passive, agglutination.

Red blood cells can be treated with formalin or glutaraldehyde and stored for prolonged periods. Coupling techniques for attaching Ag to the particles depend on adsorption by noncovalent bonds. Treatment of red cells with tannic acid, for example, permits a high density of coating protein to be adsorbed. This greatly increases the sensitivity of the agglutination reaction, so that minimal concentration of 0.01 μg of Ab/mL is detectable. Figure 4.15 depicts an indirect agglutination reaction carried out in microwells.

Latex particles have also been used widely as passive carriers for adsorbed carbohydrate or soluble protein Ags. *Latex fixation* (agglutination) tests, for example, have been employed to detect rheumatoid factors in persons with rheumatoid arthritis. (Rheumatoid factor is an auto-Ab [more often 19S IgM but may also be 7S IgM, IgG, or IgA] directed against self-IgG [Fc region].) Human IgG is adsorbed to latex particles, and the particles are then allowed to react with serum samples and appropriate controls. If auto-Abs (rheumatoid

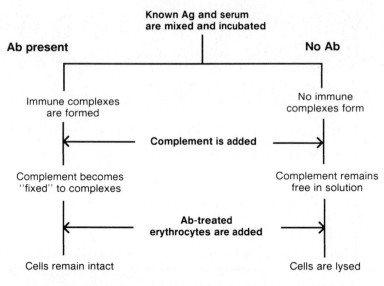

Known Ag and serum
are mixed and incubated

Ab present | | **No Ab**

Immune complexes
are formed

No immune
complexes form

Complement is added

Complement becomes
"fixed" to complexes

Complement remains
free in solution

**Ab-treated
erythrocytes are added**

Cells remain intact

Cells are lysed

Interpretation of results

Positive complement fixation

Fixation of complement by immune
complexes, when Ab is present
removes it from solution.
Complement is, therefore, not available
to bind to Abs on treated cells in
final incubation.

Negative complement fixation

Lysis of Ab-treated cells in
final incubation indicates that
complement was available.
This means that serum sample
used in first incubation
did not have Ab.

FIGURE 4.16 Complement fixation test. In this example, a known Ag is being used to detect Abs in a serum sample. The test is based on the fixation of complement, if the Ab is present, and the lack of fixation, if the Ab is absent. An indicator system is used to determine whether complement fixation has occurred.

factors) are present, they react with IgG determinants on the latex particles and agglutinate or "fix" them.

Complement Assays

The complement system consists of at least 20 immunologically distinct plasma proteins, capable of reacting with each other and with Ab (see chapter 6, Complement and its Role in Immune Responses). Complement may be bound or fixed to certain Abs complexed with Ag (either free or membrane bound). The amount of complement bound is proportional to the concentration of Ab present. Following activation (fixation) on the surface of certain cells, bacteria or viruses, a series of interactions can lead to a range of biological activity including lysis. *Complement-mediated lysis* of target cells may be measured in a variety of ways. Lysis can be followed by monitoring the release of cell components (such as hemoglobin from red cells) or the

loss of membrane integrity by failure of cells to exclude vital dyes. A number of Ag-Ab assays involve complement fixation and/or lysis. Two examples follow.

Complement Fixation Test

Any complex of a complement-activating Ab with soluble Ag can be assayed by complement fixation. It is a sensitive technique that has been widely used to detect Abs, for both research and clinical laboratory diagnosis. In this assay, a fixed amount of the test Ag is incubated with a series of serum samples at varying dilutions. Limiting amounts of complement are then added. If Ab is present in the serum samples, immune complexes form and "consume" complement. The mixture is then added to a suspension of Ab-treated red blood cells, which are observed for lysis, evidenced by the release of hemoglobin (fig. 4.16). This assay is based

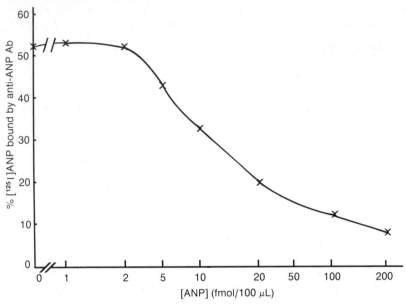

FIGURE 4.17 RIA standard curve. Increasing concentrations of unlabeled Ag (e.g., the cardiac hormone, atrial natriuretic peptide [ANP]) are added to tubes containing fixed quantities of ^{125} I-labeled Ag (*Ag) and specific Abs. The amount of *Ag bound to Ab, at various concentrations of unlabeled Ag, is determined and plotted to establish a standard curve. Part of the curve is linear and can be used to determine the Ag in samples.

on the principle that complement that has been fixed in one Ag-Ab reaction is unavailable for a second Ag-Ab reaction. Reduced red blood cell lysis indicates the presence of specific Ab in the samples. Ab concentrations in unknown samples can be determined by comparison with an appropriate standard curve using known Ab.

Complement-Mediated Lysis

Cytolysis mediated by complement can be used as an assay for Abs that have become bound to specific Ags on the surface of target cells. Only Abs of the complement-activating classes (IgM and most IgG subclasses) are detectable. Serum samples (of several dilutions) to be tested for Ab are incubated with a fixed number of target cells displaying that Ag. For example, we could assay for Ab against major histocompatibility complex (MHC) alloantigen on lymphocytes. Complement is then added, and cell lysis is measured by observing the percentage of lymphocytes that take up a vital dye, such as trypan blue. The degree of lysis is a function of the Ab's concentration, if Ab is limiting.

Radioimmunoassay

RIA techniques are highly specific and can measure Ags at picogram (10^{-12} gm) levels. They have been used to measure a variety of serum proteins (including Igs), hormones, drugs, and any other compound to which an Ab can be produced. This remarkable methodological breakthrough was introduced by **Berson** and **Yalow** in 1960, and recognized with the award of a Nobel Prize to Yalow some years after Berson's death.

The general technique is based on the competition of radiolabeled, known Ag and unlabeled, unknown Ag for specific Ab in solution or attached to a plate or tube (solid phase). To establish an assay, Ab must be produced to the known Ag and the Ag radiolabeled [*Ag] (e.g., with ^{125}I). A standard curve is established by adding fixed amounts of *Ag, specific Ab, and increasing concentrations of known unlabeled Ag to a series of tubes, or wells, in a plastic microtiter plate. Following incubation, the amount of *Ag bound to Ab is determined, after separation from free *Ag, in a gamma spectrometer. The standard, or calibration, curve is the graphic representation of the amount of bound *Ag plotted as a function of various known Ag concentrations (fig. 4.17). If a serum sample being

Origins of Radioimmunoassays

Measurements of the concentrations of many bioactive substances, such as hormones, are routinely accomplished by means of RIAs. These assays are performed fairly rapidly; they require only small amounts of sample, and large numbers of samples can be evaluated simultaneously. However, this was not always the case.

Interest in measuring the levels of biologically relevant substances has a long history. For substances that are present in milligram quantities, or greater, numerous chemical and biochemical techniques have been available. However, for substances present in the submilligram range, techniques have been limited. This is the case for many regulatory substances.

As recently as the early 1960s, bioassays were the method of choice and, in some instances, the only method available for assessing the concentration of many hormones, neurotransmitters, and other significant biologically active substances. Bioassays can be extremely sensitive. However, they require a biological test system and inherently are difficult to calibrate. Moreover, they are cumbersome to perform.

The development of RIAs, and their subsequent exploitation for a wide range of applications, arose as an attempt to test a hypothesis concerning insulin degradation in maturity-onset diabetes and not as an attempt to generate a more sensitive tool for measuring insulin itself.

While attempting to study the metabolism of radioactively labeled insulin, Berson, Yalow, and their colleagues noted a curious phenomenon. Individuals who had received insulin treatment, for a variety of reasons, displayed slower disappearance of the labeled insulin than did persons who had not been exposed to insulin injections. They considered that this was the result of binding of the injected insulin to Abs produced by prior exposure to insulin. They subsequently developed highly sensitive radioisotopic techniques to detect the insulin-Ab complexes. The culmination of their effort was the development of the RIA.

In retrospect, it seems surprising that the original attempts to publish the results of the pioneering RIA experiments met with skepticism and resistance from immunologists. Nevertheless, the validity and value of RIAs has ben more than amply demonstrated since that time, as evidenced by the extensive dependence upon this technique in both clinical and research laboratories. In addition, the scientific community expressed its appreciation and acknowledged Rosalyn Yalow's contribution in the development of this powerful tool by awarding her the Nobel Prize in 1977.

Yalow, R. S. Radioimmunoassay, a probe for the fine structure of biological systems. *Science* **200**:1236, 1978.

---

tested contains specific Ag for the Ab, then there is competition with *Ag. This appears as reduction in the amount of *Ag bound in the complex. Accordingly, the concentration of Ag in the sample can be determined from the standard curve.

Enzyme-Linked Immunoassay

Enzyme assays are similar to radioimmunoassays, in principle, and are almost as sensitive. However, they employ an enzyme rather than a radioactive label.

Enzyme immunoassays have become very popular in view of their high sensitivity, safety, economy, and the simple instrumentation requirements. One of the more widely used enzyme immunoassays is known as the *enzyme-linked immunosorbent assay (ELISA)*. In this assay, enzyme can be covalently linked to either Ab or Ag. The ELISA can be used to detect and determine concentrations of Ag or Ab (fig. 4.18).

To measure Ab in a human serum sample, for example, a known specific Ag is adsorbed or fixed to wells in a plate (solid phase). Ab standards, controls,

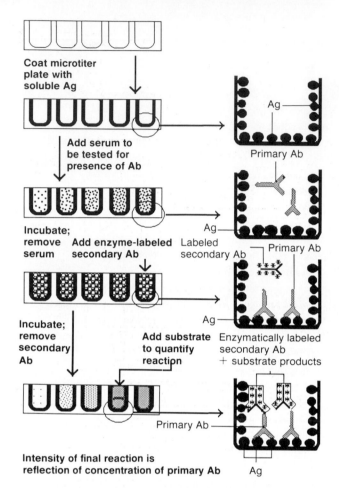

Coat microtiter plate with soluble Ag

Add serum to be tested for presence of Ab

Incubate; remove serum

Add enzyme-labeled secondary Ab

Incubate; remove secondary Ab

Add substrate to quantify reaction

Intensity of final reaction is reflection of concentration of primary Ab

Ag

Primary Ab

Ag

Labeled secondary Ab

Primary Ab

Ag

Enzymatically labeled secondary Ab + substrate products

Primary Ab

Ag

FIGURE 4.18 Enzyme-linked immunosorbent assay (ELISA). Serum samples are allowed to react with Ag-coated wells. If Ab is present, it binds to the Ag. If the Ab is human, regardless of the specificity, it may be detected by Ab generated versus human Igs. The secondary Ab, which has been labeled with enzyme, is added to the wells and will bind to primary Ab, if present. A substrate is then added to detect the presence of the enzyme. The intensity of the reaction (color), and dilution scheme employed, reflect the concentration of Abs in the samples.

and samples, conceivably containing the specific primary Ab, are added. Following incubation, the plate is washed and an enzyme-labeled secondary Ab, directed against human Ig (anti-Ig), is added. The enzyme-labeled anti-Ig binds to the primary Ab, if present. An appropriate substrate can then be added, and enzyme activity (color development) can be measured (optical density) and related to the primary Ab concentration by comparison with standards.

The ELISA can also be used to determine affinity of functional Abs. This is accomplished by comparing the results of ELISA performed in the presence and absence of diethylamine. Since diethylamine inhibits binding of low-affinity Abs to Ag, the degree to which Ag binding occurs in the assay reflects the extent to which high-affinity Abs are present. The relative affinities of several subclasses of Abs for an Ag can be ranked through their performance in the presence of diethylamine.

An adaptation of the ELISA known as an *enzyme-linked immunospot (ELISpot) assay* has recently been introduced. This assay employs the same principles of the ELISA, namely the generation of an Ab-Ag complex whose presence is detected by an enzymatic product. One important application of the ELISpot assay is the detection of cells producing particular Abs or cytokines. In this application, cells are cultured in microculture wells that have been precoated with Abs against the substance of interest. After suitable culture time has elapsed, the cells are removed and the wells are washed. Next, the enzyme-linked secondary Ab is added to each well and reaction product sought. Wells in which reaction product occurs indicate wells in which cells producing the substance of interest were cultured.

Western Blotting

Proteins (Ags) can be readily separated in gels by electrophoresis or isoelectric focusing. However, characterization of the separated Ags has been more difficult. A technique known as *Western blotting* has helped resolve this problem. Western blotting is analogous to Southern blotting, for isolated DNA, and Northern blotting, for isolated RNA. In this technique, proteins that have been separated in a gel are transferred to membranes, such as nitrocellulose, by electrophoresis. The transferred Ags are then treated, or probed, with appropriate polyclonal, or monoclonal, Abs. If the primary Ab probe is capable of reacting with a separated Ag, a complex forms and becomes immobilized on the nitrocellulose membrane. A labeled secondary Ab (anti-Ig) is then applied to the membrane. The anti-Ig binds to the immobilized primary Ab, if any is present. Either radioactive or enzyme labels can be used to visualize the complexes formed. Western blot assays are used in the diagnosis of acquired immune deficiency syndrome (AIDS).

Immunofluorescence

Coons introduced fluorescent Ab techniques in the 1940s. These techniques were received with much interest and excitement. He showed that fluorescent dyes can be attached to Ab (without affecting their specificity), permitting their ready detection, when attached to an Ag associated with a cell. Immunofluorescence (IF) is now used extensively to detect cell and tissue Ags as well as Abs to cells and tissues, including autoAbs. IF is essentially a histochemical technique.

Fluorescence is the emission of light of one wavelength, while the molecule absorbs light of another wavelength, at a higher energy level. Fluorescein isothiocyanate (FITC), for example, is a commonly used fluorochrome that binds covalently to proteins (Abs). It absorbs maximally at 490 to 495 nm and emits light (green color) at 517 nm. Fluorescence can be observed in a fluorescence microscope, which contains a high intensity UV light source (mercury lamp). The microscope is fitted with excitation filters to produce a wavelength that causes fluorescence activation and barrier filters to remove interfering wavelengths of light. With an epi-illuminated system (fig. 4.19), the excitation beam is focused directly on the specimen through the objective lens. The fluorescent light emitted from the specimen is then transmitted to the eye through a dichroic mirror. Fluorescence can be combined with transmitted light for phase contrast examination of cells or tissues. In this case, a tungsten light source is added to the fluorescence microscope. This permits us to carefully discriminate between cells that are or are not fluorescing.

Basic fluorescence-staining techniques are either direct or indirect (fig. 4.20). However, modifications of these basic staining techniques have been developed. With direct IF, Abs conjugated with a fluorescent label are added directly to a frozen tissue section or viable cell preparation. If the Ag of interest is displayed in the tissues, or on the surface of certain

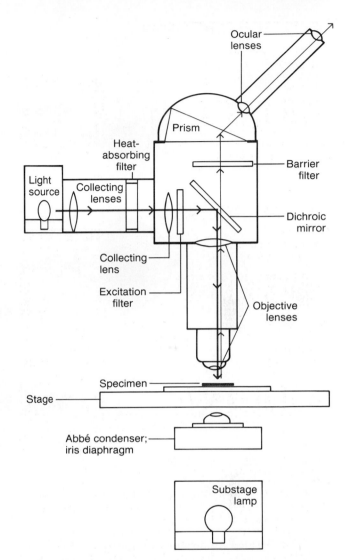

FIGURE 4.19 Fluorescence microscope. A light beam is passed through the excitation filter (producing a wavelength capable of fluorescence activation) onto the cell or tissue specimen. This is known as epi-illumination. Fluorescent light is emitted from the specimen and transmitted to the eye through the dichroic mirror. A barrier filter screens out wavelengths other than those emitted by the fluorochrome label attached to the specimen. (A fluorochrome absorbs light at one wavelength and emits light at another.) To observe clearly cells or tissues that are not fluorescing, a transmitted light source may be attached (as seen on routine microscopes).

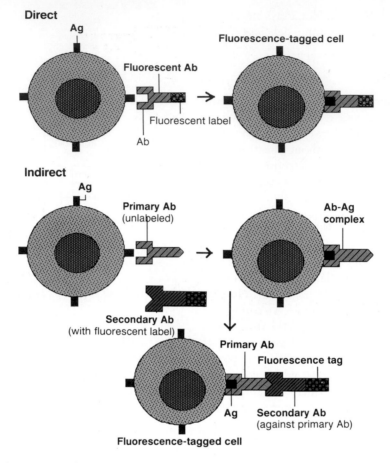

FIGURE 4.20 Direct and indirect immunofluorescence. In the top panel, Ab has been conjugated with fluorochrome and allowed to react directly with surface Ag, for visualization. In the bottom panel, specific human Ab becomes bound to surface Ag. The bound primary Ab is then detected by a fluorescent-labeled secondary Ab, which has been generated against human Ig.

cells, the labeled Ab becomes bound and can be visualized by fluorescence microscopy. All cells can be visualized, for comparison, by switching to transmitted light. In contrast, indirect IF permits detection of unlabeled primary Ab that has become bound to an Ag on a cell surface. This is accomplished by treatment with labeled secondary Ab, which is an anti-Ig that binds to the primary Ab. Indirect IF is a convenient method for detecting auto-Ab that has bound to membrane Ags *in vivo,* for example. The indirect technique can be used to evaluate an array of serum samples. It has a distinct advantage over direct IF by eliminating the need to purify and individually label each specific primary Ab population.

Biotin-Avidin Assays

Avidin is a glycoprotein derived from egg albumin, which has a very high affinity for the vitamin biotin, and does not bind to other substrates. Biotin can be easily coupled to Igs (Abs). Avidin can be labeled with fluorochromes, enzymes, or radioactive chemicals and then allowed to react with the biotin-coupled Igs. Since avidin forms strong bonds with the biotin molecules, the Ig label can be intense. If secondary Abs are labeled, using the biotin-avidin system, they can be efficiently employed in indirect IF, ELISAs, and RIAs, as described earlier.

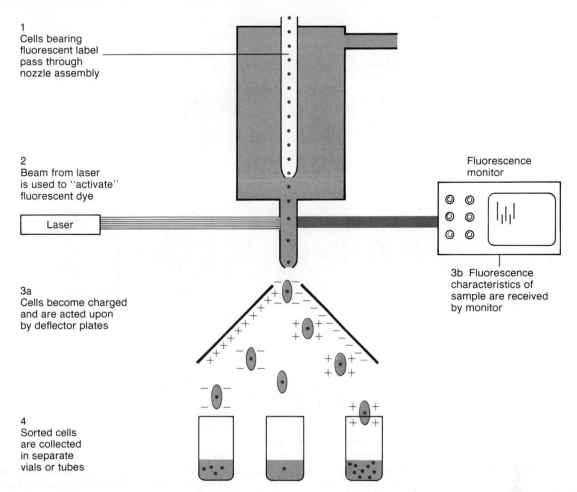

1 Cells bearing fluorescent label pass through nozzle assembly

2 Beam from laser is used to "activate" fluorescent dye

Laser

Fluorescence monitor

3b Fluorescence characteristics of sample are received by monitor

3a Cells become charged and are acted upon by deflector plates

4 Sorted cells are collected in separate vials or tubes

FIGURE 4.21 Fluorescence-activated cell sorter (FACS). A cell suspension of white blood cells is prepared and allowed to react with MAbs against a cell surface Ag, for example, CD4 molecules. The washed sample is introduced into the sample chamber and the cells are sorted and isolated as in steps 1 to 4. See plate 3 for examples of distribution profiles generated by a FACS.

Immunophotoelectron Assay

Abs may be labeled with electron-dense molecules for the detection of Ags in thin sections by electron microscopy. Electron-dense molecules, such as ferritin and gold, absorb electrons, which can be emitted when submitted to light of short wavelengths. The emitted electrons can be used to form images. This permits visualization of labeled Ab bound to tissue Ags. Gold-labeled secondary Abs, with particle labels (to a variety of animal species and class specific Igs) of varying sizes are commercially available.

Fluorescence-Activated Cell Sorting

Cells can now be analyzed and isolated on the basis of their distinct surface Ags, their size, or both by a process known as flow cytometry. Flow cytometers are instruments that can analyze properties of single cells as they pass through an orifice at high velocity. These instruments measure light scatter, volume, and fluorescence. One class of flow cytometers is designed solely to analyze these characteristics. Another class of cytometers, albeit more expensive, is designed to separate or sort cells as well as analyze their characteristics. An example of the latter type of cytometer is the fluorescence-activated cell sorter (FACS) (fig. 4.21).

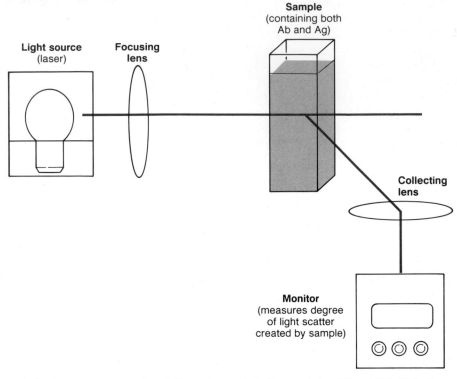

Light source
(laser)

Focusing lens

Sample
(containing both Ab and Ag)

Collecting lens

Monitor
(measures degree of light scatter created by sample)

FIGURE 4.22 Laser nephelometry. Immune complexes inherent in serum samples, or formed in samples by the addition of Ag or Ab, can be detected by exposure to the laser beam of a nephelometer. The degree of light scatter is measured by an electronic detector and digitally recorded as 0% to 100% RLS when compared with low- and high-scatter standards. RLS is proportional to the concentration of immune complexes.

FACSs can analyze and sort lymphocyte subpopulations, as identified by fluorescein-labeled MAbs, for example. In order to accomplish this, a suspension of leukocytes is incubated with labeled MAbs against CD4 helper cells. The washed sample is then introduced into the sample chamber of the cytometer, and the cells are forced through a nozzle in a liquid jet (surrounded by a sheath of saline). With vibration at the nozzle tip, the stream breaks up into droplets. The size of the droplet can be regulated so that each *contains a single cell.* The cells pass in front of a laser beam, which excites the fluorescent dye (which is monitored by fluorescence detectors) and light is scattered (which is also monitored). Droplets that emit appropriate fluorescent signals are electrically charged in a high-voltage field between deflection plates and separated into collection tubes. Thus, CD4 helper cells can be separated from other leukocytes of the suspension on the basis of the fluorescence of the bound MAbs. In certain applications, light scatter can provide signals for electrically charging droplets to achieve separations based on cell size.

Laser Nephelometry

Nephelometry has been used to detect Ags and immune complexes in serum and other biological fluids. This technique measures light that is scattered from the main beam of a laser light source (fig. 4.22). Determination of Ag concentration is performed by addition of constant amounts of optically clear specific antiserum to varying amounts of Ag. These samples, containing the immune complexes, are then placed in cuvettes and exposed to the laser beam of a nephelometer. The particles in solution (e.g., immune complexes) cause the light to be scattered. The number of particles in solution determines the degree of scatter that is produced; light scatter is slight when passing through a sample with few particles but great when passing through a sample containing many. The degree of light scatter is measured in a photoelectric cell and recorded as relative light scatter. The concentration of Ag, or immune complex, can be determined by comparison to standards and controls. Circulating immune complexes in serum can be measured by insolubilization (e.g., by the addition of polyethylene glycol) followed by relative light scatter determinations.

EFFECTS OF ANTIGEN-ANTIBODY INTERACTIONS

The effects of Ag-Ab interactions in the host are normally beneficial. Among the beneficial effects of Ag-Ab interactions are (1) initiation of immune responses, (2) neutralization of toxins and viruses, and (3) activation of complement. However, some interactions can be damaging. This occurs in immune-complex disorders.

Beneficial Effects

Initiation of Immune Responses

The most important natural physiological consequence of the interaction of Ag with Ab is the initiation of a specific humoral immune response. When Ag binds to the Ig receptors on B lymphocytes, differentiation and replication follows, with the formation of Ab-secreting plasma cells and specific populations of memory cells.

Neutralization of Toxins and Viruses

When Abs raised against toxins are allowed to react with the toxin's antigenic determinants, they may block toxic sites. Alternatively, Abs might bind to portions of the toxin that bind to the target cell. In either case, binding of Ab to toxin neutralizes its toxicity. Abs that neutralize toxins are called antitoxins. Abs engendered against viral Ags can complex with surface determinants on contact with free virus and prevent the virus

from binding to host cell receptors. Viral activity/infectivity is thus neutralized.

Activation of Complement

When an Ag and an Ab (of certain classes) form a complex in the presence of complement, a number of critical events follow (described in detail in chapter 6, Complement and its Role in Immune Responses). In brief, if the event occurs on the surface of a cell or virus, the cell or virus may be lysed or become phagocytized. Fragments of complement can be released as a result. These fragments can induce dilation and increased permeability of blood vessels, as part of an inflammatory response (see chapter 8). Under other circumstances, chemotactic factors might be generated that attract leukocyte combatants to regions of infection. The importance of complement activation for protection against infectious disease has been dramatically demonstrated from studies of disease susceptibility in those suffering complement deficiencies.

Antigen-Antibody Complexes and Fc Receptors

Many different cell types possess receptors for Ab that has complexed to Ag. The receptor is specific for a site on the Fc region of the Ig and is called the Fc receptor. Some lymphocytes can express Fc receptors for all the Ig classes, while certain subsets of lymphocytes may be class restricted. Many cells expressing Fc receptors exert cytotoxic effects on Ab-coated cells following binding to the Fc sites. These cells include killer (K) cells, natural killer (NK) cells, monocytes/macrophages, and neutrophils (see chapter 8 for further discussion). Phagocytes, possessing receptors, can also exhibit enhanced phagocytosis of target cells upon Fc binding.

Immune-Complex Disorders

The interaction of Ag with Ab to form immune complexes is not always beneficial to the host (see chapters 13 and 16). A number of diseases are associated with high levels of small, circulating immune complexes detectable in the serum and deposited in tissues (table 4.3). For example, deposition of circulating immune complexes in the renal glomeruli are responsible for kidney malfunction. Circulating immune complexes

TABLE 4.3 Some Human Diseases Associated with Immune-Complex Formation and Deposition

Infections	
Microbial Infections	*Parasitic Infections*
Bacterial and spirochetal	Leishmaniasis
Acute poststreptococcal glomerulonephritis	Malarial nephrotic syndrome
Lepromatous leprosy	Onchocerciasis
Mycoplasmal pneumonia	Schistosomiasis
Subacute bacterial endocarditis	Trypanosomiasis
Syphilis	
Viral	
Acute viral hepatitis	
Infectious mononucleosis glomerulonephritis	

Malignancies	
Solid Tumors	*Leukemias/Lymphomas*
Carcinomas of breast, colon, or lung	Acute lymphoblastic leukemia
Malignant melanoma	Chronic lymphocytic leukemia
	Hodgkin's disease

Autoimmune Disorders
Hashimoto's thyroiditis
Rheumatoid arthritis
Systemic lupus erythematosus

Miscellaneous	
Celiac disease	Hepatic cirrhosis
Dermatitis herpetiformis	Sickle cell anemia
Essential mixed cryoglobulinemia	Ulcerative colitis

Drug Reactions
Penicillinamine nephropathy
Serum sickness

Source: Stites, D. P., Stobo, J. D., and Wells, J. V. (eds.). *Basic and Clinical Immunology*. 5th ed. Lange Medical Publications, Los Altos, Calif.

have become deposited in other sites. Among these sites are the choroid plexus of the brain, walls of blood vessels, skin, and joints. Consequences of deposition of immune complexes in these sites include neurological and cardiovascular disorders and arthritis.

The damage arising from circulating immune complexes is extremely complex, and certainly not well understood. Simply put, deposited complexes can fix complement and attract cells that release hydrolytic enzymes destructive to normal tissues and cells. When these events occur as a controlled response to an insult, as outlined earlier, beneficial results are obtained. However, when they occur inappropriately, as in immune-complex disorders, the results can be catastrophic.

SUMMARY

1. The formation of an antigen-antibody complex occurs as a result of multiple noncovalent bonding between an epitope and the contact residues of an antibody-binding site. [p. 89]
2. Multiple bonds include hydrogen bridges, charged group attractions, van der Waals forces, and hydrophobic bonds. [p. 89]
3. Antibody affinity refers to the strength of binding between an antibody-binding site and an epitope. [p. 89]
4. Avidity refers to the strength of binding of a multivalent antigen with antibody possessing at least two combining sites or with antiserum containing antibodies of different specificities. [p. 89]
5. Two simple and useful ways of determining affinity constants are equilibrium dialysis and solid-phase radioimmunoassay. [pp. 89–94]
6. Antibody specificity refers to the ability of the molecule to discriminate between the antigenic determinant that stimulated its production, and other determinants. [p. 94]
7. High-affinity antibodies are more specific than low-affinity antibodies, and more contact points between the ligand and binding site are involved. [p. 94]

8. Crossreactivity often implies that an antiserum, containing antibodies engendered against a particular antigen, reacts with a different antigen. This may occur as a result of shared identical antigenic determinants, or related determinants. [pp. 94–95]
9. Specific antibodies may distinguish differences in structure, charge, optical configuration, and conformation of an antigenic determinant. [p. 95]
10. Precipitin reactions, in liquids or gels, can be used to quantify and compare antibodies and antigens. However, the antigen must possess more than one determinant and the antibody must be divalent, or multivalent, for a precipitate to form. [pp. 97–102]
11. Agglutination reactions can be direct, or indirect, and are sensitive techniques for identifying antigens displayed on cells, if known antibodies are available, or for measuring antibodies, if antigen-specific cells are available. [pp. 102–105]
12. Complement fixation is a sensitive technique to measure antibodies that is based on the principle that complement fixed in one antigen-antibody reaction is unavailable for a second antigen-antibody reaction. [pp. 103–104]
13. Complement-mediated lysis may be used to identify, or deplete, cells displaying antibodies bound to surface antigens. Following binding to the complexed antibody, activated complement damages the cell membrane (lysis). [p. 104]
14. Radioimmunoassay is perhaps the most sensitive technique available for detecting and quantifying antigen. This technique is based on the competition of radiolabeled known antigen and unlabeled unknown antigen for specific antibody in liquid or solid-phase assays. [pp. 104–105]
15. Enzyme-linked immunoassay is used to detect and quantify antibody (or antigen) and is almost as sensitive as radioimmunoassay. It has the advantage of not requiring expensive instrumentation or the precautions needed with radioactive labels. [pp. 105–106]

16. Western blotting involves transferring proteins, separated in gels, to membranes, such as nitrocellulose, for enhanced characterization. The protein antigens are detected on the membrane by primary antibody, and visualized with labeled secondary antibody. [pp. 106–107]

17. Immunofluorescence can be used to detect cell and tissue antigens as well as antibodies to cells and tissues, including autoantibodies. Fluorescence-staining techniques can be direct, in which the primary antibody is labeled, or indirect, in which the secondary antibody is labeled. [pp. 107–108]

18. Biotin-avidin assays depend upon high-affinity interaction between avidin and biotin. Biotin, a vitamin, is coupled to an antibody that is allowed to react with target cells. Avidin, derived from egg albumin, is radiolabeled and allowed to react with biotin-tagged antibody. This technique offers a powerful system for intense labeling of secondary antibodies, and enhanced detection of primary antibody. [p. 108]

19. Immunophotoelectron assays use electron-dense labels, such as gold, conjugated to secondary antibodies for visualizing antigens in thin sections of tissues by electron microscopy. [p. 109]

20. Flow cytometers are instruments for analyzing properties of single cells as they pass through an orifice at high velocity. Light scatter, volume, and fluorescence can be measured. Fluorescence-activated cell sorters are capable of isolating cells identified by fluorescent labels. [pp. 109–110]

21. Laser nephelometry may be used to measure light scattered as the result of immune complexes placed in the main beam of a laser light source. The degree of light scatter can be related to the concentration of antigen-antibody complexes in the sample. [pp. 110–111]

22. The effects of antigen-antibody interaction that occur in the host normally contribute to homeostasis when the body is perturbed by agents of disease and are thus beneficial. On the other hand, in certain diseases circulating immune complexes form and may be damaging following deposition in critical tissues. [pp. 111–113]

READINGS

Anderson, C. L., and Looney, R. J. Human leucocyte IgG Fc receptors. *Immunology Today* **7**:264, 1986.

Axelsen, N. H. (ed.). *Handbook of Immunoprecipitation in Gel Techniques.* (*Scandinavian Journal of Immunology* **10**), (Supplement). Blackwell, Oxford, 1983.

Coons, A. H., Creech, H. J., and Jones, R. H. Immunological properties of an antibody containing a fluorescent group. *Proceedings of the Society of Experimental Biology and Medicine* **47**:200, 1941.

Geysen, H. M., Tainer, J. A., Rhodde, S. J., et al. Chemistry of antibody binding to a protein. *Science* **235**:1184, 1987.

Herzenberg, L. A., Sweet, R. G., and Herzenberg, L. A. Fluorescence activated cell sorting. *Scientific American* **234**:108, 1976.

Hill, E., and Matsen, J. Enzyme-linked immunosorbent assay and radioimmunoassay in the serologic diagnosis of infectious diseases. *Journal of Infectious Diseases* **147**:258, 1983.

Hudson, L., and Hay, F. C. *Practical Immunology.* Blackwell, Oxford, 1989.

Johnstone, A., and Thorpe, R. *Immunochemistry in Practice.* Blackwell, Boston, 1987.

Karush, F. The affinity of antibodies: range, variability, and the role of multivalence. In *Immunoglobulins J* (Vol. 3). *Comprehensive Immunology* series, Plenum Press, New York, 1977.

Landsteiner, K. *The Specificity of Serological Reactions.* (Rev.) Harvard University Press, Cambridge, 1945.

Leiserson, W. Fluorescence cell sorter techniques. In *Immunological Methods* (Vol. 3). Academic Press, Orlando, Fla., 1985.

Marrack, P. New insights into antigen recognition. *Science* **235**:1311, 1987.

Rose, N. R., Fiedman, H., and Fahey, J. L. *Manual of Clinical Laboratory Immunology.* American Society of Microbiology, Washington, D.C., 1986.

Spinger, T. A. *Hybridoma Technology in the Biosciences and Medicine.* Plenum Press, New York, 1985.

Stites, D. P., Stobo, J. D., and Wells, J. V. (eds.). *Basic and Clinical Immunology.* Appleton and Lange, Los Altos, Calif., 1987.

Turgeon, M. L. *Immunology and Serology in Laboratory Medicine.* C. V. Mosby Co., St. Louis, 1990.

Verdin, E. M., Maratos-Flier, E., and Kahn, C. R., et al. Visualization of viral clearance in the living animal. *Science* **236**:439, 1987.

Waldmann, T. A. Monoclonal antibodies in diagnosis and therapy. *Science* **252:** 1657, 1991.

Weir, D. M., Herzenberg, L. A., Blackwell, C., et al. *Handbook of Experimental Immunology,* 4th ed. C. V. Mosby Co., St. Louis, 1985.

Yalow, R. S. Radioimmunoassay: a probe for fine structure of biologic systems. *Science* **200**:1236, 1980.

5 Antibody Production, Regulation, and Diversity

OVERVIEW

Specificity and memory are two properties of an adaptive immune system that evolved to protect us against disease-causing organisms. Encounter with foreign antigen can trigger specific defensive reactions characterized as humoral and cell-mediated immune responses. Execution of immune responses depends upon coordinated interplay among several components, which include instigating antigenic signals, responding cells (e.g., antigen-presenting cells, B cells, and T cells), and the products of these cells. This chapter explores the several dimensions involved in expressing humoral immune responses. Differentiation and activation of B cells are described. In addition, the organization of the genes involved in the production of specific antibodies is examined. Furthermore, mechanisms for producing an enormous diversity of specific antibodies from this gene pool are surveyed.

CONCEPTS

1. Lymphocytes possess receptors that trigger specific immune responses following binding of antigenic determinants for which they have specific affinity. Humoral immune responses, which lead to antibody production, are expressed by B lymphocytes.

2. Exposure to antigen induces humoral immune responses having immediate (primary) and prolonged (secondary) consequences that differ quantitatively and qualitatively.

3. Humoral immune responses to most antigens involve interactions of antigen-presenting cells, T helper cells, and B cells. B cells develop into antibody-secreting plasma cells or long-lived memory cells. Modulation of humoral immune responses is achieved by T suppressor cells, genes, antibodies, immune complexes, cytokines, and neuroendocrine products.

4. The body's preformed diverse antibody repertoire is programmed by three families of immunoglobulin genes. Separate genes encode the variable and constant regions of immunoglobulin molecules. Variable regions are encoded by two (light chain) or three (heavy chain) DNA segments, which are rearranged and joined during antigen-dependent differentiation of B cells.

5. Antibody diversity is achieved through recombination of variable germline genes, junction diversity, somatic hypermutation, and the random pairing of heavy and light immunoglobulin chains.

Following challenge by foreign antigen (Ag), our bodies react defensively to rid us of this insult. This occurs whether the Ag encountered appeared in the form of an invading organism (bacterium or animal parasite), a foreign product (e.g., pollen or toxin), or in some other form. Characteristically, our responses, which involve activation of the immune system, are defined as either humoral or cell mediated. These two classes of responses are examined separately; humoral immune responses are considered here and cell-mediated responses are discussed later (see unit 3).

Examination of the humoral immune response is undertaken in two parts. First, antibody (Ab) production and its regulation are explored. This discussion focuses on the respective roles and activities of specific cells that participate in humoral immune responses to foreign Ags. Second, the ability to generate diverse Abs, each unique for a particular Ag, is examined and its significance considered. This is achieved through discussions of the organization of genes encoding immunoglobulin (Ig) molecules and changes they undergo during B cell differentiation.

■ ■ ■ ■ ■ ■ ■ ■ ■

ANTIBODY PRODUCTION
Primary Humoral Responses

When Ag first encounters the immune system, it binds specifically to cells displaying complementary Ag receptors. This "selection" of potential responder cells represents the first step in activation of an immune response. These cells are stimulated to divide, thereby providing a pool (or clone) of effector cells and memory cells. This is known as clonal selection (see chapter 3, Effectors of Humoral Immunity, for additional discussion of this model). Ag-selected and expanded clones of effector B cells produce populations of circulating Abs, which are reactive with the epitopes of the Ag. The response might also take the form of a cell-mediated immune response, when T cells are selectively activated (discussed in chapter 9). Most immune reactions display both types of response.

Following Ag challenge, a **biphasic Ab response** occurs (fig. 5.1). Characteristically, there is a lag period when Ab is not detectable, followed by an exponential stage in which Ab concentrations rise markedly. A plateau with stabilized Ab concentration is subsequently reached, followed by a period of decline when Ab is cleared from the serum or is catabolized. Soon after exposure to Ag, there is a *primary Ab response*. During this time, avid *IgM* Abs are produced. After a brief delay (lag period), IgM levels rise (exponential stage) to a maximum (plateau) then fall (decline stage). A *secondary Ab response* follows. This response, initiated at the same time, displays a longer lag period before detectable Ig levels appear. In addition, the exponential phase is longer and leads to the generation of greater quantities of Abs. This is reflected in the higher Ab titer measurable in the serum of the challenged individual. During this second phase, the Abs produced are predominantly *IgG*. The peak quantities of IgG produced during this response can be more than 10 times that of the peak IgM levels achieved.

The characteristics of the primary humoral response can be affected by several factors. For example, the actual time frame depends on the nature of the Ag and the metabolic rate of the responding organism. In mammals, the entire biphasic response to an initial exposure to Ag might occur over a period of five to six weeks (as depicted). In anuran amphibians (e.g., frogs), this response might require an even longer interval. Moreover, among some organisms, the response might include only IgM and occur over a period of 30 days or more (see chapter 21, Comparative Immunobiology, for further discussion).

Secondary Humoral Responses

In subsequent encounters with the same immunogen, the response might differ qualitatively and quantitatively from the first, since memory cells are involved. Immune memory B cells are long-lived (they can live for years in humans) with the ability to react upon second contact with the original Ag by a more rapid

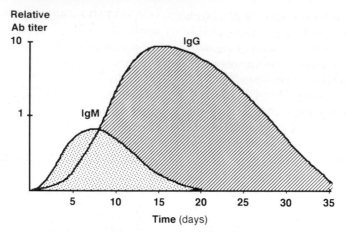

FIGURE 5.1 Primary humoral response. Exposure to foreign Ag yields a biphasic response. The first phase is associated with production of IgM, followed by production of IgG. The second phase is characterized by a reduction in serum Ab level. The time frame portrayed is illustrative only; the actual time-course might be more rapid or slower, depending upon the immunogen used and the conditions of challenge.

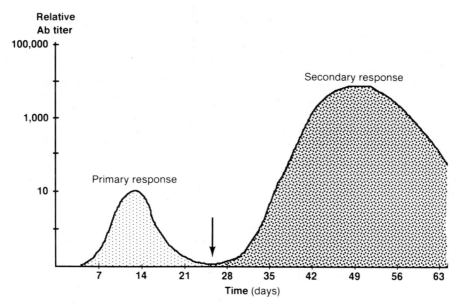

FIGURE 5.2 Secondary humoral response. Exposure to a previously encountered Ag yields a biphasic response comprised principally of IgG. In this response, the second phase produces substantially larger quantities of Ab. Re-exposure to Ag occurs at about 25 days and is marked by an *arrow*.

and stronger response. The **anamnestic** (memory) response is the result of the many more *specific clones of memory B cells* elicited by the preceding antigenic stimulation. When an individual or animal is exposed to the immunogen a second time, the response has a shorter lag period, an extended plateau, and a slower decline. In addition, the Ab levels are much higher (fig. 5.2). Differences in maximal serum IgG concentrations of 10- to 100-fold between primary and secondary humoral responses are not uncommon.

The anamnestic response consists almost entirely of IgG molecules. The binding efficiency of Abs generated in a secondary response is normally much greater than those produced following primary challenge. This is especially true when a low Ag dose is given to elicit a secondary response. Under these conditions, the few Ag molecules are preferentially bound to only B cell receptors with a high affinity for the ligand, and then clonally expanded. The average affinity of the induced Abs is thereby increased in the secondary response, and this is known as **affinity maturation.** Consequently, the *specificity of these Abs for a particular epitope is more discriminatory* than those formed during the primary humoral response.

B CELL DIFFERENTIATION

Differentiation of B cells is accomplished through two sequential processes. The first, known as **Ag-independent differentiation,** gives rise to mature B cells that are competent to engage in humoral immune responses. The second, referred to as **Ag-dependent differentiation,** is characterized by activation and differentiation of mature B cells into active, Ab-producing cells or memory cells. Two means of Ag-dependent differentiation are recognized: (1) in response to T-independent Ags and (2) in response to T-dependent Ags. The relationship between Ag-independent and Ag-dependent forms of differentiation is represented in figure 5.3.

Distinct differentiation-inducing microenvironments are occupied during both Ag-independent and Ag-dependent differentiation of B lymphocytes. Bone marrow, secondary lymphoid tissues, blood and lymph are compartments that influence B cell behavior. These environments contain cytokines, Igs, complement factors, inflammatory products, and neuroendocrine elements produced by several cell types that cooperate in the expression of humoral immune competence.

Antigen-Independent Differentiation

As a result of Ag-independent differentiation, *virgin B lymphocytes are formed from multipotent hematopoietic stem cells* of the bone marrow. During this period of differentiation in an inducing microenvironment, **germ-**

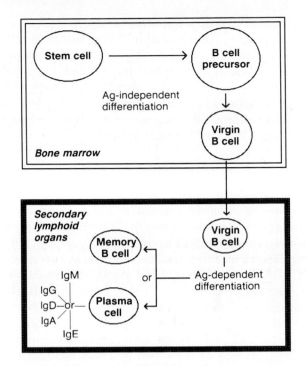

FIGURE 5.3 Differentiation of B cells. B cell precursors are derived from a stem cell. Through Ag-independent differentiation in a B cell environment, these cells acquire the competence to function as B cells (virgin B cells). They can then migrate to secondary lymphoid organs, where they can differentiate into active B cells through Ag-dependent differentiation, when acted upon by Ag. This can lead to the production of Ab-secreting plasma cells capable of secreting any class of Ig. Alternatively, memory cells can arise that will respond rapidly and more strongly upon subsequent encounter with this same provoking Ag.

line Ab gene rearrangements occur in a carefully ordered sequence—for example, V_H genes are rearranged before V_L genes. (See Production of Diverse Antibodies below for details.)

Once somatic recombination of germline genes has occurred, Ab molecules are synthesized and anchored to the cell membrane. These cells then display Ag receptors of monomeric IgM and are called B_μ cells. This population displays the entire repertoire of Ag-binding specificities possessed by an individual before Ag exposure, with a single cell expressing only one specificity. Virgin B_μ cells then differentiate into mature B cells that express both IgM and IgD receptor molecules with identical variable (V) regions. B cells that reach this stage are now *immunocompetent,* for they can respond to Ag stimulation. These mature B cells are designated $B_{\mu+\delta}$ cells. Ag-dependent differentiation occurs when $B_{\mu+\delta}$ lymphocytes respond to bound Ag and appropriate signals, thereby developing into large dividing blast cells. Additional discussion of Ag-independent differentiation of B cells can be found in chapter 20, Development of Immunity.

Antigen-Dependent Differentiation

Definitive B cells can be induced to further mature and become functionally expressive. These maturational changes, unlike those leading to the formation of virgin B cells, are **dependent upon exposure to Ags.** This Ag-dependent differentiation proceeds in two stages: (1) activation and (2) proliferation and differentiation. Ags act as specific signals that activate particular B cells (possessing complementary receptors). In addition, nonspecific signals are also provided by other cells to promote and modulate the differentiation of activated B cells. Aspects of these two processes are described separately in the following sections.

B Cell Activation by T-Independent Antigens

B cells can be activated by Ags independent of interaction with T cells. Ags that act in this fashion are known as T-independent Ags (in contrast to T-dependent Ags, which require intervention of T cells [discussed below]). T-independent Ags usually are polymeric, with repeating identical antigenic determinants (such as lipopolysaccharide), which are usually slowly degraded. They can *stimulate B cells directly by crosslinking surface receptors for Ag.* The reaction is not restricted by molecules of the major histocompatibility complex (MHC) (discussed in greater detail in unit 3). In addition, they apparently do not require the specific signal systems necessary for thymus-dependent Ags. At low concentrations, some T-independent Ags stimulate Ag-specific receptors, while at higher concentrations they act as polyclonal activators or mitogens. Low-affinity Abs are normally formed in response to T-independent Ags.

Ag interaction with membrane-bound surface Ig (mIg) receptors triggers a cascade of reactions that produce changes in the cell membrane, cytoplasm, and nucleus (fig. 5.4). Briefly, the following events occur. The membrane depolarizes leading to an influx of extracellular Ca^{2+}. This, in turn, contributes to the activation of three membrane-associated response pathways: (1) stimulation of guanylate cyclase with the production of cyclic guanosine monophosphate (cGMP); (2) activation of phospholipase C with the subsequent generation of diacylglycerol (DAG) and inositol triphosphate (ITP); and (3) activation of phospholipase A_2, which promotes the metabolism of arachidonic acid (formation of prostaglandins and leukotrienes). ITP, DAG, Ca^{2+}, and cGMP are substances that act as second messengers in the activation of several cellular systems. These factors are responsible for increasing the metabolic activity of the activated B cells. Specifically, these intracellular messengers activate protein kinases that promote the first steps of activation: (1) entry into G_1, (2) production of IL-2 and other growth factors, (3) increased expression of interleukin 2 (IL-2) receptors (IL-2Rs), and (4) increased expression of MHC class II molecules. Passage into the S phase of the cell cycle, with subsequent DNA replication and cellular proliferation, is apparently regulated by events mediated through IL-2Rs.

Ag binding to mIg leads to crosslinking of mIgs, followed by capping (migration of Ag-mIg complexes to a polar position on the cell). Subsequently, the resting B cell is induced to enter the cell cycle and to express surface receptors for B cell growth and differentiation factors (BCGFs and BCDFs). Among these are receptors for several ILs, Fc receptors (FcRs), and receptors designated as CD19, CD21, CD22, and CD23. Expressed receptors allow activated B cells to respond to several cytokines (e.g., interferons [IFNs], tumor necrosis factor [TNF], lymphotoxin [LTX], IL-1, IL-2, IL-4, and IL-6). (See chapter 9, Effectors of Specific Cellular Immunity for further discussion of cytokines.)

Most cytokines act as BCGFs and BCDFs promoting B cell proliferation and differentiation and,

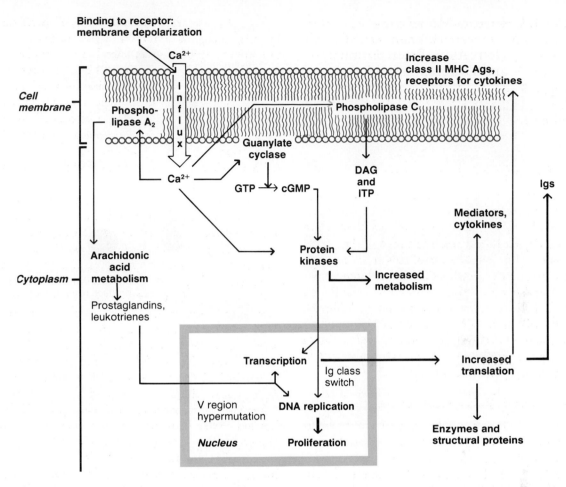

FIGURE 5.4 B cell responses to antigenic activation. Binding of Ag to appropriate B cell receptors triggers a series of responses. These lead to alterations in membrane function and expression of additional receptors, modifications of intracellular metabolism, and changes in gene expression. These lead to increased responsiveness to extracellular signals, proliferation and clonal expansion, and Ab production and secretion.

thus, clonal expansion. For example, binding of IL-1 and IL-4 to their receptors and of the undefined ligand for CD23 leads to progression through the early stages of the cell cycle (i.e., G_0–S). Moreover, binding of IL-2, IFN-γ, and perhaps IL-5 promote proliferation (completion of the cell cycle), and IL-2 and IFN-α promote differentiation. However, not all receptor-mediated input to activated B cells has a positive effect.

Whereas ligand binding to CD22 and CD21 (a receptor for C3d, a product of the complement system [discussed in chapter 6]) potentiates progression of activated B cells through the cell cycle, binding of IFN-γ to its receptor or of ligand to CD19 and FcRs shortly after activation inhibits this progression.

In the absence of inhibition, these cells undergo events characteristic of B cell differentiation

TABLE 5.1 Factors Modulating Antigen-Dependent B Cell Activation, Proliferation, and Differentiation

Factor	Influence on B Cell Behavior
Ag	Induces mIg crosslinking and capping phenomenon; induces expression of receptors for BCGFs and BCDFs
IL-4, IL-6	Stimulate transition from G_0 to G_1 (entry into cell cycle) or early events in G_1
BCGFs	Promote transit through cell cycle; are responsible for clonal expansion; favor somatic hypermutation (?)
IL-1	Augments proliferation response; acts in mid-G_1
BCDFs	Promote exit from cell cycle and expression of Ab-secreting function; influence Ig class switch selection (?)
IL-2, LTX, TNF	Modulate proliferation and differentiation
IFNs	Modulate proliferation and possibly B cell differentiation

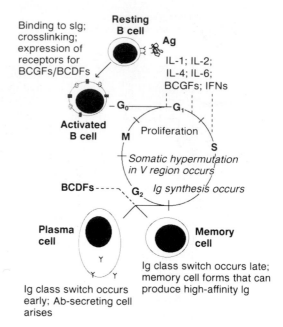

FIGURE 5.5 Activation of B cells by T-independent Ags. Binding of Ag to specific receptors (surface Igs) activates B cells. This triggers entry into the cell division cycle. Cytokines (e.g., IL-1, IL-2, IL-4, IL-6, and IFNs) help promote this. Other cytokines, like IL-2 and BCGFs, further promote cell division. This leads to clonal expansion of activated B cells. Cells that are induced to undergo terminal differentiation early by BCGFs undergo class switching early (if switching occurs). These become Ab-secreting plasma cells. Those that do not receive this signal early continue to repeat this divisional cycle. During each cycle, the opportunity exists to modify V regions through somatic mutation.

(discussed later). Although activation is induced in the absence of overt T cell participation, B cell differentiation is not without influence from T cells. In fact, T cells are instrumental in promoting both proliferation and differentiation following antigenic exposure through the numerous lymphokines that they produce (table 5.1 and fig. 5.5).

B Cell Activation by T-Dependent Antigens

Most Ags (immunogens) that stimulate the production of Abs are not T independent, but rather are T dependent. They *require interaction of two or three distinct cell types in effecting a humoral immune response to an immunogen.* These cells include Ag-presenting cells (APCs), T helper (T_H) cells, and B cells. In this triad, each cell plays a specific role. B cells are Ag-responsive cells that

proliferate and differentiate into Ab-producing plasma cells. T_H cells (phenotypically CD4) provide growth and differentiation factors for B cells. APCs facilitate T and B cell interaction by acquiring and processing Ag for presentation to T cells in immunogenic form. The interaction of these cells for the induction of Ab formation is illustrated in figure 5.6.

This stimulation of B lymphocytes requires a combination of specific and nonspecific signals. Specific stimulation of B cells is accomplished by interaction between an Ag and mIgs expressed by the B cell, while nonspecific signals are provided by cytokines and other cofactors. The epitopes of the Ag that participate in specific B cell activation are distinct from those that trigger T cell help. Consequently, cells involved in a T-dependent Ab response to a foreign substance recognize at least two parts of an Ag.

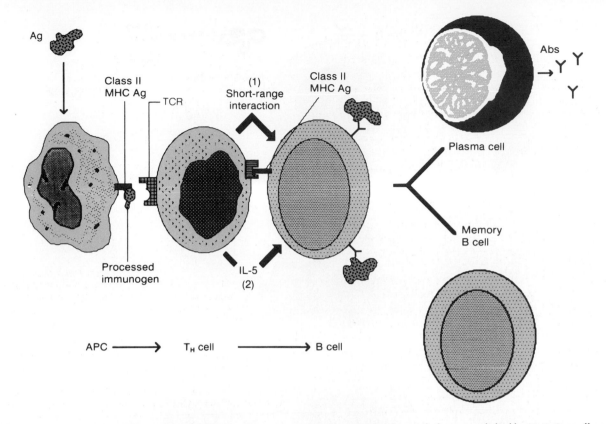

FIGURE 5.6 Activation of B cells by T-dependent Ags. T-dependent activation of B cells can occur in either of two ways, following presentation of Ag to T cells by APCs. (*1*) This can be accomplished by short-range interaction between T and B cells. (*2*) Alternatively, this might be accomplished by IL-5. Regardless of which means is used, B cells are stimulated to proliferate and differentiate into Ab-producing plasma cells and memory cells.

The specific changes induced in B cells that are activated by T-dependent Ags are the same as outlined earlier for T-independent Ags.

Antigen Processing and Presentation Nonspecific APCs might take up Ag in the periphery (i.e., away from lymphoid centers like the spleen or lymph nodes). The Ag becomes internalized and is processed. Different determinants are returned to the cell surface. These immunogenic determinants are transported to lymphoid organs. There they are presented by the APCs to T$_H$ cells which, in turn, "help" in stimulating the B cells. Thus, APCs facilitate T/B cell interactions. Alternatively, soluble Ag might bind directly to specific B lymphocytes by means of an accessible conformational epitope. These B cells might act, in turn,

as APCs themselves. Conventional APCs, such as macrophages or dendritic cells, do not recognize Ags specifically. However, B cells have specific Ag receptors, which can enhance their ability to recognize and present Ag to T cells. After binding to mIgs, multivalent Ags are internalized, partially degraded, and the antigenic fragments recycled to the B cell surface. The displayed determinants are associated with MHC class II Ags, then are presented to T lymphocytes (fig. 5.7). T cells appear capable of recognizing quite small antigenic fragments, while B cells often recognize larger, conformationally intact epitopes. Since the B cell response is focused largely against conformational determinants, which might be easily lost on processing, Ag presentation by B cells might be a common occurrence.

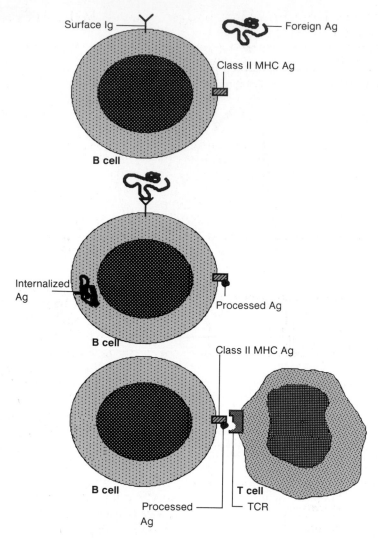

FIGURE 5.7 Ag presentation by B cells. Surface Igs specific for a particular Ag can bind it, then cause it to become internalized. Following processing, antigenic determinants can then be presented, in association with class II MHC Ags, to T cells. Through this association, B cells can function as APCs for T cell activation.

APCs display immunogens (Ags) that possess two domains. The first is an *epitope* capable of binding to the *paratope* of a T$_H$ cell receptor. The second is an *agretope* that is intimately associated with a class II MHC molecule. The T cell Ag receptor (TCR) consists of transmembrane proteins that bind Ag. The TCR is noncovalently associated with five additional integral membrane proteins (designated CD3) that transduce signals following Ag binding (see chapter 9 for further discussion of the TCR and MHC restriction). The part of the MHC molecule that binds to the epitope determines the orientation of the immunogen and is called a *desetope*. The part of the MHC molecule recognized by the T$_H$ cell is designated the *histotope*. (These domains are summarized in table 5.2 and schematically represented in fig. 5.8.) The processed Ag then reacts

TABLE 5.2 Functional Domains of Immunogen, Class II MHC Antigen, and T Cell Receptor

Domain	Location	Functional Definition
Epitope	Immunogen	Region recognized by TCR (in conjunction with class II MHC Ag); region against which Ig is specific
Paratope	TCR	Region that recognizes epitope of immunogen and histotope of class II MHC Ag
Agretope	Immunogen	Region recognized by class II MHC Ag of APC (name derives from *Ag recognition* region)
Desetope	Class II MHC Ag	Region that recognizes agretope of immunogen and determines its orientation for presentation to T cell (name derives from *determinant selection* region)
Histotope	Class II MHC Ag	Region recognized as ''self'' by TCR

Relationship of these regions to each other is depicted in figure 5.8.

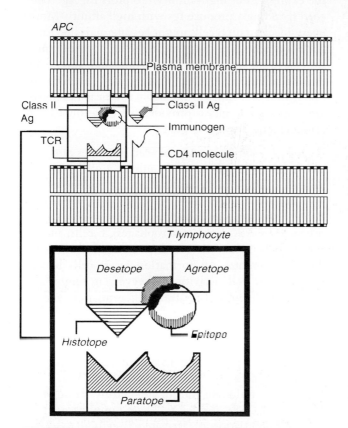

FIGURE 5.8 Immunogenic domains. Interactions between APCs and T cells that lead to immunological activation involve interactions of the foreign Ag, class II MHC Ag, and TCR. Interactions occur between portions of these molecules that display appropriate specificity. These domains are defined in table 5.2.

with TCRs that recognize both the epitope and the class II Ag. Interaction between the T cell and the APC is stabilized by bonds formed between CD4 molecules on T_H cells and a nonpolymorphic area of the MHC class II molecules of the APC.

In addition to Ag presentation to T cells, APCs also interact physically with B cells during the early stages of humoral immune responses. Recent studies have demonstrated that Ig production by activated B cells is reduced in cultures containing only T and B cells. Restoration of Ig production is still not achieved by the further addition of lymphokines (to supplement for their reduced production in the absence of APC/T cell interaction). Only in the presence of accessory cells does Ig production reach maximal levels. This effect can be achieved even when the APCs used are fixed (not physiologically active) monocytes.

The Role of T Cells T_H cells are essential for all IgG, IgA, IgD, and IgE responses, but they may be important for only certain IgM responses. They can cooperate only with APCs and B lymphocytes with which they share class II MHC determinants, recognized as self. T_H cells are activated by reactions with antigenic determinants and IL-1, IL-6, and TNF produced by activated APCs. Ag-activated T_H cells provide a variety of lymphokines that promote subsequent B cell proliferation and differentiation.

...ells progress through a series of changes ...acteristic of Ag-dependent differentiation. These are *similar whether activation has been induced by T-independent or T-dependent Ags.* By following one of two alternative differentiation pathways, activated B cells produce short-lived **plasma cells** or long-lived **memory cells.** What factors are specifically responsible for a particular cell becoming a plasma cell or a memory cell are not known. However, it has been proposed that activated cells become memory cells, rather than Ab-secreting plasma cells, if the strength of the differentiation signal is not strong enough to reach the threshold for complete differentiation. Nevertheless, many activated B cells do, of course, become plasma cells. *During this differentiation, class switching in Ig gene expression occurs* (discussed later in this chapter). Although this might lead to the expression of a different class, or subclass, of Ab, it **does not involve a change in Ag-recognition specificity.**

Progeny lymphocytes in the clones derived from activated B cells display receptors of the *same specificity as the parent cell.* Those lymphocytes that become plasma cells produce and secrete Abs of the same Ag-recognition specificity as displayed by the surface Ag receptor of the activated precursor B cell. This process takes about a week and eight to 10 cell generations. Moreover, the progeny lymphocytes also include clones of memory cells, which can also display the same Ag-recognition specificity as their lymphocyte precursors. However, lymphocytes are subject to hypermutation, which can be triggered by reaction with Ag, giving rise to higher affinity Ab (discussed in detail later in this chapter). These cells can develop into a second wave of plasma cells and memory cells upon subsequent encounter with Ag. They are responsible for the more rapid and more intense response to previously encountered foreign Ag.

Differentiation Pathways Two general differentiation pathways are open to naive B cells: early or delayed differentiation. Differentiation is often associated with switching in the class of Ig produced. Thus, early differentiation of B cells in a primary humoral response represents early class switching. Cells that make this switch in Ig class early become Ab-secreting plasma cells early. These cells produce Ig with relatively low affinity for Ag. Cells that delay class switching might progress through several cell division cycles. During this time, hypermutation of genes in the V region can occur. In addition, cells that become memory cells are believed to arise in this manner.

B cells that differentiate into plasma cells early do so at a time when Ag concentration is usually high. These cells have been found to have low-affinity receptors for Ag and correspondingly produce low-affinity Abs. In contrast, B cells that do not become activated and differentiate into plasma cells until later in the humoral response react at a time when Ag concentration is fairly low. Their activation depends upon the expression of high-affinity receptors for Ag. They correspondingly produce Igs with high affinity. Moreover, since certain B cells might become activated early, but not differentiate until late in the humoral response, they have the opportunity to pass through several additional divisional cycles. This greatly increases the opportunity for somatic mutation, since each each passage through S phase provides an occasion for rearrangements among Ig genes.

Role of Cytokines Ag-induced responses of B cells can involve both direct and indirect T cell help and include a variety of signals initiated by binding of soluble ligands to B cell receptors. Nonspecific signals for B cell activation and differentiation are soluble factors produced by APCs (e.g., macrophages), B cells, and T_H cells which include IL-1 and IL-2 (fig. 5.9). IL-1 indirectly promotes Ab formation by B cells by enhancing T_H cell activity. However, it might also directly augment proliferation, differentiation, and Ab production.

In addition, two classes of T_H cell, discriminated by the lymphokines or ligands they produce, can participate in promoting the humoral immune response. T_{H1} cells produce and secrete IL-2, IL-3, TNF, IFN-γ, granulocyte-monocyte–colony-stimulating factor (GM-CSF), and LTX. These lymphokines promote differentiation of activated B cells that secrete IgM, IgG2a, and IgG3. T_{H2} cells produce and release IL-3, IL-4, IL-5, GM-CSF, and TNF, which support proliferation of quiescent B cells and their differentia-

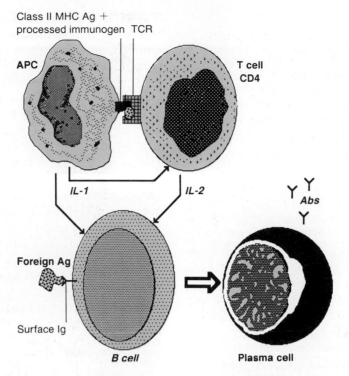

FIGURE 5.9 Nonspecific influences on B cell activation and differentiation. B cells that have been activated by Ag can be influenced nonspecifically by cytokines. In particular, IL-1 from macrophages and IL-2 from T_H cells promote proliferation of activated B cells and assist in their clonal expansion.

tion into cells that secrete IgM, IgG1, and IgG3. The direct influence and involvement of T_H cells is more prevalent in secondary humoral immune responses than in primary humoral immune responses.

REGULATON OF ANTIBODY PRODUCTION

The relative ability of each individual to respond to the antigenic universe is inherited to a large extent. However, numerous environmental factors (e.g., diet, disease, and life-style) can influence our immune capacity. Homeostatic mechanisms control the size, nature, and duration of ongoing humoral and cell-mediated immune responses. Lymphocytes that are specifically activated by Ag proliferate and differentiate to become Ab-forming cells, effector T cells, or memory B and T cells. However, lymphocytes neither reproduce in un-

controlled fashion nor continuously produce increasing quantities of Abs or lymphokines. A decline in functional expression follows primary and secondary immune responses. Hence specific immune responses must be down-regulated in some fashion. Several mechanisms operate to modulate immunological expression (table 5.3). Positive regulators include Ags (sometimes in their native form, at other times processed) and cytokines (e.g., IL-1, IL-2, BCGF/BCDF) from macrophages and helper/inducer T ($T_{H/I}$) cells. In addition, complement components and immune complexes can stimulate immune responses. Negative regulators, discussed later, include formed Abs, immune complexes, suppressor factors (from suppressor [T_S] cells), and Ig idiotype networks (Abs against Abs). In addition, changes in neural and endocrine status can modulate immunological expression in either positive or negative fashion.

TABLE 5.3 Some Regulators of Immunological Expression

Regulator	Action and Effect on Immune Response
Positive Regulators	
Antigens	
Native (limited)	Bind to mIg, trigger humoral response
Processed (broad)	Presented to T cells; bind to TCRs, can lead to expression of humoral or cellular immune responses, or both
Complement components	Bind to complement receptors; stimulate T cells to augment humoral or cellular immune responses, or both
Cytokines	Released by macrophages (IL-1) or T$_H$ cells (IL-2, BCGFs, BCDFs); potentiate proliferation and differentiation of B or T cells, with augmented humoral or cellular responses
Immune complexes	At high Ab:Ag ratio, bind to Fc receptors of APCs and promote T cell activation
Negative Regulators	
Formed antibodies	Bind to circulating Ag; block access to sIg; diminishing continued stimulation
Immune complexes	At low Ab:Ag ratio, bind to B cells and reduce humoral response
Suppressor factors	Released by T$_S$ cells; block activation of B or T cells, limiting humoral or cellular responses
Anti-antibodies	Network of antiidiotype Abs that bind to and inactivate primary Abs

TABLE 5.4 Genes Influencing Immunological Expression

Category	Role in Immune Response
Genes for Surface Receptors	Required for initial activation—no response possible in absence; recognize antigenic determinants as necessary first step in humoral or cellular immune responses
Immune Response Genes	Affect quality and extent of immune responses
MHC (class I)	Mediate activation and expression of T$_C$ cells leading to cytotoxicity in cellular immune responses, or T$_S$ cells effecting negative immune regulation
MHC (class II)	Mediate activation and expression of T$_H$ cells with potentiation of humoral and cellular responses, or T$_D$ cells with mediation of delayed hypersensitivity
Non-MHC	Affect metabolism of APCs influencing Ag processing and presentation; affect cellular and humoral immune responses

Genetic Control

Two broad categories of genes contribute to the control of immune responses (table 5.4). The first category of genes, receptor genes, encoding B and T cell Ag recognition receptors, determine whether or not a response to a particular foreign or self-determinant is possible. Gaps in the B or T cell repertoire, because an individual lacks a receptor for a specific antigenic determinant, might account for a failure to respond in particular cases. The second category, immune response (Ir) genes, influence the quality and extent of the possible immune response. This category is composed of two types of genes. Ir genes either can be part of the MHC or be unrelated to it (see chapter 7 for further discussion of histocompatibility genes). Ir genes of the MHC, which encode class II molecules, primarily influence responses involving T$_H$ and sensitized T (T$_D$) cells, while those that encode class I molecules, principally control T$_S$ and cytotoxic T (T$_C$) cell responses. Non-MHC Ir genes appear to encode several products that might influence both arms of the immune response. There are numerous Ir gene loci (MHC and non-MHC) that influence the level of the immune response to any particular Ag.

Ir Genes Encoding MHC Class II Molecules

Genes encoding class II MHC molecules have stimulated a great deal of interest, and their function is perhaps better known than any of the other Ir genes. Using synthetic polypeptides, McDevitt and colleagues challenged inbred mice possessing a variety of MHC haplotypes (a set of linked genes on the same chromosome). High, low, and intermediate Ab responses to the same immunogen were observed in these mice. These differences in Ab responses depended, in part, on the particular haplotype inherited by the mice. Subsequent studies have shown that strain differences, which mapped to the I region (encoding class II molecules) of the MHC, correlated with the levels of Ab response observed. Moreover, MHC gene control appears to be quite specific. A single amino acid substitution, within the epitope of a synthetic polypeptide, can affect the response of certain mouse strains.

Ir MHC class II products are believed to *act at the stage when Ag is processed or presented.* Thus, they influence cell interactions and the activation process. This action appears to be primarily focused on $T_{H/I}$ cells. However, signals for activation of T_D cells are also influenced by the nature of the class II gene product associating with stimulating Ag. Several factors enter into expression of this influence by MHC class II molecules. First, the ability of a potentially immunogenic Ag to associate with an MHC molecule depends on the nature of the unique MHC-binding site or desetope. Structurally distinct desetopes of class II molecules, formed in individuals of different haplotypes, might vary in their complementary association with the agretope of an Ag. Second, if association for a particular Ag is poor, then recognition by T_H cells for the composite epitope and histotope might be affected. Consequently, the immune response might be poor or nonexistent. For example, malfunctioning class II–restricted T_H cells might not provide the proper, or optimal, signals for B cell activation for a normal humoral response. Similarly, $T_{H/I}$ cells, incapable of perceiving MHC "altered" Ag, might not provide help for full activation of T_C cells.

Ir Genes Encoding MHC Class I Molecules

Ir gene products also regulate activation of T_C and T_S cells. However, these cells display a dependence upon MHC class I products. The nature of the binding site or desetope of the MHC product, as genetically determined, can influence the association of Ag, via the agretope, for presentation to T_C cells. This is qualitatively similar to that observed for MHC class II–associated presentation of Ag to T_H cells. For example, failure of T_C cells to normally recognize the composite of the T cell determinant associated with the MHC determinant prevents activation. This parallels the role of MHC class II products in the activation of T_H or T_D cells.

Those responses that display an apparent dependence upon class II MHC gene products are considered MHC class II restricted. This applies to T_H and T_D cells, almost exclusively. MHC class I restriction, therefore, describes those responses in which there is an apparent dependence upon class I MHC gene products for activation. Class I restriction applies to T_C or T_S cells.

Non-MHC Ir Genes

Several genes that do not encode Ag receptors, class I, or class II MHC molecules, also affect the functioning of cells involved in immune responses. These genes are found on several different chromosomes. Their products appear to affect metabolic activity of APCs. Some studies have shown differences in macrophages from strains of mice that respond well or poorly to particular T-dependent Ags. Macrophages of poor responders processed Ag less efficiently than macrophages of high responders. Products of non-MHC Ir genes are believed to be responsible for expression of these differences.

Antibody Feedback

The humoral response is controlled, in part, by Ab production itself. This appears to be negative feedback regulation that is highly specific (fig. 5.10). On the one

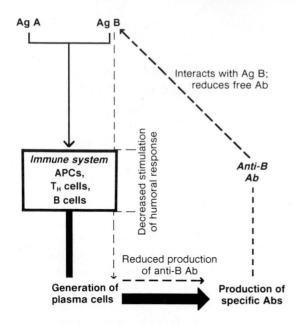

FIGURE 5.10 Feedback regulation of Ab production. Activation of B cells by Ag leads to production of Abs specific for those Ags. For example, Ag B stimulates to the production of anti-B Abs. Subsequently, the Abs reduce the concentration of that Ag. This diminishes stimulation of further production of that specific Ab. Eventually, Ag B is completely removed, and no further stimulation of the production of anti-B Ab occurs. These interactions, however, have no effect on the level of Ag A or its influence in stimulating Ab (anti-A) production.

hand, removal of blood from an immunized (vaccinated or clinically exposed) individual can increase Ab synthesis. On the other hand, passive administration of specific Ab can suppress the induction of an immune response to a specific Ag, without affecting responses to other Ags. Ab, commonly IgG, can bind to Ag, thereby preventing the Ag from binding to receptors of T_H cells or B cells, including those serving as specific APCs. A small amount of Ag, not neutralized by Ab, could still remain. These molecules might bind to high-affinity receptors on lymphocytes. Thus, although the Ab response may have been dramatically down-regulated as a result of Ab feedback, low levels of high-affinity Abs might still be produced. This mechanism has two effects. It diminishes total Ab output; but at the same time, it contributes to the preferential appearance of high-affinity Abs. Regulation by endogenous Ab may also require an intact and available Fc portion of secreted Ab. In this case, lymphocyte ac-

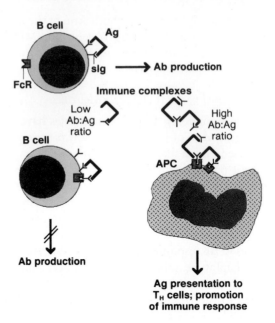

FIGURE 5.11 Influence of immune complexes on immune responses. Ag characteristically triggers an immune response, for example, Ab production. However, Ag that is complexed with Ab has differential effects on immune responses. At low Ab:Ag ratios, suppression of Ab production can occur. Under these conditions, immune complexes can bind to both mIg (Ag) and FcRs (Ab) of the B cells. This suppresses Ab production. In contrast, at high Ab:Ag ratios, immune responses can be stimulated. This occurs through binding to FcRs on APCs that leads to activation of T_H cells and subsequent enhancement of immune responses.

tivation might be inhibited by crosslinking of Ag and FcRs by the Ab. This might be a contributing mechanism to the induction of tolerance (see chapter 10).

Regulatory Immune Complexes

Preformed immune complexes with low Ab:Ag ratios can suppress B cell activation. This can be accomplished by crosslinking Ag and FcRs (fig. 5.11). In contrast, preformed immune complexes with high Ab:Ag ratios can enhance a response. In this case, activation is achieved by binding to the FcRs of APCs. This leads to crosslinking of FcRs, which appears to be an important step in activation. This, in turn, leads to Ag presentation to T cells. Stimulation and promotion of an immune response can then follow. This is a common means of inducing hypersensitivity reactions (see chapter 13 for further discussion).

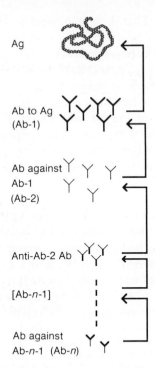

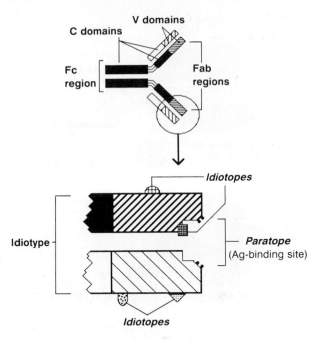

FIGURE 5.12 Idiotype network. Ag triggers Ab production. The Abs produced (Ab-1) not only react against the Ag, but they also serve as Ags themselves. This triggers the production of a second level of Abs (Ab-2). In turn, these Abs react against Ab-1 but serve to induce anti-Ab-2 Ab. And so the process continues. However, at each step, the concentration of Ab available to provoke formation of an anti-Ab is less than in the preceding step. As a result, a level is eventually reached at which there is insufficient Ab produced to provide an antigenic signal.

FIGURE 5.13 Idiotype. An idiotype consists of a set of epitopes associated with the V regions of an Ab molecule. Each individual epitope is designated an idiotope. Idiotopes can be associated with the paratope or lie outside it.

Idiotypic Regulation

Some years ago Jerne proposed that Ab production in a humoral immune response might be regulated by the production of anti-Abs. Specifically, this suggested that the Abs generated in response to Ag could provoke the production of Abs against themselves. In turn, these secondary Abs would neutralize and down-regulate the original humoral response. This physiological auto-immune mechanism for the regulation of an immune response was designated an **idiotype network** (fig. 5.12). Jerne defined an idiotype as "a set of epitopes displayed by the variable regions of a set of antibody molecules." Each individual idiotypic epitope becomes known as an idiotope (Id). Within this model, each Fab arm of an Ab molecule possesses one paratope (Ab-

combining site) and a small set of Ids (fig. 5.13). Jerne's idiotype network model contained three important features:

1. Lymphocytes can respond either positively or negatively to a recognition signal. A positive response leads to cell proliferation, cell activation, and Ab secretion. A negative response results in tolerance and suppression.
2. Ab molecules can recognize Ags, but can also be recognized as Ags.
3. The generation of antiidiotype Abs displays a step-down feature that eventually terminates the ongoing response. This means that at each step, the amount of anti-Ab required is less than in the previous step. Eventually, the amount of Ab needed is returned to normal (nonstimulated) levels, at which point the humoral response is extinguished.

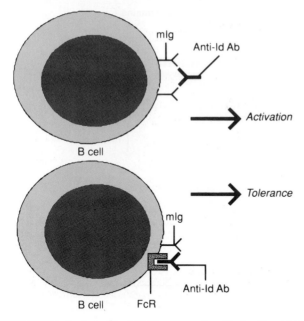

FIGURE 5.14 Actions of anti-Id Abs. Abs against Ids that lie within a paratope can crosslink mIgs. In so doing, they can activate the affected B cell. On the other hand, Abs against Ids lying outside a paratope can interact with mIg through their Fab region and with Fc receptors of the same B cell. In this configuration, Ab production is suppressed. The result is tolerance.

This model has received experimental verification. Indeed, B lymphocytes have been shown to be capable of recognizing and responding to idiotypes of Abs and Ab receptors on lymphocytes.

For any given idiotype, some Ids may lie within the paratope and others outside. Since an Ab molecule binds to a single antigenic determinant (an epitope/Id), then an anti-Id Ab binds to the paratope only if the Id lies within it. In this case, the anti-Id might substitute for the epitope (internal image) of a traditional Ag. As Ag, anti-Id can either stimulate or depress the immune response. What dictates which of these two paths is followed remains to be determined. Since anti-Ids are theoretically present in the receptor repertoire of the naive animal, their concentrations, in secreted form, must increase as a result of immunogenic challenge if they are to serve either as immunogens or tolerogens (fig. 5.14). Anti-Ids can activate lymphocytes by crosslinking Ag receptors on lymphocytes (since they have at least two binding sites). Alternatively, they can inhibit activation by crosslinking

Ag and FcRs. That these two opposite actions are possible has been experimentally demonstrated. For example, two different subclasses of IgG, exhibiting the same anti-Id specificity, have been shown to either stimulate or suppress immune responses in mice. This might relate to the binding affinity of the FcR for the Fc region of one isotype over the other.

Antiidiotypes can also recognize receptors of T_H cells and other T cell subpopulations. The TCR, although not an Ig, possesses an idiotype that is a collection of idiotopes associated with the V region of the α, β heterodimer. T and B cells might share Ids associated with their receptors. T cells have been shown to react with anti-Id Abs. In some instances, that has resulted in blocked functional expression. In other instances, anti-Id Abs have stimulated T cells. This stimulation appears to be analogous to B cell stimulation by antiidiotypes, rather than Ag. Antiidiotypic T_S cells might influence Ab responses by reacting with the Ids of an Ig receptor on B lymphocytes (see below).

T Suppressor Cells

T and B cell activity can be regulated by T_H and T_S cells. Both cell types are stimulated during a normal immune response. They play a continuous homeostatic role in regulation of the response. T_H cells collaborate with B cells, providing positive signals for T-dependent humoral responses. $T_{H/I}$ cells also provide positive signals for the generation of effector T cells (T_C, T_D, and T_S). T_S cells, on the other hand, provide negative signals. These signals limit, or inhibit, the development of Ab-producing cells and of T effector cells (T_H, T_C, T_D, and T_S). T_S cells can also prevent suppression (inactivation). Those T_S cells that prevent the inactivation of $T_{H/I}$ cells are called *contrasuppressor* T cells.

Several different T_S cells and suppressor circuits have been described (table 5.5). Some populations of T_S cells are Ag specific, targeting T_H and B cells (T_{S1}) or T_D cells (T_{S3}). Other T_S cells are idiotype specific (T_{S2}), acting on B cells. Ag-specific T_{S1} cells (phenotypically CD8) can bind directly to Ag on T_H and B cells. In addition, T_S cells might carry antiidiotypic determinants that can bind directly to B cells bearing the complementary idiotype. If this occurs, activation

TABLE 5.5 T Suppressor Cell Subpopulations

Subpopulation	Actions on Immune Response
T_{S1}	Causes Ag-specific suppression of cellular and humoral immune responses; blocks activation of T_H or B cells
T_{S2}	Causes idiotype-specific suppression of humoral immune responses; blocks activation of B cells
T_{S3}	Causes Ag-specific suppression of delayed-type hypersensitivity responses; inactivates T_D cells

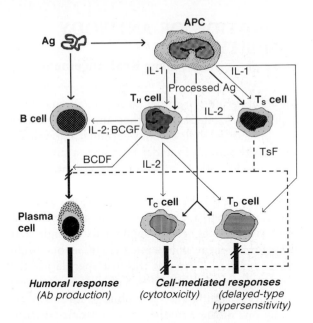

FIGURE 5.15 Regulation of immune responses: an overview. Ag can trigger both humoral and cell-mediated immune responses. Expression of these responses is promoted through the action of cytokines (*thin solid lines*) derived from APCs (IL-1) and T_H cells (IL-2, BCGF, BCDF). In addition, immune responses can be suppressed (*dashed lines* and *hatch marks*) by the products of activated T_S cells (TsF). The final pathway of activation leads not only to specific effector responses (*depicted*) but can lead also to the formation of memory cells (*not shown*).

of B cells is blocked. T_{S3} cells can bind directly to T_D cells causing inactivation. T_S cells release **suppressor factors** (TsF) that promote most of the functions. For most suppressor cells there are no clear-cut MHC restrictions, as exist for T_H, T_C, and T_D cells.

Synopsis

The immune response, then, is regulated by two major classes of factors: positive factors that promote the expression of cellular or humoral immunity and negative factors that diminish or suppress immunological expression. Figure 5.15 presents a schematic outline of some of the interactions involved in modulating the expression of immune responses. This diagram does not presume to illustrate all interactions that exist, but rather intends to highlight major interactions that lead to the expression of cell-mediated or humoral responses to challenging Ag.

Ag binding to mIg on B cells can induce their activation. In addition, processed Ag presented, in MHC-restricted fashion, to T cells can lead to their activation. This interaction with T cells can give a boost to the humoral response (T_H influence on B cell proliferation and differentiation). On the other hand, this interaction between APCs and T cells can ultimately suppress response by stimulation of T_S cells. Moreover, products of the immune response itself can exert negative influence on further expression of a response (e.g., Ab feedback or idiotype network). The presence

of receptors with specificity appropriate to the stimulating Ag dictates which cells can be affected by the Ag. Ir gene products then influence interactions among APCs, T_H, B cells, and T effector cells. In turn, cytokines from these activated cells further modulate cellular behavior and expression following activation. The balance of interactions among these several components of this system ultimately determines the quality and extent of the response evoked.

In addition to foreign Ags, immunological responses can also be triggered by reactions to tissue damage and injury, whether caused by foreign substances or other means. This can be seen in the stimulation of immune responses by complement components (see chapter 6). However, interplay between the immune responses and inflammation is bilateral. Immunological processes can also provoke inflammatory reactions when tissues become damaged (see chapters 8 and 13 for further discussion).

GENERATION OF ANTIBODY DIVERSITY

Theory of Germline Gene Rearrangement

When myeloma proteins (pure Igs) were first sequenced, it became clear that both light (L) and heavy (H) chains varied markedly in their amino-terminal regions, but not in their carboxy-terminal regions. For many it was difficult to understand how a single gene might encode both V regions and constant, or conserved (C), regions of either H or L chains.

In 1965 Dreyer and Bennett proposed that the V and C regions of a single Ig chain might be encoded by two different genes, as opposed to a single gene coding for an entire polypeptide chain, as one might normally expect. This was the first speculation that genes might be "split." They envisioned the possibility that many different V germline genes existed and that any one of these might become associated with a single C region gene at the DNA level. They predicted that these Ab genes were brought together during B cell differentiation. Their proposal became known as a **recombinational germline theory.** Recent studies using a host of methods, including recombinant DNA techniques, have confirmed and extended this hypothesis to permit a rather clear account of the organization and expression of Ig genes, which follows.

Immunoglobulin Genes

Genetic analysis of Ab genes has been carried out by following the inheritance of allotypic, isotypic, and idiotypic markers (described in chapter 3) on Ig molecules. Somatic cell hybridization techniques have been used to determine the chromosomal location of Ig genes.

For example, murine B lymphocytes may be fused to another mammalian cell line to form unstable hybrids, whose chromosomes are randomly lost. The DNA of each hybrid cell line is then probed with radiolabeled complementary, or copy, DNA (cDNA) corresponding to kappa (κ), lambda (λ), or H chain regions for the presence of complementary H or L chain

TABLE 5.6 Organization of Germline Genes For Ig L and H Chains

Chain Class/ Family	Number of Genes for Region			
	V	J	C	D*
L chain				
κ	>200	5	1	–
λ	<100	5	Several	–
H chain	>300	5	3–4†	10–20

*D regions are absent in L chains.

†In H chains, there are three to four C gene domains: γ, α, δ, and μ and ϵ.

Ig genes (fig. 5.16). By correlating loss of a particular mouse chromosome with loss of a particular Ig gene, we can determine the chromosomal location of gene families.

Using this approach, it became clear that *three unlinked families of genes* encode H and L chains and are located **on separate chromosomes.** Each family consists of a cluster of gene segments capable of encoding V regions (V genes) separated from one or more genes capable of encoding C regions (C genes). One of these families in humans encodes H chains (located on chromosome 14); one encodes κ L chains (on chromosome 2); and one encodes λ L chains (on chromosome 22). In the mouse the H, κ, and λ genes are deployed on the twelfth, sixth, and sixteenth chromosomes, respectively. A general summary of these gene families is presented in table 5.6.

Hybridization experiments conducted by **Tonegawa** and others in the 1970s revealed that V region and C region gene segments were separately encoded and located on distinct DNA fragments in embryonic cells, but on the same fragment in mature plasma cells (fig. 5.17). These studies suggested that DNA rearrangements must have occurred during maturation and differentiation of B lymphocytes. These rearranged DNA segments were destined to be expressed as specific monospecific receptors by Ab-forming plasma cells. From the collection of gene segments available in each family, several may be specifically

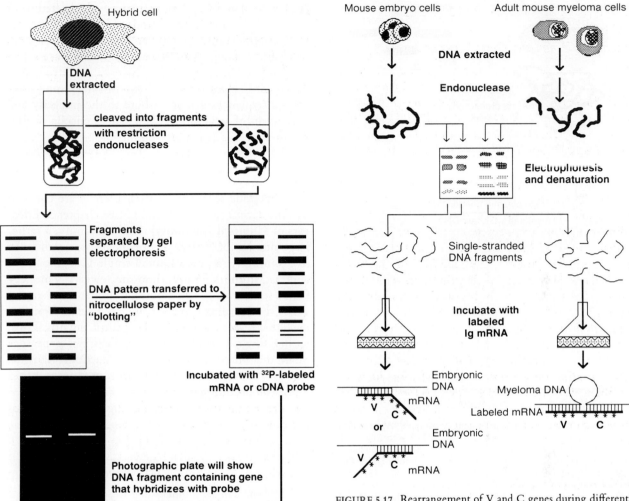

FIGURE 5.16 Southern blotting to detect Ig genes. Extracted DNA, from a hybrid cell line, was cleaved into fragments with restriction enzymes. DNA fragments were separated, according to size, by gel electrophoresis and denatured to form single-stranded DNA molecules. A replica of the DNA fragments in the gel was made by blotting gel to nitrocellulose paper. A radiolabeled probe of mRNA (or cDNA), known to encode λ, κ, or H Ig chains, was then allowed to hybridize with complementary DNA, if present. Autoradiographs permit detection of Ig genes of hybrid cells that hybridize with the radiolabeled probe.

FIGURE 5.17 Rearrangement of V and C genes during differentiation. Extracted germline DNA (from mouse embryos) and differentiated DNA (from myeloma cells) were cleaved with restriction enzymes. Fragments were separated by electrophoresis, denatured to yield single-stranded fragments, and extracted. Fragments were hybridized with κ chain radiolabeled probes (mRNA), derived from myeloma cells. The entire mRNA molecule (encoding V and C regions) or only the 3' half of mRNA (encoding the C region) was employed. Results showed that mRNA for Ig L chain hybridized to germline DNA by its V region to one DNA fragment and by its C region to a totally separate DNA fragment. In contrast, the same mRNA hybridized to both V and C regions in a single DNA fragment from fully differentiated cells.

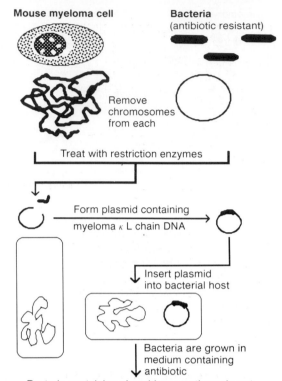

Mouse myeloma cell

Bacteria (antibiotic resistant)

Remove chromosomes from each

Treat with restriction enzymes

Form plasmid containing myeloma κ L chain DNA

Insert plasmid into bacterial host

Bacteria are grown in medium containing antibiotic

Bacteria containing plasmid grow, others do not
(have antibiotic-resistant gene and κ L chain gene);
cloning of these bacteria leads to amplification of κ L chain gene

FIGURE 5.18 Cloning of specific Ig genes. Mouse DNA (from myeloma cells producing κ L chains) and plasmid DNA were "cut" with restriction enzymes to form cohesive ends. (A plasmid is an autonomously replicating piece of extrachromosomal circular DNA. Plasmids will reproduce in many bacteria.) The κ L chain gene was inserted into a plasmid containing an antibiotic-resistance marker, with a ligase enzyme. Susceptible bacteria were then artificially transformed with the hybrid plasmids, which reproduce along with the bacteria. Bacterial cells containing recombinant DNA molecules were selected, based on their ability to grow in media containing the antibiotic.

joined to encode an entire Ig chain, L or H, as described below. It should be noted that genes of one family are never intermingled with genes of either of the other families.

With the advent of recombinant DNA technology, it became possible to clone specific Ig genes (fig. 5.18). Sufficient quantities of specific DNA segments could be obtained, permitting analysis of their organization. Studies of DNA sequence showed that discontinuous segments existed that did not code for peptides. Some noncoding segments were deleted from the DNA before transcription and others from the mRNA after transcription. Intervening sequences deleted before transcription became known as spacers, and those deleted after transcription are called introns. Expressed sequences are named exons. Intervening noncoding sequences can contribute to the integrity and expression of structural genes, which encode chains, but their role is essentially unknown.

Light Chain Gene Organization

Three peptide segments in each L chain are encoded by *three distinct genes,* V, J, and C (see chapter 3, Effectors of Humoral Immunity). In the κ family, a rather large number of V gene segments are separated from five joining (J) segments and a single C segment. By contrast, in the λ family, there are fewer V gene segments (only two in the mouse), a similar number of J genes, but several C genes. V and J gene segments encode V regions and C genes encode C regions. Thus, each L chain is encoded by three distinct gene segments that must be joined to form a functional Ab gene.

Joining of Gene Segments

During the process of differentiation of a pluripotent stem cell into a mature Ag-reactive B cell, DNA rearrangements take place. Within the κ family, for example, *one of the many V gene segments will become joined directly to one of the J gene segments.* Subsequently, this *V-J segment will be joined to the C segment* to create a **functional Ab gene** (fig. 5.19). The joining of these segments is brought about through the activity of recombinase enzymes, discovered in 1989 by David Baltimore and colleagues. DNA between the V and J segments being joined is excised and lost during this rearrangement.

Each germline V_κ gene contains a region encoding the V segment and a leader sequence (designated as "L" in figs. 5.19–5.22, and 5.24). The leader sequence encodes a "leader peptide" that controls passage of new protein products across the rough endoplasmic reticulum. The leader peptide is cleaved and removed before the Ig molecule is secreted. The *V segment* (second exon) encodes the first 95 N-terminal amino acids of the V region of the Ig L chain. The *J*

Tailor-Made Monoclonal Antibodies

T he pioneering work of Kohler and Milstein in producing hybridomas has given rise to entirely new areas of immunodiagnosis and immunotherapeutics. It is now possible to produce monoclonal antibodies (MAbs) for use as probes and as potential therapeutic agents. However, there are numerous technical problems that make production of therapeutic human MAbs generally unsatisfactory. On the other hand, murine MAbs can be more readily produced. But therapeutic use of murine MAbs also has its shortcomings. In particular, since murine MAbs are foreign proteins to a human recipient, they can stimulate Ab production.

A means of circumventing this problem has been developed. Recombinant DNA technology and transfection have been combined to enable Ig genes to be manipulated so that Abs can be "tailor-made."

Through these procedures, desired Ig genes, from mice or humans, can be isolated, cloned, and recombined. The tailor-made genes can then be inserted into suitable vectors and transfected into myelomas. The resulting products have been called **transfectomas.**

For example, V regions of mouse Ig genes can be removed and spliced to C region human Ig genes. These are next inserted into a plasmid and are inserted into a suitable bacterial host. The copies of mouse-human H chain plasmid are then transfected into myeloma cells that are not normally producing Ig. New chimeric Ig molecules, with murine V and human C domains, are synthesized and secreted. These chimeric MAbs can be administered to human hosts.

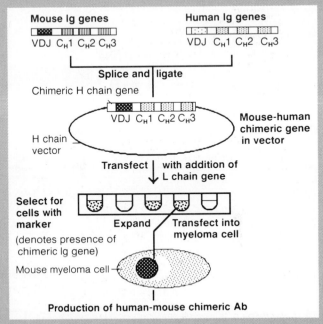

FIGURE 5.A Producing hybrid Abs.

Aguila, H. L., Pollock, R. B., Spiro, G., et al. The production of more useful monoclonal antibodies. *Immunology Today* **7**:381, 1986.

Boulianne, G. L., Hozumi, N., and Shulman, M. J. Production of functional chimeric mouse/human antibody. *Nature* **312**:643, 1984.

segments, consisting of five alternative forms, encode the remaining 12 or more amino acids of V region L chains. All segments are separated by short introns. In contrast, the single C region is preceded by a long intervening sequence.

As a result of this rearrangement, a transcriptional promoter site for the gene (which lies upstream [5'] to the leader sequence) is brought within activational distance of an enhancer region found within major introns of L chain loci. Both the promoter (where RNA polymerase actually initiates transcription) and the enhancers contain clusters of sequence elements (octanucleotides) that constitute binding sites for nuclear proteins that can recruit RNA polymerase to the region. Activated enhancer permits transcription of the rearranged gene. During primary transcription, V and J segments remain separated from the C segment (by perhaps 2.5 kilobase pairs). In addition, a gap (0.2 kilobase pairs) occurs between the leader sequence and the V-J exon. These intervening sequences are removed

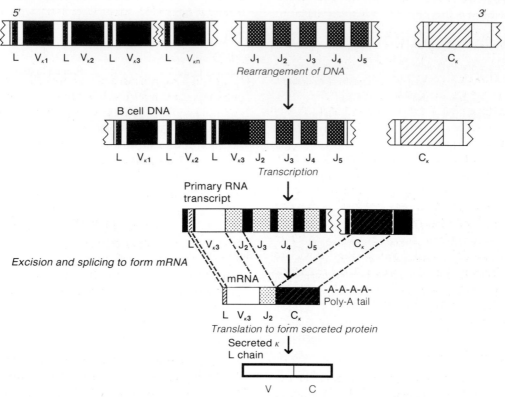

FIGURE 5.19 Recombination of V-J gene segments. During differentiation of pluripotent stem cells, one of the five alternative J segments, for example J_2, becomes joined to one of the several hundred V segments, for example $V_{\kappa 3}$. The rearranged genes are still separated by introns in the primary transcript. The intervening sequences are then removed by RNA splicing, and functional mRNA is formed for translation and subsequent secretion of κ L chains.

from the primary gene transcript by a splicing process, enabling the leader sequence, V-J exon, and C exon to be joined. With the formation of a functional mRNA, translation of a complete L chain can occur.

Recognition Signals for V-J Joining

Analysis of DNA sequences has revealed that a set of conserved nucleotides border germline V and J segments. These special sequences of DNA occur at the site where V-J fusion takes place and may provide recognition signals to facilitate the joining process.

After each V_κ segment is a heptamer with an identical sequence (5′ CACAGTG 3′), followed by a spacer of 11 or 12 nucleotides of unconserved sequence. The spacer is followed by a nonanucleotide (5′ ACAAAAACC 3′), or its analogue. Preceding the J segments there are two *signal sequences* complementary to those following the V segments. First, a nonanucleotide (5′ GGTTTTTGT 3′) occurs, then a spacer of 23 or 24 nucleotides, which is followed by the heptanucleotide (5′ CACTGTG 3′). When two segments can join, one always has a 11- or 12-nucleotide-long spacer between its conserved heptanucleotide and nonanucleotide, while the other has a 23- or 24-nucleotide-long spacer.

Interestingly, the lengths of the spacers between the heptamers and the nonamers correspond to one (11 base pairs) or two (23 base pairs) turns of the

DNA helix. The conserved, inverted complementary sequences are believed to provide *recognition signals* for joining a V_κ segment to a J_κ segment. Several models have been proposed to explain the recognition process, which involve recently described recombining enzymes controlled by a recombination activating gene. These models suggest that *melding of a single V and J segment results in the loss of intervening sequences,* as well as all V and J segments in between, *by an excision or a looping-out process.*

Stem and loop models for this process are depicted in figure 5.20. In the stem model (fig. 5.20*a*), it is proposed that the two heptamers and the two nonamers base pair forming a stem. Although this does not occur in the loop model (fig. 5.20*b*), the heptamers and nonamers are believed to provide recognition sequences, which might serve as binding sites for endonucleases that mediate the process. Advocates submit that a binding enzyme could adhere to both recognition signals, drawing together the ends to be spliced and excising the stem or the loop (fig. 5.21).

Nonuniform Recombinations

Amino acid sequences of L_V chain domains can be predicted if the nucleotide sequences of the V and J regions are known. However, when corresponding L chains were actually sequenced, greater variability was observed at the position where V-J joining took place than was expected. It became clear that the precise site at which V and J gene segments join can vary somewhat, relative to the heptamer-nonamer recognition sequences. As a consequence, several different nucleotide sequences can be generated at the junction of the V and J segments involving the codon for the ninety-sixth amino acid. Thus, different, or additional, amino acids can be generated at this position. Since the ninety-sixth amino acid lies within the third hypervariable region, or CDR3 (see chapter 3, Effectors of Humoral Immunity) this amino acid contributes to Ab diversity. Accordingly, junctional diversity can contribute significantly to the generation of Ab diversity. Although there may be a number of variable functional rearrangements of V and J gene segments due to joining flexibility, not all rearrangements are productive. A correct reading frame must be preserved and, if not, a termination codon may be generated giving rise to nonfunctional lymphocytes.

Allelic Exclusion

Nearly 70% of human Abs and over 95% of mouse Abs carry κ chains. Apparently κ genes are rearranged first and, only when such arrangements are unproductive, is the λ family rearranged. This may explain the predominance of κ chains in Abs produced by either species. In any event, Ab-producing B cells, or plasma cells, *rearrange only one effective V-J recombination during differentiation* from the pluripotent stem cell. The B lymphocyte expresses either the maternal or paternal copy of its two inherited L chain alleles, never both. After functional rearrangements have occurred, enzymes responsible for the rearrangements are apparently turned off by termination signals. In this regard, mature B cells possess unexpressed L chain genes in unrearranged germline configuration.

Multiple V_κ Genes

Multiple germline V_κ genes exist as sets of genes within the family. The mouse κ gene family may have over 300 V_κ gene segments, which may, as earlier noted, join during B cell differentiation with any of the four functional J_κ segments ($J_{\kappa 3}$ acts as a pseudogene). This, therefore, may permit a minimum of 1,200 recombination possibilities and, of course, as many antigenically distinct chains to be formed.

The V gene repertoire, for the κ gene family in humans, is also estimated to be in the hundreds, but with five functional J_κ joining regions rather than four. There are fewer V genes in the human λ family and only two in the mouse. Collectively, however, these gene rearrangements contribute dramatically to L chain variability and, as such, to Ab diversity.

Heavy Chain Variable Region Diversity

H chain diversity is generated by mechanisms quite similar to those previously described for L chains. Here, too, there are many V genes in the H chain gene family (perhaps over 300), which may encode the leader and

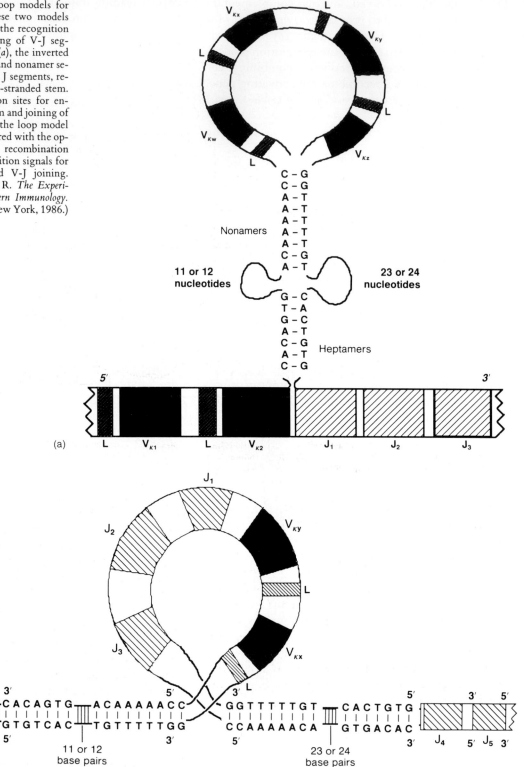

FIGURE 5.20 Stem and loop models for V_L-J_L recombination. These two models have been used to explain the recognition process involved in melding of V-J segments. In the stem model (*a*), the inverted complementary and nonamer sequences, next to the V and J segments, recombine to form a double-stranded stem. This establishes recognition sites for enzymatic excision of the stem and joining of the V and C segments. In the loop model (*b*), each strand remains paired with the opposite strand, permitting recombination enzymes to bind to recognition signals for excision of the loop and V-J joining. (Adapted from Clark, W. R. *The Experimental Foundations of Modern Immunology.* John Wiley & Sons, Inc., New York, 1986.)

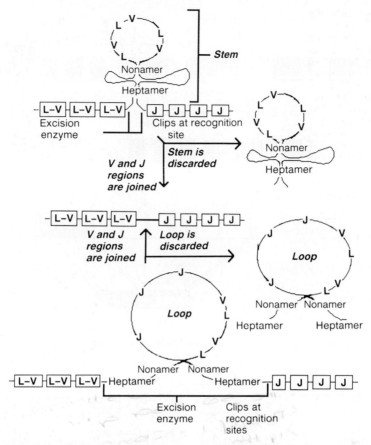

FIGURE 5.21 Recognition sequences act as sites for binding protein. Recognition sequences for joining V-J segments serve as binding sites for excision/recombination proteins. Enzymes may adhere to both recognition signals, drawing them together for splicing and excising the stem or loop.

the main region to the ninety-fifth residue, as seen for L chains. There are also a number of functional J_H segments (four in mice, five in humans), which may encode part of the CDR3 and all of the last framework region (FR4) described for L chains. The process is, however, somewhat more complex, since 10 to 20 short DNA segments, known as D, or diversity, segments (see chapter 3, Effectors of Humoral Immunity), are located between the V_H and J_H segments. D segments encode two to 14 amino acids in the third hypervariable region, or complementarity region 3 (CDR3), and, therefore, are critically involved in determining the specificity of an Ab.

Joining of V_H-D_H-J_H Genes

Diversity segments are flanked on each side by the same heptamer and nonamer signal sequences separated by one turn spacers of 11 base pairs as described for V-J segments in L chains. Mechanisms for joining three H chain gene segments are similar to those proposed for L chains (fig. 5.22; compare with fig. 5.19). To form a functional H chain gene, *one D segment, randomly selected, is first joined to a J_H segment*. Then a *second DNA recombination event joins a V_H to the D-J_H segment*. As with L chain genes, each V exon has a promoter followed by a leader peptide adjacent to each V exon. In addition, there is an enhancer (a conserved octamer) in

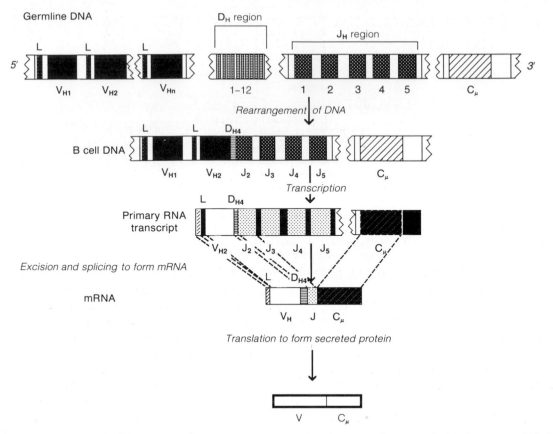

FIGURE 5.22 Recombination of V_H-D_H-J_H segments. During differentiation of pluripotent stem cells, a D_H segment, J_H segment, and V segment, in this example D_{H4}, J_{H2}, and V_{H2}, become joined. The rearranged genes are then transcribed (primary transcript). A second transcription follows, whereby introns are removed and mRNA is formed and translated into specific Ig H chains.

the intron between the J and C segments. Following the second DNA rearrangement, the promoter of the chosen V segment is brought nearer (within two kilobase pairs) the enhancer (a conserved octamer, ATGCAAAT). This strategy apparently activates the enhancer, leading to an enhanced level of gene expression.

These gene segments obviously contribute significantly to the generation of hypervariability in the V regions. When three segments of DNA randomly join to encode the entire H chain V region, they enhance the recombination possibilities. Thus, if there were 300 V_H, 12 D, and four alternative J gene segments, and one of each becomes randomly associated during differentiation, 14,400 different chains could be formed ($300 \times 12 \times 4$). However, there is apparently a greater chance of incorrect assembly of V-D-J segments, resulting in nonproductivity, than in the assembly of V-J sequences in L chains. It is of interest, in this regard, that the first DNA rearrangements in the differentiation of stem cells into mature B cells is the assembly of H chain genes. Nevertheless, it is only after both chains are expressed in the cytoplasm that complete Ab molecules appear.

Nonuniform Recombinations

Germline V, D, and J gene segments may not join at exact splice points, as noted for L chain genes (V and J). Each of the genes may use several frames of

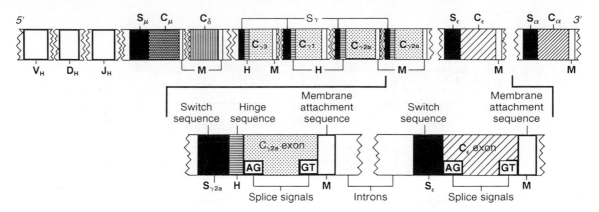

FIGURE 5.23 Arrangement of genes encoding C_H chains. C region genes are arranged over six kilobases downstream (3') from the recombined V-D-J segment. Each C gene, except that for δ, has an upstream (5') S sequence next to it. δ genes may use the same S sequence as the μ gene.

recombination, thereby producing several amino acid sequences from a single gene and, thus, generating further Ab diversity. In H chains additional sequence diversity is created at the V-D and D-J junctions by enzymatic introduction of bases, called N sequences, which are not in the germline. Consequently, flexibility of V-D-J joining is expected to contribute significantly to the generation of Ab diversity.

Heavy Chain Constant Gene Organization

Constant Region Genes

H chains have three (γ, α, and δ) or five (μ and ε) C domains (C_H), as previously described. Each isotype and homology region is encoded by genes separated by intervening sequences or introns. Thus, C_H genes are composed of multiple exons in contrast to L chain constant domain (C_L) genes. Interestingly, all of the *different classes and subclasses of Igs use the same set of V region genes*. Thus, if the class or subclass is changed, only the C region is switched. This was first suspected from sequence studies of IgM and IgG Abs from multiple myeloma patients, which exhibited identical V regions. Moreover, when IgM and IgD are displayed on a B lymphocyte membrane simultaneously, they exhibit the same Ag specificity, suggesting possession of identical V regions.

The C_H exons are arranged in a definite pattern downstream (3') from the J gene segments along the DNA chain (fig. 5.23). Upstream (5') to the μ gene is a switch (S) sequence, or recombination site, which is repeated 5' to all of the other C region genes, with the exception of the δ segment. It appears that all Ig H chain isotypes are synthesized in two forms, membrane and secreted. Accordingly, each C_H segment at its 3' end possesses one or more exons (labeled "M" in fig. 5.23) that code for a hydrophobic C terminus that anchors membrane-bound Abs to the membrane.

Rearranged DNA segments are assembled by RNA splicing and removal of intervening sequences. Donor (GT) and acceptor (AG) splice signals at the ends of intervening sequences are required for RNA splicing and, if absent, a gene segment may be nonfunctional.

Membrane-Bound and Secreted Immunoglobulin

All classes of Ig can be synthesized in membrane-anchored or secreted form, as a result of differential RNA processing. Each form has identical amino acid sequences up to their carboxyl termini, where they diverge. The last 41 amino acid residues of the membrane-bound forms are replaced by 20 different amino acid residues in the secreted form.

IgM, for example, exists either as a monomeric membrane receptor (m) on B lymphocytes or in pentameric form, which is secreted (s). The $C_μ$ gene contains both the complete $μ_s$ sequence and an additional separated coding segment containing the

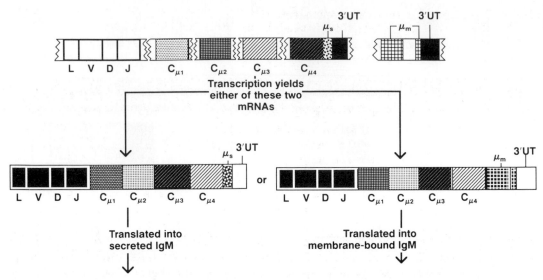

FIGURE 5.24 Formation of secreted and membrane-bound IgM. A single C region locus, encoded by C_μ domains 1, 2, 3, and 4, can form secreted or membrane-bound C_μ chains. A single exon, for either the secreted or membrane terminus, is spliced during the primary transcription process to the $C_{\mu 4}$ domain. Two forms of mRNA, identical except for the μ_m or μ_s sequences, are then translated into membrane-bound IgM or secreted IgM.

μ_m-specific membrane-anchoring sequence. During processing of μ transcripts, either the μ membrane (μ_m) sequence is selected and spliced to the $C_{\mu 4}$ domain to make μ_m mRNA or the μ secreted (μ_s) sequence is chosen to make μ_s mRNA (fig. 5.24). Binding of Ag to membrane IgM brings about alteration in RNA processing and the production of the secreted form of IgM. However, how this occurs remains unclear.

The nucleotides 5′ to the $C_{\mu 4}$ secreted terminus are GT and the two nucleotides 5′ to the beginning of the M exon are Ag, making an RNA splice site. Twenty hydrophilic carboxy-terminal amino acids of the μ_s chain are encoded by a short μ_s gene segment contiguous with the $C_{\mu 4}$ exon. Two exons located approximately 1,850 base pairs to the 3′ side of the $C_{\mu 4}$ domain encode the 41 amino acid residues of the hydrophobic membrane portion of the μ_m chain.

Alternative production of a μ_m versus a μ_s mRNA can be controlled by the site of transcription termination and the addition of poly-A to one of the two alternative sites. When polyadenylation occurs at the site immediately downstream from the $C_{\mu 4}$ segment, μ_s mRNA is produced. On the other hand, if the transcript is extended to the poly-A site immediately downstream from the μ_m exons, then RNA splicing produces μ_m RNA.

Heavy Chain Class Switching

During differentiation from pluripotent stem cells, B lymphocytes reach a stage, while still immature, when they produce surface IgM. Somewhat later, they produce both surface IgM and IgD and subsequently become capable of switching to the production of IgG, IgA, or IgE. When a B lymphocyte reacts with an Ag, its differentiating progeny may switch from producing one Ab class or subclass to another so that the resulting clone of cells gives rise to several different H chain isotypes. Significantly, each of these H chain classes may be successively associated with the same V_H genes on the same chromosome within a given cell. There are two mechanisms of class switching: one mechanism involving differential RNA splicing and the other DNA recombination.

The first mechanism of class switching is limited to shifting from IgM to IgD. In giving rise to Ig H chains, a given V-D-J exon might be joined to a C region of any class—for IgM, this class is μ. Mature Ag-reactive lymphocytes, prior to activation, express

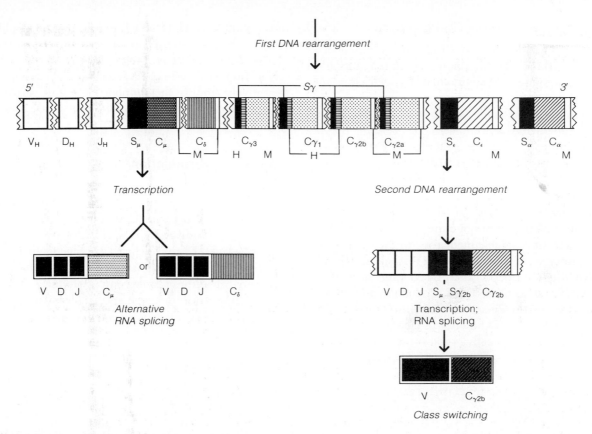

First DNA rearrangement

5′   Sγ   3′

V_H D_H J_H S_μ C_μ C_δ $C_{\gamma3}$ $C_{\gamma1}$ $C_{\gamma2b}$ $C_{\gamma2a}$ S_ϵ C_ϵ S_α C_α

M   H   M   H   M   M   M

Transcription

Second DNA rearrangement

V   D   J C_μ or   V   D   J C_δ

V   D   J S_μ $S_{\gamma2b}$ $C_{\gamma2b}$

Alternative
RNA splicing

Transcription;
RNA splicing

V $C_{\gamma2b}$

Class switching

FIGURE 5.25 H chain class switching. δ Genes can use the same S signal as μ (S_μ) genes. Either C_μ or C_δ, or both, can be produced by alternative RNA splicing (depicted in *left panel*). Subsequently, a B cell can switch to another H chain class, for example γ 2b, by a second DNA rearrangement (*right panel*). All introns are removed by RNA splicing.

both membrane-bound IgM and IgD. This means that some V-D-J segments have joined to C regions for class μ, while other segments have joined to C regions for class δ. Since exons encoding C_δ lie downstream from C_μ exon, differential RNA splicing in long transcripts enables the C_δ exon to be used in place of C_μ for translation of H chains.

Switching to Ig classes other than IgD involves recombination in the switch regions of the H chain C region genes. This type of class switching involves a rearrangement of an assembled V_H-D_H-J_H gene from its original position upstream of C_μ to a site upstream to one of the other C_H genes (fig. 5.25). In this process, the enhancer element remains in the same location relative to the gene's transcriptional promoter that it occupied before the switch took place. This mechanism for Ig class switching is predominantly ac-companied by deletion of genes 5′ to the expressed C_H gene. Therefore, in perhaps most instances, once a cell has switched to a particular Ig class it can no longer switch back to another class encoded upstream to the expressed isotype. However, exceptions have been noted. In these instances, it is believed that genes are not deleted.

Sequence analyses of DNA have shown that homologous switch sites are located two or three kilo-base pairs upstream, or on the 5′ side, of each C region which mediate the switching process. These are composed of tandemly arranged short repetitive units composed of base pair repeats (e.g., GAGCT and GGGT for the switch site 5′ to the C_μ gene). It is thought that the repetitive nature of the switch regions displayed in front of each C region gene may promote homologous recombinations.

Regulation of Heavy Chain Class Expression

It has been known for some time that T_H lymphocytes may determine the Ab isotype produced during an immune response. An individual T_{H2} cell clone may provide the signals for the expression of multiple isotypes by B cells. If Ag-activated B lymphocytes are simultaneously stimulated by certain isotype-determining T cell clones, then preferential production of a particular Ab class may occur.

Evidence from clonal population studies suggests that T cells may either select B cells precommitted to one isotype or directly induce isotype switching. Whether or not a single T cell clone might produce distinct soluble mediators for the induction of each isotype is unknown. Nevertheless, T cell–derived IL-4 (formerly called B cell stimulating factor or BCGF) can enhance IgG1 production and suppress production of IgG2b and IgG3. Although the mechanisms are largely unknown, it is clear that cloned T_H cells can signal B cells, promoting either heterogeneous or restrictive expression of H chain isotypes.

PRODUCTION OF DIVERSE ANTIBODIES

Our immune system, and those of other mammals, may actually produce 10^8 to 10^{10} different kinds of Ab molecules. The enormous Ab repertoire generated affords each individual with a preformed capability to respond to an antigenic universe. A variety of mechanisms contribute to such impressive diversity.

Somatic Recombination and Junctional Diversity

Combinatorial joining of a small number of germline genes, coupled with the flexibility of joining sites between segments, can serve as the major contributors to Ab diversity. Apparently, only a few germline Ig genes account for a large number of structurally distinct L and H chains. Since any L chain may randomly pair with any H chain, a large number of different Ag-specific Abs may be generated from a very small pool of germline genes. Assuming, for example, 1,200 different L chain (300 V × 4 J) and 14,400 different H chain (300 V × 12 D × 4 J) possibilities, it would be possible, by random pairing, to produce approximately 1.7×10^7 (1,200 L × 14,400 H) different Ab molecules. Imprecise joining of gene segments could conservatively amplify this number 10-fold, if variability of only two different amino acids is assumed for each junction.

Somatic Hypermutation

Extensive somatic mutation of V region genes can follow their rearrangement in the B lymphocyte. Direct evidence for the occurrence of point mutations as contributors to Ab diversity was provided by Tonegawa and colleagues. They sequenced a V gene segment from a mouse myeloma (designated H2020) λ L chain, and compared it with an embryonic germline λ L chain. The mature myeloma gene segment was found to be identical to the embryonic germline gene segment, with the exception of two base changes. Comparison of the amino acid sequence in the gene products showed that they differed by two residues, as a result of the base changes. This is of interest since recently it has been shown that a single amino acid substitution in a complementarity-determining region (CDR) can cause a very substantial increase in Ab affinity. (See chapter 5 for details.)

Further evidence for somatic hypermutation has been derived in part from studies of families of MAb generated in response to a single Ag in a single animal. Large numbers of closely related Ab were generated in the course of the immune response. Using hybridoma technology, these Abs were deduced to be the products of a single Ab-forming B cell clone. Analysis of the nucleic acid sequences encoding the MAbs produced confirmed that rearranged H and L chain V region genes accumulate large numbers of base changes during the course of the immune response.

The process of somatic mutation can be triggered when B cells expressing low-affinity Ab receptors are activated by Ag. Following Ag binding, the B cell can terminally differentiate into an IgM-secreting plasma cell. Alternatively, it might undergo class switching and secrete a new class of Ig. On the other hand, if the B cell did not fully differentiate following interaction with Ag, it might become a memory cell. The memory cell might be the primary target cell for the hypermutation of rearranged L and H V genes.

Milstein and coworkers showed that IgM and IgG made during the first seven days after immunization did not exhibit somatic mutations. However, Abs made 14 or more days after exposure to Ag displayed significant numbers of base changes. It is believed that the process of somatic mutation is continuously active during cell division. However, all of the base changes do not arise during a single cell division, but rather occur sequentially during successive cell divisions. Estimates of mutation rates of 10^{-3} to 10^{-4} changes per base pair may occur in a cell division (based on the assumption that cells are doubling every 17 to 18 hours), providing maximal sequence diversity. The high rate of somatic mutation appears to act concomitantly on the H and L chain V regions expressed initially in response to Ag. Somatic mutation may cease as the B cell differentiates into a plasma cell that is secreting Ab. Thus, the frequency of mutations in the V region of dividing myeloma or hybridoma cells is very low. Ab with increasingly higher affinities may be formed as progressive somatic mutations occur. These Abs exhibit an "improved fit" for the Ag. Cells displaying high-affinity Igs as membrane receptors are selectively stimulated by Ag to proliferate and differentiate.

Hypermutation certainly generates additional Ab diversity. Many now believe that generation of high-affinity Abs depends largely on somatic hypermutation of rearranged germline Ig V region genes. This is called affinity maturation, and it occurs in B cells following Ag activation.

S U M M A R Y

1. The primary humoral response following antigen challenge is characterized by a lag (delay) phase, an exponential rise in antibody concentration, a plateau, and a phase of antibody decline. IgM is the initial immunoglobulin isotype followed by switching to another immunoglobulin class, usually IgG. [p. 117]

2. The secondary humoral response to immunogen is more rapid and pronounced because of memory cells generated during the primary response. In addition, antibodies formed in a secondary response have higher affinity for antigen than those derived in a primary response. They are almost entirely IgG. [pp. 117–119]

3. Two forms of B cell differentiation are recognized: antigen independent and antigen dependent. Antigen-independent differentiation leads to the production of antigen-responsive cells, while antigen-dependent differentiation gives rise to antibody-producing cells. [pp. 119–120]

4. T-independent antigens are usually polymeric antigens that are capable of activating B cells without interaction with T helper cells and antigen-presenting cells. [p. 120]

5. During activation, a variety of intracellular changes can be observed in lymphocytes. These include (a) metabolic changes, providing second messengers for transduction of extracellular signals into intracellular responses; (b) membrane changes, as exemplified by expression of lymphokine surface receptors and increased expression of MHC molecules; and (c) nuclear changes, leading to proliferation and specific expression (e.g., antibody or lymphokine production). [pp. 120–122]

6. Activation by T-dependent antigens includes participation of B cells, antigen-presenting cells, and T helper cells. Distinct determinants on antigen is used to activate B cells and T cells. B cells recognize epitopes in the nonprocessed antigen, while T cells recognize epitopes after processing by antigen-presenting cells. Both antigen-presenting cells and T cells provide cytokines that promote and modulate differentiation of activated B cells. [pp. 122–125]

7. Activated B cells can proliferate and differentiate into either (a) antibody-producing plasma cells or (b) long-lived memory cells. Differentiation into active plasma cells during primary humoral responses often is associated with switching in

the class of immunoglobulin produced. How soon after activation this occurs can affect antibody affinity (early class switching is associated with low affinity, whereas late switching is associated with high-affinity antibody). Differentiation into memory cells provides a population upon which secondary humoral responses depend. [pp. 126–127]

8. Humoral immune responses are regulated by numerous factors. The most significant regulators are immune response (Ir) genes, antibody, and immune complexes produced in response to antigen, idiotype networks, T_S cells, and the neuroendocrine system. [p. 127]

9. Some immune response genes are part of the MHC. These genes act at the stage when antigen is presented to the T cell. The genetically determined binding site of the MHC molecule plays a critical role in determining whether or not a response occurs. [pp. 128–129]

10. Formed antibody and immune complexes, with low antibody-antigen ratios, can down-regulate a humoral response by preventing antigen binding to receptors or by crosslinking antigen and Fc receptors. [pp. 129–130]

11. Antiidiotypic antibodies can activate lymphocytes by crosslinking antigen receptors. Alternatively, they might inhibit activation by crosslinking antigen and Fc receptors. Which result is produced might be related to the binding affinity of the Fc receptor for the Fc region of one isotype over another. [pp. 131–132]

12. T_S cells can be antigen specific or idiotype specific. They provide negative signals that limit, or inhibit, the development of antibody-producing cells and T effector cells, respectively. [pp. 132–133]

13. Each human being produces virtually millions of different kinds of antibodies, which are displayed as monospecific receptors on B lymphocytes. These antibodies are produced by three unlinked families of immunoglobulin genes, which encode heavy and light chains (κ and λ) and are located on separate chromosomes (14, 2, and 22, respectively in humans). [pp. 134–136]

14. Each light chain is encoded by three distinct gene segments designated V (variable), J (joining), and C (constant). Joining of V and J segments takes place during the process of differentiation of a pluripotent cell into a mature antigen-reactive B lymphocyte. When V-J segments are transcribed, they become joined to a C segment by a process known as splicing to form functional mRNA, permitting translation of a complete light chain. [pp. 136–138]

15. Recognition signals for V-J joining may serve as binding sites for recombining proteins that mediate the process. They consist of a set of conserved nucleotides that border germline V and J segments at the site where V-J fusion occurs. Flexibility in the precise site of V-J joining may contribute significantly to antibody diversity due to nonuniform recombinations. [pp. 138–139]

16. B cells, destined to become plasma cells, rearrange only one effective V-J recombination during differentiation from the pluripotent stem cell. Allelic exclusion restricts expression to either the maternal or paternal copy of its light chain alleles. [p. 139]

17. Any one of the multiple germline V_κ genes may join any one of the four functional J genes. This permits a large number of recombination possibilities, and an equally large number of antigenically distinct light chains may be formed. [p. 139]

18. Heavy chain diversity is generated by mechanisms quite similar to those observed for light chains. The process is somewhat more complex, however, since 10 to 20 short DNA segments, known as D (diversity) segments, are located between the V and J segments. The recombination possibilities are accordingly much greater. [pp. 138–143]

19. Heavy chain constant genes are composed of multiple exons that encode the three or four constant domains. C_H genes are arranged in a definite pattern downstream from the J segments, and each is preceded by a switch region with the exception of the δ segment. [p. 143]

20. All heavy chain classes are synthesized in two forms, membrane and secreted. A C_H gene contains both the complete class sequence and an additional separated coding segment containing the membrane-anchoring segment. During processing of transcripts either sequence is selected and spliced to the C_H 3 or 4 domain to make the appropriate mRNA. [pp. 143–144]

21. Class switching may occur during differentiation of pluripotent stem cells and following antigen stimulation of mature B lymphocytes. It involves a rearrangement of an assembled V-D-J gene from its original position in front of C_μ to a site upstream of one of the other C_H genes. Regulation of heavy chain class switching is regulated by factors produced by T_H cells. [pp. 144–146]

22. Diversity of Ig chains is generated by combinatorial joining of a small number of germline genes, nonuniform joining of variable region segments, and the occurrence of somatic hypermutations. Since any light chain may randomly pair with any heavy chain, an enormous number of diverse antibody molecules are produced. [pp. 146–147]

READINGS

Abas, A. K. A reassessment of the mechanisms of antigen-specific T-cell-dependent B-cell activation. *Immunology Today* **9**:89, 1988.

Akira, S., Okazaki, K., and Sakano, H. Two pairs of recombination signals are sufficient to cause immunoglobulin V-(D)-J joining. *Science* **238**:1134, 1987.

Baltimore, D. Gene conversion: Some implications for immunoglobulin genes. *Cell* **24**:592, 1981.

Callard, R., and Turner, M. Cytokines and Ig switching: evolutionary divergence between mice and humans. *Immunology Today* **11**:200, 1990.

Cambier, J. Lymphocyte subsets and activation. *Current Opinion in Immunology* **1**:220, 1988.

Clark, E. A., and Lane, P. J. L. Regulation of human B-cell activation and adhesion. *Annual Review of Immunology* 9:97, 1991.

French, D., Laskov, R., and Scharef, M. The role of somatic hypermutation in the generation of antibody diversity. *Science* **244**:1152, 1989.

Gordon, J., and Guy, G. R. The molecules controlling B lymphocytes. *Immunology Today* **8**:339, 1987.

Hozumi, N., and Tonegawa, S. Evidence for somatic rearrangement of immunoglobulin genes coding for variable and constant regions. *Proceedings of the National Academy of Science* (USA) **73**:3628, 1976.

Huse, W., Sastry, L., Iverson, S., et al. Generation of a large combinatorial library of the immunoglobulin repertoire in phage lambda. *Science* **226**:1275, 1989.

Jerne, N. K. Towards a network theory of the immune system. *Annals of Immunology* (Pasteur Inst.) **125C**:373, 1974.

Katz, D. D. Antigen presentation, antigen-presenting cells and antigen processing. *Current Opinion in Immunology* **1**:213, 1988.

Lanzavecchia, A. Antigen-specific interaction between T and B cells. *Nature* **11**:537, 1985.

Marx, J. Key piece found for immunology puzzle? *Science* **246**:1561, 1989.

Meek, K. Analysis of junctional diversity during B lymphocyte development. *Science* **250**:820, 1990.

Neuberger, M., and Cook, G. The expression of immunoglobulin genes. *Immunology Today* **69**:278, 1988.

Oettinger, M. A., Schatz, D. G., Gorka, C., et al. RAG-1 and RAG-2, adjacent genes that synergistically activate V(D)J recombination. *Science* **248**:1517, 1990.

Ritter, M., and Larché, M. T and B cell ontogeny and phylogeny. *Current Opinion in Immunology* **1**:203, 1988.

Rooijen, N. Direct intrafollicular differentiation of memory B cells into plasma cells. *Immunology Today* **11**:154, 1990.

Schwartz, R. Immune response (Ir) genes of the murine MHC. In *Advances in Immunology* (Vol. **38**). Academic Press, New York, 1986.

Shiiba, K., Stohl, W., Gray, J. D., et al. A novel role for accessory cells in T-cell-dependent B cell differentiation. *Cellular Immunology* **127:**458, 1990.

Sinclair, N. R., and Panoskaltsis, A. Antibody response and its regulation. *Current Opinion in Immunology* **1:**228, 1988.

Staudt, L. M., and Lenardo, M. J. Immunoglobulin gene transcription. *Annual Review of Immunology* 9:373, 1991.

Taussig, M. J. The genetics of antibody V regions. *Immunology Today* **8:**356, 1987.

Taussig, M. J., Sims, M., and Krawinkel, U. Regulation of Ig-gene rearrangement and expression. *Immunology Today* **10:**143, 1989.

Tonegawa, S. Somatic generation of antibody diversity. *Nature* **302:**575, 1983.

Vitetta, E. S., Berton, M. T., Burger, C., et al. Memory B and T cells. *Annual Review of Immunology* 9:193, 1991.

Weaver, C., and Unanue, E. The costimulatory function of antigen-presenting cells. *Immunology Today* **11:**49, 1990.

Complement and its Role in Immune Responses

6

OVERVIEW

Among the body's weapons for defense against foreign cells is a group of serum proteins that constitute the complement system. The biological effects of this system are diverse and include cell lysis, stimulation of smooth muscle contraction, mast cell degranulation, neutrophil chemotaxis, and activation of phagocytes. The means through which activation of the complement system is achieved and its interactions with other components of the immune system are the focus of this chapter.

CONCEPTS

1. Two pathways of complement activation exist: one is antibody dependent while the other is not. However, both converge at a common point to achieve their final effects.

2. Complement activation can lead to cell lysis and mediation of inflammation, serving to attract phagocytic cells and to enhance phagocytosis (opsonization).

3. The consequences of complement activation can be beneficial (e.g., lysis of microbes) as well as deleterious (e.g., immune-complex inflammatory damage).

4. There is an association of genetic complement deficiencies with certain disease states (e.g., absence of C5–C8 associated with neisserial infections).

Blood contains a group of serum proteins that can act in conjunction with the cells of the immune system to eliminate foreign cells. Once activated, the complement system can bring about a variety of responses. For example, it can initiate an inflammatory response or cause the destruction of bacteria, parasites, virus-infected cells, or red blood cells. In addition, it can facilitate the clearance of dead cells and immune complexes.

The complement system is composed of several unique plasma proteins. There are three separate **activation triggers** for this system. These are (1) Ab binding to a cell surface, (2) formation of immune (Ab-Ag) complexes, and (3) a carbohydrate component of a microbe's cell membrane. There are two **activation mechanisms** through which these proteins execute their roles. These two mechanisms separately function in the *classical pathway* and the *alternative,* or *properdin, pathway.* The classical pathway requires the presence of Ab for activation. It depends upon immunological memory and previous exposure to Ag. In contrast, the alternative pathway does not need Ab and can be triggered by the mere presence of bacterial or viral components. For example, the lipopolysaccharide (LPS) layer of a gram-negative bacterial cell wall is enough to activate alternative complement components. In this regard, the alternative pathway appears to be more primitive. Both activation mechanisms generate a cascade of active molecules that can initiate inflammatory and phagocytic events, as well as the terminal event of cell lysis.

During the late nineteenth century, complement was discovered by several investigators, including Nuttall, Buchner, and Erhlich. They found that a heat-labile factor present in serum was needed for bactericidal activity. In addition, their investigations revealed that killing of microbes also depended upon a *heat-stable factor,* called "amboceptor" (now identified as Ab), which bound to the bacteria. Addition of the heat-labile substance appeared to bind to the "amboceptor" and caused lysis of the microbe. The *heat-labile substance* was labeled "complement" since it seemed necessary to complete the lytic reaction.

The conclusions reached in the late nineteenth century still hold today. However, we now realize that the complement system is more than a series of reactions that complete an immune response. Rather, it is a pathway that can be directly responsible for effecting the expression and amplification of a number of biological responses, which include inflammation and phagocytosis. This chapter introduces the two complement cascades, explores the resulting biological consequences of complement activation, and discusses the regulation of this system.

■ ■ ■ ■ ■ ■ ■ ■ ■ ■

THE CLASSICAL COMPLEMENT PATHWAY

The classical complement pathway involves the coordinated activity of several proteins. Briefly, activation of this pathway requires first the presence of Ab, either as immunoglobulin (IgG or IgM) bound to cell-surface Ag or as an Ag-Ab immune complex. Serum protein, C1, binds to the Ab. This interaction results in the sequential activation of C4, C2, and C3 and leads to the formation of complex cleaving enzymes. The activation of C5, C6, C7, C8, and C9 then completes the cascade and results in the formation of the C5–C9 **membrane attack complex (MAC),** which can lyse the cell. In addition, cleavage products with anaphylatoxic (histamine-releasing) and chemotactic (for phagocytes) activity are produced. This system is regulated at different levels and involves several plasma and membrane-associated proteins. Precisely controlled cycles of activation and inactivation are regulated in order to maintain homeostasis.

Proteins of the Classical Complement Pathway

There are eleven proteins that comprise the classical complement pathway (table 6.1). All are designated by "**C**" followed by a number, but additional symbols appear as well. The nomenclature of the native com-

TABLE 6.1 Proteins of the Classical Complement Pathway

Protein	Serum Concentration (μg/mL)	Physical Characteristics		Immunological Function
		Molecular Weight	Sedimentation Rate	
C1				Stabilizes immune complexes
C1q	75	410,000	11.0S	Binds to Fc portion of Ab (IgG, IgM) molecules
C1r	34	190,000	7.0S	Links C1q and C1s; enzymatically activates C1s
C1s	30	87,000	4.1S	Enzymatically activates C4 and C2
C2	25	115,000	5.5S	Cleaved into C2a and C2b; C2b, with C4b, enzymatically activates C3 (C3 convertase)
C3	1,500	180,000	9.5S	Cleaved to C3a and C3b—C3a has anaphylatoxic, chemotactic, and opsonic properties; C3b forms C5 convertase and when associated with C4b2b has opsonic properties
C4	450	210,000	10.0S	Cleaved into C4a and C4b—C4a has anaphylatoxic properties; C4b binds C2b and can neutralize viruses
C5	75	190,000	8.7S	Cleaved into C5a and C5b—C5a is phagocyte chemoattractant and has anaphylatoxic properties; C5b binds avidly to membranes and initiates MAC
C6	60	128,000	5.7S	Serine protease—forms part of MAC
C7	60	121,000	5.6S	Forms part of MAC
C8	80	163,000	8.0S	Forms part of MAC
C9	58	79,000	4.5S	Forms part of MAC

Complement system is heat labile, being inactivated by heating at 56°C. However, not all components of classical pathway display similar lability. C1 and C2 are especially heat labile; they can be inactivated within a few minutes at 56°C. C3, C4, C6, and C8 are less heat labile; they require 20 to 30 minutes at 56°C before inactivation results.

plement components has changed over the years. Currently, the following rules for identifying complement components apply:

1. Inactive components are described as C1, C2, and so forth.
2. Activated forms are designated by placing a bar over the number, for example, C2 represents activated C2 (which is actually C2b).
3. Since activation of components C2–C5 occurs through proteolysis with the generation of subcomponents, the larger proteolytic fragment (associated with target cell plasma membranes) is designated as "b," while the smaller, released fragment is designated as "a." (The only exception to this third rule was the original designation of C2a and C2b, which has now been altered to concur with the nomenclature of the other components.)

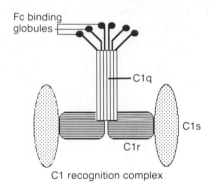

Fc binding
globules

C1q

C1s

C1r

C1 recognition complex

FIGURE 6.1 Complement C1 protein. This figure provides a representation of the structure of the C1 molecule. The globular heads of C1q interact with immunoglobulin, while the stemlike tail region provides binding sites for the two C1r subunits. C1r is the serine esterase activator of C1s and is the physical link between C1q and C1s.

The Sequence of Reactions

There are several sequential reactions in the classical complement pathway. In following these reactions from initial activation to cell lysis, **three phases** or stages can be identified. These are (1) a *recognition* phase, during which the complement system becomes activated; (2) an *enzymatic* phase, which is characterized by amplification of complement activation; and (3) an *attack* phase, during which cell destruction actually occurs.

The Recognition Phase

The classical pathway is initiated when the inactive *C1 serum protein interacts with the Fc portion of either cell-bound Ig (IgG or IgM) or an immune complex.* The C1 protein is composed of three proteins: C1q, which binds to the Fc portion of the Ab molecule; C1s, which can enzymatically cleave the next complement component, C4; and C1r, which acts as a bridge connecting C1q to C1s (fig. 6.1).

Although only one IgM-bound molecule is necessary to fix the C1 complex, two molecules of IgG bound in close proximity are required for activation to occur. The **C1 recognition complex** needs calcium

to form the inactive unit, C1, consisting of one molecule of C1q and two molecules each of C1r and C1s. In response to bound Ab, C1q connects with Ab receptor sites located on the Fc portions of two adjacent Ab molecules. These receptor sites are exposed when the Ab binds to the Ag. After binding to the sites, C1q undergoes a conformational change, which causes C1r to activate itself by limited self-cleavage. *Autoactivation of C1r creates an enzymelike activity, which now sees C1s as its substrate. Activation of C1s by cleavage gives rise to its ability to cleave the next two complement proteins in this sequence, namely, C4 and C2. C̄1̄s̄ (also referred to as C1 esterase) initiates the assembly of the next two proteins by enzymatic activation of binding sites on C4 and C2 (fig. 6.2).

The Enzymatic Phase

Activation of C4 and C2 (the proteins were numbered prior to discovery of the initiation sequence, hence C4 precedes C2 in activation) involves the cleavage of a specific peptide bond in each molecule, resulting in the dissociation of peptide fragments, C4a and C2a (C4a has anaphylatoxic activity), and the *exposure of a binding site in the larger fragment,* C̄4̄b̄2̄b̄. The C̄4̄b̄ peptide binds to the cell membrane, while C̄2̄b̄ attaches itself to the C̄4̄b̄ fragment. This C̄4̄b̄2̄b̄ complex is enzymatically active, requires magnesium ions, and is called *C3 convertase* since it can bind and cleave the next inactive complement component in the sequence, C3. The proteolytic actions of C1 esterase and C3 convertase are focused on the α chains of C4 and C3, respectively (fig. 6.3)

Activation of C3 initiates the generation of a second convertase enzyme. This occurs when C3 is cleaved into C3a and C3b. The larger C̄3̄b̄ fragment attaches to both the cell membrane and C̄4̄b̄2̄b̄ complex, while the smaller fragment, C3a, is released to the body fluids. C3a has opsonization properties. C̄4̄b̄2̄b̄3̄b̄ is termed *C5 convertase* (or *C3/C5 convertase*), and its newly created catalytic site now accommodates C5, the next component in the sequence. The creation of C3/C5 convertase concludes the enzymatic phase, following activation of the C1 complex.

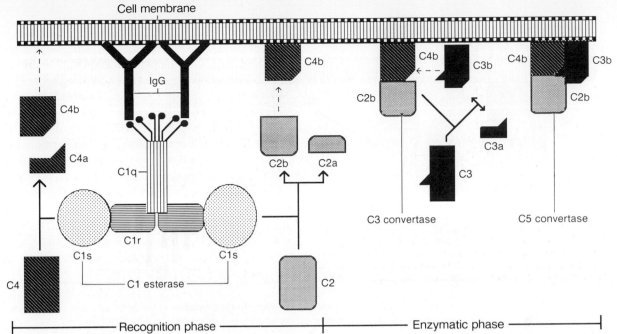

FIGURE 6.2 Initial reactions of the classical complement pathway. This diagram shows assembly of complement components C1–C3. C1 binds to Ab already bound to the cell surface, creating a C1 recognition site. This leads to the formation of an enzymatic site on the target cell surface, where C4, C2, and C3 bind. Membrane-bound components are C1, C4b, C2b, and C3b, while fragments C4a, C2a, and C3a are released and can diffuse away from the site. *Note:* The latest terminology is used to describe activation of C2. C2a refers to the small released fragment, while C2b refers to the larger membrane-bound component. This is the reverse of the original designations appearing in earlier studies.

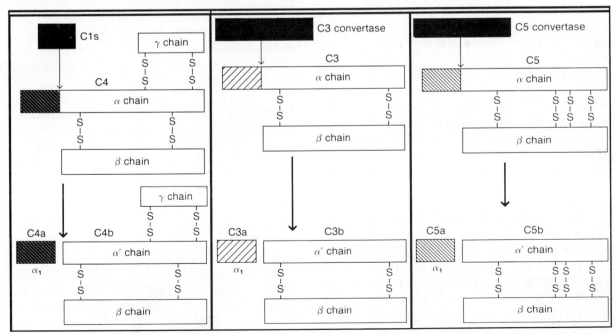

FIGURE 6.3 Proteolytic cleavage of C4, C3, and C5. This diagrammatic representation shows the polypeptide subunit structure of C4, C3, and C5 and the fragments generated by the action of their respective esterase activators: C1s for C4, C3 convertase for C3, and C5 convertase for C5. The larger fragments—C4b, C3b, and C5b—are membrane bound, while the smaller components—C4a, C3a, and C5a—are released and can migrate from the site.

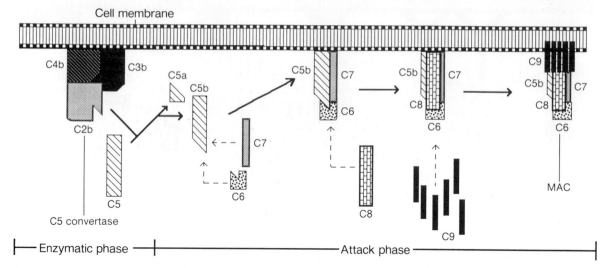

FIGURE 6.4 Terminal reactions of the classical complement pathway. Activation of C5 is portrayed on the *left*. This leads sub- sequently to the formation of the MAC at a site distinct from the recognition and enzymatic sites, shown on the *right*.

The Attack Phase

This now initiates the last phase of the classical pathway, or the attack phase. It begins when C3/C5 convertase cleaves C5 into two products, C5a and C5b (fig. 6.4). C5a, which is a powerful chemoattractant of neutrophils and monocytes and has anaphylatoxic activity, is released when formed. On the other hand, C5b attaches to the cell membrane. The binding of C5b leads to the uncovering of a binding site for C6 and C7 on the molecule, producing a stable complex, C5b67. This trimolecular complex attaches to the membrane surface and enables C8 to bind. Once incorporated, C8 binds several C9 molecules. The fully assembled C5b6789 is a stable complex that can *produce a lesion in the plasma membrane* causing cell lysis (fig. 6.4).

These assembled C5–9 components are referred to as the MAC, and its ability to lyse depends on the proper polymerization of C9 units. The C9 protein units (approximately 10 to 18) attach to the C5–8 base to form a long, hollow tube (fig. 6.5). This membrane-bound appendage creates a membrane pore, or lesion, that is approximately 100 Å in diameter (fig. 6.6). This *creates a transmembrane channel* which, with

the displacement of membrane constituents by polymerization of C9, can cause cell death through membrane damage. In addition, secondary effects produced by the MAC contribute to cell death. For example, pores in the outer membrane created by the MAC might permit degradative enzymes in the area to enter and destroy cellular organelles, and constituents or extracellular ions might enter and initiate improper metabolic cascades. All of these effects can contribute to target cell death.

The effectiveness of complement-mediated lysis depends on the target, be it a bacterium, a virus, a nucleated cell, or an erythrocyte. Certain organisms have developed interesting ways to circumvent cell death by complement. For example, certain strains of *Salmonella minnesota* seem to escape destruction because of an extra long cell wall component (LPS chain), which can prevent insertion of C8 and C9. In contrast, vaccinia virus produces a secretory protein that can neutralize C4b, thereby inactivating the complement cascade. Nucleated cells, in general, are relatively resistant to complement killing due to their ability to remove MACs from their surfaces by endocytotic or exocytotic mechanisms. In addition, the formation of

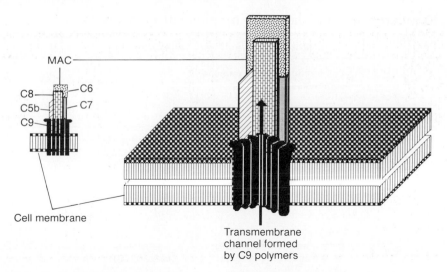

MAC

C8 — C6
C5b — C7
C9

Cell membrane

Transmembrane
channel formed
by C9 polymers

FIGURE 6.5 Membrane attack complex (MAC). This representation is the subunit architecture of the MAC. The transmembrane channel is formed by C5b, C6, C7, C8, and 10 to 18 polymerized molecules of C9.

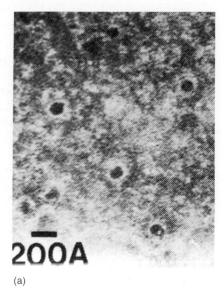

(a)

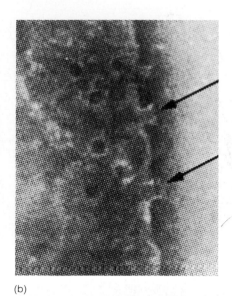

(b)

FIGURE 6.6 Transmembrane channels produced by complement. (*a*) View from above (scale bar, 200 Å, is provided). (*b*) Lateral view shows insertion of the MAC into the cell membrane (*at arrows*). (From Tranum-Jensen, J., Bhakdi, S., Bhakdi-Lehnen, B., et al. Complement lysis: ultrastructure and orientation of the C5b–9 complex on target sheep erythrocyte membranes. *Scandinavian Journal of Immunology* **7:**45–56, 1978, fig. 1c, 7b. Blackwell Scientific Publications Limited.)

TABLE 6.2 Regulators of the Classical Complement Pathway

Stage	Regulator*	Action
Recognition Phase	**Cell-bound IgG, IgM; Immune complexes**	Bind C1q, activating C1r and C1s; *initiate recognition phase*
	C1 inhibitor	Causes dissociation of C1r and C1s from Ab-bound C1q; *blocks entry to enzymatic phase*
Enzymatic Phase	C1s	Acts enzymatically on C4 and C2 to yield C4b2b (C3 convertase); *initiates enzymatic phase*
	C3 convertase	Enzymatically acts on C3 with resultant formation of C4b2b3b (C5 convertase); *mediates progression of enzymatic phase*
	C5 convertase	Enzymatically acts on C5; *sets stage for attack phase*
	C4 binding protein (C4BP); Decay-accelerating factor (DAF)	Competitively inhibits binding of C2b to C4b; acts like C4BP; *interrupts enzymatic phase*
	Factor I (C3 inactivator, conglutinogen-activating factor)	Degrades C4b to C4c and C4d; inactivates C3 convertase; also inactivates C5 convertase by degrading C3b to C3f and iC3b; *blocks transit to attack phase*; N.B. assistance of cofactor is required by Factor I
	Carboxypeptidaselike serum enzymes	Neutralize chemotactic and anaphylatoxic activities of complement products (C3a, C5a)
Attack Phase	C5b	Attaches to membrane and initiates formation of MAC; *initiates attack phase*
	S protein	Binds soluble C5–C7 complex; prevents lysis of ''bystander'' cells; limits scope of damage to surrounding tissues

*Regulators *not* part of the complement pathway, or derived therefrom, are in boldface print.

MACs are not necessarily fatal to the cell if it possesses an effective mechanism that can repair or compensate for the initial damage.

In summary, the reactions of the classical complement cascade can be divided into three phases: (1) activation of Cl, (2) the formation of C3/C5 convertase (the enzymatic phase), and (3) the assembly of the MAC (the attack phase).

Regulation of Complement Activity

The classical complement cascade must be carefully regulated. This series of events must be of limited duration in order to prevent the complete consumption of inactive complement components in the serum. In fact, there are regulatory proteins for each stage in the classical pathway (table 6.2). *Certain of these regulators exert positive effects.* These are mostly derived from the reactions of the classical pathway itself (discussed above) and drive the reactions toward cell destruction. *Other regulators exert a negative effect on the classical pathway.* These bring about the rapid destruction of activated complement factors generated during the cascade.

The first stage of complement activation is the formation of recognition complex, $\overline{C1}$. The protein responsible for the inactivation of $\overline{C1}$ is a protease inhibitor called **C1 inhibitor.** Its main function is to combine with activated C1 by binding to sites of $\overline{C1r}$ and $\overline{C1s}$, causing these subunits to dissociate from Ab-bound C1q. The dissociated complex consists of one molecule each of C1r and C1s and two molecules of C1 inhibitor. In this way, C1s is physically removed from the membrane site and cannot proceed to cleave C4 and C2. Thus, C1 inhibitor effectively halts the generation of C3/C5 convertase and the MAC. This inactivation is rapid (10 to 20 seconds) and effective enough to inhibit any spontaneous activation of plasma C1 by nonspecific activators, such as heparin.

The *inactivation of C3/C5 convertase* is accomplished in two stages. In the first stage, activity is lost by dissociation of C2 from cell-bound C4. This dissociation is promoted by **C4-binding protein (C4BP)** and **decay-accelerating factor (DAF).** Both are proteins that can attach to C4 near the C2-binding site, thereby competitively inhibiting C2 binding to C4. In the second stage, the generation of C3 convertase is blocked. This occurs through the further degradation of C$\overline{4b}$ into the inactive fragments C4c and C4d. This is accomplished by the cleavage enzyme, Factor I (also called C3 inactivator, or conglutinogen-activating factor). This is the same enzyme that inactivates C5 convertase by splitting membrane-bound C3b into C3f and iC3b (inactive C3b). **Factor I** requires a cofactor. There are three proteins that might act as cofactors: *factor H* (from the alternative pathway [see below]), *membrane cofactor protein,* and *CRI* (a complement receptor). Thus, without the ability to cleave C5, the third phase of the complement cascade is halted, and the synthesis of the MAC cannot be executed.

There are also **carboxypeptidaselike enzymes** in serum that have been shown to destroy the anaphylatoxic and chemotactic activities of C3a and C5a by cleaving them into inactive fragments. These enzymes do nothing to halt the lysis of the target cell, but they negate the biological effects of the powerful inflammatory agents, C3a and C5a.

The other problem of complement activation is damage to surrounding cells, usually host cells. This can happen when the complex, C$\overline{5b67}$, is released from the target cell membrane and inserts into host cell membrane. Rapid activation of C8 and polymerization of C9 ensues and can result in the destruction of host tissue. We must keep in mind that complement activation is an **amplification process.** The activation of

one C1 molecule results in binding 30 molecules of C4, which can generate up to 200 bound C3 molecules. Consequently, there are many molecules of C5 to initiate formation of the MAC. The binding is not always tight, and a few units can dissociate and randomly reassociate on host cell membranes, causing lysis of innocent bystander cells. However, a protective mechanism has evolved that ensures that this is not a major consequence of complement activation. There are a group of plasma proteins, called *S proteins* and lipoproteins, that are endowed with C5b67 binding activity. S protein binds only to soluble C5b67 units, not to cell-bound C5b67 units. Since the resulting SC5b67 complex cannot reinsert itself into any cell membrane, lysis of host bystander cells is blocked.

THE ALTERNATIVE OR PROPERDIN PATHWAY

The alternative or properdin pathway can be activated in the complete absence of Ab. Nonimmune activators, such as repeating polysaccharide units or the LPS found on the cell walls of some microbes, can activate this pathway. The alternative pathway differs from the classical pathway in that it has substitutes for the early acting C1, C4, and C2 components. Therefore, it can directly initiate the reactions of the late-acting C3–C9 components. It also differs in that it provides an immediate line of defense that does not require immunological memory.

Proteins of the Alternative (Properdin) Pathway

The proteins of the alternative pathway are similar to those of the classical pathway, produce similar enzymes, and cause formation of a MAC. This pathway converges at the C3 utilization step of the classical complement pathway. In addition, the alternative pathway has factors that can be activated with protein fragments generated that are capable of binding to acceptor surfaces (table 6.3). Thus, activation of complement via the alternative pathway provides a natural system of defense against infectious agents.

TABLE 6.3 Additional Proteins Occurring in the Alternative (Properdin) Pathway

Protein	Serum Concentration (μg/mL)	Physical Characteristics		Immunological Function
		Molecular Weight	Sedimentation Rate	
Factor B* (C3 proactivator)	200	93,000	5.9S	Is precursor for serine esterase that acts on C3
Factor D (C3 proactivator convertase)	1	24,000	2.5S	Acts on C3bB to yield active C3/C5 convertase
Factor H	470	150,000	6.0S	Blocks binding between B and C3b; dissociates Bb from C3bB complex; makes C3b susceptible to action by Factor I
Factor I (C3b inactivator)	34	88,000	5.5S	Inactivates C3b
Factor P (properdin)	20	220,000	5.4S	Enhances activity of alternate pathway's C3/C5 convertase

*Factor B is heat sensitive; an earlier designation of this component was "heat-labile factor."

The Sequence of Reactions

The alternative pathway is functionally a **two-phase system** in which six proteins participate. The first phase is *initiation*. During this phase, particle-bound C3b acts like the C1 recognition complex. The second phase is *amplification* driven by a positive feedback loop involving bound C3b, Factor B, and Factor D (fig. 6.7).

The Initiation Phase

The key to understanding the first phase is found in the structure of C3. C3 is a two-chain molecule. Upon cleavage, a highly reactive thiol-ester group is exposed on the C3b fragment. This reactive group can be attacked by water, by the surface of an organism, or by foreign substances to which it might bind. If the acceptor surfaces are chemically suitable, interaction with C3b can occur and the alternative pathway can be activated.

There are a wide variety of pathogens that can be recognized within minutes after they come in contact with plasma. Organisms sensitive to attack by the alternative pathway include bacteria, fungi, certain viruses and virus-infected cells, and certain tumors and parasites. C3b bound to these foreign surfaces can interact with plasma protein Factor B. Factor B then is cleaved into membrane-bound fragment Bb and soluble fragment Ba, through the action of an enzyme called Factor D. The newly formed $\overline{\text{C3bBb}}$ is a C3/C5 convertase. Since Factor B ultimately activates C3, but must first be converted to Bb, it is referred to as C3 proactivator. Similarly, Factor D is known as C3 proactivator convertase because it converts Factor B from its inactive to its active form.

The Amplification Phase

An amplification process begins as $\overline{\text{C3bBb}}$ converts more C3 to C3b. The newly generated C3b binds more factor B. This positive feedback cycle continues until the membrane surface is saturated with $\overline{\text{C3bBb}}$. The result is *opsonization* (enhanced engulfment) of the cell or particle by neutrophils. In addition, the soluble C3a that is released upon cleavage of C3 has *anaphylatoxic activity*, which can initiate an inflammatory response. The C3 convertase can bind additional C3b to produce

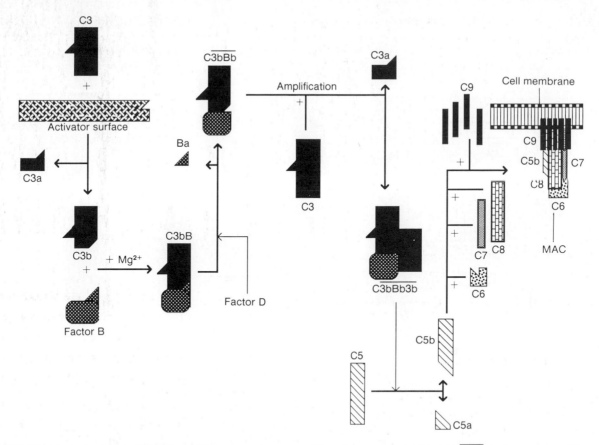

FIGURE 6.7 Alternative (properdin) pathway. This schematic represents the molecular events of alternative pathway activation. Initiation results from the hydrolysis of the thiolester in C3, which produces a C3 convertase molecule that can interact with Factor B.

The subsequent generation of $\overline{C3bBb}$, in the presence of Factor D, can mediate a positive feedback amplification that results in further C3b deposition and C5 convertase formation. C5–C9 can then join the cascade and form the MAC.

C5 convertase ($\overline{C3bBb3b}$), which, in turn, activates the terminal lytic complement sequence, C5–C9.

Thus, activation of either the classical or alternate complement pathways leads to formation of C3 convertases ($\overline{C4b2b}$ or $\overline{C3bBb}$). Cleavage of C3 and binding of C3b to C3 convertases results in the formation of C5-converting enzymes ($\overline{C4b2bC3b}$ or $\overline{C3bBb3b}$). The two pathways converge in their activation of C5 by cleavage to C5a and C5b. This is followed by the association of $\overline{C5b}$ with C6, C7, C8, and C9 to form the MAC, which mediates lysis of target cells in both pathways (fig. 6.8).

Regulation of the Properdin Pathway

The alternative pathway is also precisely regulated (fig. 6.9). Inhibition of the pathway is achieved by Factors H and I, while stimulation is mediated by a plasma protein called properdin. This pathway can be artificially stimulated by a poison, cobra venom factor (CoVF).

Factor H is a β-globulin that regulates the alternate pathway by binding to C3b in the fluid phase or when attached to a nonactivator surface. Once bound, it blocks access of Factor B to C3b, dissociates

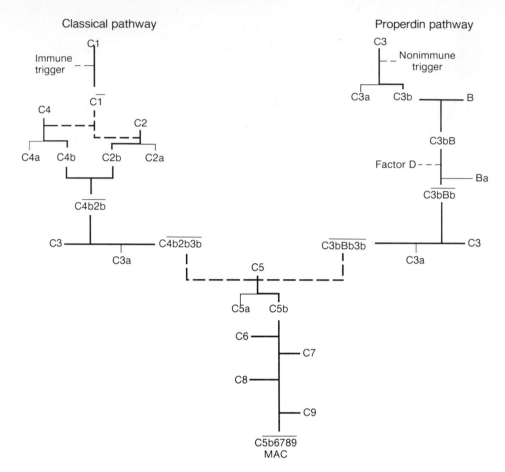

FIGURE 6.8 Convergence of classical and alternative complement pathways. The steps leading to the formation of C3 convertase differ in the two pathways. The formation of the MAC ($\overline{\text{C5b6789}}$) is the same for both since both pathways produce C5 convertase.

Bb from the active complex, $\overline{\text{C3bBb}}$, and makes C3b susceptible to cleavage by Factor I. These properties of Factor H allow it to inactivate the enzymatic capability of the C3/C5 convertase and to regulate the amplification of the lytic sequence initiated by C5. On the other hand, **Factor I** (or C3b inactivator) is a regulatory enzyme that can cleave and inactivate C3b and C4b when these activated complement components are associated with their cofactor, Factor H. Once $\overline{\text{C3b}}$ is inactivated, it can no longer form C3 convertase. Thus, the amplification process unique to the alternative pathway is blocked.

Factor P, or **properdin,** is a serum protein that functions as an enhancing regulator of the alternative pathway C3/C5 convertase. It was the first component of the alternative pathway to be identified. The pathway was initially named after it because purified properdin caused experimentally induced complement activation through this mechanism.

Properdin has two forms: native and activated. Native properdin, in plasma, can bind to $\overline{\text{C3bBb}}$ and undergoes a conformational change that activates it. Activated properdin can (1) bind directly to bound and nonbound C3b, (2) stabilize C3/C5 convertases,

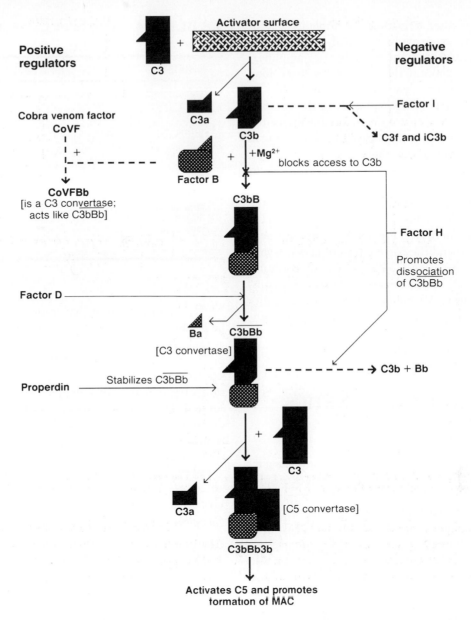

FIGURE 6.9 Regulation of the properdin pathway. The alternative pathway can be both positively and negatively regulated. The positive regulators stimulate events in the early stages of the pathway, leading to production of C5 convertase. Negative regulators act to inhibit the generation of C5 convertase.

and (3) induce further activation of complement components indirectly by extending the half-life of C3bBb. It enters the activation sequence only after amplification begins. It promotes the positive feedback loop mainly by slowing the dissociation of the highly reactive C3bBb. The ensuing explosion of the complement cascade ensures that foreign organisms in the blood are rapidly destroyed and cleared before they can multiply and further invade the body.

CoVF is a protein found in the venom of cobras. This protein activates complement and lyses erythrocytes. It can combine with Factor B to form the complex CoVF-Bb, which is equivalent to C3/C5 convertase. This activates the terminal complement sequence C5–C9 and the passive lysis of erythrocytes. The interaction between CoVF and Factor B is catalyzed by Factor D, which cleaves Factor B in the complex to Bb. Thus, CoVF behaves like C3b in its ability to activate C3 and the later components of the complement system. Unfortunately, the venom seems resistant to the action of the inactivators of the alternative pathway, Factors H and I.

PRODUCTION AND GENETICS OF COMPLEMENT
Production

The liver is responsible for the production of several complement proteins. However, hepatocytes are not the sole producers since several of the complement proteins appear to be synthesized by other cells, including macrophages, fibroblasts, and several types of mucosal epithelial cells (table 6.4). For example, although C3 is mainly produced by hepatocytes, it also can be synthesized by macrophages when stimulated by the phagocytic process. Normal plasma levels of C3 result from hepatocyte synthesis, but C3 synthesis also occurs at the site of local inflammation, facilitating host defense. Moreover, the complement proteins are not all synthesized at the same rate. This is reflected in the widely varying serum concentrations of these proteins, from 1 μg/mL for Factor D up to 1,500 μg/mL for C3.

TABLE 6.4 Sources of Complement Proteins

Proteins	Source
Classical Pathway	
C1	Epithelium and fibroblasts
C3, C4, C6, C7, C8, C9	Liver
C1, C2, C3, C4, C5	Macrophages (stimulated by phagocytic events)
C1 inactivator	Liver
Alternative Pathway	
Factors B, D, H, I, P	Macrophages (stimulated by phagocytic events)

Thus, we know that complement proteins can be produced at several sites, but not to the same extent at each. In addition, we know that these proteins are produced at different rates, even from the same source. On the other hand, our understanding of the regulation of production of complement proteins is more limited. For example, regulation of complement production by the liver appears to be separate from the regulation of complement production at other sites in the body. However, the nature of the control has not yet been defined.

Genetics
Complement Protein Genes

Complement proteins are specified by autosomal codominant genes. Genes for C2, Factor B, and C4 are located within the major histocompatibility complex (MHC) and are considered class III Ags of the MHC locus. Like MHC class I and II genes, the class III (complement) genes are highly polymorphic (allelic variation). The class III region is located on the human sixth and murine seventeenth chromosomes and is inherited as a single unit (complotype). In the human MHC (human leukocyte—associated [HLA] complex), C2, Factor B, and C4 form a gene cluster lying

TABLE 6.5 Chromosomal Location of Identified Complement Genes

Gene Coding for	Maps on Chromosome Number	
	Human	Mouse
C2	6	17
C4	6	17
Factor B	6	17
C3	19	6
Factor H	1	Unknown
C4-binding protein	1	1 or 3
CR1	1	1 or 3

close to the HLA-B locus. Known chromosomal locations of complement genes appear in table 6.5. (Further discussion of the MHC is presented in chapter 7.)

In contrast, C1, C3, C5, C6, C7, C8, and C9 are not linked to the MHC region. Mapping of several of the complement genes to specific chromosomes has been accomplished through population genetic studies, using marker variants of the complement proteins. Tracing the electrophoretic variants of C3 mapped it to chromosome 19 in humans and chromosome 6 in mice.

With the advent of recombinant DNA technology, progress has been made toward understanding the genomic relationship of these genes to one another. For example, studies of polymorphisms and homologies between complement proteins of the HLA region showed that, in humans, the order of the complement genes was C2, Factor B, C4A, and C4B. Thus, it was determined that a curious genetic phenomenon existed in the inheritance of C4. C4 is coded for by two tandem genes, C4A and C4B. Therefore, there are two isotypes of C4, which can be equally expressed in the same individual. Certain C4 variants (e.g., null alleles) occur more frequently in autoimmune diseases, particularly those involving defects in the processing of immune complexes, such as systemic lupus erythematosus (SLE). Perhaps this polymorphism of C4 ensures interaction with a wide range of chemical structures, both self-Ags and those on pathogens. However, in the case of null allele C4 variants, one of the tandem proteins is not expressed, which apparently leaves the person more susceptible to autoimmune disease.

Chromosomal assignment of all the complement genes is not complete. Nevertheless, once cDNA (copy DNA or complementary DNA) probes become available, mapping the other unmapped genes should be accomplished using techniques like *in situ* hybridization. In this technique, radioactively labeled complement-cDNA probes can be hybridized to specific areas on a chromosome. By identifying where these hybridizations occur, localization of the gene site on a particular chromosome will be possible.

In addition to mapping complement genes, some of the complement proteins have been grouped according to sequence similarity with each other. C1r and C1s are closely related both structurally and functionally. They have marked sequence homology, and they interact with each other in the C1 complex. In addition, C6 and C7 are structural homologs and share functional properties since both interact with C5b and C8 in the formation of the MAC. Thus, these and other recent findings provide a strong foundation for further studies of the complement genes and the molecular genetic basis for the many functional activities of the complement proteins. Insights gained through these studies will contribute to additional understanding of the function of this system in immune regulation, inflammation, and other host-defense reactions.

Genes for complement regulators

Loci for regulator molecules (Factor H, C4BP, and CR1) are tightly linked on chromosome 1 in humans. These factors have a common structural element, a terminal repeat sequence, which is shared by a number of other proteins that interact with C3b or C4b (i.e., Factor B, C2, C1s, and C1r). Thus, there seems to be a superfamily of C3b/C4b-binding proteins that contains this repetitive unit. This may be the result of multiple gene duplication and relocation of an ancestral DNA segment in a complement protein that occurred early in the phylogenetic lineage of complement.

THE BIOLOGICAL CONSEQUENCES OF COMPLEMENT ACTIVATION

The biological consequences of complement activation are not limited to cell lysis. Some of the *protein fragments generated during complement activation can have diverse effects.* Among the activities mediated by complement fragments are contraction of smooth muscle, release of histamine from mast cells and platelets, enhanced phagocytosis, chemotaxis of phagocytes, and activation of lymphocytes and macrophages. A summary of biological activities mediated by complement is presented in table 6.6.

Anaphylaxis

Proteolytic cleavage of C3 and C5, in either the classical or alternative pathway, generates two potent mediators of inflammation, **C3a** and **C5a.** The main biological activity of these two polypeptides is *anaphylaxis.* Specifically, these anaphylatoxic fragments cause histamine release from mast cells and basophils. The direct action of these anaphylatoxins and the secondary effect of histamine release can affect the activity of smooth muscle. Among the consequences that might be encountered are contraction of the uterus, trachea, arteries, atrium of the heart, and intestines. This biological property, termed *spasmogenicity,* accounts for the ability of these molecules to induce an anaphylactic response in animals (see chapter 13, Hypersensitivity, for additional discussion of anaphylaxis).

Mast cells and basophils possess receptors for C3a and C5a. Binding of C3a or C5a to these receptors causes these cells to release histamine. However, the anaphylatoxins are controlled by a serum enzyme, carboxypeptidase N, called *anaphylatoxin inhibitor,* which removes the carboxy-terminal arginine from

TABLE 6.6 Biological Activities Mediated by Complement

Complement Component	Activities
C3a	Promotes histamine release; increases vascular permeability; stimulates smooth muscle contraction; is immunosuppressive
C3b	Activates properdin pathway; promotes immune adherence; enhances opsonization; enhances Ab production
C4a	Displays anaphylactic activity
C4b	Promotes immune adherence; enhances phagocytosis; enhances Ab production
C5a	Augments immune responses; promotes histamine release; increases vascular permeability; stimulates smooth muscle contraction; promotes chemotaxis of phagocytes and release of lysosomal enzymes
C567	Promotes chemotaxis of leukocytic phagocytes

C3a and C5a. Removal of this terminal amino acid from these complement fragments inactivates them. Consequently, they can no longer induce histamine release from mast cells or directly stimulate smooth muscle.

In addition to spasmogenicity, histamine release induced by the anaphylatoxins has effects on inflammation. In particular, histamine can increase vascular permeability, producing edema. Furthermore, C5a, the more potent of the anaphylatoxins, has other, more direct, inflammatory consequences. These are exerted on certain white blood cells—namely, neutrophils and monocytes. These target cells have C5a receptors on their membranes. **C5a** can exert a series of unique effects on these blood cells and thus promote their participation in the events of acute or chronic inflammation. The cellular responses of neutrophils and monocytes to C5a include (1) *degranulation* and *lysosomal enzyme release,* (2) *cell adherence,* and (3) *chemotactic migration* (fig. 6.10). Thus, the generation of C5a at a

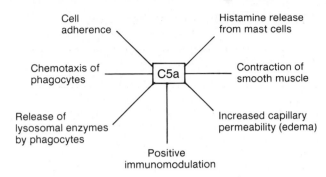

FIGURE 6.10 Biological activities promoted by C5a.

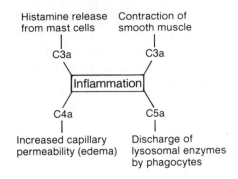

FIGURE 6.11 Events of inflammation mediated by complement by-products.

localized site can promote adherence of granulocytes to the endothelium, induce their chemotactic migration into the site (which is also exhibited by the ternary complement complex C$\overline{5b67}$), and prime these cells to release inflammatory molecules. All of these responses are important in promoting host defense (see chapter 8 for additional discussions).

Another complement fragment that has weak anaphylactic activity is **C4a.** It is weakly spasmogenic and increases vascular permeability. The spasmogenic activity of C4a is also controlled by serum carboxypeptidase N, which results in the rapid destruction of serum C4a.

It has been suggested that the anaphylatoxins also have **immunomodulatory properties.** They are believed to play a role in enhancing or suppressing the host's immune response. For example, once C5a binds to macrophage cell membrane receptors, ligand-receptor binding interactions cause these cells to produce the enhancing regulatory cytokine, interleukin 1 (IL-1). On the other hand, it appears that C3a can bind to suppressor T lymphocytes, leading to suppression of polyclonal Ab production. Thus, **C5a** can serve as a *positive immunomodulator,* whereas **C3a** can act as an *immunosuppressor.*

In summary, the acute inflammatory response is characterized by symptoms of redness, pain, swelling, and heat due to the action of C4a, C3a, C5a, and histamine. The primary goal of inflammation is to set into motion a series of events that result in the elimination of foreign and damaged cells, protecting the host against further injury. The inflammatory response can

be mediated by the anaphylatoxins and their byproducts. Figure 6.11 summarizes the events of inflammation that can be mediated by the anaphylatoxins and their byproducts.

Opsonization

Complement helps to regulate immune-complex aggregation and clearance. Within the circulation, complement can inhibit the aggregation of 10 times as many immune complexes as it solubilizes. In addition, complement contributes to clearance of immune complexes by phagocytes such as macrophages, monocytes, and neutrophils. Since these cells all possess stable surface receptors for C3b, such as CR1, if immune complexes have activated the complement system, the C$\overline{3b}$ bound to them facilitates their recognition and ingestion by these phagocytes. In addition, C$\overline{4b}$ can also facilitate phagocytosis by leukocytes, but is not as powerful as C$\overline{3b}$.

This facilitated phagocytosis is referred to as **opsonization.** In this process, C$\overline{3b}$, which coats the particle, is known as an *opsonin* (which is Greek meaning "to prepare food"). Opsonization is an important process in host defense. Opsonization occurs when cells, viruses, or immune complexes are made ready for enhanced phagocytosis by becoming coated with C$\overline{3b}$ or C$\overline{4b}$. For example, bacteria in the bloodstream would activate the alternative pathway and generate C$\overline{3b}$, which would coat the bacteria. This leads to binding of bacteria to phagocyte C3 receptors and the subsequent clearance of the bacteria by phagocy-

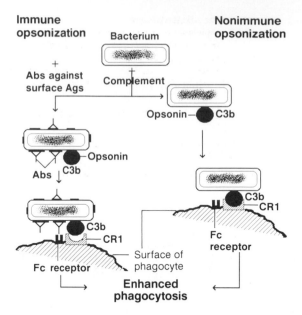

FIGURE 6.12 Mechanisms of opsonization. Enhanced complement-mediated phagocytosis can occur either in the presence or absence of Ab. Opsonization occurs in the presence of Ab when the Fc and CR1 receptors bind Ab and C3b bound to a bacterium. In contrast, nonimmune opsonization requires only that opsonin (C3b) bound to a bacterium becomes associated with the phagocytic CR1 receptor.

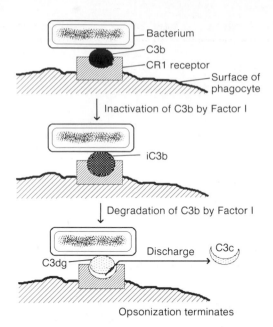

FIGURE 6.13 Degradation of C3b by Factor I. The phagocytic receptor CR1 can bind complement C3b. C3b can be degraded in a two-step process by Factor I; the first is the inactivation of C3b to iC3b (which is opsonic), while the second is the degradation of iC3b to C3dg and C3c (which are not opsonic), with subsequent release from the complex.

tosis (fig. 6.12). This can take place in either the presence or absence of Ab. Viruses, soluble immune complexes, and tumor cells are opsonized and removed by the same mechanism.

Opsonic C$\overline{3b}$ can be generated on particles by either the classical or alternative complement pathways. Fixed C$\overline{3b}$ can be converted by Factor I into *iC3b* (inactive), which is itself an important opsonin with affinity for two types of phagocyte receptors. Coating particles with either C$\overline{3b}$ and iC3b can cause them to bind to phagocytic receptors and subsequently stimulate phagocytosis. C4b and *iC4b* can act in a similar manner, but the strength of binding is considerably weaker than that of fixed C3. Nevertheless, fixed C4 plays a complementary and supporting role in opsonization. Particles coated with both iC4b and iC3b have an enhanced rate of phagocytosis. Factor I can further degrade iC3b into the degradation products C3dg and C3c (and iC4b into C4d and C4c), which terminates the opsonization effect (fig. 6.13).

Complement-Dependent Viral Neutralization

Part of the body's natural defense against viral attack is the production of Abs, which can bind to the surface of the infecting virus. This, in turn, can activate complement, which could neutralize the virus. In fact, the complement system appears to play an important role in neutralizing viruses since it can be activated against certain viruses and virus-infected cells in the absence of Ab. Thus, the complement system seems to represent a surveillance system operative against viruses on first and second exposure (table 6.7).

Viral neutralization can be accomplished by the complement system through four mechanisms: (1) viral aggregation, (2) coating of viral surfaces, (3) lysis of virally infected cells, and (4) activation of inflammatory cells (fig. 6.14).

In complement-dependent *viral aggregation,* complement deposition on viral surfaces can cause clumping of viruses, neutralizing them, thus pre-

TABLE 6.7 Methods of Complement-Dependent Viral Neutralization

Complement Pathway	Antibody Dependence	Encounter with Virus	Examples of Virus or Virus-Infected Cells Attacked
Classical	Ab independent	First exposure	Retroviruses; Sindbis and Newcastle disease viruses
	Ab dependent	Second exposure	Most DNA and RNA viruses; most virus-infected cells
Alternative	Ab independent	First exposure	EBV*; Sindbis virus; cells infected with EBV or measles

*EBV, Epstein-Barr virus.

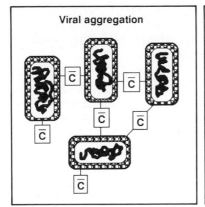

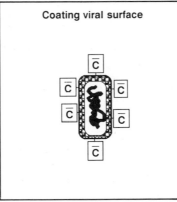

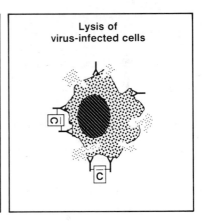

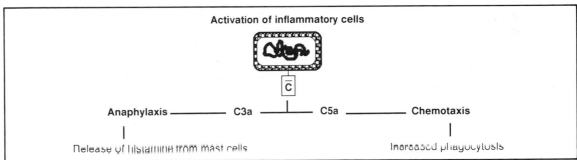

FIGURE 6.14 Mechanisms of viral neutralization by complement. This schematic representation shows the complement-dependent molecular processes, which can lead to viral neutralization. These include viral aggregation and coating of viral surface to reduce the number of infectious viral particles, destruction of virus-infected cells by lysis, and the activation of inflammatory events that can lead to phagocytosis and intracellular virus destruction.

venting invasion of host cells. Neutralization can also be accomplished when complement components coat the surface of the virus, impairing the ability of the virus to attach to the surface of a host cell and infect it. Complement can also coat virus-infected cells, which might interfere with viral maturation. Complement-mediated *lysis of virus-infected cells* can occur with or without Ab attachment, by means of either the classical or alternative complement pathway. In addition, phagocytes with complement receptors can be attracted to these complement-coated virus-infected cells. Activation of these phagocytes initiates engulfment and inflammatory processes. In fact, the host response to viral infections, which includes headaches, fever, and muscle pain, can result from the release of inflammatory agents like histamine. Thus, the consequence of complement interaction with viruses represents a broad-based defense system, which can back up specific humoral and cellular immune responses to viral attack.

Some viruses (e.g., herpes simplex, Epstein-Barr, and vaccinia viruses) produce substances that can counteract the effects of complement. For example, herpes simplex viruses possess a coat glycoprotein that acts as a C3b receptor. This allows herpes simplex virus to modulate the activity of the alternative complement pathway. In addition, a major secretory protein of vaccinia virus contains 38% amino acid identity with C4BP, which enables it to affect activation of the classical complement pathway.

Interaction with Other Mediator Systems

$C\overline{3b}$ can initiate other side reactions during complement fixation. Receptors for $C\overline{3b}$ (e.g., CR1 and CR2) have been found on B cells and platelets. *Ab synthesis* can be stimulated when $C\overline{3b}$ binds to B cells. Moreover, C3 appears to be required for the induction and maintenance of B memory cells. Furthermore, there is evidence that C3d can act as a progression factor, potentiating cell cycle progression (G_0–G_1–S) of Ag-activated murine B cells. Should $C\overline{3b}$ bind to platelets, *thrombus formation* can occur. Adherence of $C\overline{3b}$-coated particles (such as immune complexes) to platelets causes

their aggregation and degranulation. This leads to secretion of vasoactive factors (e.g., histamine and serotonin) and can promote *local inflammation*. Since T cells and NK cells express C3 receptors, C3 might have a role in stimulating *lymphocyte-mediated cytotoxicity*.

In addition to lymphocytes and platelets, complement components can also interact with humoral mediators of hemostasis (fig. 6.15). For example, complement proteins can interact with the *fibrinolytic system*. This process regulates blood clotting by digesting the clot matrix, fibrin. The fibrinolytic system consists of a series of enzymes that generate plasmin, a fibrinolytic enzyme. Plasmin can also activate C1 and C3, and is inhibited by C1 inactivator. Thus, plasmin can be generated, and complement subsequently activated, during certain stages of inflammation. C1 inhibitor can block further clot dissolution by inhibiting plasmin.

Complement can also interact with the *kinin-generating system*. Kinins (e.g., bradykinin) are peptides that can mediate acute inflammatory reactions and contraction of smooth muscle. Kinins are derived from precursors by the action of proteolytic enzymes called kallikreins. In the complement system, C1 inhibitor can inhibit kallikreins, thereby preventing the conversion of kininogen to kinin. In addition, kallikreins can destroy C1 activity by cleavage of the C1s subunit. This aborts the complement cascade.

COMPLEMENT DEFICIENCIES

Most deficiencies of the complement system appear to be due to inborn errors of metabolism. In humans, genetic defects have appeared affecting all the complement proteins. There are four types of inherited complement abnormalities: homozygous deficiency, heterozygous deficiency, dysfunctional proteins, and allotypy. Inherited deficiencies of the *early complement components* (C1, C4, C2, and C3) are frequently associated with immune and rheumatic disorders, whereas deficiencies of *late complement components* (C5, C6, C7, and C8) are linked with recurrent (*Neisseria*) infections (table 6.8). Genetic deficiencies in complement pro-

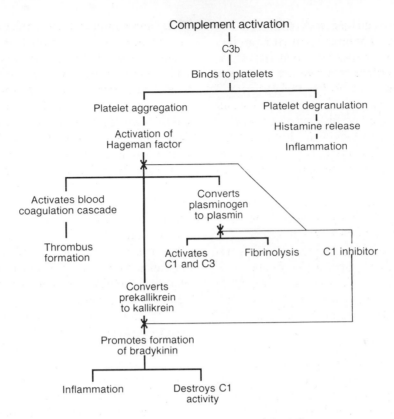

FIGURE 6.15 Interactions between the complement system and blood coagulation. The complement system can interface with the blood coagulation cascade, the fibrinolytic system, the kinin-generating system, and the inflammatory response in several ways. Certain of the more important positive and negative (with ✕ interrupting the pathway) interactions are depicted.

teins can be demonstrated using gel electrophoresis of serum proteins and DNA restriction enzyme techniques to detect protein polymorphisms.

Deficiencies of the complement system described in humans are numerous and are associated with several pathological conditions. Those involving C1 include C1q in combined immune deficiency states, C1r deficiencies associated with infections and lupus-like symptoms, C1s with SLE. Deficiencies in other early complement components are associated with lupuslike symptoms (C4 deficiency), with SLE and increased susceptibility to infections (C2 deficiency), and with recurrent infections of the GI tract and skin (C5 deficiency). Deficiencies of late complement components appear to be associated with increased suscepti-

bility to infections. For example, deficiencies of C3 are found in individuals with severe pyogenic infections (especially of the respiratory tract), deficiencies of C6 are associated with disseminated gonoccocal infection and recurrent meningococcal meningitis, deficiencies of C7 are marked by recurrent *Neisseria* infections, and deficiencies of C8 predispose to disseminated gonococcal infections and neisserial meningitis. In marked contrast, the majority of individuals with deficiencies in C9 do not seem more susceptible to disease than other individuals in the general population.

Deficiencies of regulatory complement proteins have also been characterized and have been found to be quite similar. For example, deficiency of C3b inactivator (Factor I) is coupled with recurrent bacterial

TABLE 6.8 Disease States Associated with Deficiencies of Specific Complement Proteins

Pathway	Protein	Disease State
Classical		
	C1q	Combined immune deficiency states
	C1r	Lupuslike syndromes; infections
	C1s	SLE; infections
	C2	SLE; infections
	C3	Infections
	C4	Lupuslike diseases
	C5	Infections (*Neisseria*)
	C6	Infections (*Neisseria*)
	C7	Infections (*Neisseria*)
	C8	Infections (*Neisseria*)
	C9	None
Alternative		
	C3	Infections
	Factor D	Infections
	Properdin	Infections
Regulatory proteins		
	C1 inhibitor	Hereditary angioneurotic edema
	Factor I	Infections

infections, and deficiency of C1 inhibitor is associated with hereditary angioneurotic edema (recurrent episodes of localized edema, especially of the respiratory tract). Properdin deficiency predisposes to recurrent infections, while Factor D deficiency is associated with increased bacterial infections.

We might ask, What is the role of these inherited complement component abnormalities in predisposing to disease? The high incidence of recurrent infections can be explained by recognizing the importance of the complement cascade in eliminating invading organisms. For example, the pathology of hereditary angioedema in C1 inhibitor deficiencies can be seen when we consider the consequence of increased levels of activated C1. Such an increase would cause exhaustion of C4 and C2 levels, and increase activity in the fibrinolytic and kinin-generating systems. The result would be increased production of mediators

(e.g., bradykinin) that enhance vascular permeability and, ultimately, edema. However, the nature of the association between complement deficiencies and immune disorders, like SLE, is still not clearly elucidated. Since C4 and C2 play a role in the clearance of immune complexes, their failure to clear these complexes normally from the circulation could account for the subsequent expression of immune-comples disorders like lupus. There also seems to be a link between C4 and C2 deficiency and HLA-DR3 and DR2 alleles, which suggests that immune response genes may be closely linked to those of HLA. Therefore, the HLA-linked complement deficiencies might also be linked to immune response genes. These might express themselves as immunologically mediated diseases. Thus, complement deficiencies associated with SLE might only represent markers for a subset of individuals with lupus.

IMMUNOLOGICAL TESTS FOR COMPLEMENT

The *measurement of complement levels* in the serum can be accomplished by a simple assay, which measures the proportion of sensitized erythrocytes that are lysed as a function of the amount of complement added. This assay is based on the one-hit theory of hemolysis, which states that a single lesion in an erythrocyte, induced by Ab and complement, is sufficient for lysis. The *hemolytic unit of complement (CH_{50} unit)* is defined as that amount of complement that lyses 50% of sensitized erythrocytes under defined standardized conditions. Reduced hemolytic activity (fewer CH_{50} units/mL of serum) might be indicative of (1) recent activation of the complement cascade, (2) degradative consumption of complement, or (3) failure to produce some complement component(s) because of a genetic defect. This assay has several uses which include monitoring the clinical course of immune-complex disease and screening for genetic deficiencies of complement components.

In the **complement fixation test** (see fig. 4.16), the ability of complement to lyse red blood cells is used as a way to *measure serum Ab levels*. It is based

The Role of Complement in Disease

Usually, complement activation is one way that the body protects itself against injury and invasion. However, in certain pathological conditions, these same complement defense mechanisms may be responsible for tissue destruction and progression of a disease state. Examples of this can be found in certain immune-complex diseases, for example, the autoimmune disorders of rheumatoid arthritis, SLE, and autoimmune hemolytic anemia.

The appearance of auto-Abs can trigger an Ab response which might produce the formation of Ag-Ab complexes. These immune complexes can trigger complement activation. In autoimmune disease, the complement system actually operates in the same way as it does to defend the body against microbial invasion. Thus, if an Ab binds to a self-Ag on an erythrocyte or a platelet or glomerular basement membrane, the complement cascade is activated, causing the pathological destruction of the person's own erythrocytes, platelets, or kidney. Furthermore, a rapid buildup of immune complexes can overwhelm the protective role of the complement system in the clearance of immune complexes. This could lead to deposition of immune complexes in tissues, causing inappropriate local inflammatory responses and the destruction of tissues in which the complexes are lodged.

In the majority of individuals with immune-complex disease, the complement system is functionally normal. Unfortunately, this very appropriate response to immune-complex deposition enhances the inflammatory response and adversely affects cell membranes. The pathophysiology of joint destruction in rheumatoid arthritis, or glomerulonephritis in SLE, or hemolysis in autoimmune hemolytic anemia, can be attributed, in part, to the complement response and the ensuing damage inflicted by inflammation.

Thus, in autoimmune disease, the cytotoxic, anaphylactic, and opsonic functions of complement are directed against normal tissues through auto-Ab activation of the classical pathway. A normal function of complement is the safe disposal of circulating immune complexes with the macrophage phagocytic system. But in autoimmune disease, a chronic high level of immune complexes exhausts the normal supply of complement and reduces the quantity of complexes cleared. This can lead to deposition of immune complexes into small blood vessels, which can lead to vasculitis. More complete understanding of how the complement system is regulated may lead to future therapies in which the complement response might be selectively curtailed in autoimmune disease.

Atkinson, J. P., Kaine, J. L., Hollers, V. M., et al. Complement and the rheumatic diseases. In *Immunobiology of the Complement System.* Ross, G. D., (ed.). Academic Press, Inc., Orlando, Fla. 1986.

Schifferli, J. A., Ng, Y. C., and Peters, D. K. The role of complement and its receptor in the elimination of immune complexes. *New England Journal of Medicine* 315:488, 1986.

on the fact that activated complement components can be used only once, then they are used up or "fixed" and can be replenished only by the further addition of complement. The test consists of two parts: (1) Ag and test serum (containing no complement) are incubated with guinea pig serum that has complement, and then (2) an indicator system of Ab-coated sheep red blood cells is added. If lysis of the indicator system occurs, it is a negative result, meaning that complement was not fixed since the specific Ab was absent from the test serum. On the other hand, if the indicator system is not lysed, it is a positive result since the complement had to be fixed by the Ab in the test serum that was specific for the test Ag.

Techniques for the *measurement of complement components* consist of hemolytic assays based on immune hemolysis, and the preparation of erythrocytes sensitized with Ab-carrying complement components (e.g.,

EAC1, EAC4). The basic principle in measuring a single component of the complement system is to make that component limiting by supplying an excess of the remaining components. For example, in the titration of C1, EAC4 cells are added to the diluted serum, then C2 is added, followed by C3–C9. The number of lesions per erythrocyte can be correlated with the original concentration of C1 in the test serum. Alternatively, immunochemical methods can be used to measure separate components. Specific antisera can be raised to isolated complement components, which then can be quantified by a variety of immunological assays.

S U M M A R Y

1. Complement is a sequential, multimolecular system of plasma proteins, which can be activated by a variety of immunological (e.g., IgG and immune complexes) and nonimmunological stimuli (e.g., polysaccharides). Complement activation can proceed via two different pathways, the classical pathway, which is triggered by immunological memory, or an alternative pathway, which requires no immunological trigger. [p. 152]

2. The classical complement pathway is activated by IgG and IgM containing immune complexes and is composed of eleven distinct plasma proteins, which are identified numerically as C1 (q, r, s) and C2–C9. [pp. 152–159]

3. The alternative complement pathway is activated by plant, fungal, and bacterial polysaccharides and lipopolysaccharides. It is composed of six plasma proteins identified as Factors D, B, H, I, P (properdin), and C3. In addition, C5–C9 can be recruited to attack membrane surfaces, as in the classical pathway. The C3–C9 components are thus common to both pathways. [pp. 158–164]

4. The biosynthesis of complement components occurs mainly in the liver, but macrophages can produce components at the site of infection. [p. 164]

5. The genes for C4, C2, and Factor B are class III genes located within the MHC. The other gene loci are scattered throughout the genome. [pp. 164–166]

6. Activation of either complement pathway produces several biological effects. These include (a) irreversible damage to biological membranes associated with complement-dependent cytolysis; (b) deposition of molecules on the surfaces of particles under complement attack, resulting in particle opsonization and clearance; and (c) production of potent mediators of inflammation. [pp. 166–170]

7. In general, congenital deficiencies of complement components result in an increased susceptibility to infection. Deficiencies of C2, C1r, or C4 are associated with the immune-complex disease, systemic lupus erythematosus, whereas C1 inactivator deficiency is associated with hereditary angioedema. [pp. 170–172]

8. Immunological tests involving complement can measure (a) complement levels in serum, (b) antibody levels in serum, and (c) individual complement component levels in serum. [pp. 172–174]

R E A D I N G S

Alsenz, J., Bork, K., and Loos, M. Autoantibody-mediated acquired deficiency of C1 inhibitor. *New England Journal of Medicine* **316:**1360, 1987.

Bentley, D. R., and Porter, R. R. Isolation of cDNA clones for human complement component C2. *Proceedings of the National Academy of Science* (USA) **81:**1212, 1984.

Burger, R. Complement research: the impact of molecular genetics. *Immunology Today* **7:**27, 1986.

Carroll, M. C. Molecular genetics of the fourth component of human complement. *Federation Proceedings* **46:**2457, 1987.

Klaus, G. G. B., and Humphrey, J. H. A reevaluation of the role of C3 in B-cell activation. *Immunology Today* **7:**163, 1986.

Kotwal, G. J., Isaacs, S. N., McKenzie, R., et al. Inhibition of the complement cascade by the major secretory protein of vaccinia virus. *Science* **250**:827, 1990.

Kristensen, T., D'Eustachio, P., Ogata, R. T., et al. The superfamily of C3b/C4b-binding proteins. *Federation Proceedings* **46**:2463, 1987.

Liszewski, M. K., Post, T. W., and Atkinson, J. P. Membrane cofactor protein (MCP or CD46): newest member of the regulators of complement activation gene cluster. *Annual Review of Immunology* **9**:431, 1991.

Morgan, B. P. *Complement: Clinical Aspects and Relevance to Disease.* Academic Press, London. 1990.

Pangburn, M. K. Alternative pathway of complement. *Methods of Enzymology* **162**:639, 1988.

Ross, D. R. (ed.). *Immunobiology of the Complement System.* Academic Press, Inc., Orlando, Fla., 1986.

Schifferli, J. A., Ng, Y. C., and Peters, K. D. The role of complement and its receptor in the elimination of immune complexes. *New England Journal of Medicine* **315**:488, 1986.

Schur, P. H. Inherited complement component abnormalities. *Annual Review of Medicine* **37**:333, 1986.

Stoppa-Lyonnet, D., Tosi, M., Laurent, J., et al. Altered C1 inhibitor genes in Type 1 hereditary angioedema. *New England Journal of Medicine* **317**:1, 1987.

Teisner, B., Brandslund, I., Folkersen, J., et al. Factor I deficiency and C3 nephritic factor: Immunochemical findings and association with *Neisseria meningitidis* infection in two patients. *Scandinavian Journal of Immunology* **20**:291, 1984.

Weismann, H. F., Bartow, T., Leppo, M. K., et al. Soluble human complement receptor type I: in vivo inhibitor of complement suppressing post-ischemic myocardial inflammation and necrosis. *Science* **249**:146, 1990.

Cellular Immunity

Cellular, or cell-mediated, immunity represents the second major arm of the immune system. In cellular immunity, the immune response is mediated by direct cellular participation in the defensive reactions. This unit explores the bases for cellular immunity. Chapter 7, Histocompatibility Systems, outlines the genetic background upon which cellular immune mechanisms depend. In particular, this includes a discussion of the genetic basis upon which self/nonself discrimination depends and the influence of immune response genes on the expression of cellular immunity. The cells that are responsible for actually expressing cell-mediated immune responses are examined in chapter 8, Effectors of Nonspecific Cellular Immunity, and chapter 9, Effectors of Specific Cellular Immunity. These chapters examine effector cells from the perspectives of antigen-nonspecific and antigen-specific immunological responses. Last, chapter 10, Immune Tolerance and Suppression, examines modulation of immunological responsiveness, with particular emphasis on expressing nonresponsiveness to self-antigens or foreign antigens.

CHAPTER 7

Histocompatibility Systems

OVERVIEW

The composition and function of major and minor histocompatibility systems are selectively described. The roles of these obligatory systems in self-governance of (1) immunological cell interactions controlling immune capacity, (2) disease susceptibility, and (3) transplantation are identified. In addition, the influence of minor lymphocyte stimulatory genes is described.

CONCEPTS

1. Two types of histocompatibility genes exist: (a) major histocompatibility genes that exist in clusters on a single chromosome and (b) minor histocompatibility genes that are dispersed throughout the genome.

2. Major histocompatibility genes control self/nonself, cell-surface recognition systems required for appropriate lymphocyte responses (class I and II) and synthesis of certain complement components and stress-related proteins (class III). Class I molecules impose specific restrictions on cell-mediated responses, while class II molecules govern our capacity to exhibit humoral and, to some extent, cell-mediated responses.

3. Foreign minor histocompatibility gene products may stimulate chronic, slow, intense forms of graft rejection, rather than acute, rapid responses as seen in major histocompatibility systems.

4. Minor lymphocyte stimulatory genes, which are distinct from histocompatibility genes, regulate some aspects of functional expression of activated lymphocytes.

In 1948 George Snell introduced the expressions histocompatibility gene and histocompatibility antigen (Ag). At this time tissue and organ transplantation from one person to another to replace diseased organs was almost invariably unsuccessful. It became apparent that a graft from one individual to another unrelated individual of the same species, known as an allograft, simply could not be permanently tolerated. Grafts between outbred mice were similarly unsuccessful. Grafts between members of different species (*xenografts*) were even more discouraging. On the other hand, grafts between identical twins (*isografts*), or from one part of the body to another (*autografts*), were usually tolerated. In an attempt to elucidate the genetic basis of graft rejection, investigators became interested in histocompatibility gene products that determine resistance or rejection. Later it became clear that these gene products participate not only in transplantation rejection, but are significantly involved in regulating immune responsiveness involving cell-to-cell interactions and, in turn, susceptibility to a number of diseases.

■　■　■　■　■　■　■　■　■　■　■

BACKGROUND

A gene is a portion of DNA that contains information necessary to produce a specific protein molecule or, at least, part of a protein molecule. The specific site of location for any gene in a chromosome is referred to as its locus, and is, therefore, represented twice since chromosomes are paired. Two genes at a particular locus, on matched or sister chromosomes, control one particular trait or characteristic and are called alleles. In humans, paired chromosomes commonly carry different alleles. If each gene is expressed, in a heterozygous situation, they are said to be codominant and two different gene products, or allo-Ags, are produced.

In 1933 Haldane proposed that, during transplantation, an immune reaction was directed against specific allo-Ags displayed on cell membranes of the donor, but absent in the recipient. To prove this it was necessary to show that different individuals possess unique gene products (i.e., allo-Ags), which can stimulate an immune response in those lacking these same gene products. Furthermore, it was necessary to show that such a response could result in graft rejection. The eventual development of inbred (syngeneic) strains of mice permitted an animal model for extensive study of histocompatibility systems.

Today it is recognized that the number of different permutations and combinations of major and minor genes governing histocompatibility is immense, and extremely important immunologically. Everyone on earth, with the possible exception of identical twins, has a personal set of **histocompatibility genes** and gene products (as glycoprotein allo-Ags on cell surfaces) that are not exactly identical to those of anyone else. Our histocompatibility type is as distinct as our fingerprints. These genetically defined Ags, some of which are found on the surface of all body cells, serve to *discriminate self from nonself.*

Inbred Mouse Strains

In early studies on transplantation, only outbred animals, from randomly bred colonies, were available. These animals contained alleles that were homozygous as well as heterozygous. The need for genetically uniform animals, for more controlled experimentation, became obvious.

Since mice possess short gestation periods, and produce relatively large litters, various strains were developed by sister-brother matings. Such inbred matings eventually led to overall homogeneity, and a single allele tended to become fixed for each gene. Subsequently, several hundred inbred strains of mice have been developed. The availability of inbred strains has provided an opportunity to produce unique strains that differ from one another by only a small portion of a single chromosome. Such strains are said to be *congenic,* since they share all genes (background alleles) except those located at a particular locus. Usually a congenic strain is selected for an allele of a single gene called the *differential gene.* Congenic strains are produced by selective breeding, and repeated backcrossing (fig. 7.1). Congenic strains are designated by the abbreviation of the background strain and donor strain (that contributed the new histocompatibility locus) separated by a period. Thus, an **A.B** mouse represents a congenic

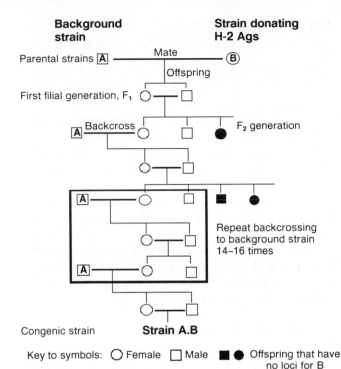

Background strain

Strain donating H-2 Ags

Parental strains Ⓐ ——— Mate ——— Ⓑ

Offspring

First filial generation, F₁ ○—□

Ⓐ Backcross ○—□ ● F₂ generation

○—□

Ⓐ ○—□ ■ ● Repeat backcrossing to background strain 14–16 times

○—□

Ⓐ ○—□

○—□

Congenic strain **Strain A.B**

Key to symbols: ○ Female □ Male ■ ● Offspring that have no loci for B

FIGURE 7.1 Production of a congenic mouse strain. Mice of strain "**A,**" possessing background genes, are bred to mice of strain "**B,**" possessing desired H-2 genes. Skin from F₁ hybrids cannot be grafted to strain **A** mice since they carry one "b" allele for each histocompatibility locus. When F₁ mice are backcrossed to strain **A** mice, some of the offspring may be homozygous for the "a" allele at all H loci. These mice may be selected for elimination from the progeny since a graft of their skin will not be rejected by strain **A** mice. By extensive backcrossing, progeny that do not possess b alleles are removed. Progeny that retain b alleles, after repeated backcrossings, may express a/b at only one locus. Mice, homozygous (b/b) at the locus, are obtained by mating (a/b × a/b) and are selected by their ability to reject a strain **A** skin graft. Such congenic mice (**A.B**) possess the genetic background of strain **A** mice and the donated H-2 locus from strain **B** mice.

strain carrying background genes of the A strain and a homozygous pair of histocompatibility genes derived from the B strain.

In addition to differential histocompatibility alleles, congenic strains can differ in alleles of other genes. Strains differing only by the allele of a single gene are called *coisogenic*. Such strains can be derived from selective breeding of inbred animals in which a point mutation has been identified. A number of tech-

niques are available to screen mice for mutated genes that determine histocompatibility.

In brief, inbred strains that differ from one another by only a small portion of a single chromosome and share background alleles are said to be congenic. Strains differing by the allele of a single gene are called coisogenic.

Immunological Detection of Alloantigens

With the development of inbred, congenic, and mutated strains of mice, genetic differences could be detected by immunological analysis of the allo-Ags or gene products. Cell-surface allo-Ags could be identified by a variety of immunological techniques employing specific antibodies (Abs) or effector cells (lymphocytes). For example, cells from one inbred strain (donor) that possessed an allo-Ag of interest might be given to another strain (recipient) not possessing that particular gene product. The recipient would respond to the foreign allo-Ag by synthesizing specific anti-allo-Abs and by expanding allospecific clones of effector cells. Here, then, were tools that could be used to detect specific allo-Ags, determine their distribution on cells and tissues in the animal, and contribute to their isolation and characterization.

Histocompatibility Antigens

Since congenic pairs of inbred strains differed by alleles of a single histocompatibility gene, graft rejection between the pair occurred in response to a single Ag or even a single epitope (antigenic determinant). Two groups of histocompatibility gene products (allo-Ags) were now recognized. These were seen as major or minor histocompatibility Ags that stimulated either acute, rapid, intense forms of graft rejection (major) or chronic, slow, less intense responses (minor). (Additional discussion of transplantation reactions can be found in chapter 19.)

The genes encoding these proteins were found to occur in clusters. Subsequently, these clusters of genes became known as major and minor histocompatibility complexes, responsible for transplantation Ags. Major histocompatibility genes are located on a single chromosome, whereas minor histocompatibility genes are scattered throughout the genome. In the mouse, for example, 15 of the 20 chromosome pairs contain minor histocompatibility genes, whereas the components of the major histocompatibility system are restricted to chromosome 17.

The first **major histocompatibility complex** (**MHC**) to be characterized was that of the mouse. It was designed the **H-2 complex** and details of its organization were published by Gorer in 1936. Fourteen years passed before the next MHC system, the *B complex* of the chicken, was characterized by Briles and associates. Before the close of the next decade, initial details of the human MHC, called the **HLA system,** were determined and reported by Dausset in 1958. Since then, the MHCs of many species have been characterized. Among mammals two general patterns seem to exist: (1) the murine pattern found among rodents (chiefly mice and rats, accounting for approximately 40% of all mammalian species) and (2) the HLA-like pattern found among most other mammals (e.g., dogs, cats, pigs, cows, sheep, and nonhuman primates). We examine these two models of MHC organization in more detail in the following pages.

In recent years it has become evident that histocompatibility genes and their Ags are involved in a variety of functions in addition to graft rejection. In the 1960s, it was suggested that the MHC genes that we possess play a role in our ability to respond immunologically. Selected strains of inbred mice, each with a distinct MHC, were shown to respond strongly, weakly, in an intermediate fashion, or not at all to the same Ag.

Following the work of Benacerraf and McDevitt showing the influence of the MHC on immune responsiveness, Zinkernagel and Doherty in the 1970s demonstrated **MHC restriction** of humoral and cell-mediated responses to Ag. (This topic is treated in greater detail later in this chapter.) *The need for an Ag-reactive cell to recognize a marker of self,* a product of an MHC gene, *as well as a foreign Ag* became evident in an increasing number of observed cell-to-cell interactions. Moreover, the cluster of genes making up the MHC in an individual, and the gene products identifiable on that individual's cells (histocompatibility type), determine susceptibility to a variety of diseases.

MURINE MAJOR HISTOCOMPATIBILITY COMPLEX
Arrangement of MHC Genes

Mice of an inbred strain have the same MHC genes and are homozygous at all gene loci, making them ideal subjects for studying histocompatibility. The genes of the murine MHC occur in the region designated as the **H-2 complex.** The H-2 complex is a linked series of genes in a small segment of *chromosome 17.* Proximal to this region (nearer the chromosome's centromere) is a related complex designated **T1a.**

H-2 Complex

The H-2 complex is comprised of *four major regions* known as **K, I, S,** and **D,** each defined by a number of recombinants (fig. 7.2). The **I region** has several subregions, which are divided into eight subdivisions, while the **S** and **D regions** each have at least two subdivisions. Each region or subregion is believed to contain one locus, but may contain more. For example, there may be over 60 distinct genes assigned to the H-2 complex. A minimum of two dozen genes are known. Their products are designated according to structure and function as class I, II, or III molecules.

It is principally, but not exclusively, the H-2 gene products that regulate the processes of *transplantation, immune responsiveness,* and *aspects of complement synthesis.* These products, however, may serve more than one function.

Each gene of the H-2 complex possesses multiple alleles, usually inherited as a block on a given chromosome and designated the H-2 haplotype. Two H-2 haplotypes make up an animal's H-2 genotype, which would be identical in an inbred mouse. In outbred mice the two haplotypes may be totally or partially distinct. There are over 200 known inbred strains of mice exhibiting different H-2 haplotypes, designated by lowercase letter superscripts. Haplotypes of several representative inbred and inbred congenic strains of mice are shown in table 7.1.

T1a Complex

To the right, or downstream, of the D region is the Tla complex. This complex contains several alleles. The products of these genes are very *similar to class I*

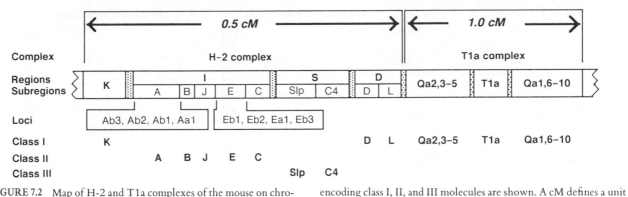

FIGURE 7.2 Map of H-2 and T1a complexes of the mouse on chromosome 17. The H-2 complex is composed of four major regions (K, I, S, and D), each defined by a number of recombinants. Genes are assigned to specific points along the chromosome, permitting a genetic map to be constructed showing loci. Genes of the MHC- encoding class I, II, and III molecules are shown. A cM defines a unit of a genetic map. A cM corresponds to the distance between two genes that recombine with a frequency of 1%, that is, in 1% of the animals comprising the population. *Note:* H-2 and T1a regions are not represented in true scale.

molecules of the H-2 complex. These genes may share in the functions of the H-2 complex.

Distribution of MHC Antigens

The K and D regions of the H-2 complex encode class I Ags found on all nucleated cells, erythrocytes, and platelets. They are present in particularly high concentrations on leukocytes. In contrast, the I region encodes class II Ags, which are found only on B lymphocytes, monocytes, macrophages, epithelial cells, and spermatozoa. Class III Ags may be formed in, and displayed on, macrophages, and bound, under certain conditions, to lymphocytes, neutrophils, erythrocytes, and platelets.

Specificity of MHC Antigens

As with most membrane-surface Ags, portions of molecules exposed on the surface of a cell display a number of epitopes or antigenic determinants (fig. 7.3). Allo- Ags possess unique epitopes peculiar to their haplotype (*private specificities*), but they may share epitopes with Ags of other haplotypes (*public specificities*). This is portrayed in figure 7.4.

Each haplotype of an inbred strain produces Ags which can stimulate an immune response in strains possessing a haplotype lacking that Ag or unique epitopes within that Ag. This can be exploited as

TABLE 7.1 H-2 Haplotypes of Common Mouse Inbred and Congenic Inbred Strains

Strain	H-2 Haplotype*	MHC Region†							
		K	Ia	Ib	Ij	Ie	Ic	S	D
Inbred									
B10	H-2ᵇ	b	b	b	b	b	b	b	b
C57BL/6	H-2ᵇ	b	b	b	b	b	b	b	b
C57BL/10	H-2ᵇ	b	b	b	b	b	b	b	b
BALB/c	H-2ᵈ	d	d	d	d	d	d	d	d
DBA/Z	H-2ᵈ	d	d	d	d	d	d	d	d
NZB	H-2ᵈ	d	d	d	d	d	d	d	d
C3H	H-2ᵏ	k	k	k	k	k	k	k	k
CBA	H-2ᵏ	k	k	k	k	k	k	k	k
Congenic Inbred									
B10.DZ (Donor = DBA/Z Background = B10)	H-2ᵈ	d	d	d	d	d	d	d	d
BALB.B10 (Donor = B10 Background = BALB/c)	H-2ᵇ	b	b	b	b	b	b	b	b

*H-2 haplotype designations for the several strains of mice listed.
†H-2 haplotype appearing in each MHC region.

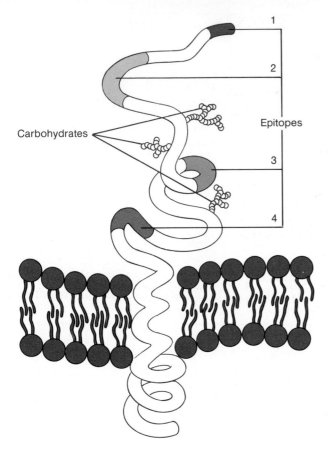

FIGURE 7.3 Exposed epitopes of a histocompatibility Ag in a cell membrane.

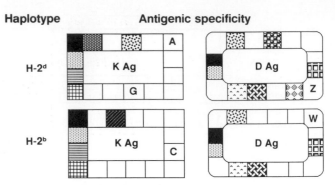

Haplotype	Antigenic specificity		

Key to symbols:
Patterns depict **public specificities**
Letters represent **private specificities**

FIGURE 7.4 H-2 public and private specificities. Antigenic determinants of class I molecules may be shared with other class I molecules or haplotypes (*depicted by patterns*) and are designated **public specificities.** Antigenic determinants that are unique for a particular class I molecule and haplotype (*depicted by letters*) are termed **private specificities.**

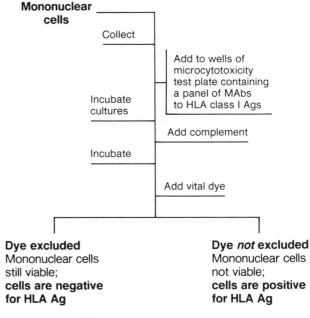

FIGURE 7.5 Cell/tissue typing of HLA class I Ags with MAbs. Mononuclear cells to be tested are mixed with a panel of MAbs specific for a variety of class I Ags. Complement is added that becomes fixed if one of the MAbs combines with the HLA Ag of the mononuclear cell. Subsequently, the cell bearing the immune complexes becomes damaged, permitting a vital dye to enter. The mononuclear cell expressing the class I molecule is thus identified by MAb that is specific for a known HLA Ag.

a diagnostic or analytical tool; for example, for the production of Abs that are **monospecific for the epitope** in question (monoclonal Abs [MAbs]; see chapter 3 for further details). Thus, MAbs can be obtained against the unique epitopes for discrimination. A panel of different MAbs has been developed that permits *serological tissue typing.* These can be used to identify a wide range of class I MHC determinants (fig. 7.5). Class II Ags can be detected by measuring their ability to stimulate allogeneic lymphocytes to divide in a *mixed lymphocyte culture (MLC,* fig. 7.6).

Class I Antigens

Class I Ags (fig. 7.7) are considered "classical transplantation" Ags. Each is a membrane-bound glycoprotein of 45,000 daltons (45 kD), consisting of a single

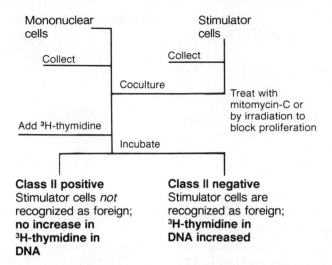

Class II positive
Stimulator cells *not*
recognized as foreign;
**no increase in
³H-thymidine in
DNA**

Class II negative
Stimulator cells are
recognized as foreign;
**³H-thymidine in
DNA increased**

FIGURE 7.6 Typing of HLA class II Ags by the MLR. A panel of inactivated stimulator cells (lymphocytes), exhibiting known class II Ags, are mixed with mononuclear cells to determine their HLA types. If class II molecules of a potential stimulator cell differ from those of the sample, a response follows involving DNA synthesis, which is easily monitored. If, on the other hand, class II molecules of a stimulator cell are identical to those of the cells being typed, no response occurs. In this way HLA Ag on the sample cells is readily identified.

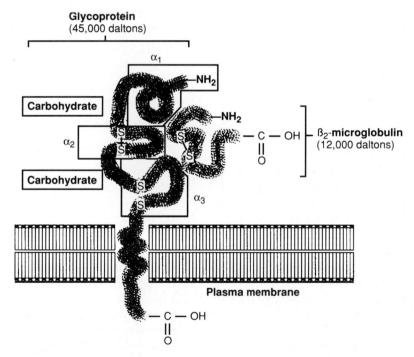

FIGURE 7.7 Structure of class I Ags. Three external domains (α_1, α_2, and α_3) and a cytoplasmic domain make up the heavy polypeptide chain that is encoded by the MHC. The α_1 and α_2 domains display specific antigenic determinants, and each contains an attached carbohydrate unit. The lighter chain is β_2-microglobulin, which is not encoded by the histocompatibility complex. The β_2 domain appears to be critically involved in the expression of the class I molecule.

peptide chain noncovalently linked to a smaller molecule. This second molecule is a protein (12 kD) called β_2-microglobulin.

The gene for β_2-microglobulin is not part of the MHC, but is located on chromosome 2. Genes of the K region and D region, with two subregions (D and L), and the T1a region, with 11 subregions (Qa2,3–5, T1a, Qa1,6–10), encode class I molecules. About 30 of these genes map to the Qa and T1a regions, which lie to the right of the H-2D, L region on mouse chromosome 17.

Class I genes in the H-2K and H-2D, L regions encode cell-surface polypeptides that are found on almost all cell types, are highly polymorphic, and are involved in signaling effector T cells during cell-mediated immunity. *Class I genes within the Qa and T1a regions* exhibit low polymorphism, encode Ags displayed primarily on hemopoietic cells, and are not required for cell-mediated immunity.

Both *K and D regions,* however, encode strong transplantation Ags. These class I molecules are capable of provoking strong cell-mediated responses as well as Ab responses. Each class I Ag bears many antigenic determinants, some unique (private specificity) and some shared with other class I Ags (public specificities). Cytotoxic T (T_C) cells involved in recognition and acute rejection of foreign tissue grafts respond to unique epitopes of H-2K, H-2D, and H-2L Ags on foreign cells. In cooperation with T helper (T_H) cells, they destroy foreign cells.

In addition to transplantation reactions, class I Ags are involved in immune surveillance, for example relating to viral infection. During many viral infections, host T_C cells recognize viral Ags on cell surfaces. However, recognition of self class I MHC Ags (H-2 K/D) is also required for interaction of T_C cells with virally infected cells. Effector T cells must recognize both the foreign viral Ag and the host MHC Ag during the initiative and destructive phases (fig. 7.8). Effector T cells will not destroy cells of a different haplotype infected with the same virus; thus, they exhibit **haplotype-restricted killing.** A similar system may be operative in the detection and elimination of trans-

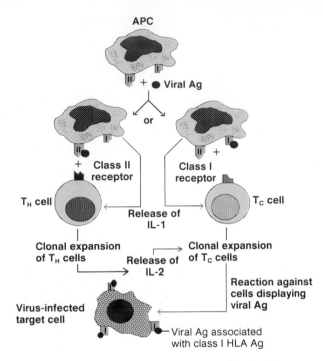

FIGURE 7.8 MHC restriction. APCs, or virus-infected cells, present viral Ag in association with self class I molecules, recognized by cytotoxic (T_C) cells, and class II molecules, recognized by helper (T_H) cells. Binding of the class I molecule/viral Ag complex to T_C cell receptors stimulates expansion of cytotoxic cells. Binding of the class II molecule/viral complex to T_H receptors stimulates expansion of helper cells. The response may be amplified by the release of interleukin 1 (IL-1) from APCs and interleukin 2 (IL-2) from both T cell subsets. T_C cells will recognize and destroy only target cells expressing both self class I molecules and viral Ag.

formed cells that must display self-MHC Ags to be destroyed by effector T cells. This *requirement that both the foreign Ag and the host MHC Ag be present* is known as **MHC restriction.**

Class I Ags encoded by the T1a region are found on immature cortical thymocytes, serving as markers of *T cell differentiation,* and on some T leukemic cells. Qa Ags are found on B and T lymphocytes and on stem cells in the bone marrow. They are not strong transplantation Ags, and they do not apparently restrict cell-to-cell interactions, as seen for K and D Ags. To date the function of the T1a complex is not clear.

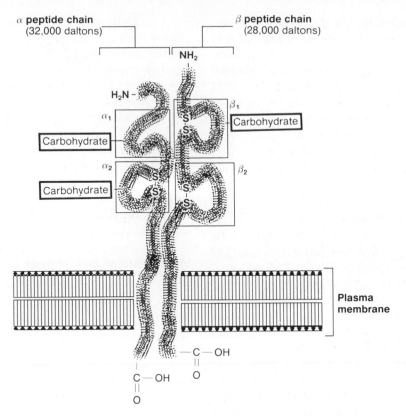

FIGURE 7.9 Structure of class II Ags. Class II Ags consist of two peptide chains, α and β, which are noncovalently bonded together. Each chain possesses two globular domains. Antigenic determinants are located primarily within the β chain.

Class II Antigens

Class II Ags are glycoproteins consisting of two noncovalently linked α and β peptide chains with molecular weights of 32 and 28 kD, respectively. Each chain contains two extracellular domains (α_1, α_2 or β_1, β_2), a connecting peptide, a transmembrane region, and a cytoplasmic tail (fig. 7.9).

The I region is divided into five subregions. I-A, I-B, I-J, I-E, and I-C, with eight alleles encoding class II Ags: Ab3, Ab2, Ab1, Aa1, Eb, Eb2, Ea, and Eb3, arranged in this order on chromosome 17 (see fig. 7.2). Two types of I molecules exist, which are composed of either $A_a A_b$ or $E_a E_b$ chains. These Ags are involved in a number of immunological events.

Antigen-presenting cells (APCs) display I region Ags (Ia), in a restricted manner, analogous to MHC restriction (seen on p. 182 for class I Ags). T_H cells responding to APCs must recognize a given Ia Ag presented together with a foreign Ag. On secondary Ag challenge, the T_H cell recognizes the foreign Ag when it is presented with the initially recognized self-Ia Ag.

Ia Ags also control interaction between T_H cells and B cells or T_C cells and between T suppressor (T_S) cells and other T cells. Delayed-type hypersensitivity (mediated by T_D cells) is also controlled in large measure by I region gene products. Thus, class II molecules are concerned with T_H, T_S, *and* T_D recruitment.

Many genes of the I region and their subregions and subdivisions dramatically influence our ability to mount an immune response to an Ag. Consequently, they are sometimes referred to as **immune response (Ir) genes.** Since these genes, and their products (Ia Ags), may vary from one mouse strain to another, so does their immune capacity.

Class III Antigens

Genes in this region control the level of at least two major proteins known as **C4,** the fourth component of complement, and **Slp,** a sex-limited protein. C4 is a three-chain glycoprotein containing an α, a β, and a γ chain with molecular weights of 93, 77, and 32 kD, respectively. Two antigenic variants of C4, C4a and C4b, are commonly found bound to cell membranes. The role of C4 in the complement system is discussed in chapter 6, Complement and its Role in Immune Responses. The Slp locus encodes a sex-linked protein expressed only in males of certain strains of mice. Males of strains capable of producing Slp do so only after puberty. Female mice of the same strain possess Slp genes but do not produce the Ag unless treated with the male hormone, testosterone. The function of this MHC molecule is unclear. In addition, a gene locus, provisionally designated RD, has been identified between the B_f and C4/Slp loci. The RD gene encodes a 42 kD protein with unusual periodic structure and, as yet, no defined function. Class III molecules are considered transplantation Ags.

MAJOR HISTOCOMPATIBILITY COMPLEX IN HUMANS (HLA)

Nearly forty years ago **human leukocyte–associated (HLA) Ags** were discovered that provided strong transplantation Ags, similar to the H-2 complex in mice. Thus, Ags of the HLA system were of critical interest in relation to organ transplantation, and attempts were made to identify and "match" donor Ags as nearly as possible with those of the recipient. Codification of the reaction patterns of thousands of different anti-HLA allo-Abs has helped delineate the system.

Today such Ags may also be of interest in paternity testing, other questions of heredity, and in the field of anthropology. Certain diseases are closely related to specific HLA Ags, permitting relative disease risks and absolute risks to be determined in accord with a particular HLA type. Characterization of HLA type may even be helpful in clinical diagnosis.

Although HLA Ags are prominently involved in transplantation phenomena, they also play a major regulatory role in cell-to-cell interactions and immune responses involving obligatory self-recognition. The broad functional responsibilities of class I, II, and III Ags of the HLA system are very similar to those described in the murine H-2 system.

Arrangement and Nomenclature of HLA Genes

Every few years an International Workshop, sponsored by the World Health Organization (WHO), meets to update the description of the organization and nomenclature of the human MHC. Obviously, this is a very active area of research and new information is being reported almost continuously. The entire human MHC is known as the **HLA complex.** It occupies a segment of somewhat less than 4 centimorgans (cM) on chromosome 6. The HLA complex, showing the regions containing HLA loci, is depicted in figure 7.10.

The major domains of the HLA complex can be subdivided into regions reflecting the MHC class to which the gene products belong. Genes encoding class I proteins are located near the end (telomere) of chromosome 6; those encoding class II products appear near the centromere; and those encoding class III products occupy an intermediate position between these two regions. (This organization differs from the murine H-2 complex in which class I genes occur closer to the centromere than do class II genes.) Each region, in turn, contains several identified loci, each encoding a particular product. These loci are either (1) expressed genes, which produce functional MHC products; (2) pseudogenes, which are homologous to expressed genes occurring elsewhere in the genome; or (3) genes of unknown status, which means that no known role for the gene product is currently available.

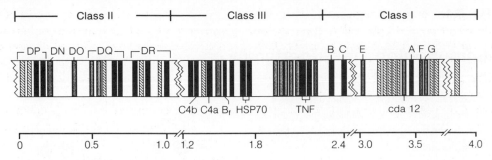

FIGURE 7.10 Human major histocompatibility HLA complex. A genetic map of the HLA gene complex located on chromosome 6 is represented. The chromosome's orientation places the centromere to the left. Loci designated A, B, C, E, F, and G encode class I Ags; DN, DO, DP, DQ, and DR encode class II Ags; and C4a and C4b and B_f encode class III Ags. In addition loci encoding selected other products (cda 12, HSP70, and TNF) are represented. Expressed genes are depicted by *solid bars,* while those of unknown status are portrayed by *stippled bars.* In contrast, pseudogenes are represented by *hatched bars.* Distance along the chromosome is approximate and is given in cM. (From Altman, D. M., and Trowsdale, J. Major histocompatibility complex structure and function. *Current Opinion in Immunology.* 2:93, 1989.)

The region encoding **class I** Ags contains three expressed genes (HLA-A, B, C), four genes of unknown status (HLA-E, G, F, and *cda*12), and eight pseudogenes. The HLA-D region, which encodes **class II** Ags, contains several subdomains, which account for seven expressed genes, four genes of unknown status, and five pseudogenes. The region encoding **class III** Ags contains nine expressed genes, seven genes of unknown status, and one pseudogene. This region also encodes a cytokine (tumor necrosis factor, TNF) and stress-induced proteins, designated HSP70 (for "70 kD heat-shock protein").

TNFs have diverse effects on target tissues involved in inflammation and wound healing (see chapter 8 for further discussion). These effects include activation of macrophages and stimulation of interleukin 1 (IL-1) production, stimulation of fibroblast proliferation, and regulation of the production by liver cells of acute-phase proteins (proteins involved in early stages of inflammation). There are more than nine proteins in the HSP70 family, which is one of several families of proteins that are sensitive to various forms of stress and trauma. The other HSP families are HSP110, HSP90, HSP60, and HSP20. Some HSP70 proteins are present in normal cells, where they apparently play a role in the maturation of newly synthesized proteins, including IgG. Certain of these proteins are increased, while others are not affected by stress. Yet other HSP70 proteins are produced only in response to stress. HSP70s also have been found on the surfaces of macrophages and B cells, but not T or natural killer (NK) cells.

At each locus, one of several alternative forms of a gene may be formed. Alleles at a particular locus are designated by the locus and a number. For example HLA-B1 is the number 1 allele at the HLA-B locus. Tentatively assigned alleles are designated by a w (for workshop) placed before the number, such as HLA-Bw4. When the assignment is officially confirmed, the w is dropped.

Since we inherit one chromosome (with a combination of alleles at each locus) from each parent, we have two haplotypes. HLA genes are codominant; thus, both alleles at a given locus are expressed and two complete sets of HLA Ags can be detected on cells. Since the HLA system is extremely polymorphic, there may be a very large number of alleles at each locus. For example, there are over 30 distinct alleles at the HLA-B locus.

Distribution of HLA Antigens

Class I Ags are present *on all nucleated cells.* Although these molecules are distributed more or less homogeneously in the cell membranes, their concentrations in each cell varies considerably in different tissues and

The Immunoglobulin Superfamily

Homology has been found to exist between the two classes of MHC Ags, class I and class II (panel *a* in fig. 7.A). This includes the α_3 domain of the class I Ag and the α_2 and β_2 domains of the class II Ag. In addition, homology also exists between these domains and the β_2-microglobulin associated with the class I MHC Ag.

Homologies like this that occur in different proteins strongly suggest a common ancestry for the molecules. Thus, the two classes of MHC Ags would be expected to have arisen from a common, or similar, precursor through evolutionary development.

However, studies of the sequences of other significant immunological proteins have demonstrated yet other homologies. As might be expected, homologies were found between constant domains of the various immunoglobulin classes. More strikingly, however, was the discovery that homologies also existed between these domains and the homologous regions of the MHC Ags (panel *b*). Furthermore, the Thy-1 (murine) and CD3 (human) Ags also display homologies with these protein sequences.

All of these distinct molecules share responsibility for immune response. In addition, each, in some way, functions in Ag recognition. Since these diverse proteins have all been derived, through evolution, from a common ancestor, they are related—that is, they are all members of the same family. The "familial" relationship among this broad range of distinct proteins is considered to constitute the immunoglobulin superfamily.

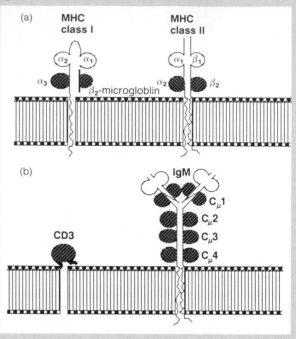

FIGURE 7.A Immunoglobulin superfamily. Domains (regions) of molecules in this superfamily that display substantial sequence identity (similar amino acid sequences) are indicated by *shading*. (From Hood, L., Steinmetz, M., and Malissen, B. Genes of the major histocompatibility complex of the mouse. *Annual Review of Immunology* **1**:529, 1983.)

Hood, L., Steinmetz, M., and Malissen, B. Genes of the major histocompatibility complex of the mouse. *Annual Review of Immunology* 1:529, 1983.

organs. Few class I molecules are present on spermatozoa, for example. Concentrations of these Ags are relatively greater on immature cells, especially developing blood cells. The highest concentration of class I molecules occurs on lymphocytes, representing about 1% of the membrane proteins. In addition, antigenic and/or mitogenic stimulation of lymphocytes causes increased expression of these molecules. In individuals heterozygous at the three loci (HLA-A, B, and C) as many six distinct class I molecules can be displayed on the cell membrane.

Class II Ags are found only *on B lymphocytes, activated T lymphocytes* (resting T cells in small quantities), *macrophages, monocytes, Langerhans' cells, some epithelial cells, spermatozoa, and myeloid stem cells.* The concentration of class II molecules varies in different cells and is usually greater in less differentiated cells, as with class I Ags.

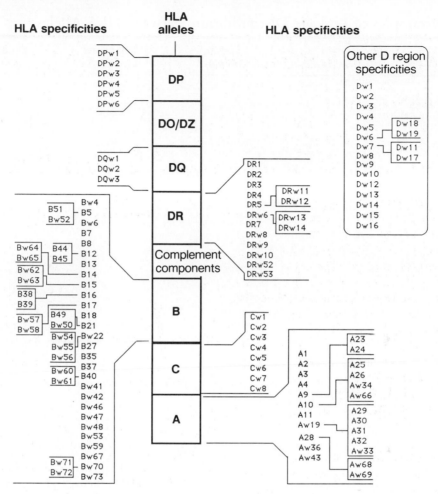

FIGURE 7.11 Recognized HLA Ags. This figure lists some of the recognized HLA Ags that have been detected by serological tests or MLRs.

Class III Ags may be formed in, and displayed on, *macrophages* and bound under certain conditions to lymphocytes, neutrophils, erythrocytes, and platelets.

HLA Specificities and Linkage Disequilibrium

The number of distinct antigenic specificities at each HLA subregion, detectable either serologically or by *mixed lymphocyte reaction (MLR)*, is large in a human population (fig. 7.11). With random matings, the frequency of finding a given allele at one HLA locus, together with a given allele at a second HLA locus, should simply be the product of the frequencies of each allele in the population. Thus, if 15% of the population possess HLA-B5 Ag and 10% of the population possess HLA-A3, then 1.5% might predictably possess B5 linked to A3 on the same chromosome. However, certain combinations of alleles are found with a frequency far greater than expected (table 7.2). This phenomenon is called **linkage disequilibrium.** It has been suggested that a given haplotype might have a selective advantage in the environment. It has also been suggested that inbreeding, or random drift, might be involved, but mechanisms that might account for linkage disequilibrium are unclear.

TABLE 7.2 Examples of Linkage Disequilibrium between HLA Alleles

Haplotypes	Gene Frequency	Expected Linkage*	Observed Linkage*	Disequilibrium† (Δ × 1,000)
A1/B8				
European caucasoids	14.9%/8.2%	0.0122	0.0641	51.9
Japanese	0.5%/0.1%	0.0001	0.0026	2.5
A3/B7				
European caucasoids	11.6%/8.8%	0.0102	0.0283	18.1
A26/Bw38				
European caucasoids	3.7%/2.5%	0.0009	0.0055	4.6
A26/Bw51				
Blacks	3.8%/1.4%	0.0005	0.0081	7.6
B7/Cw4				
Blacks	8.9%/15.9%	0.0142	0.0339	19.7
B8/DR3				
European caucasoids	9%/12%	0.011	0.0723	61.3
B15/Cw3				
Blacks	3.0%/9.2%	0.0028	0.0132	11.4
European caucasoids	4.8%/10.1%	0.0048	0.0299	25.1
Japanese	9.3%/26.9%	0.0250	0.0509	25.9

*Linkages are calculated by multiplying gene frequencies of individual alleles. For example A1/B8 has frequencies of 14.9% and 8.2%; thus, $0.149 \times 0.082 = 0.0122$. *Expected linkages* are derived by calculation; *observed linkages* are actual values within the population. (Values are rounded to the fourth decimal place.)

†*Disequilibrium* reflects difference between observed and expected linkages between dissimilar alleles. For example, for A1/B8 these values are 0.0122 and 0.0641; thus, $0.0641 - 0.0122 = 0.0519$. When multiplied by 1,000, this yields 51.9.

Class I Antigens

Human class I Ags are encoded in the HLA-A, B, and C regions. They are glycoproteins consisting of a protein chain of approximately 40 to 45 kD and a single carbohydrate side chain of about 3 kD. The glycosylated chain is noncovalently associated with a nonglycosylated peptide known as β_2-microglobulin, of about 12 kD. The Ags can be identified with MAbs and dissociated from the cell membrane with detergents. The protein chain can be divided into intracellular, intramembrane, and extracellular portions. The extracellular portion can be subdivided further into three domains, as seen in murine systems (see fig. 7.7). The α_1 region spans residues 1 to 90; the α_2 residues 91 to 180; and the α_3 residues 181 to 272.

β_2-microglobulin is bound to the α_3 domain on the outer side of the membrane. The β_2-microglobulin does not form part of the antigenic site of the HLA Ag; but it is, nevertheless, necessary for the expression of the class I Ag. That is, it is apparently needed for the transport of the molecule to the cell surface and anchorage in the membrane.

From sequence studies, it appears that HLA epitopes occur on the α_1 and α_2 domains. Class I molecules in living cells undergo constant turnover involving the shedding of old molecules and the synthesis of new ones. Treatment of cells with protein inhibitors results in a loss of class I Ags. Some molecules are internalized. Some shed molecules, however, appear in the serum, and it has been suggested that these play a role in the prevention of autoimmunity by blocking receptors of autoreactive lymphocytes.

Class II Antigens

Class II Ags, the products of HLA-D and D-related genes, consist of two distinct transmembrane polypeptide chains (α and β), which are joined by noncovalent forces (see fig. 7.9). The larger portions of each are extracellular, and only the smaller portion of each chain is intracellular. The α chain has a molecular weight of

34 kD, and the β about 28 kD. Each chain carries a complex-type oligosaccharide. These are analogous to the murine Ia molecules and sometimes are referred to as human Ia-like molecules. The β chain is more variable than the α chain and, as such, expresses the antigenic determinants or epitopes of the Ag. The detection of HLA-D molecules and their allelic variants may be identified by their ability to stimulate an MLR when cells expressing different class II Ags are cocultured. Alloantisera may also be used, with some restrictions, to identify class II molecules.

Class III Antigens

Complement components C2, C4, and B_f are included as class III molecules, as seen in the murine H-2 complex. The structure and major role of these components is discussed in chapter 6, Complement and its Role in Immune Responses. In addition, a provisionally designated RD locus, encoding an unusual 42 kD protein, occurs between the B_f and C4 loci. Class III Ags, as with other molecular products of the HLA complex, can serve as transplantation Ags. These Ags are probably those expressed on the surfaces of macrophages (see above). Products of C2, C4, and B_f alleles are expressed codominantly, as are other allo-Ags.

CLINICAL SIGNIFICANCE OF THE MAJOR HISTOCOMPATIBILITY COMPLEX
MHC and Graft Rejection

Rapid graft rejection of foreign cells, tissues, or organs is the result of an immune response of the recipient to specific MHC Ags present on the surface of the grafted cells, but absent from the recipient. The **histocompatibility Ags** elicit a predominantly cell-mediated response. *Class I MHC molecules stimulate T_C cells. Class II MHC molecules may stimulate T_H cells,* which, in turn, amplify the generation of specific effector T and B cells. Effector T cells may invade the graft along with macrophages and either directly or indirectly (via soluble factors) cause tissue damage during first-set graft rejection (occurs following first exposure to tissue from a particular donor). Abs, nevertheless, are generated against foreign MHC products and can participate in second-set graft rejection (occurs following second exposure to tissue from a particular donor). Transplantation is discussed in detail in chapter 19, Transplantation Immunology.

HLA and Disease Association

The association of certain HLA Ags with various diseases has received considerable attention in recent years. Several of these diseases are of unknown cause, involve immunological abnormalities (e.g., autoimmunity), and do not appear to affect reproduction. While the associations are primarily statistical, it is generally agreed that they may represent a biologically relevant finding. Such associations are determined by identifying the HLA type of patients with a particular disease and comparing these with the HLA types of a random panel of unaffected individuals from the same ethnic groups and geographic areas. The association may be quantified by calculating the **relative risk** that an individual has of developing the disease, if possessing the disease-associated HLA Ag. Relative risk can be determined in accord with the following formula:

$$RR = \frac{p^+ c^-}{p^- c^+}$$

where: p^+ = patients with the HLA Ag
c^- = controls lacking the HLA Ag
p^- = patients lacking the HLA Ag
c^+ = controls with the HLA Ag

Several HLA types and disease associations, with relative risks, are given in table 7.3.

It is also possible to carry out linkage analysis and map disease-linked genes. For example, it has been shown, using recombinant DNA technology, that the DNA sequences of HLA genes in individuals with these diseases differ from those of normal individuals. Such studies suggest that genes adjacent to HLA genes encoding the marker Ags may be unique in affected individuals, predisposing them to certain diseases. Mechanisms accounting for disease susceptibility relating to HLA Ags have not been defined.

TABLE 7.3 Diseases Associated with HLA Ags

Disease	HLA Allele(s)*	Relative Risk†
Dermatological		
Psoriasis	A1	2
	B13	9
	Bw37	8
	Cw6	4
Endocrine		
Addison's disease	Dw3	9 (6)
Congenital adrenal hyperplasia	B47	15
Graves' disease	B5	4
	B8	3
	Bw35	5
	Dw3/DR3	6 (4)
Hashimoto's thyroiditis	Dw5/DR5	3
Juvenile-onset diabetes	Dw3/DR3	3
mellitus	Dw4/DR4	6
Gastrointestinal and Related		
Celiac disease	B8	9
	Dw3/DR3	73 (11)
Chronic hepatitis	B8	9
	Dw3/DR3	14 (5)
Hematological/Lymphoproliferative		
Acute lymphoblastic leukemia	A2	1
Chronic myelocytic leukemia	A2	39
Chronic lymphocytic leukemia	B18	5
Hemochromatosis	A3	9
Hodgkin's disease	A1, A11, B8, B15	≤8
Neuromuscular		
Multiple sclerosis	A3, B7, Bw2	2
	Dw2/DR2	4
Myasthenia gravis	B8	4 (3)
	Dw3/DR3	3
Rheumatological and Connective Tissue		
Acute anterior uveitis	B27	10
Ankylosing spondylitis	B27	88
Juvenile arthritis	B27, Dw5,	4
Reiter's syndrome	Dw8, B27	37
Rheumatoid arthritis	Dw4/DR4	4
Systemic lupus erythematosus	Dw3/DR3	6

*Where more than one allele can be associated with disease with same relative risk, these alleles are all listed on same line. Where sources disagree on allele designation, these alleles are represented separated by "/", as for example Dw4/DR4.

†Where more than one estimate of relative risk has appeared, higher risk is given first and lower follows in ( ).

PRIMARY FUNCTIONS OF THE MAJOR HISTOCOMPATIBILITY COMPLEX

Although the products of the MHC may be clinically significant in the transplantation process, clearly this is not their primary function. The *primary function of the various products of the MHC is to serve as an Ag-specific, mandatory, strict system of self-governance for the cell-to-cell interactions of T cell subsets, B cells, and APCs.* The allo-Ags of the MHC are **essential for the immune recognition of self.**

Immune Response Genes Control Antigen-Specific Responses

Studies using inbred strains of animals have shown that the relative capacity to mount an immune response to an antigen is inherited. Most genes that influence resistance and susceptibility to microbial and parasitic diseases are either linked to the MHC or map within it. However, some influential genes are independent of the MHC, and many are located on different chromosomes (see Minor Lymphocyte Stimulatory Genes below).

Humoral responses may be controlled by genes different from those influencing cell-mediated reactions. Genetic control of immune responses to specific antigenic determinants has been demonstrated for nearly 50 different Ags in murine models. Any one Ag may express a large number of epitopes, or antigenic determinants. Moreover, it has been shown that the response to each determinant is often controlled independently. Thus, immune response control appears to be very specific. In this respect, an animal might be a good responder to a given determinant and a poor responder to another. Studies with synthetic polypeptides show that an animal may be capable of discriminating among determinants of a single amino acid substitution. Responses under immune response control require T_H cells (expressing differentiation Ag CD4) and the immune response effect may be quantitative (low and high responders) or qualitative (responders and nonresponders).

Class II molecules are Ir gene products of the HLA-D region. They are generally *presented as self-Ags to T_H cells* by APCs, *in association with foreign Ags.* The

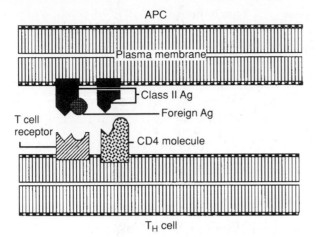

FIGURE 7.12 Recognition of Ag by human helper CD4 cells. Foreign Ag is recognized by CD4 helper cells only when it is associated or complexed with "self" class II molecules. Binding of the complex to the T cell receptor is apparently enhanced by accessory association of other self class II molecules with CD4 molecules adjacent to the T cell receptor.

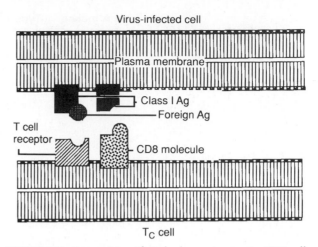

FIGURE 7.13 Recognition of Ag by human cytotoxic CD8 cells. Foreign Ag is recognized by CD8 cytotoxic cells only when it is associated with "self" class I molecules. Binding of the complex to the T cell receptor is apparently enhanced by accessory association of other self class I molecules with CD8 molecules adjacent to the T cell receptor.

foreign Ag-MHC complex yields a unique specificity requiring unique recognition. Dembic and associates suggested that two immune response (Ir) gene products may be expressed on a cell and are needed for response to a single antigenic determinant. In this model, both T cell MHC receptors and CD4 molecules on helper cells act as recognition units (fig. 7.12).

Thus, the **associative recognition hypothesis** proposes that Ir gene influence of immune responses is mediated during Ag presentation. It suggests that certain Ir gene products may associate very well with some Ags (high responders), not very well with other Ags (low responders), and perhaps not at all with still other Ags (nonresponders). A spectrum of responses to a single Ag, displaying a variety of epitopes, occurs. A spectrum of responses to a single antigenic determinant may also occur. Accordingly, the response to a given Ag is *restricted by the class II Ags* encoded by the **Ir genes** of the host or potential responder.

MHC Restriction

Recognition of Ags by regulatory (helper) CD4 lymphocytes is restricted by class II HLA molecules. The nature of the Ir genes possessed, therefore, largely defines a host's capacity to exhibit a humoral or cell-mediated response, as seen above. On the other hand,

CD8 lymphocytes, which may exhibit cytotoxic cell functions, are restricted by class I HLA molecules. Cell interactions involving *MHC restriction,* thus, are *not actually confined to either of the main T cell subsets.* However, by convention, the phenomenon has had an assumed reference to class I self-Ag restriction, unless otherwise defined.

Class I molecules are involved in MHC-restricted cell-mediated immunity. Cytotoxic responses to virus-infected cells, and autologous cells exhibiting membrane-altered or exogenous Ag, are MHC restricted. *MHC restriction implies that stimulator cells and target cells **must** possess identical class I molecules* recognizable to responding effector cells. Thus, a specific clone of T_C cells responds to a foreign Ag only if it is presented by cells carrying class I self-Ags identical to its own, as seen in the murine system. Similarly, the T_C cells induced lyse and destroy only target cells that possess both the foreign Ag and class I self-Ags. Significantly, MHC restriction may prevent saturation of T cell receptor (TCR) sites with free Ag, before target cells may be engaged, since T_C cells bind Ag in association with class I molecules. Recognition of foreign Ag in association with class I molecules (fig. 7.13) is believed to be analogous to recognition of the foreign Ag/class II self-Ag complex (see fig. 7.12). However, in either case, the matter has not been clearly resolved.

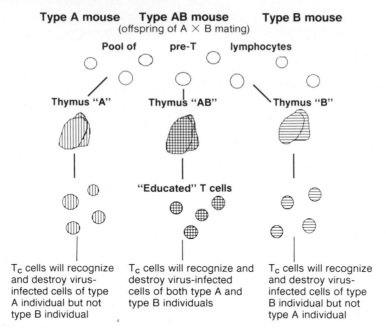

Type A mouse **Type AB mouse** **Type B mouse**
(offspring of A × B mating)

Pool of   pre-T   lymphocytes

Thymus "A"   Thymus "AB"   Thymus "B"

"Educated" T cells

T$_C$ cells will recognize and destroy virus-infected cells of type A individual but not type B individual

T$_C$ cells will recognize and destroy virus-infected cells of both type A and type B individuals

T$_C$ cells will recognize and destroy virus-infected cells of type B individual but not type A individual

FIGURE 7.14 MHC self-education. T cells learn to discriminate between self and nonself Ags in the thymus. This has been demonstrated by introducing immature T cells (bone marrow) of F$_1$ hybrids (A × B) into mice of A, B, and AB haplotypes. Recipient mice, whose own T cells have been inactivated, are then challenged with virus. Results show that T cells, with genome AB, recognize as self either A or B, or both A and B, depending on the haplotype of the thymus in which T cells developed. This is based on T cell recognition and lysis of virus-infected cells from each MHC type.

MHC Self-Education

Remarkably, immature T cells *learn to discriminate between self and nonself determinants in thymus tissue,* independent of Ag. This involves interaction between hemopoietic (or lymphocyte) precursor cells and the stroma of the thymus gland. During this process, positive and negative interactions occur. Through positive selection, cells capable of recognizing MHC Ags within the thymic stroma are selected for continued survival through means that remain undefined. However, if this recognition might lead to activation of an immune response, negative selection brings about the elimination of these cells. Thus, *self-recognition is achieved through selection for immature T cells displaying an affinity for self-MHC Ags expressed by cells within the thymic stroma.* Hypotheses of how these interactions might lead to continued cell survival or death are explored in chapter 10. Nevertheless, it is clear that interactions between immature T cells and the stromal cells of the thymus are important to self-discrimination. This has been established through two kinds of experiments: (1) allowing lymphocytes to mature in a host thymus and (2) transplanting thymic rudiments to athymic mice.

If immature lymphocytes are introduced into a host, thymic education is determined by the host's genotype (fig. 7.14). Immature lymphocytes of one haplotype migrate to the thymus of their host (of a different haplotype), where they undergo Ag-independent differentiation. Subsequently, mature T cells can be challenged with virus-infected cells. If these cells express Ags of the same haplotype as the thymus in which they matured, MHC-restricted lysis occurs. However, if the cells express other Ags, recognition as self is not possible and lysis does not occur.

Alternatively, embryonic thymic rudiments can be transplanted into neonatal athymic (nude) mice. Hemopoietic cells from the host subsequently populate the implanted thymic tissues. Following Ag-independent differentiation of lymphocytes, the mice are challenged with skin grafts. Grafts from mice isogeneic to either the host mouse or the thymus donor are tolerated. On the other hand, grafts from other strains of mice are rejected. These experiments demonstrate that recognition of self is conditioned by exposure to the thymic environment. In addition, the latter experiment demonstrates that the genetic identity of the lymphocytes themselves also plays a role in self-recognition.

MINOR HISTOCOMPATIBILITY ANTIGENS

Both major and **minor histocompatibility (mH)** genes give rise to allo-Ags that may evoke an allograft response, resulting in the rejection of a graft (see chapter 19, Transplantation Immunology). In the former instance, a histoincompatible reaction is more rapid and intense than in the latter. In murine systems, graft rejection in response to mH products occurs usually within several weeks to several months. In some instances, however, rejection may not occur for more than a year. As seen in the MHC, the function of gene products is varied, extensive, and not restricted to transplantation phenomena. Similarly mH gene products probably perform a variety of biological functions (albeit mostly uncharacterized).

In mice, less than 100 distinct mH genes have been described, but some investigators suggest that there may be nearly 1,000. The *genes are scattered throughout the mouse genome,* in contrast to genes of the MHC.

Responses to tumor cells or skin grafts have been used to demonstrate products of mH genes. The immunogenicity of different allo-Ags is related to the time it takes for a graft to be rejected. In some instances, the effect of several mH Ags is cumulative, whereby several different Ag-specific clones are activated. Accordingly, MHC matching alone may be quite inadequate in preventing graft rejection.

Examples of Minor Histocompatibility Antigens

Within highly inbred strains of mice, grafts from males to females may be rejected. At least one mH Ag is located on the male Y chromosome in mice and the gene product (H-Y Ag) is found on most nucleated cells, and on half of the spermatozoa. Since females do not possess a Y chromosome, T_C cells of a female may recognize the H-Y Ag of an isogeneic male as foreign, when presented in association with an identical class I MHC molecule. Thus, the graft rejection may be MHC restricted. A skin-specific (Skn) mH Ag may induce skin graft rejections involving both Abs and specific T_C lymphocytes. The Ag is found on epidermal cells and brain cells, but not on lymphocytes. Some mH Ags, however, have been described that are expressed on lymphocytes, that may give rise to an MLR and elicit graft rejection.

Minor Histocompatibility Antigens in Humans

Very little is known about mH Ags in humans. Nevertheless, evidence suggests that although mH Ags remain undefined, for the most part, they play a role in graft rejection. Graft rejections (e.g., renal) have been observed even in cases with a complete HLA match. Abs so generated would not bind to HLA antigens, but they would bind to certain lymphocytes, which may be displaying mH Ags. In addition, an H-Y Ag, analogous to the murine H-Y Ag, has been described. This mH Ag induces a cell-mediated response in females resulting in rejection of the male graft (e.g., skin).

Minor Lymphocyte Stimulatory Genes

Ags encoded by the MHC are strong activating determinants when presented to members of another strain (e.g., allogeneic or xenogeneic). In addition, it has been known that stimulation of isogeneic cells can occur in mixed lymphocyte cultures (MLCs). Since all cells in these cultures are MHC-related, stimulation of the response is not induced by histocompatibility differences. Stimulation has been attributed to mH genes designated **minor lymphocyte stimulatory (Mls)** genes.

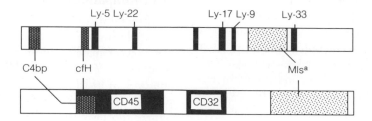

Human chromosome 1q

FIGURE 7.15 Location of Mls[a]. The map location for Mls[a] is portrayed relative to selected other loci on mouse chromosome 1 and human chromosome 1q. Loci for Ly-5, Ly-9, Ly-17, Ly-22, and Ly-33 encode the respective lymphocyte surface Ags in mice. Loci for CD32 and CD45 encode the respective lymphocyte surface Ags in humans. C4bp encodes complement component 4 binding protein while cfH encodes complement Factor H. (From Festenstein, H., Kimura, S., and Biasi, G. Mls and tolerance. *Immunological Reviews.* **107:**29, 1989.)

Neither the nature nor the functions of Mls products are known. Nevertheless, Mls gene products, like *Staphylococcus* enterotoxins, are considered **super-Ags.** This means that Mls gene products can stimulate a larger number of T cells (10%) than most Ags (about 1%). Moreover, this stimulation occurs in a distinctive manner. While foreign Ags interact with the Ag-recognition site of the TCR during T cell activation, super-Ags interact with a portion of the β chain of the TCR outside the Ag-recognition site. Despite this feature, T cell activation by Mls gene products displays class II MHC restriction.

Four distinct Mls haplotypes have been characterized, which are designated Mls[a], Mls[b], Mls[c], and Mls[d]. These four haplotypes appear to be the consequence of only two distinct genes, Mls[a] and Mls[c]. Mls[d] is believed to represent the presence of *both* Mls[a] and Mls[c], whereas Mls[b] is believed to represent the null state in which products of *neither* gene are present.

The presence of Mls[a] and Mls[d] is associated with strong stimulation of lymphocyte proliferation in MLCs, while Mls[c] is only weakly stimulatory. In contrast, Mls[b] does not lead to stimulation of lymphocyte proliferation in MLCs. Rather, the presence of Mls[b] is associated with the generation of T_C cells. A further distinction between Mls[b] and Mls[a] is that Mls[a] leads to an activation of T_S cells, while Mls[b] does not. This is believed to have potential significance for the induction of self-tolerance. These responses appear to be Mls specific and MHC restricted (class II).

The Mls system is believed to be analogous to the MHC, although possessing many fewer genes. In mice, Mls[a] maps to chromosome 1 while the location of Mls[c] is unknown. In mice, Mls[a] maps adjacent to several genes specifying immunologically significant products (fig. 7.15). Mls gene products are believed to be expressed by macrophages, B cells, and possibly erythroid cells, but *not* T cells.

S U M M A R Y

1. A gene is a portion of DNA containing information needed to produce a specific protein molecule, completely or in part. Alternate forms of a gene at a specific locus on sister chromosomes that control a single characteristic are called alleles. Paired chromosomes commonly carry different alleles, and if each gene is expressed two different alloantigens are produced. [p. 178]

2. Inbred strains that differ from one another by only a small portion of a single chromosome and share background alleles are said to be congenic. Strains differing by the allele of a single gene are called coisogenic. [pp. 178–179]

3. Two groups of transplantation antigens are recognized, which are encoded by major and minor histocompatibility genes. Major histocompatibility genes are located on a single chromosome, whereas minor histocompatibility genes are scattered throughout the genome. [pp. 179–180]

4. The murine MHC is known as the H-2 complex and contains a linked series of genes comprising four major regions: K, I, S, and D. Proximal to this region is a T1a complex. [p. 180]

5. H-2 gene products consist of class I, II, and III molecules, which mainly, but not exclusively, regulate the processes of transplantation, immune responsiveness, and aspects of complement synthesis. [p. 180]

6. Class I molecules are found on all nucleated cells, whereas class II molecules are found only on B lymphocytes, monocytes, macrophages, epithelial cells, and spermatozoa. [p. 181]

7. Alloantigens possess unique epitopes peculiar to their haplotype (private specificities), but they may also share epitopes with antigens of other haplotypes (public specificities). [pp. 181–182]

8. Class I antigenic determinants can be detected by serological tissue typing with monoclonal antibodies, while class II determinants can be detected by mixed lymphocyte reactions. [pp. 181–182]

9. Class I MHC antigens are required for the interaction of cytotoxic T cells with virus-infected or transformed cells. [pp. 182–184]

10. Class II MHC antigens, encoded by immune response (Ir) genes, dramatically influence our ability to mount an immune response by affecting T cell help, suppression, and recruitment. [pp. 185–186]

11. Class III antigens control the level of two major proteins known as C4, the fourth component of complement, and Slp, a sex-limited protein. [p. 186]

12. The MHC in humans is known as the HLA complex. Major regions include HLA-A, B, and C, which encode class I antigens; HLA-D, containing four closely linked clusters of genes, which encode class II antigens; and HLA-C4, C2, and B$_f$, which encode class III antigens. [p.000]

13. The association of certain HLA antigens with various diseases involving immunological abnormalities has been observed. [p. 191]

14. The primary function of the various products of the MHC is to serve as an antigen-specific, mandatory, strict system of self-governance for the cell-to-cell interactions of T cell subsets, B cells, and antigen-presenting cells. [pp. 192–195]

15. Minor histocompatibility antigens, foreign to a recipient, may collectively evoke tissue rejection within several weeks to several months. [p. 195]

16. Minor lymphocyte stimulatory genes exist which are responsible for modulating responses from MHC-related lymphocytes. The nature and role of the gene products remains unknown. Nevertheless, they possess distinctive features characterizing them as superantigens. [pp. 195–196]

READINGS

Abe, R., and Hodes, R. J. Properties of the Mls system: a revised formulation of Mls genetics and an analysis of T-cell recognition of Mls determinants. *Immunological Reviews* **107**:5, 1989.

Altmann, D. M., and Trowsdale, J. Major histocompatibility complex structure and function. *Current Opinion in Immunology* **2**:93, 1989.

Beckmann, R. P., Mizzen, L. A., and Welch, W. J. Interaction of Hsp70 with newly synthesized proteins: implications for protein folding and assembly. *Science* **248**:850, 1990.

Bodmer, J. G., Marsh, S. G. E., and Albert, E. Nomenclature for factors of the HLA system. *Immunology Today* **11**:3, 1989.

Dalgleish, A. G. The T4 molecule: function and structure. *Immunology Today* **7**(5):142, 1986.

Dembic, Z., von Boehmer, H., and Steinmetz, M. The role of T-cell receptor alpha and beta genes in MHC restricted antigen recognition. *Immunology Today* **7**(10):308, 1986.

Festenstein, H., Kumura, S., and Biasi, G. Mls and tolerance. *Immunological Reviews* **107**:29, 1989.

Figueroa, F., Gutknecht, J., Tichy, H., et al. Class II Mhc genes in rodent evolution. *Immunological Reviews* **113**:27, 1990.

Figueroa, F., and Klein J. The evolution of MHC class II genes. *Immunology Today* **7**(3):78, 1986.

Guillet, J-G., Lai, M-Z., Briner, T., et al. Immunological self-nonself discrimination. *Science* **235**:865, 1987.

Kroener, G., Bernot, A., Béhar, G., et al. Molecular genetics of the chicken MHC: current status and evolutionary aspects. *Immunological Reviews* **113**:119, 1990.

Litwin, S. D., Scott, D. W., Flaherty, L., et al. (eds.). *Human Immunogenetics: Basic Principles and Clinical Relevance.* Marcel Dekker, New York, 1989.

Lechler, R. I. MHC class II molecular structure—permitted pairs? *Immunology Today* **9**:76, 1988.

Levi-Strauss, M., Carroll, M. C., Steinmetz, M., et al. A previously undetected MHC gene with an unusual periodic structure. *Science* **240**:201, 1988.

Malissen, B. Transfer and expression of MHC genes. *Immunology Today* **7**(4):106, 1986.

Marrack, P., and Kappler, J. The antigen-specific, major histocompatibility complex–restricted receptor on T cells. In *Advances in Immunology.* Dixon, F. J. (ed.). Academic Press, Inc., Orlando, Fla., 1986.

Marrack, P., and Kappler, J. The staphylococcal enterotoxins and their relatives. *Science* **248**:705, 1990.

Marx, J. Histocompatibility restriction explained. *Science* **235**:843, 1987.

Mills, K. H. G. Processing of viral antigens and presentation to class II-restricted T cells. *Immunology Today* **7**(9):260, 1986.

Moller, E., and Moller, G. *Genetics of the Immune Response,* Plenum Publishing Co., New York, 1983.

Nepom, G. T. MHC genes in HLA-associated disease. *Current Opinions in Immunology* **2**:588, 1990.

Patrusky, B. A biological imperative. *MOSAIC* **21**(3):2, 1990.

Salaün, J., Bandeira, A., Khazaal, I., et al. Thymic epithelium tolerizes for histocompatibility antigens. *Science* **241**:1471, 1990.

Schwartz, R. H. Immune response genes of the murine major histocompatibility complex. In *Advances In Immunology.* Dixon, F. J., (ed.). Academic Press, Inc., Orlando, Fla., 1986.

Sherry, B., and Cerami, A. Cachectin/tumor necrosis factor exerts endocrine, paracrine, and autocrine control of inflammatory responses. *Journal of Cell Biology* **107**:1269, 1988.

Stites, D. P., Stobo, J. D., and Wells, J. V. (eds). *Basic and Clinical Immunology,* Appleton and Lange, Norwalk, Conn., 1987.

Wassom, D. L., Krco, C. J., and Child, C. S. I-E expression and susceptibility to parasite infection. *Immunology Today* **8**(2):39, 1987.

Zaleski, M. B., Dubiski, S., Niles, E. G., et al. *Immunogenetics.* Pitman Publishing, Inc., Marshfield, Mass., 1983.

CHAPTER 8

Effectors of Nonspecific Cellular Immunity

OVERVIEW

Cell-mediated immune responses are mediated by specific and nonspecific effectors. Immunologically nonspecific effectors include a diverse array of cell types, for example, natural killer cells, macrophages, and granulocytes. These cells are responsible for innate immunity and inflammatory reactions. The major forms of inflammatory response are defined and compared and the events of acute inflammation are explored. In addition, the importance of repair is discussed.

CONCEPTS

1. Innate immunity is provided by several diverse cell types that respond in an immunologically nonspecific fashion to infective agents, transformed cells, and damaged tissues.

2. Inflammation is a natural consequence of many antigenically nonspecific cell-mediated immune responses.

3. The events of an inflammatory response involve the interplay between (a) affected (damaged or infected) tissues, (b) the vascular system, and (c) effector cells (chiefly leukocytes) and their products.

4. Full restoration of homeostasis often requires repair or wound healing.

I nfections or injuries provoke responses that can be limited to specific sites or widespread throughout the body. Certain of these responses are immediate and generalized, whereas others occur more slowly and are focused on unique characteristics (determinants) of the insulting agent. The rapid, generalized responses represent nonspecific defenses against infection or injury and are executed by antigen-nonspecific (Ag-nonspecific) effectors of immunity. A systematic pattern of reactions, referred to as inflammation, is often associated with these responses. In addition to immunological defense, the events of the inflammatory response provide the potential for repairing damage. Since these generalized responses are expressed quite early in development, being available to the fetus, they are responsible for much of what is called innate immunity. Generalized (Ag-nonspecific) immune responses are distinct from responses that are Ag specific—antibody (Ab) production, on the one hand, and activation of effector T cells, on the other. Moreover, effectors of Ag-nonspecific immune responses are different from effectors of Ag-specific immune responses. Nevertheless, interactions between these effectors can (and often do) occur.

This chapter examines nonspecific immune responses. This is undertaken in two parts, through exploration of (1) the cells responsible for Ag-nonspecific immune responses and (2) inflammatory responses. Chapter 9 discusses Ag-specific effectors of cell-mediated immunity.

■ ■ ■ ■ ■ ■ ■ ■ ■ ■

INNATE IMMUNITY

Immunity is mediated by humoral and cellular effectors. Certain immune responses are Ag specific. They are provoked by unique determinants of the Ags, and the effectors (Abs or T cells) produced are Ag specific. In contrast, other immune responses can be evoked by infectious agents or injury in a generalized, Ag-nonspecific manner. These responses are not induced by unique determinants. In addition, the effectors produced (or activated) *recognize conserved,* rather than unique, *determinants.* The former responses require selection of effectors of appropriate specificity for clonal

expansion before an effective response can be observed. On the other hand, nonspecific immune responses can employ any and all nonspecific effectors. Specific selection and clonal expansion are not required. Consequently, nonspecific immune responses display more rapid activation following encounter with the challenging agent.

In addition, Ag-specific responses depend upon maturation of B and T cells capable of recognizing the unique determinants on the provoking Ags. As a result, expression of Ag-specific immune responses changes with progressive maturation of the immune system during development (see chapter 20 for additional discussion). The ability to execute Ag-nonspecific immune responses is present before birth and is less dependent upon maturity of the immune system. In fact, in some mammals, Ag-nonspecific immune responses are the only fully developed immunological defenses available to the neonate and thus provides innate immunity. Thus, **innate immunity** can be defined as *rapidly evoked, generalized defense* provided by effectors that are *activated in an Ag-nonspecific manner.*

Recognition and Mediator Systems

As already mentioned, effectors of innate immunity are not activated by unique determinants of particular Ags for which they possess complementary receptors. Consequently, all cells of a particular type (see below) are equally capable of reacting against a provoking agent. Nevertheless, activation of these effectors is triggered through specific recognition systems. However, these systems recognize conserved, rather than unique, determinants. In addition, mediation of functional expression of these effector cells is achieved through similar recognition systems.

The recognition and mediation systems of Ag-nonspecific effector cells fall into four categories: (1) complement receptors (CRs) and Fc receptors (FcRs), (2) cell adhesion molecules (CAMs), (3) cytokine receptors, and (4) receptors for other (sometimes undefined) ligands. These receptors interact with ligands that activate the effectors cells expressing these receptors. In addition, CAMs and cytokine receptors interact with ligands that promote functional expression by activated effector cells. Some

TABLE 8.1 Representative Recognition and Mediation Systems Used by Nonspecific Mediators of Cellular Immunity

Receptor or Mediator Family	General Characteristics or Features	Example	Cells Which Express Them
CRs	Recognize products of complement activation		
	e.g., C3b, C4b	CR1	Mφs, granulocytes
	C3bi	CR3, CR4	Mφs, granulocytes, NK cells
	C3d	CR5	Granulocytes, platelets
	C3a, C4a	C3a/C4aR	Eosinophils, monocytes
FcRs	Recognize Fc domain of Igs (members of class III recognize IgG)		
	Induces phagocytosis	FcγR III-1	Granulocytes
	Induces ADCC reaction	FcγR III-2	Mφs, NK cells
CAMs	Surface adhesion molecules that interact with carbohydrate moieties of ligand		
	Participates in attachment to vascular endothelium	MEL-14	Granulocytes
	Cooperates in contact guidance and chemotaxis	Leu-CAMb	Granulocytes
	Stabilizes adherence to target cells	Leu-CAMa Leu-CAMc	Lymphocytes, Mφs
Cytokine receptors	Mediate response to particular cytokines		
	e.g., IL-2	IL-2R	Mφs, NK (LAK) cells
	IL-3	IL-3R	Eosinophils, NK cells (?)
	IFNγ	IFN-R	Mφs, LAK cells
	TNF	TNF-R	Mφs, granulocytes

This list identifies some of the receptors and adhesion molecules found on nonspecific mediators of cellular immunity. Other receptors for complement products, Fc domains of Abs, CAMs, and cytokines also appear on these cells.

features of these surface recognition and mediation systems are outlined in table 8.1.

Complement and Fc Receptors

Numerous cells possess *receptors for products of complement activation*. Nine separate receptors, each displaying different specificities, have been characterized. Most recognize products of the classical complement pathway (see chapter 6). Six of these receptors recognize products of C3 activation, while two others recognize either C1q and C5a. In addition, one receptor recognizes factor H.

The major FcRs expressed by Ag-nonspecific effector cells are type III *receptors that recognize the Fc domain of IgG*. They are designated as FcγR III. Two classes of FcγR III have been identified in these effector cells. FcγR III-1 are expressed by granulocytes, while FcγR III-2 are expressed by macrophages (Mφs) and natural killer (NK) cells. FcγR III-2 are transmembrane receptors that mediate *Ab-dependent cellular cytotoxicity* (ADCC) reactions. In contrast, FcγR III-1 are glycosyl-phosphatidylinositol-linked molecules that mediate transmembrane signaling following Ab binding. Although it is not precisely known how they activate granulocytes, FcγR III-1 do not mediate ADCC reactions.

Genes for FcγR III have been mapped to chromosome 1. In humans, two genes for FcγR III-2 and one for FcγR III-1 have been found. On the other hand, in mice one gene for FcγR III-2 has been found on chromosome 1, but no gene for FcγR III-1 has yet been found.

Through these receptors, activation of Ag-nonspecific (using CRs) and Ag-specific (FcRs) humoral immune responses can lead to general recruitment of the Ag-nonspecific cellular effectors described below.

Adhesion Molecules

CAMs represent a diverse group of surface Ags that are used for ligand-specific attachment and interaction. For example, CAMs play prominent roles in (1) *adherence to vascular endothelium,* (2) *chemotactic guidance,* and (3) *attachment and stabilization in target cell killing.*

The common CAMs expressed by leukocytes are considered to constitute a family, designated the *Leu-CAM family.* Leu-CAMs are considered part of the integrin family. Leu-CAMs are heterodimers composed of a β chain, common to all leukocytes, and an α chain, which varies in a cell type–specific fashion. The common β chain is recognized by specific monoclonal Abs (MAbs) and is designated CD18. MAbs against individual α chains are designated CD11a (on lymphocytes), CD11b (on granulocytes), and CD11c (on monocytes and Mϕs). Members of the Leu-CAM family can be more specifically identified by noting their CD11 type. Accordingly, Leu-CAMa represents the CD18/CD11a heterodimer expressed on lymphocytes, Leu-CAMb the CD18/CD11b heterodimer on granulocytes, and Leu-CAMc the CD18/CD11c heterodimer found on monocytes and Mϕs.

Leu-CAMa appears to play a role in attachment of NK cells to target cells in NK cell killing (discussed below). Leu-CAMb seems to play a role in emigration of granulocytes from the blood and into extravascular tissues (extravasation) in inflammation. Expression of this adhesion molecule appears to be up-regulated (more expressed) following granulocyte activation, while the expression of another surface Ag, MEL-14, is down-regulated (less expressed). This latter adhesion molecule seems to play a role in attachment to vascular endothelium prior to extravasation.

Cytokine Receptors

All cells express *receptors for biological response modifiers* to which they are sensitive. These include receptors for hormones, neurotransmitters, and growth factors.

For cellular effectors of immune responses, these also include receptors for the various cytokines generated during immune responses, whether Ag specific or nonspecific. Binding of ligand to these receptors leads to altered responses in the affected cells. This can be expressed in altered sensitivity to ligand binding or modulated response on the part of the stimulated cell. Thus, in contrast to the former receptors that are clearly involved in cellular activation, the cytokine receptors seem to play a more significant role in mediating functional expression of effector cells, once activated.

For example, a transition from expression of low-affinity to high-affinity receptors for interleukin 2 (IL-2) can be observed following activation of NK cells. This is accompanied by increased responsiveness of NK cells to IL-2. This can lead to enhanced NK cell killing. Similar enhancement of functional expression by Mϕs or granulocytes can be observed following exposure to a variety of cytokines (e.g., interferon [IFN] and tumor necrosis factor [TNF]). Among the effects of exposure to TNF are augmented phagocytosis and killing by granulocytes and increased cytokine production by Mϕs.

Other Receptors

Other receptors are probably also involved in the initial activation of effectors of Ag-nonspecific immune responses. These include receptors for bacterial lipopolysaccharide, lectins, and other determinants expressed predominantly by infective agents. These are probably conserved determinants, as suggested by immune responses displayed by phylogenetically more ancient organisms (see chapter 21).

Effectors of Innate Immunity

Innate immunity possesses both humoral and cell-mediated components. The major effector of Ag-nonspecific (innate) humoral immunity, the complement system, has already been discussed (see chapter 6). Effectors of cell-mediated immunity that exhibit precise immunological specificity and immunological memory are restricted to T cell populations. (these are examined in greater detail in chapter 9). However, several other cell types, which *do not express immunological specificity or memory,* also are involved in cell-mediated innate immunity. This diverse group includes NK cells, Mφs, neutrophils, eosinophils, basophils, mast cells, and platelets. They provide immunological protection through (a) phagocytosis and pinocytosis of foreign cells (and products), (b) direct or indirect lysis of cells recognized as nonself, or (c) a combination of these two methods.

Natural Killer Cells

Because of their ability to directly lyse certain kinds of tumor cells and virus-infected cells, cells displaying NK activity have stimulated much interest in recent years. NK activity is characterized by *spontaneous, non-MHC-restricted* lysis of target cells. Cells of different phenotypes, and even different lineages, can display NK activity. Often they are all termed NK cells, regardless of their origins. Nevertheless, the predominant cell type exhibiting NK cytolytic activity is a **non-T/non-B lymphocyte.**

NK cells appear to be present as a unique, antigenically distinct population of *large granular lymphocytes (LGLs).* They can be identified and enumerated using MAbs specific for differentiation Ags on their surface. These Ags include determinants designated CD11b, CD16, CD56 (formerly NKH-1), CD57 (formerly HNK-1), and NKH-2. More recently, a particular γδ variant of T cell receptor (TCR) has been found on lymphocytes displaying NK activity that are associated with epithelium (e.g., in the skin and gut). The **γδ TCR** is composed of γδ chains rather than αβ chains, which constitute TCRs of T cells (see chapter 9 for further discussion). Although a precise role for γδ TCRs has yet to be determined, it is proposed that they play a role in discriminating alterations to self-Ags rather than recognition of foreign Ags.

LGLs can be separated from other mononuclear cells by centrifugation through a gradient of Percoll®. These nonadherent, nonphagocytic cells lack classic fine immunological specificity (and memory) exhibited by cytotoxic T (T_C) cells. However, they possess the innate ability to recognize and kill, or lyse, various tumor cells, virally infected cells, and certain microorganisms. Reynolds and Ortaldo proposed that this population be termed "null," or "N," cells (lymphocytes) to distinguish them from other cell types exhibiting NK activity. The following discussion is

TABLE 8.2 Summary of Non-T/Non-B Lymphocyte Functions

Category	Function
Influence on hemopoiesis and immune expression	Regulates growth and differentiation of hemopoietic stem cells; regulates cell-mediated immunity; regulates antibody response; acts as natural suppressor cell; produces cytokines
Involvement in infectious disease resistance	Participates in control of infections by viruses, bacteria, fungi, and parasites (intracellular and extracellular)
Involvement in tumor and transplantation immune phenomena	Inhibits development of primary tumors and metastases; is involved in organ transplant rejection; is involved in development of graft-versus-host disease
Participation in autoimmune and related phenomena	Contributes to some forms of aplastic anemia and neutropenia; potentiates autoimmune and neurological disease; contributes to some forms of diabetes, is involved in several gastrointestinal diseases

Source: Reynolds, C. W. and Ortaldo, J. R. Natural killer activity: the definition of a function rather than a cell type. *Immunology Today* **8**:172, 1987.

restricted to this cell type, commonly referred to as NK cells.

LGLs can be found in the bone marrow and circulating in the blood. In addition, they are found in several lymphoid tissues, particularly the spleen and lymph nodes. Moreover they are associated with several other organs. The most significant of these are the gallbladder, liver, intestines (lamina propria), lungs, respiratory tract, and uterus.

Function of NK Cells   Several functions have been ascribed to NK cells (table 8.2). Although the mechanisms through which these functions are performed might not be characterized in all instances, it appears that cell-to-cell contact is involved in many, if not most, functions. NK cells have been observed binding to potential target cells through direct membrane-to-membrane contact between NK cell and glycoprotein target cell structures. Carbohydrate moieties might be expressed in increased density on target cells, making them sensitive to NK cells. Spontaneous lysis of the target cell eventually follows in the absence of MHC restriction, Abs, or complement. NK cells, in contrast to T_C cells, can thus lyse allogeneic as well as syngeneic target cells.

NK cells can produce a large variety of cytokines including IFNs, ILs, and lymphotoxins (LTXs). In addition, NK cells may serve as critical components of the body's spontaneous natural surveillance system against tumor cells that arise at primary and metastatic sites.

Activated Killer Cells   The cytotoxic activity of NK cells can be augmented both *in vitro* and *in vivo* by cytokines such as IL-2 and IFN. IFN-activated NK cells can directly lyse several target cells. They can also be recruited by T cells during specific adaptive responses to tumor Ags. In addition, they may participate as innate protectors against infectious agents of disease, such as viruses, certain fungi, and animal parasites. NK cells that are stimulated by lymphokines to display enhanced activity are known as lymphokine-activated killer (LAK) cells.

In addition to cytokine receptors, NK and LAK cells possess FcγR III-2, which enables them to be recruited to exhibit ADCC reactions, as well as direct spontaneous cytotoxicity.

The Cytolytic Process   NK cells are believed to induce cytolysis through two mechanisms: (1) perforin-induced cytolysis and (2) apoptosis. **Perforin-induced cytolysis** is accomplished through the creation of membrane channels that lead to target cell destruction. The events of this mechanism are outlined below. In contrast, **apoptosis** entails nuclear degeneration followed by cytolysis. How nuclear degeneration is induced by interaction between the NK cell and the target cell to which it binds remains unknown. Nevertheless, nuclear degeneration is believed to be the primary result of this interaction, with cytolysis following as an inevitable consequence of cell death. This process resembles programmed cell death observed during embryonic development.

Perforin-induced cytolysis appears to be achieved through a cyclical process comprised of four basic stages. The stages of this killing cycle are (1) specific binding to the target cell, (2) activation of the NK cell, (3) target cell killing, and (4) detachment and recycling of the NK cell.

Attachment to the target cell appears to be *mediated by Leu-CAMa.* These NK Ags specifically recognize conserved carbohydrate determinants expressed by the target cell. Interaction between Leu-CAMa and the target cell determinants creates stable contact between the two cells.

Interaction of surface receptors with the target cell initiates a series of changes in the NK cell that constitutes **activation.** For example, the cytoplasm may undergo rearrangement within minutes after binding to the target cell. The granules and Golgi apparatus, which become enlarged, are repositioned between the nucleus and the target cell. Moreover, the membranes and cytoplasm of the effector cell and target cell become interlocked to enlarge the contact area. The NK cell's cytoplasmic granules, containing lytic enzymes and soluble toxic factors, now can be delivered (exocytosed) to the target cell. In the presence of Ca^{2+}, these factors polymerize on the target cell membrane and form transmembrane pores similar to those generated by complement (C5–C9). These cytotoxic pore-forming proteins, which bear some sequence identity to C9, are called *perforins* or *cytolysins.*

Perforins can be activated by Ca^{2+}. **Cytolysis of the target cell** occurs when the integrity of the plasma membrane is violated and small ions and other solutes are allowed to exchange through these new pores. The granules of NK cells also contain protease-resistant proteoglycans. Proteoglycans are highly negatively charged molecules consisting of long, unbranched, sulfated, polysaccharide chains bound to a core protein. These molecules might protect the NK cells from self-destruction, or autolysis, when perforin is secreted.

The NK cell subsequently **detaches** from the killed target cell and is free to seek out another target cell. Thus, a single NK cell can destroy, or kill, multiple target cells without itself being destroyed, or damaged, in the process. In addition, NK cell killing is unidirectional; all activities are focused on the target cell, with no reciprocal effects being experienced by the NK cell.

Evaluating NK Cell Killing   The cytotoxic function of isolated NK cells may be examined by cytotoxicity testing against certain tumor cell lines. For example, this can be demonstrated using erythroleukemia cell line K562. If these cells are incubated in the presence of ^{51}Cr, the isotope is taken up by the erythroleukemic cells. Following addition of NK cells, erythroleukemic cells are destroyed, causing release of ^{51}Cr into the medium.

Macrophages

The mononuclear phagocyte system is briefly characterized in chapter 2, Cells and Tissues of the Immune System. The major cell of this system is the monocyte/ Mϕ. Mϕs are derived from pluripotent stem cells in the bone marrow, as are all blood cells. Progenitor cells differentiate into monocytes, which enter the bloodstream. Here they have a circulating half-life of approximately one day. They then leave the blood and enter the tissues, where they develop into Mϕs to live for perhaps several months. Mϕs can also be formed from division of immature Mϕs *in situ,* but probably most are derived from emigrating monocytes. During inflammatory responses, both the influx of blood monocytes and the local proliferation of tissue Mϕs is significantly increased. On occasion, Mϕs can fuse to form giant cells.

Mϕs are actively motile, adherent, and intensely phagocytic. In addition, they can be activated by lymphokines, such as immune IFN. Mϕs display a variety of Ags and receptors. For example, they express class II MHC Ags. Mϕ receptors with significant roles in immune responses include FcγR III-2, CRs, LeuCAMc, and receptors for lymphokines. Although Mϕs can bind, ingest, and degrade almost any type of Ag, they lack receptors that recognize unique epitopes.

Cells of the mononuclear system are found in the bone marrow, where they are produced, and in the blood, where they circulate. They are also normal constituents of connective tissues, lungs, serous cavities, liver, bone, the nervous system, joints, spleen and other lymphoid tissues. In these tissues, Mϕs are often identified by specific names. For example, they are called alveolar phagocytes (lungs), microglia (central nervous system), reticular cells (bone marrow and lymphoid organs), or Kupffer cells (liver). During inflammation, macrophages can be found in any tissue.

Migration of Macrophages   Once monocytes emigrate from the bloodstream and differentiate into Mϕs, they become capable of random and specifically directed migration into and through tissues. Specifically directed migration occurs in response to chemotactic stimuli, released, for example, from Ag-stimulated T cells. Other chemotactic factors include activated B cells, complement factors, bacterial products, and several other proteins released from cells. Orientation of Mϕs is apparently determined by the concentration of chemoattractant. For example, if lymphokine is presented, Mϕ migration will be in the direction that the lymphokine is most concentrated. Migration may be inhibited as well. This can be accomplished by Mϕ migration-inhibiting factor (MIF), also released from activated T cells, and plasmin, a protein capable of dissolving fibrin blood clots. During inflammatory reactions, the rate of Mϕ migration can be increased by chemical stimuli released into the microenvironment. In contrast, Mϕ migration may be adversely affected in certain disease states.

Phagocytosis   Mononuclear phagocytes exhibit nonimmune and immune phagocytosis. This process consists of several steps: (1) recognition of and attachment to the particle to be phagocytosed, (2) actual engulfment, (3) killing and digestion, and (4) postdigestion disposal of remnants. The major events of this process are schematically outlined in figure 8.1.

Recognition and **attachment** (fig. 8.1a) in immune phagocytosis is *mediated by the FcγR III-2, CR5 (which recognizes C3d), and CD35 (CR1, which recognizes C3b)* on the phagocytes. These receptors become attached to immune complexes and complement bound on opsonized target particles. During phagocytosis, foreign particles are bound to either spe-

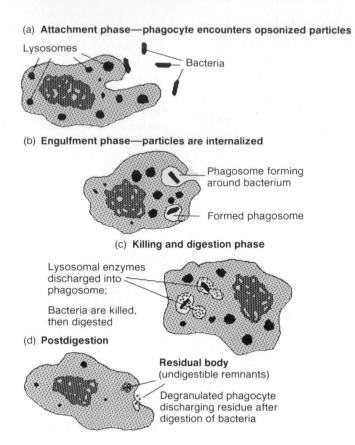

(a) **Attachment phase—phagocyte encounters opsonized particles**

Lysosomes

Bacteria

(b) **Engulfment phase—particles are internalized**

Phagosome forming
around bacterium

Formed phagosome

(c) **Killing and digestion phase**

Lysosomal enzymes
discharged into
phagosome;

Bacteria are killed,
then digested

(d) **Postdigestion**

Residual body
(undigestible remnants)

Degranulated phagocyte
discharging residue after
digestion of bacteria

FIGURE 8.1 Major events of phagocytosis. The major steps in the ingestion, killing, and digestion of bacteria that constitute the process of phagocytosis are shown diagrammatically in these four panels.

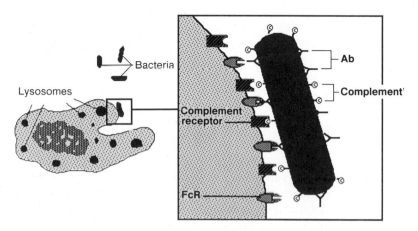

Bacteria

Lysosomes

Ab

Complement'

Complement
receptor

FcR

FIGURE 8.2 Attachment of opsonized substances through Fc and complement receptors.

cific or nonspecific receptors (fig. 8.2) and then surrounded by the cell membrane to form a phagocytic vesicle (see chapter 6, Complement and its Role in Immune Responses, for further discussion of opsonization). Alternatively, soluble macromolecules might be pinocytosed in a similar fashion. FcRs and CRs enable Mφs to recognize particles coated, or opsonized, with Ab and complement molecules. However, some Abs are cytophilic. These Abs bind to the Mφ first, then bind to the Ag on the particle to be phagocytosed. In this manner, immunological specificity for target particles is acquired. Bound soluble and insoluble materials are then ingested. Following phagocytosis, formerly interiorized receptors are reexpressed on Mφ membranes.

Engulfment (fig. 8.1*b*) is accomplished by *physical wrapping of the membrane around the particle.* This creates a phagocytic vesicle, or phagosome, which is taken into the cell. Once formed, the phagosomes are moved within the Mφ, directed by microtubules. They then fuse with lysosomes forming phagolysosomes. Next the contents become acidified and are digested (fig. 8.1*c*) by a veritable host of hydrolytic enzymes (table 8.3). Some intracellular parasites escape this fate by penetrating the phagosomal membrane, thereby gaining access to the more compatible cytoplasm of the Mφ. This strategy is used by the protozoan, *Leishmania,* which preferentially infects Mφs in the host. Other parasites are even capable of preventing the fusion of the phagocytic vesicle with a primary lysosome. (See chapter 12 for further discussion.)

Two major mechanisms of killing and digestion are used by phagocytes. One depends upon oxygen, while the other is not dependent upon oxygen. The following sequence is believed to represent the steps of **oxidative (oxygen-dependent) killing** of phagocytized microorganisms that is *mediated by the enzyme myeloperoxidase.*

1. Glycolysis supplies energy for engulfment (oxygen consumption is increased two- to three-fold).
2. NADPH oxidase becomes activated, leading to the generation of peroxide (H_2O_2).
3. The NADP made available stimulates the hexose monophosphate shunt substantially (from 1% to 10% of glucose utilization), providing increased substrate for NADPH oxidase.

TABLE 8.3 Lysosomal Enzymes of Phagocytes

Enzymes	Neutrophils	Macrophages
Glycosidases		
α-L-fucosidase	Yes	
α-1,4-glucosidase	Yes	
α-mannosidase	Yes	
α-N-acetylglucosaminidase	Yes	
β-glucuronidase	Yes	Slight
β-galactosidase	Yes	
β-N-acetylglucosaminidase	Yes	
Hyaluronidase	Yes	Yes
Lysozyme	Yes	Yes
Lipases		
Acid lipase	Yes	Yes (?)
Phospholipase	Yes	Yes (?)
Nucleases		
Ribonuclease	Yes	
Deoxyribonuclease	Yes	
Phosphatases		
Acid phosphatase	Yes	Abundant
Alkaline phosphatase	Yes	
Phosphatidic acid phosphatase	Yes	
Phosphoprotein phosphatase	Yes	
Proteases		
Cathepsins B, C, D, E	Yes	Cathepsin C (?) Yes
Collagenase	Yes	Yes
Elastase	Yes	
Kininase	Yes	
Kininogenase	Yes	
Miscellaneous Substrates		
Aryl sulfatases A and B	Yes	
Esterases	Yes	Abundant
Peroxidase	Yes	Modest Amounts

4. The H_2O_2 generated interacts with myeloperoxidase, and possibly intracellular halide (Cl^-), to cause bacterial killing. In this final step, toxic oxidants (for example, hypochlorite [bleach]) can be produced, which can chemically disrupt the microbial surface wall, leading to its eventual death. This sequence is outlined in figure 8.3.

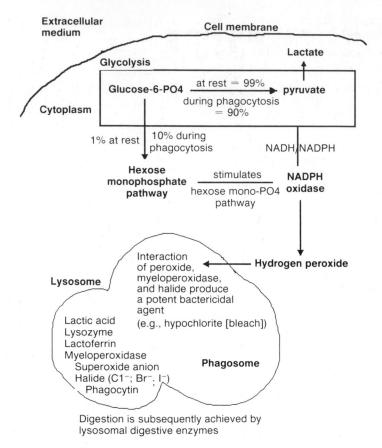

FIGURE 8.3 Steps of microbial killing by phagocytes. The intracellular events in microbial killing are summarized. Note that peroxide is produced in the cytoplasm and acts in the phagosome in conjunction with halide ions and lysosomal products. Digestion is accomplished separately.

A second oxidative mechanism exists that is *not dependent on myeloperoxidase.* Through this mechanism, microbes are destroyed by the direct effects of H_2O_2, superoxide ions (O_2^-), reactive singlet oxygen radicals ($O\bullet$), and hydroxyl ions (OH^-). Since Mϕs lack myeloperoxidase, this is their principal means of microbial killing.

Alternatively, killing can be accomplished through a **non-oxygen-dependent mechanism.** The *lysosomal cationic proteins* and *lactoferrin* are implicated in this microbicidal mechanism. Peroxide generation is not a part of this process. The cationic proteins are most active in an alkaline environment, as exists within the phagosome shortly after its creation. If the microorganisms engulfed are gram-negative bacteria, these proteins have an opportunity to cause serious damage to the cell wall before the pH shifts downward into an acidic range. Since lactoferrin can bind iron, it might bring about microbial death by depriving the bacteria of iron, which is a necessary element for their survival. This binding of iron by lactoferrin can occur at either high (alkaline) or low (acidic) pH.

As the particle is reduced by the hydrolytic enzymes to its component building blocks (amino acids, simple sugars, fatty acids, etc.), they simply diffuse, or are transported, across the vesicle membrane into the cytoplasm (fig. 8.1*d*). While the events of microbial killing can sometimes be oxygen dependent, the actual digestive phase of phagocytosis is oxygen independent. After digestion is complete, a shriveled depleted vesicle, called a residual body, is all that remains. The nondigestible residue that remains here can then be discharged through exocytosis (a "reverse engulfment").

Macrophage Secretions   Mononuclear phagocytes provide immune protection in two ways. The first, as discussed above, is through their phagocytic/pinocytic capabilities. The second, and perhaps equally important, manner is through their secretions. Through FcRs, phagocytosis can be enhanced (as described above). In addition, FcRs permit Mϕs to exhibit ADCC. The damage inflicted on targeted cells, such as cancer cells, by Mϕs during ADCC depends on the actions of secretory products released.

Dozens of products may be secreted by Mϕs/monocytes, depending upon their status. These include a host of enzymes active at neutral and acidic pH. Among these enzes are plasminogen activator (which dissolves clots), lysozymes (which digest bacteria), and collagenases and acid hydrolases (which act on tissue products). Mϕs also produce and secrete several critical plasma proteins, including coagulation proteins and complement components. In addition, Mϕs secrete a variety of *bioactive substances*. These can be placed into three categories: (1) reactive metabolites of oxygen like H_2O_2; (2) bioactive lipids such as prostaglandins (PGs); and (3) factors regulating cell activities, for example, IL-1, IFN, and angiogenesis factor (which promotes vascularization of tissues). Of these substances, lysosome and complement components can be secreted regardless of the activation state of the Mϕ. In contrast, secretion of the other products depends upon appropriate stimulation. These triggers include activation of specific receptors, endocytosis, and alterations in tissue pH and oxygen tension.

The secretory products released by Mϕs critically influence the inflammatory response at many steps (discussed later in this chapter). Mϕ secretions provide an intricate regulatory network that bears critically on host resistance to infection. For example, to provide a simplified generalization, secretory products from activated Mϕs can inhibit the proliferation of cancer cells (IFN) or cause their cytolytic destruction (secreted enzymes).

Activated Macrophages   Mϕs can be activated by lymphokines produced by Ag- or mitogen-stimulated lymphocytes and by complement components. When this occurs, they become morphologically and functionally modified. This enables activated Mϕs to be easily distinguished from their nonactivated relatives. Activated Mϕs increase in size and become metabolically more active. They are more adherent to glass, spread more rapidly, and display increased rates of phagocytosis and pinocytosis. In addition, activated Mϕs release increased amounts of their protein secretions, H_2O_2, and PGs. As a result, they are dramatically more microbicidal and more tumoricidal than quiescent Mϕs.

Macrophages as Antigen-Presenting Cells   Mϕs can affect immune responses in numerous ways. As discussed above, **Mϕs can process and present Ags** to lymphocytes involved in both humoral and specific cell-mediated immune responses. For example, Mϕs can produce and release IL-1. This cytokine can promote the differentiation and expression of both T and B cells. In addition, Mϕs can interact more directly with T cells. This occurs when Mϕs act as antigen-presenting cells (APCs). However, in order to efficiently accomplish this, *T cells and Mϕs must display identical MHC Ags*. It should be noted, however, that not all influences from Mϕs have a positive effect on lymphocytes. Under certain conditions, Mϕs can suppress lymphocyte proliferation nonspecifically. This can occur when they release complement cleavage products, PGE, and IFN at critical periods. This role is explored in greater detail in the following chapter.

Granulocytes and Platelets

Other nonspecific effectors of cell-mediated immunity include a group of cells characterized by the presence of distinguishing cytoplasmic granules, the granulocytes, and extremely active cytoplasmic fragments, called blood platelets. The granulocytes can be classified by the nature of the specific granules that they possess as basophils, eosinophils, or neutrophils.

Neutrophils   Neutrophils are derived from the pluripotent stem cells located in the bone marrow. Their primary function is that of *phagocytosis of foreign, aber-*

rant, or dead cells and *pinocytosis of pathological immune complexes.* They can also exhibit ADCC. These cells are especially capable of rapid activation and mobilization in response to chemotactic stimuli, such as bacterial products or activated components of complement (C5a). A variety of receptors (Fc, C3b,d and C5a) are increasingly displayed following activation. During the early stages of inflammation (discussed later in this chapter), arising from infectious and/or immune-complex disease, neutrophils are the most prominent cell type. At an inflammatory site, they bind, ingest, or lyse (and in essence remove) the foreign or aberrant target.

Eosinophils　In contrast to neutrophils that are active primarily in inflammation, eosinophils *participate chiefly in allergic reactions and parasitic infections.* During certain allergic conditions (chapter 13, Hypersensitivity), and during certain parasitic infections (chapter 12, Immunity to Infectious Diseases), the numbers of eosinophils can increase dramatically. Through their phagocytic/pinocytic potentials, eosinophils can engulf and remove immune complexes and can inactivate certain allergic mediators. Eosinophils possess FcRs and can mediate ADCC. They respond to chemotactic factors released by T-cells that have been activated by helminthic (worm) antigens. They can bind to worm larvae (e.g., schistosomulae) coated with IgG, degranulate and release toxic proteins that are damaging to the parasites. They also respond to chemotactic products released by basophils and mast cells. For example, eosinophils can release enzymes (e.g., histaminase) that inactivate pharmacologically active mediators of Type I hypersensitivity reactions (e.g., histamine) that have been secreted by basophils and mast cells.

Basophils/Mast Cells　Basophils and mast cells, like eosinophils, are *active in allergic reactions.* They possess prominent, randomly distributed basophilic granules that contain eosinophil chemotactic factors and pharmacological mediators of Type I hypersensitivities (chapter 13, Hypersensitivity). These granules release their contents when stimulated with allergens that specifically bind to IgE (and crosslink these molecules) that has become attached to the basophil through high-affinity FcRs (designated FcɛR, since they bind IgE). Basophils also have FcγRs (which bind IgG) and re-

ceptors for complement components C3a, C3b, and C5a, suggesting a capability to exhibit ADCC, phagocytosis, and chemotaxis.

Platelets　Platelets are derived from megakaryocytes in the bone marrow. They possess small granules, surface FcɛRs and FcγRs, and class I MHC Ags. Platelets are not only *important in blood clotting,* but they are also critically involved in *hypersensitivity reactions and the inflammatory process.* They can release permeability-increasing substances, such as histamine, following aggregation and degranulation. Platelets can be induced to aggregate and degranulate by platelet-activating factor (PAF), immune complexes, and complement factors (C3a, C5a). PAF is produced by a variety of cells, for example, basophils and mast cells, following interaction with allergens or immune complexes and complement factors.

INFLAMMATORY RESPONSES

Inflammation is a *generalized (nonspecific) response to infection, wounding, or trauma.* Its existence as an adaptive response has been known for some time. For example, a term appears in the Smith Papyrus (written about 1600 B.C., but believed to be derived from a source written between 3000 and 2500 B.C.) denoting the existence of "a hot thing" associated with wounds. The Greeks of Hippocrates' time (460–380 B.C.) used the term *phlegmoné* ("the burning thing"), and the Romans used the term *inflammatio* (from which we derive inflammation) to describe this response.

　　A general knowledge of the characteristics of inflammation seems to have been acquired by the ancient Greeks. Although the Romans did little to expand on this knowledge, Celsus (circa A.D. 170–180) catalogued the major features of an inflammatory reaction. These are carried down even today as the **four cardinal signs** of inflammation: *rubor* (redness), *tumor* (swelling), *calore* (heat), and *dolore* (pain). A **fifth feature** was subsequently added, *functio laesa* (disturbed or altered function). This last sign (or symptom) is believed to have been added by Virchow in his *Cellular Pathology* (published in 1858), but is most frequently attributed to Galen (A.D. 130–200).

　　These cardinal signs of inflammation reflect certain of the immediate reactions that occur after

TABLE 8.4 Classification of Inflammatory Reactions

Type	Characteristics	Examples
Based on Duration		
Acute	Has short duration—hours or days; site is occupied by phagocytes (neutrophils in early stages, MφS after first day)	Small cut; pinprick
Chronic	Is long lasting—weeks to years; site is occupied by mononuclear cells (typically MφS and lymphocytes)	
Fibrous	Is marked by production of abundant fibrous material	Chronic pyelonephritis
Serous	Displays slow accumulation of clear exudate	Tuberculous infection of the lung
Suppurative	Is characterized by formation of abscess with great abundance of neutrophils	*Staphylococcus* infection
Granulomatous	Has local accumulation of mononuclear cells (MφS lymphocytes, fibroblasts)	Tuberculosis; leprosy; syphilis
Based on Cellular Activities		
Nonimmunological	Is typified by accumulation of inflammatory cells triggered by physical (or other) cause of tissue damaged	Pinprick; paper cut
Immunological	Occurs when products of immune response lead directly to increased vascular permeability or to cell death and trigger inflammation	Hypersensitivity reactions (e.g., systemic lupus erythematosus)

injury. They are common to all inflammatory responses. These manifestations are caused locally by changes brought about by the insult. The vasodilation (expansion of blood vessels) and increased blood flow contribute to the visible reddening of the affected area and the increase in heat perceived. Local swelling is produced by the loss of fluid from the vasculature to the wound area. The formation of a blister is perhaps the most striking and common manifestion of this phenomenon. The pain that we experience is caused by stimulation of nerve fibers by biologically active products of tissue destruction and of cells participating in the inflammatory process. Last, the affected tissues do not behave typically. This disturbance of routine function might be extremely subtle in the case of a small wound (e.g., a pinprick or small cut) or quite dramatic after severe injury (e.g., a bone fracture).

There are **two objectives** to an organism's response to infection or traumatic injury. The first objective is *elimination of the source of the infection or injury and any damaged tissue*. The second objective is *restoration of tissue integrity*. The inflammatory response is the process, an active reaction on the part of the organism, that seeks to achieve the first objective. Wound healing, or tissue repair, is the term used to describe those events designed to accomplish the second objective. Since there is a continuum linking these two processes in many instances, it can appear somewhat artificial to separate them. A distinction is being made, nevertheless, in order to stress the two major phases of this response: the reaction to infection or traumatic insult and repair of any damage produced.

Inflammatory responses can be classified according to the duration of the reactions to injury. Thus, acute inflammation refers to a short-lived response while chronic inflammation denotes a reaction that occurs over a longer period of time. Alternatively, inflammatory responses can be categorized by the types of cellular activities associated with them. In this regard, we can describe nonimmunological and immunological inflammatory reactions. Each of these can be further subdivided. Table 8.4 provides a sample scheme for classification of inflammatory reactions.

Throughout much of this discussion, reference is made to wounding or trauma as a trigger for the inflammatory response. These are not the only means of provoking this pattern of reponse, however; bacterial infections can produce these exact reactions as well.

The Acute Inflammatory Response

Within a few hours of sustaining tissue damage, the body has responded with the characteristic changes leading to redness, swelling, and pain in the affected area. These early events are essentially the same regardless of the nature of the insult: physical damage, bacterial infection, or immunological damage. These early changes were recognized a century ago, as reflected in Julius Cohnheim's *General Pathology*, published in 1889. In this treatise, the initial events of inflammation were characterized as involving (a) alterations in blood vessel size and blood flow, (b) increased vascular permeability, and (c) emigration of leukocytes into the tissues.

Local tissue damage triggers a series of events that involve vascular changes and leukocyte activation (fig. 8.4). Damaged cells discharge their contents, causing increased acidity in their local microenvironment. This local perturbation leads to a generation of bradykinin, which, in turn, acts on blood vessels, nerves, and mast cells. The immediate consequences of this stimulation are the release of PGs and leukotrienes by capillary cells and leukocytes, of substance P by nerves, and of histamine by mast cells. These set into motion the ensuing responses that we recognize as an inflammatory reaction. The ultimate consequences of these events appear as *altered blood flow* (redness and heat), *increased vascular permeability* (swelling), and *stimulation of nerve endings* (pain).

Vascular Alterations

The long-recognized initial events of inflammation are changes in the vasculature. These are of two types: (1) changes within the vascular system and (2) altered exchange between the vascular system and the interstitial fluid. These events constitute what can be called the **transudative phase** of the inflammatory response because of the alterations of the transudate (defined below) occurring at the site of injury.

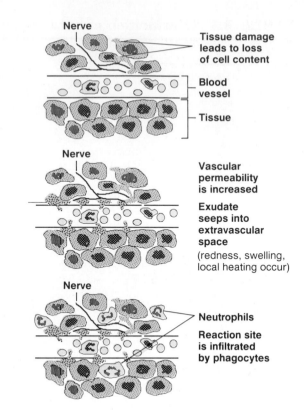

FIGURE 8.4 Initiation of inflammatory reactions. The major vascular and leukocytic responses that provide the hallmark of inflammation are depicted.

Increased Blood Flow The first type of alteration leads to increased blood flow through the affected region. Mediated by vasoactive substances such as histamine and serotonin (which can be released by mast cells and platelets), the vessels dilate. The vasodilation that is induced enables local blood flow to be increased. Consequently, the characteristic reddish color of the inflamed site appears. In a sense, this effect occurs within the vascular system.

Increased Vascular Permeability However, the vascular system is being affected in other ways that impact on the interstitial fluid. This second alteration leads to increased vascular permeability. The capillary endothelium provides a barrier to exchange between the blood and the extravascular compartments. Under normal conditions, a fluid ultrafiltrate is produced by the intravascular hydrostatic pressure. This ultrafiltrate

TABLE 8.5 Substances that Increase Vascular Permeability

Class	Substance	Source	Effects
Bioactive amines	Histamine	Mast cells/basophils; platelets	Induces smooth muscle contraction, causing vasodilation and increased permeability; stimulates pain response
	Serotonin	Platelets; mast cells/basophils	Has effects similar to histamine
Polypeptides/proteins	Kinins	Plasma α-globulin (as precursors)	Have effects similar to histamine
	Anaphylatoxins	Cleavage of components of complement	Indirectly act on vessels; provoke histamine release from mast cells
	Substance P	Nerves	Increases permeability
	Neurotensin	Nerves	Causes vasodilation
	Cationic proteases	Neutrophils; platelets	Increase permeability
Lipids	Leukotrienes	Leukocytes	Produce slow and prolonged contraction of smooth muscle, causing increased permeability
	PGs, A, E, F, I	Neutrophils; vascular endothelium	Cause vasodilation; increase permeability; enhance response to histamine/kinin (PGE)

is protein poor (less than 0.2%), and is called a *transudate.* Under the influence of these vasoactive substances, the capillary endothelium becomes less effective as a filtration barrier. Consequently, larger solutes are able to pass through with the filtrate. In addition, they can appear in substantial quantities. This new filtrate, called an *exudate,* can have protein content that is greater than 5%. This increased fluid loss is responsible for the swelling (edema, accumulation of fluid in tissues) associated with inflammation.

Agents that increase vascular permeability (table 8.5; also discussed below) produce their actions very rapidly and acutely. The increase in vascular permeability occurs immediately upon application of the substance and subsides within 15 to 30 minutes. This is designated a histamine-type response. It appears that the principal target is the venule. Here, smooth muscle cells are stimulated to contract. This causes them to pull apart slightly, thereby creating small gaps in the blood vessel wall through which the exudate seeps.

In contrast, vascular leaking that is produced by direct vascular injury might have variable onset, but it will be of longer duration. If the injury is mild, formation of an exudate might be somewhat delayed. In severe injury, leakage is essentially immediate. Nevertheless, in either case, exudation persists until the integrity of the vascular wall is restored.

The exudates produced at inflammatory sites can be categorized on the basis of their composition. Serous exudates are cell free and suggest mild inflammation only. Purulent exudates are cell rich, usually neutrophils, and usually reflect a bacterial infection. Hemorrhagic exudates are also rich in cellular content, but generally denote severe vessel damage. Fibrinous exudates are characterized by deposits of polymerized fibrin, typically on serous surfaces such as the pericardium or pleura.

Leukocytic Responses

A second important aspect of the inflammatory response is the reaction of leukocytes. This involves emigration from the blood into the inflammatory site and active phagocytosis in cleansing the area of debris. These events constitute the **cellular phase** of an inflammatory response.

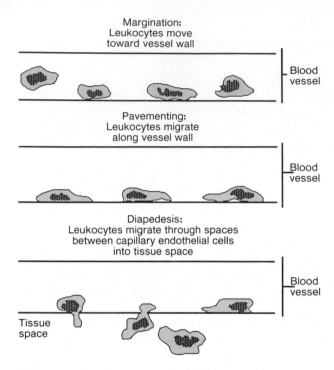

Margination:
Leukocytes move
toward vessel wall

Blood
vessel

Pavementing:
Leukocytes migrate
along vessel wall

Blood
vessel

Diapedesis:
Leukocytes migrate through spaces
between capillary endothelial cells
into tissue space

Blood
vessel

Tissue
space

FIGURE 8.5 Leukocyte infiltration of inflammatory site. The sequence followed by leukocytic phagocytes in their emigration from the blood into the tissue spaces is diagrammatically portrayed in the accompanying panels.

Infiltration   In order to be effective in removing debris (or bacteria) from a wound site, leukocytes must emigrate from the vascular channels and into the tissue spaces. The infiltration and accumulation of leukocytes at an inflammatory site is accomplished in three stages: margination, pavementation, and diapedesis (fig. 8.5).

Margination involves translocation of leukocytes from the blood to the walls of the blood vessels. As blood flows through the vessels, leukocytes will occasionally make contact with the vessel wall. *Pavementation* occurs when these cells adhere, or stick, to the vessel wall. The mechanism used to achieve this adherence is not clear, but it appears that Ca^{2+} is important for it to occur successfully. The pavemented leukocytes next migrate on the inner blood vessel surface until they encounter a site through which they can pass. This will be a point of contact between two endothelial cells. The leukocytes can next insinuate themselves between the interendothelial junctions, thereby leaving the vascular system and gaining access

to the extravascular tissue space (extravasation). This process of leukocyte emigration through the blood vessel wall is called *diapedesis.*

As these events occur, changes in the expression of surface markers of granulocytes can be observed. For example, MEL-14, which mediated adhesion to vascular endothelial cells, is rapidly (within 4 minutes) down-regulated. In contrast, Leu-CAMb (which is implicated in extravasation) expression appears to be enhanced.

Typically in inflammation, the cells that accumulate at the site of injury are phagocytes. In the early stages of an acute inflammatory response (the first few hours), neutrophils are the principal cell type. As the reaction proceeds longer, they are replaced as the principal cell type by Mϕs. However, this picture can be altered by the conditions responsible for the response. For example, following the injection of serum into the pleural cavity of rats, the maximal number of neutrophils was achieved within 4 to 6 hours. The numbers of Mϕs progressively increased between 6 to 18 hours, and by 48 hours, there were only Mϕs present. If living bacteria (*Klebsiella pneumoniae*) were injected instead, then neutrophils predominated thoughout the period of observation (24 hours) with few Mϕs being present.

Why should there be such a difference? The apparent answer is that particular cells are attracted to the site of injury. Thus, products from the site of injury act as specific signals activating and guiding leukocytes with appropriate receptors to where they are needed. This *chemically directed migration* of leukocytes to the site of injury is called chemotaxis. The substances responsible for "luring" leukocytes are called chemoattractants.

There are numerous chemotactic factors; some are listed in table 8.6 (discussed further in a later section). These include bacterial products, substances released by vascular damage, products of tissue damage, products of the complement system, and even products of leukocyte activity. There does not appear to be an easily discerned common denominator among these subtances. It is obvious that the leukocytes recognize the signal because of specific receptors that they possess. How these cells are able to determine the direction of migration remains unclear; nevertheless, there is evidence of an extremely sensitive ability to measure

Measuring Chemotaxis

Success of the inflammatory reaction depends upon removal of the cause of increased vascular permeability. This might be in the form of cellular contents from damaged cells, invading bacteria, or some other damaging agent. Since a common means of eliminating these materials is by phagocytosis (with subsequent killing and digestion), it becomes necessary to have a means of directing phagocytes to the site of injury. This is typically achieved by chemoattractant substances. These can arise from the damaged tissues or from cells acted upon by these products.

Whether a substance, or tissue product, can serve as a chemoattractant and how powerful an attractant it is can be determined. A common technique makes use of a chemotactic chamber (depicted in fig. 8.A).

A substance that is chemotactic, when placed in the lower chamber, causes a greater number of phagocytes to migrate into the filter than does a nonchemotactic agent. In addition, the rate of migration through this filter might be increased.

Chemotactic agents can be compared to each other in this same way. More potent chemotactic factors cause more phagocytes to enter the filter or cause them to migrate further in a shorter period of time than do weaker agents.

This same technique can be used to determine if phagocytes have impaired chemotactic responsiveness. If cells from a patient fail to respond to a chemotactic substance while cells from a healthy individual react, there is evidence for impaired chemotactic responsiveness or migration ability.

In addition to drawing phagocytes to the site of injury, it is desirable to keep them there so that they can perform their function. This is accomplished by a lymphokine called MIF. Its action can be demonstrated by observing its effects on Mϕ migration out of the end of a capillary tube (depicted in fig. 8.B).

Mϕs normally migrate away from the tip of the capillary, creating a halo zone. When their migration is inhibited, this zone is diminished.

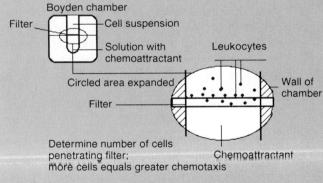

FIGURE 8.A Demonstration of chemotactic activity.

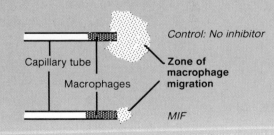

FIGURE 8.B Demonstration of MIF.

TABLE 8.6 Chemotactic Factors

Chemoattractant	Responding Cells
Bacterial or viral products	Granulocytes (all classes); monocytes/Mφs
Byproducts of blood coagulation (e.g., fibrin degradation products)	Neutrophils
Collagen fragments	Neutrophils
Kallikrein (kinin-generating enzyme)	Neutrophils; basophils/masts cells; monocytes/Mφs
PGE₁	Neutrophils
Components of complement system (especially C3 and C5 fragments)	Granulocytes (all classes); monocytes/Mφs
Cationic enzymes (from lysosomes of neutrophilic granulocytes)	Monocytes/Mφs
Lymphokines	Granulocytes (all classes); monocytes/Mφs; lymphocytes

concentration differences. Using stationary neutrophils in slide-coverslip preparations, directed movement can be demonstrated in a chemotactic gradient. The neutrophils apparently can detect a difference in the number of molecules across their own dimensions.

Phagocytosis Merely directing leukocytes to, and accumulating them at, a site of injury or infection is not sufficient to resolve any problem that might exist. These cells must then perform a function. Characteristically, the function that is performed is phagocytosis. **Metchnikoff** first observed phagocytosis as a defensive strategy in invertebrates in 1882. He later (1892, *Lectures on the Comparative Pathology of Inflammation*) elaborated on this role of phagocytes as a major defensive strategy among all animals from the simplest (protozoans) to the most complex (mammals). (Further comparisons of defensive and immunological strategies across evolutionary lines can be found in chapter 21, Comparative Immunobiology.)

   The essential events in the process of phagocytosis (attachment, engulfment, and digestion) have already been outlined (refer to fig. 8.1).

Mediators of Inflammation

The events of inflammation do not occur spontaneously nor haphazardly. They represent a well-orchestrated composite of vascular, leukocytic, and local tissue reactions. This is achieved through the actions of chemical messengers, or mediators. These substances can be classified as exogenous mediators or endogenous mediators. *Exogenous mediators* are foreign substances such as bacterial products. *Endogenous mediators* are products of the damaged tissue, the blood and vascular tissues, and leukocytes.

Plasma/Serum Factors The plasma provides an immediate line of defense following damage to vascular integrity. This is accomplished through the activities of several plasma proteins and calcium (fig. 8.6). These substances comprise the *plasma-clotting factors* and are responsible for hemostasis, or blood clotting. In addition, a component of this system (Hageman factor, Factor XII) activates the pathway for *kinin* production (fig. 8.7). In turn, both of these pathways can interact with the *complement* system.

   There exist, therefore, complex interactions among the coagulation, kinin-generating, and complement activation pathways (fig. 8.8). These components lead to alterations in vascular permeability (see table 8.5) and leukocyte infiltration (see table 8.6).

   In addition, there are several plasma proteins, known as the **acute-phase proteins** (table 8.7), that vary in concentration during inflammation. These can be classified as early acute-phase proteins, which are derived from Mφs, and late acute-phase proteins, which are derived from the liver.

   The Mφ-derived *early acute-phase proteins* include IL-1 (formerly called endogenous pyrogen [EP]), glucocorticoid-antagonizing factor (GAF), TNF, and serum amyloid A inducer (SAAI). IL-1 (EP) has systemic effects, leading to fever generation (see below). In addition, IL-1 stimulates IL-6 production, modulates expression of the acute-phase response, and affects the proliferation and expression of other cells involved in the inflammatory response. GAF and TNF are two related, but separable, factors produced within a few hours of appropriate injury. GAF blocks the glucocorticoid induction of certain liver enzymes. TNF, named because of its ability to mediate hemorrhagic necrosis

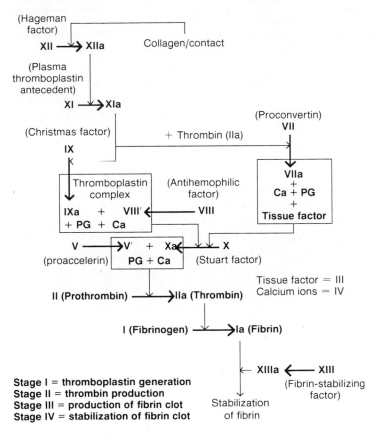

Intrinsic pathway　　　　　**Extrinsic pathway**

(Hageman factor)
XII ⟶ XIIa　　Collagen/contact

(Plasma thromboplastin antecedent)
XI ⟶ XIa

(Christmas factor)　　+ Thrombin (IIa)　　(Proconvertin)
IX　　　　　　　　　　　　　　　　VII
K

Thromboplastin complex　　(Antihemophilic factor)
IXa + VIII′ ⟵ VIII
+ PG + Ca

VIIa
+
Ca + PG
+
Tissue factor

V ⟶ V′ + Xa ⟵ X
(proaccelerin)　PG + Ca　(Stuart factor)

Tissue factor = III
Calcium ions = IV

II (Prothrombin) ⟶ IIa (Thrombin)

I (Fibrinogen) ⟶ Ia (Fibrin)

XIIIa ⟵ XIII
(Fibrin-stabilizing factor)

Stabilization of fibrin

Stage I = thromboplastin generation
Stage II = thrombin production
Stage III = production of fibrin clot
Stage IV = stabilization of fibrin clot

FIGURE 8.6 Coagulation system. The components of the blood coagulation cascade system are shown. The intrinsic pathway involves plasma-clotting proteins only, while the extrinsic pathway includes participation by tissue factors. Conversion to active forms is shown by *bold arrows;* factors serving as activators are in *light arrows.*

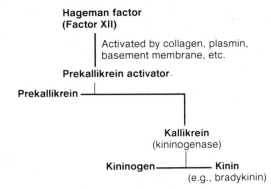

Hageman factor
(Factor XII)

Activated by collagen, plasmin, basement membrane, etc.

Prekallikrein activator

Prekallikrein

Kallikrein
(kininogenase)

Kininogen ⟶ **Kinin**
(e.g., bradykinin)

FIGURE 8.7 Pathway for kinin generation.

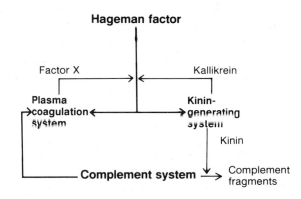

Hageman factor

Factor X　　　　　Kallikrein

Plasma coagulation system　　**Kinin-generating system**

Kinin

Complement system ⟶ Complement fragments

FIGURE 8.8 Interactions of coagulation, kinin-generating, and complement systems. Hageman factor triggers both the coagulation cascade and the kinin-generating system. In turn, each of these systems reinforces activation by Hageman factor. Moreover, the kinin-generating system interacts with the complement system. This system, in turn, interacts with the coagulation system.

TABLE 8.7 Acute-Phase Proteins

Protein	Source*	Characteristics
Albumin/prealbumin	Liver	Are large serum proteins; concentration reduced in acute phase
α-globulins (e.g., haptoglobin, α_1-antitrypsin	Liver	Are glycoproteins showing two- to four-fold increase; play various roles
Ceruloplasmin	Liver	Is glycoprotein important for copper transport; increases up to 50%
CRP	Liver	Can increase up to 300-fold; might have immunoregulatory role
Fibrinogen	Liver	Is glycoprotein-clotting factor; becomes increased
GAF	Mφ	Is protein that antagonizes production of certain liver enzymes; becomes elevated
IL-1	Mφ	Is protein that induces fever; becomes increased
SAA	Liver	Can increase up to 300-fold; is fibrillar protein
SAAI	Mφ	Induces production of SAA; may be related to CRP inducer
Transferrin	Liver	Is iron binding and transporting glycoprotein; is decreased in acute phase
TNF; cachectin	Mφ	Is glycoprotein capable of causing death of tumors; is possibly related to GAF

*Early acute-phase proteins come from Mφs; late acute-phase proteins come from liver.

of certain mammalian tumors, has several effects. For example, in conjunction with IL-1, TNF induces IL-6 production, modulates expression of the acute phase of inflammation, and induces fibroblasts and vascular endothelium to produce factors that, in turn, stimulate granulopoieis and monopoieis. This latter effect increases the numbers of granulocytes and Mφs available to participate in the inflammatory response. The last protein, SAAI, plays a role in the production of one of the late acute-phase proteins, serum amyloid A (SAA), by the liver.

The most significant of the *late acute-phase proteins* are C-reactive protein (CRP) and serum amyloid A (SAA). Both substances increase several hundred-fold during inflammation and appear to have immunosuppressive effects. Another group of proteins increases only modestly (two- to four-fold). These include haptoglobin, which reduces serum iron levels; fibrinogen (coagulation Factor I), which is the precursor of fibrin; α_1-acid glycoprotein, which potentiates clotting; and α_1-antiproteases, which reduce tissue damage. Ceruloplasmin and C3 (of complement) are increased mar-

ginally (approximately 50%). Ceruloplasmin binds copper and scavenges free radicals. The role of C3 is explored more fully elsewhere (see chapter 6).

Tissue-Derived Factors The inflammatory response is also affected by a variety of substances of tissue origin. Certain of these factors potentiate the vascular changes, others affect leukocyte behaviors, and some mediate both types of reactions.

The tissue-derived factors that mediate the increase in vascular permeability include bioactive amines, lipids, and a variety of peptides and proteins (see table 8.5). The most active of these amines are histamine and serotonin, released by both mast cells and platelets. The leukotrienes (formerly known as slow-reacting substance of anaphylaxis [SRS-A]) and the several PGs represent the major lipids released. The leukotrienes are probably produced by mast cells, while the PGs are derived from neutrophils during phagocytosis and from vascular endothelial cells. Nevertheless, both are derived as metabolites of arachidonic acid. The principal peptides and proteins affecting vascular permeability are derived from two sources: neurons and neutrophils. The neurons release substance P and neurotensin (11 and 13 amino acid peptides, respectively). Whether these neuropeptides are being used as neurotransmitters or neurohormones in affecting the vascular smooth muscle is not entirely clear. Neutrophils, and perhaps platelets, contribute cationic proteases from their lysosomes during phagocytosis. In addition to their roles in digestion of phagosomal contents, these enzymes can induce increased vascular permeability. This effect might be direct or achieved indirectly through histamine release from mast cells.

Other cellular products exert striking influences on leukocyte chemotaxis (see table 8.6) and adhesion. The chemoattractants are responsible for the infiltration into the site of injury of specific leukocyte populations. From a teleological point of view, a relationship exists between the kinds of chemoattractants produced at the site of injury and the kinds of cells that are needed to effectively respond to the cause of that injury. In addition, vascular endothelial cells release IL-8 (formerly called leukocyte adhesion inhibitor), which reduces adhesion of neutrophils to vascular endothelium. This presumably limits tissue damage that could be produced by the release of neutrophil proteases at the inflammatory site.

Phagocyte-derived factors attract not only more neutrophils, but monocytes/Mϕs, eosinophils, and basophils/mast cells as well. For example, cationic proteases released by neutrophils stimulate Mϕ chemotaxis in addition to increasing vascular permeability. The neutral proteases are able to generate chemotactic factors from C5 (complement system) and kininlike substances. These substances then can attract other neutrophils, Mϕs, eosinophils, and mast cells. Additional neutrophils are also attracted to the site of injury by as-yet-uncharacterized, serum independent factors released from the lysosomes of phagocytizing or damaged neutrophils. In addition to these neutrophil-derived factors, Mϕs also are believed to liberate substances that influence the cell populations at the inflammatory site. For example, Mϕ-like cells have been shown to produce and release a lymphocyte migration-enhancing factor (LMEF) and a lymphocyte migration-inhibiting factor (LMIF). LMEF attracts T cells to an inflammatory site, while LMIF impairs their migration from the inflammatory site after their arrival. Presumably, this enhances the opportunities for interactions between Mϕs (as APCs) and T cells, as well as the stimulatory effects of secreted lymphokines on effector cells that are at the inflammatory site.

Under circumstances in which a lymphocyte population is associated with inflammation (e.g., due to immune complexes), lymphocyte-derived chemotactic factor can be produced. This chemotactic lymphokine is responsible for attracting neutrophils, monocytes/Mϕs, basophils/mast cells, eosinophils, and additional lymphocytes to the site of injury. In addition, lymphocytes can influence phagocyte migration negatively by means of two other lymphokines. Leukocyte-inhibiting factor (LIF) and migration-inhibiting factor (MIF) inhibit the migration of neutrophils and Mϕs, respectively. Consequently, the action of these lymphokines "fixes" the phagocytes at the site of injury after they are directed there by chemoattractants. Moreover, these factors also activate the phagocytic processes of the phagocytes upon which they act.

Chronic Inflammation

The inflammatory process continues until the conditions responsible for its initiation are resolved. In most instances, this occurs fairly rapidly. However, conditions sometimes exist that lead to a long-term inflammatory response. When this occurs, a condition of **chronic inflammation** is said to exist. Chronic inflammation can arise directly or by expansion of an acute inflammatory response. Chronic inflammation can be distinguished from acute inflammation by two histological features: (1) the predominant "inflammatory" cells are *mononuclear cells* (Mϕs rather than neutrophils) and sometimes lymphocytes and eosinophils (if there is an immunological component) and (2) the presence of *granulation tissue* (young connective tissue rich in fibroblasts and newly formed capillaries).

The four forms of chronic inflammation encountered are (1) fibrous, (2) serous, (3) suppurative, and (4) granulomatous. These are classified largely by histological criteria (table 8.8).

In *chronic fibrous inflammation* there is the production of abundant fibrous tissue. Within this fibrous tissue, fibroblasts differentiate into myofibroblasts. The

TABLE 8.8 Types of Chronic Inflammation

Class	Features
Chronic fibrous	Site of inflammation possesses abundant fibrous connective tissue; fibroblasts present differentiate into myofibroblasts—their ability to contract can lead to physical distortion of injury site, causing mechanical defects
Chronic serous	Site of inflammation displays progressive swelling because of slow accumulation of clear, serumlike exudate; pleural cavities and joints are most likely affected
Chronic suppurative	Presence of accumulation of pus in abscess; progression of lesion depends upon ability of abscess to discharge its contents naturally
Chronic granulomatous	Presence of one but usually several foci of concentrated inflammatory cells about a "unit" of irritant; core contains epithelioid macrophages—this is surrounded by lymphocytes and fibrous connective tissue; is poorly vascularized or not vascularized

fibers contained in these cells are arranged in a fashion similar to that seen in smooth muscle cells. Since these myofibroblasts can be made to contract, the fibrous tissue in this form of inflammation can contract, leading to mechanical defects like stiffened joints or stenosis (narrowing) of ducts.

Chronic serous inflammation is characterized by the gradual accumulation of a serumlike, clear exudate. This form of inflammation typically occurs in serous cavities or joints in which the fluid producing membranous tissues become inflamed. One example of this type of inflammation is tuberculous infection of the pleura.

If pus (neutrophils) accumulates within a newly formed cavity, this is an abscess, which is a hallmark of *chronic suppurative inflammation.* Although neutrophils are typically associated with acute inflammation, the slow, progressive accumulation over the days or weeks necessary to establish a sizable abscess

reflects a long-standing or chronic condition. The events leading to the formation of such an abscess might be as follows:

1. Pus-producing (pyogenic) bacteria (e.g., *Staphylococcus aureus*; see chapter 12 for further discussion of microbial pathogens) enter tissues and create a focus of local "injury."
2. An acute inflammatory response occurs to counter the bacteria.
3. Within the center of the inflammatory site, necrosis (cell death and degeneration, caused by the bacteria) and liquefaction (caused by neutrophils' lysosomal enzymes) occur.
4. The abscess itself is formed by enclosure within fibrous tissue, resembling granulation tissue (see Tissue Repair, below). If the bacteria are killed off, the pus might subsequently be resorbed by Mφs or be discharged; otherwise, surgical intervention might be required to drain the abscess.

The most common form of chronic inflammation is *chronic granulomatous inflammation.* Characteristic of this form of inflammation is the occurrence of several discrete structures called granulomas. Each granuloma represents a small amount of the affecting agent surrounded by aggregates of inflammatory cells, usually Mφs and lymphocytes. Granulomas can vary in size from microscopic to approximately 1 mm in diameter. They can be caused by bacterial (e.g., syphilis) or parasitic (e.g., schistosomiasis) infections, aseptic foreign substances (e.g., asbestos), or by unknown agents (e.g., sarcoidosis). Typically, these are materials that the Mφs cannot adequately digest.

In general, granulomas have a core of epithelioid Mφs. These cells have taken on an appearance similar to that of epithelial cells. A consequence of this morphological transformation is a reduction or loss in phagocytic capacity. Intermingled with the Mφs, giant cells can be found. These cells, named because they are large and multinucleated, arise through fusion of Mφs. In addition, lymphocytes, plasma cells, or eosinophils might be associated with or surround the epithelioid core. This central mass of inflammatory cells is surrounded by a fibrotic zone. This outer zone of fibrosis is the result of collagen deposition by fibroblasts. The granuloma differs from granulation tissue (found in repair, see the next section) in that the central epithelioid core is avascular. Granulation tissue typically contains an abundance of new blood vessels.

Tissue Repair and Wound Healing

The removal of the cellular debris or infective agent that triggered the vascular and leukocytic reactions discussed above does not necessarily mark the end of the inflammatory response. Since tissue damage occurred, some form of healing or repair is necessary to restore some semblance of the original conditions. Two major processes are responsible for this reparative, or healing, phase of inflammation. These are (1) **tissue regeneration,** which involves *hyperplasia or hypertrophy of the tissues* originally damaged and (2) **fibroplasia and fibrosis,** which are *responses of fibroblasts* of the connective tissues. The balance between these two processes determines the outcome of this phase of inflammation (fig. 8.9).

Tissue Regeneration

Regeneration is the ideal reparative process to end the inflammatory response. In this process, the very tissues that sustained damage, whether by external injury (e.g., a cut) or through infection, would serve to replace what was lost. This requires that the affected tissue have within it a population of cells capable of cellular proliferation (mitosis).

With the loss of tissue because of damage, healthy cells that remain can be activated to divide. This leads to increased numbers of cells in the tissue and a restoration of tissue mass. Proliferation might be triggered by increased availability of nutrients indirectly produced by the reduction in tissue mass or by mitogenic factors released by the inflammatory cells. Macrophages and lymphocytes produce mitogenic factors that act on fibroblasts (see below). An alternative explanation for the increased proliferation observed is a reduction in the concentration of tissue-specific mitotic inhibitors produced by these same tissue cells. These substances, called chalones, have been proposed as regulators of cell division in epidermis, liver, kidney, and blood.

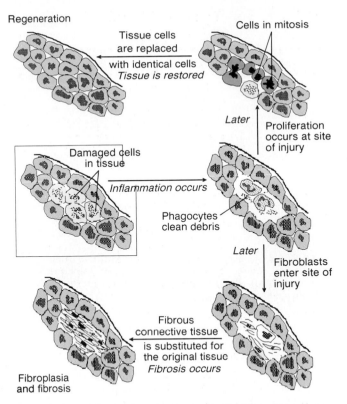

FIGURE 8.9 Healing and repair phase of inflammation. Once damaged tissue has been removed, reconstruction is necessary. This can take the form of *regeneration,* in which the tissue's own cells are used to replace the damaged cells. Alternatively, *fibroplasia and fibrosis* might be employed. This leads to a replacement of the normal tissue cells by a fibrous connective tissue scar.

Fibroplasia and Fibrosis

Tissue regeneration is not possible for all tissues. For an organ like the liver, such a response can occur. However, if nervous tissue (e.g., the brain or spinal cord) was damaged, this option does not exist. In these instances, an alternative mechanism for repair is needed. This mechanism produces a substitute for the tissue originally damaged. This tissue is called a scar. The process through which scar tissue is formed involves fibroplasia, proliferation of fibroblasts, and fibrosis, increased fiber production. (*Note*: The terms fibroplasia and fibrosis are both used to denote an increase in fibrous connective tissue.) This is how most inflammatory reactions are finally resolved.

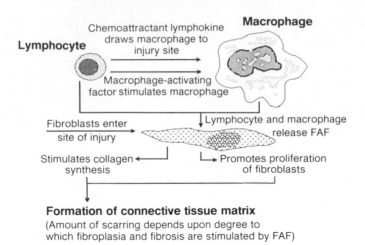

Formation of connective tissue matrix
(Amount of scarring depends upon degree to
which fibroplasia and fibrosis are stimulated by FAF)

FIGURE 8.10 Leukocyte influence on scar formation. Lymphocytes at the site of injury affect scar formation by direct influence on fibroblasts. They also exert an indirect influence on the fibroblasts through their effects on macrophages. Both effects lead to fibroplasia (fibroblast proliferation) and fibrosis (formation of matrix fibers). The extent of these activities greatly affects how much fibrous scar tissue is produced at the site of injury.

As the inflammatory response moves toward completion, the site of injury becomes highly vascularized by newly formed capillaries. These capillaries are believed to be induced by angiogenesis (blood vessel formation) factor(s) originating in the site of injury. This area, still heavily populated by neutrophils, becomes infiltrated by fibroblasts. This infiltration is apparently brought about, or enhanced, by chemotactic factors released by Mϕs and Ag- or mitogen-stimulated lymphocytes. The tissue that is produced is called granulation tissue. Although granulation tissue and granulomas both have substantial populations of inflammatory cells and fibroblasts, granulation tissue has a rich network of capillaries, whereas granulomas are avascular.

The expansion of the fibroblast population in granulation tissue also comes about through local proliferation. This is mediated by fibroblast activating factor (FAF), which is produced by Mϕs and Ag-activated lymphocytes. FAF has two effects on fibroblasts: (1) it promotes proliferation, thereby increasing the numbers of fibroblasts and (2) it also stimulates the production and release of fibroblast products (e.g., collagen) that are used in creating a fibrous network for the replacement tissue. This network is originally composed of collagen fibrils (small fibers), but as synthesis of new collagen decreases, these fibrils are re-

organized into thicker fibers. The remodeling process involves a balance between synthesis of new collagen and destruction/reassembly of old collagen. The fibers that are formed are oriented along lines of stress in the wound and strengthen the scar tissue. The interplay between collagen synthesis and destruction affects this orientation and determines the final character and appearance of the scar. These events are diagrammatically outlined in figure 8.10.

In acute inflammation, fibroplasia and fibrosis occur to a limited extent with minimal physical distortion of tissue. In chronic inflammation, fibroplasia and fibrosis can occur to a much greater extent. Substantial scarring, and permanent damage, can result. The consequences can include fibrous replacement of normal parenchymal tissues in vital organs (e.g., liver and kidneys) or narrowing of the gastrointestinal tract or blood vessels.

Systemic Aspects of Inflammation

The foregoing discussion was biased toward a local perspective. What events are occurring at the site of injury? Changes in blood flow, in vascular permeability, and in leukocyte behavior are focused on the area in which the inflammation is occurring. Nevertheless, we must remember that the human body is an integrated, coordinated whole. If something is done to alter conditions or circumstances in one area, its effects are perceived elsewhere as well, although these effects might be extremely subtle. For example, the local alteration in blood flow is associated with peripheral redistribution of blood flow. In addition, associated with the emigration of blood cells to the site of injury, there is a transient increase in the number of circulating blood cells. However, their eventual infiltration of the inflammatory site leads to a reduction in the circulating blood cell count, which must be restored. Two systemic consequences of local inflammatory reactions are worth noting: fever and hemopoiesis.

Fever

Fever occurs in association with inflammation because of the release into the blood of endogenous pyrogens, for example, IL-1. These are proteins derived from a variety of leukocytes (neutrophils, monocytes/Mϕs, and possibly eosinophils) that act on the hypothalamus in the same way that cold does. The result of this stimulation is vasoconstriction of cutaneous blood vessels (a strategy to reduce heat loss) and shivering (to generate heat). The consequence is an inappropriate increase in central body temperature, or fever. The fever subsides when normal thermoregulatory control is regained.

Hemopoiesis

The hemopoietic response that results from inflammation is somewhat more complex. If there has been blood loss, there is need to replace all cell types. A general increase in bone marrow activity follows, with erythropoiesis being the most conspicuous result. However, even if there is no blood loss, an acute inflammatory response draws phagocytes from the circulation into the extravascular tissue spaces. This leads to a reduction in leukocyte numbers, and evokes a compensatory increase in this leukocyte population.

Under ordinary circumstances, leukocytes (e.g., neutrophils) are being produced at a steady-state rate. Approximately half of the neutrophils in the circulation are actually freely circulating; the other half are in a marginated pool (i.e., associated with the blood vessel walls). When conditions evoke an inflammatory response, a demand for phagocytes is created. As we have seen above, this leads to emigration of neutrophils to the site of injury. An immediate reduction in the number of circulating neutrophils results. What then follows is an increase in the number of circulating neutrophils, a state of leukocytosis.

The leukocytosis associated with inflammation is produced by two phenomena. The first is a rapid release of neutrophils from the marginated pool to the circulating pool. This can be induced by epinephrine and exercise. Second, a reserve pool of immature neutrophils is released from the bone marrow. This can be evoked by C3 fragments and neutrophil-releasing factors (inducible by bacterial products). Both mechanisms lead to a rapid increase in the numbers of circulating neutrophils. These responses are believed to be directed at making available a large pool of neutrophils for emigration to the site of injury. However, it should be realized that immature granulocytes are less able, or are unable, to function effectively in phagocytosis and bacterial killing.

A third, but slower, mechanism for maintaining the leukocytosis is also initiated. This is a stimulation of granulopoiesis. So called colony-stimulating factors (CSFs) are produced by lymphocytes and Mϕs in association with inflammation. These substances act on bone marrow CFUs (see chapter 2) to promote proliferation and maturation of additional neutrophils. This stimulation of granulopoiesis is believed to be counterbalanced by a chalone. This proposed chalone, produced by granulocytes, would act on the granulocyte precursors to block proliferation. As more neutrophils are produced, the concentration of chalone increases and proportionally suppresses further granulopoiesis. Through this mechanism, the steady state rate of granulopoiesis would be reestablished after the inflammatory episode had passed.

Defects in Inflammatory Responses

The inflammatory response is generally beneficial. On occasion, however, undesirable results occur. This can be the consequence of defective execution of particular functions or of inappropriate responses to otherwise routine events.

Leukocytic Dysfunctions

Defective inflammation can result from quantitative or qualitative inadequacies of the leukocytes involved (table 8.9). If there are too few phagocytic neutrophils available, a condition known as neutropenia, then an effective inflammatory response might not be possible. On the other hand, an adequate number of phagocytes might be available, yet defects might arise in the execution of specific functions. In this regard, defects can affect any of the individual steps of the process: migration, chemotaxis, phagocytosis, or microbial killing.

Defects of Migration and Chemotaxis Disorders of migration and chemotaxis can prevent phagocytes from being recruited into the site of injury. An adequate population of responding cells might be provided, and an effective inflammatory response might not occur.

Problems of this nature can be traced to one of three causes:

1. Intrinsic defects in cellular locomotion that prevent cells that receive chemotactic stimulation from efficiently responding. Such defects occur in Chédiak-Higashi syndrome and with diabetes mellitus.
2. The presence of extrinsic locomotion inhibitors that interfere with chemotactic responses by intact leukocytes. Certain drugs (e.g., quinoline derivatives and phenylbutazone) and hormones (e.g., cortical steroids) exert such effects.
3. Reduced signal presentation because of deficiencies in chemotactic precursors or their premature inactivation. For example, individuals might genetically underproduce C3 or C5 and consequently have an impaired ability to generate active chemotactic factors. Such individuals would produce fewer chemotactic signals following tissue damage or infection and have a correspondingly diminished stimulation of leukocyte migration and infiltration of the site of injury or infection.

Disorders of Phagocytosis In other instances, sufficient numbers of phagocytes might be attracted to the site of injury (or infection), but might not be able to engulf and ingest the bacteria or cellular debris responsible for their presence. Such defects can result

TABLE 8.9 Leukocytic Disorders Affecting Inflammation

Disorder	Impact on Inflammatory Response
Quantitative Disorder	
Neutropenia	Ineffective response occurs because of an insufficient number of effector cells; individual phagocytes are otherwise normal functionally (can occur in drug-induced agranulocytosis and aplastic anemia, or in association with leukemia)
Qualitative Disorders	
Chemotaxis/migration	Cells are unable to recognize or respond to chemotactic signal; they are not mobilized to site of inflammation (can occur naturally in Chédiak-Higashi syndrome or be induced by variety of drugs)
Phagocytosis	Cells are unable to recognize or ingest bacteria, foreign or damaged cellular products; cells might not be able to engage lysosomes; although present at inflammatory site they are ineffective (can occur in association with agammaglobulinemia or sickle cell anemia; can be induced by variety of drugs (e.g., C3 deficiency affects opsonization; Chédiak-Higashi syndrome impairs degranulation)
Killing	Bacteria can be ingested but not killed because of deficiency in myeloperoxidase or in H_2O_2 generation; inflammatory response is ineffective because infective agent cannot be destroyed (can occur with G-6-PD deficiency, which impairs H_2O_2 generation)

from impairment of any of the steps of the phagocytic process: attachment, engulfment, and degranulation.

If Ig or C3 are underproduced, opsonization of infecting bacteria might not occur. Although present in suitable numbers, the phagocytes might not recognize the bacteria as targets. An ineffective inflammatory response might result. Such is the case in individuals with hypogammaglobulinemia (underproduction of Ig) or complement deficiencies.

Impaired engulfment and degranulation would be associated with an abortive response by the phagocyte following recognition of opsonized bacteria. Under these circumstances, phagosomes either do not form or they do not fuse with the lysosomes. In either case, killing and digestion cannot be expected. One example of a condition in which formation of phagolysosomes is impaired is Chédiak-Higashi syndrome. In addition, drugs such as morphine, and its analogues, produce defects of a similar nature.

Microbicidal Defects   Ineffective phagocytosis can also result from an inability to execute the final step of bacterial killing. This typically occurs for one of three reasons: (1) inability to generate H_2O_2, (2) peroxidase deficiencies, or (3) reduced formation of superoxide radicals. Deficiencies of glucose-6-phosphate dehydrogenase (G-6-PD) or myeloperoxidase are responsible for this type of ineffective phagocytosis. In granulomatous disease, defective microbial killing is the result of a reduced capacity to form superoxide radicals. Drugs (e.g., sulfonamides) and steroid hormones (e.g., cortisol) can have similar effects.

Synopsis

The inflammatory response provides an adaptive, and often defensive, reaction by leukocytic and tissue phagocytes. These cells are very rapidly called into action when there is violation of tissue integrity, whether as a result of physical trauma, microbial infection, or some other means. The immediate action of the phagocytes appears to have a two-fold objective. On the one hand, it clears the affected area of debris. On the other hand, the phagocytes perform an extremely aggressive role in ridding the tissue of infectious organisms. This latter, defensive function, can be performed independently of the immune system. It is an effective, albeit more primitive (see chapter 21, Comparative Immunobiology), means of preserving the integrity of the organism. However, in mammals it is not uncommon to encounter immunological participation in inflammation. This participation is more likely to occur when the inflammatory response alone does not resolve the problem or provide an adequate defense. However, the intimate intercommunication and interaction between phagocytes and lymphoid cells can also lead to circumstances in which the immune system itself triggers an inflammatory response.

In addition to its defensive aspects, the inflammatory response also has a restorative dimension. Specifically, there is a phase of "healing" and repair that concludes an inflammatory episode. Thus, not only is the threat to the individual (e.g., tissue damage, infection) overcome, but an effort is made to reestablish former conditions.

S U M M A R Y

1. Innate, or nonspecific, immune responses provide generalized defenses against infectious agents and foreign substances. They are rapidly evoked by conserved, rather than unique, determinants. Cells that contribute to nonspecific (innate) immunity include natural killer cells, macrophages and monocytes, neutrophils, eosinophils, basophils, and platelets. [p. 200]

2. Reactions of these cellular effectors are mediated by recognition systems composed of (a) complement and Fc receptors, (b) cell adhesion molecules, and (c) cytokine receptors. [pp. 201–202]

3. Natural killer cells provide a population of active cytolytic cells. Many of these cells are large granular, non-B/non-T lymphocytes. They are capable of destroying several target cells by the release of perforins, which are cytolysins that produce transmembrane pores in the target cell surface membrane. [pp. 202–205]

4. Macrophages provide a major population of antigen-nonspecific effectors. These cells function chiefly as phagocytes. In addition, they supplement this role through the production of cytokines and can function as antigen-presenting cells to stimulate specific cell-mediated immune responses. [pp. 205–209]

5. Granulocytes and platelets comprise additional populations of effectors of nonspecific cellular immunity. Granulocytes function as phagocytes, while platelets provide substances active in nonspecific humoral immunity as well. [pp. 209–210]

6. Inflammation can be recognized by four characteristic features or signs: redness (rubor), swelling (tumor), heat (calore), and pain (dolore). Occasionally, a fifth sign is added, disturbed function (functio laesa). [pp. 210–211]

7. There are two major facets to inflammation. The first is the response against the cause of injury. The second is repair. Inflammatory responses are classified as acute or chronic based on the duration of the response and the predominant inflammatory cells present at the site of injury. Further subdivision can be made on the basis of other features associated with the inflamed site. [p. 211]

8. The events of inflammation can be divided in two phases: a vascular phase and a cellular phase. During the vascular phase, local blood flow and vascular permeability are increased. These contribute to the redness, heat, and swelling associated with inflammation. During the cellular phase, leukocytes infiltrate the site of injury and interact with the cause of the injury. [p. 212]

9. The vascular changes are brought about by tissue damage and by vasoactive substances released by effector cells responding to this damage. [pp. 213–214]

10. During the cellular phase, chemotactic factors released by the damaged tissue and responding cells attract appropriate effector cells. These cells gain entry to the extravascular space through the following sequence: (a) margination, (b) pavementation, and (c) diapedesis. These events often are followed by phagocytosis. [pp. 213–216]

11. The events of inflammation are mediated by a variety of factors derived from the plasma/serum or inflammatory cells. Important plasma factors include the acute-phase proteins and components of the coagulation, kinin-generating, and complement systems. Tissue-derived factors include vasoactive factors, lysosomal enzymes, and lymphokines/monokines. [pp. 216–219]

12. Chronic inflammations are classified on histological criteria: accumulations of fibers (fibrous), serumlike fluid (serous), pus (suppurative), or granulomas (granulomatous). [pp. 219–221]

13. The repair phase of inflammation endeavors to restore the tissue after the source of the injury has been removed. It might take the form of tissue regeneration or fibroplasia and fibrosis. In order for tissue regeneration to occur, a population of cells capable of proliferation is required. The result of this form of repair is a restoration of the damaged tissue. Fibroplasia and fibrosis occur where this is not possible. This produces a replacement of the damaged tissue by fibrous connective tissue. The events of fibroplasia lead to scarring. [pp. 221–222]

14. Inflammation also can produce systemic effects which include fever and a compensatory leukocytosis and hemopoiesis. [pp. 222–223]

15. Defective inflammatory responses can occur because of neutropenia or defects (intrinsic or extrinsic) in migration and chemotaxis, or phagocytosis and microbial killing. [pp. 223–225]

READINGS

Akira, S., Hirano, T., Taga, T., et al. Biology of multifunctional cytokines: IL 6 and related molecules (IL 1 and TNF). *FASEB Journal* **4**:2860, 1990.

Densen, P., and Mandell, G. L. Phagocytosis. In *Fundamentals of Immunology and Allergy*. Lockey, R. F. and Bukantz, S. C. (eds.). W. B. Saunders Co., Philadelphia, 1987.

Gallin, J. I. Abnormal phagocyte chemotaxis: pathophysiology, clinical manifestations, and management of patients. *Reviews of Infectious Disease* **3**:1196, 1981.

Gimbrone, M. A., Jr., Obin, M. S., Brock, A. F., et al. Endothelial interleukin-8: a novel inhibitor of leukocyte-endothelial interactions. *Science* **246**:1601, 1989.

Harding, C. V., and Unanue, E. R. Cellular mechanisms of antigen processing and the function of class I and II major histocompatibility complex molecules. *Cellular Regulation* **1**:499, 1990.

Herberman, R. (ed.). *NK Cells and Other Natural Effector Cells.* Academic Press, Inc., New York, 1982.

Hill, C. P., Yee, J., Selsted, M. E., et al. Crystal structure of defensin HNP-3, an amphiphilic dimer: mechanisms of membrane permeabilization. *Science* **251**:1481, 1991.

Kishimoto, T. K., Jutila, M. A., Berg, E. L., et al. Neutrophil Mac-1 and MEL-14 adhesion proteins inversely regulated by chemotactic factors. *Science* **245**:1238, 1989.

Lydyard, P. M., and Fanger, M. W. Characteristics and functions of Fc receptors on human lymphocytes. *Immunology* **47**:1, 1982.

Movat, H. Z. *Inflammation, Immunity and Hypersensitivity: Cellular and Molecular Mechanisms.* 2d ed. Harper & Row Publishers, New York, 1984.

Oppenheim, J. J., Rosenstreich, D. L., and Potter, M. *Cellular Functions in Immunity and Inflammation.* Elsevier/North Holland, New York, 1981.

Ord, M. G., and Stocken, L. A. *Cell and Tissue Regeneration: A Biochemical Approach.* John Wiley & Sons, Inc., New York, 1984.

Ortaldo, J. R., and Hisderodt, J. C. Mechanisms of target cell killing by natural killer cells. *Current Opinion in Immunology* **2**:39, 1989.

Pattarrayo, J., Prieto, J., Rincon, T., et al. Leukocyte-cell adhesion: a molecular process fundamental to leukocyte physiology. *Immunological Reviews* **114**:67, 1990.

Qhu, N. Q., deBurin, D., Drownstein, B. H., et al. Organization of the human and mouse low affinity FcγR genes: duplication and recombination. *Science* **248**:732, 1990.

Ravetch, J. V., and Kinet, J. P. Fc receptors. *Annual Review of Immunology* **9**:457, 1991.

Reynolds, C. W., and Ortaldo, J. H. R. Natural killer activity: the definition of a function rather than a cell type. *Immunology Today* **8**:172, 1987.

Samuelson, B. Leukotrienes: mediators of immediate hypersensitivity reactions and inflammation. *Science* **220**:568, 1983.

Sayers, T. J., Mason, L. H., and Wiltrout, T. A. Trafficking and activation of murine natural killer cell: differing roles of IFN-γ and IL-2. *Cellular Immunology* **127**:311, 1990.

Sherry, B., and Cerami, A. Cachectin/tumor necrosis factor exerts endocrine, paracrine, and autocrone control of inflammatory responses. *Journal of Cell Biology* **107**:1269, 1988.

Tschopp, J., and Conzelmann, A. Proteoglycans in secretory granules of NK cells. *Immunology Today* **7**:135, 1986.

Wade, B. H., and Mandel, G. L. Polymorphonuclear leukocytes: dedicated professional phagocytes. *American Journal of Medicine* **74**:686, 1983.

Weller, P. F. The immunobiology of eosinophils. *New England Journal of Medicine* **324**:1110, 1991.

Wolpe, S. D., and Cerami, A. Macrophage inflammatory proteins 1 and 2: members of a novel superfamily of cytokines. *FASEB Journal* **3**:2565, 1989.

Ye, S., and Cheung, H. T. Regulation of lymphocyte mobility by macrophages: characterization of a lymphocyte migration inhibitory factor derived from a macrophage-like cell line. *Cellular Immunology* **122**:231, 1989.

Young, L. H. Y., Liu, C.-C., Joag, S., et al. How lymphocytes kill. *Annual Review of Medicine* **41**:45, 1990.

CHAPTER 9

Effectors of Specific Cellular Immunity

OVERVIEW

Effectors of specific cell-mediated immunity include several subpopulations of antigen-specific T lymphocytes. Certain of these cells act cytolytically against target cells, while others play central roles in modulating immune responses, both cell mediated and humoral. Cell-mediated immune responses may be involved in (1) host protection against viruses, bacteria, fungi, animal parasites, and cancer cells, (2) rejection of histoincompatible tissues, (3) hypersensitivity reactions, and (4) autoimmune disorders.

CONCEPTS

1. All antigen-specific, cell-mediated immune responses involve T lymphocytes. These cells undergo antigen-independent and antigen-dependent differentiation similar to B cells. However, antigen-dependent differentiation is triggered by processed antigens and is MHC restricted.

2. Antigen recognition is mediated through T cell receptors which possess a repertoire capable of interacting with the antigenic universe. Genes for T cell receptors display recombinatorial modification during T cell maturation.

3. Certain subpopulations of T cells become actively cytolytic following activation by antigen. Other subpopulations are stimulated to produce lymphokines, which can (a) recruit and regulate nonspecific effectors of cellular immunity, (b) stimulate the proliferation and differentiation of activated B and T cells, or (c) suppress expansion of immune responses.

Certain immune responses are provoked that are antigen (Ag) specific, yet are not executed through the generation of immunoglobulins (Igs). These responses are triggered by Ags which "select" effector cells with complementary receptors for clonal expansion. In this respect, the responses parallel those observed in activating humoral immune responses. However, in these responses, B cells are not the effector cells selected; rather, T cells are selected and activated. Thus, all precise Ag-specific, cell-mediated immune responses involve T lymphocytes and their subsets. These cells are identifiable by the **CD (cluster determinant) differentiation Ags** they display. Mice that have been thymectomized (surgical removal of the thymus), or that are genetically athymic (nude mice), either lack or have substantially reduced T lymphocyte populations. Consequently, they may not mount specific T cell responses. These mice are particularly susceptible to certain cancers and to viral and intracellular parasitic infections. Moreover, they usually fail to reject transplants of foreign cells and tissues. From this we can conclude that specific cell-mediated immune responses involving T cells occur in the body's resistance to many infectious agents (especially intracellular pathogens) and some malignant tumors. In addition, they are critically implicated in the rejection of allografts and graft-versus-host (GVH) reactions, delayed-type hypersensitivities (DTHs), certain drug allergies, and some autoimmune disorders.

■　■　■　■　■　■　■　■　■　■

CELL-MEDIATED IMMUNE RESPONSES

Cell-mediated immune responses are evoked by several factors. For example, they can be elicited in response to foreign Ags that are presented on allografts (see chapter 19, Transplantation Immunology, for further details). Alternatively, they can occur in response to inappropriately expressed Ags, as might occur during oncogenesis (tumor formation; see chapter 18, Tumor Immunology, for further discussion of this topic). Two forms of response might occur: nonspecific and specific. Nonspecific cellular immune responses are mounted primarily by natural killer (NK) cells, macrophages (Mϕs), and granulocytes. (Refer to chapter 8 for additional discussion.) These cells appear to respond to a variety of stimuli, apparently in a nonspecific manner. In particular, NK cells are peculiar in displaying natural cytotoxicity toward tumor cells. In contrast, specific cellular immune responses are conducted by T cells. In these instances, antigenic stimulation selects and activates particular cells that possess receptors with specificity for that Ag.

Ag-specific cell-mediated immune responses display parallels to humoral immune responses (table 9.1). Most notably, primary and secondary responses can be identified, each with features contrasting them. As with humoral immune responses, **primary cell-mediated immune responses** are *evoked by an initial exposure,* or contact, with a particular Ag. Foreign Ag is presented by Ag-presenting cells (APCs) to T cells, leading to their activation. T cells have Ag-specific receptors that recognize a bimolecular ligand composed of foreign Ag and a self-MHC molecule on the surface of the APC. Through the specificity inherent in the T cell receptors (TCRs), only particular cells become activated. These cells proliferate and *produce specific clones of effector T cells and memory T cells.* This process of clonal selection and expansion, in response to an immunogen, is qualitatively similar to that demonstrated by B cells. Moreover, the effector and memory cells generated each display identical Ag-recognition specificity. Several cell generations, and several days, must elapse before expression of the cell-mediated immune response can be seen. For example, rejection of first-set allografts might not be expected in less than 10 to 14 days.

A **secondary cell-mediated immune response** displays similar characteristics to a secondary humoral immune response. It is usually more pronounced and occurs more rapidly. Because of the availability of a population of specific memory cells, an increased number of effector T cells can be rapidly generated. Furthermore, these T cells can express receptors with greater binding efficiencies for the Ag. Consequently, expression of a cell-mediated response occurs sooner after challenge. Second-set allografts can be rejected within one week, in some instances.

TABLE 9.1 Parallels Between Humoral and Cell-Mediated Immune Responses

Response	Humoral	Cell-Mediated
Primary	Low specificity initial response (IgM)	Low specificity initial response
	Clonal selection and expansion of specific precursors (B cells)	Clonal selection and expansion of specific precursors (T cells)
	Expression of specific (IgG) response by effectors (plasma cells); generation of memory cells	Expression of specific response by effectors (e.g., T_H/T_D or T_C); generation of memory cells
Secondary	Activation of memory cells; rapid clonal expansion	Activation of memory cells; rapid clonal expansion
	Stronger and more rapid expression of specific (IgG) response by effector cells (plasma cells)	Stronger and more rapid expression of specific response by effector cells (e.g., T_H/T_D or T_C)

T CELL DIFFERENTIATION

The formation of T cells that are actively engaged in cell-mediated immune responses is achieved through an extensive process of differentiation. First, stem cells must undergo differentiation into Ag-responsive T cells. This is an Ag-independent process. Next, mature Ag-responsive T cells become activated and differentiate into functional effector cells. This latter series of events is Ag dependent. The general process of human T cell differentiation is outlined schematically in figure 9.1.

Antigen-Independent Differentiation

Initial differentiation of T cells progresses through two phases (see chapter 20, Development of Immunity). Both phases proceed without influence from foreign Ags. These events are Ag independent; nevertheless, they are influenced by factors in the microenvironments in which the cells find themselves. First, stem cells in the bone marrow (or fetal hemopoietic organs) undergo differentiation into T cell precursors. These cells are responsive to directing signals from the thymus, which enable them to migrate to and take up residence in the thymus.

After homing to the thymus, the precursors further differentiate to produce mature T cells. Within the thymus, several hormones act on the T cell precursors and influence their differentiation into one of the several **effector T lymphocyte subsets.** These subsets reflect the different functional roles played by T cells in immune responses and can be discriminated on the basis of the CD Ags they display (table 9.2).

T Cell Subsets

Approximately 65% of mature T cells that leave the thymus display the CD2+CD3+CD4+CD8− phenotype (**CD4+** cells), while approximately 35% display the CD2+CD3+CD4−CD8+ phenotype (**CD8+** cells). (See table 20.6 for changes in differentiation Ags during T cell differentiation.) A very small number express neither CD4 nor CD8 and consequently have a phenotype of CD2+CD3+CD4−CD8− (**CD4−CD8−** cells).

The major effector T cells that recognize and react specifically with Ag on target cells, causing their lysis, are CD8+ cells. These are called **cytotoxic T (T_C)** cells. The other CD4+ and CD8+ cells modulate inflammatory reactions and immune responses. For example, some CD4+ T cells are known as **DTH (T_D)** cells. These T cells secrete lymphokines when stimulated by Ag. Several different lymphokines can be released which, in turn, recruit and activate other leukocytes that serve as nonspecific effectors of inflammation. Both T_C and T_D effector cell subsets show a memory response and are regulated by **helper T (T_H)** (CD4+) and **suppressor T (T_S)** (CD8+) cell populations. Most T cell populations are CD4+ or CD8+ and are MHC restricted (see chapter 7, Histocompatibility Systems). In contrast, the few T cell populations that are CD4−CD8− are not MHC restricted.

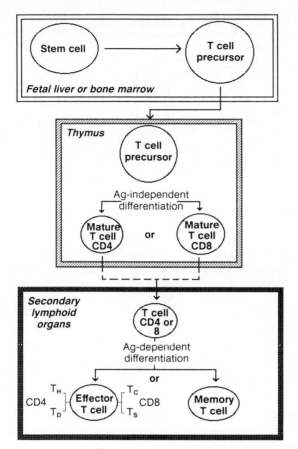

FIGURE 9.1 T cell differentiation. Differentiation of human T cells proceeds in two phases. First, T cell precursors arise from stem cells and undergo Ag-independent differentiation under the influence of the thymus. Second, mature T cells, through Ag-dependent differentiation, can be induced to become functioning effector or memory cells. A similar process occurs in other mammals; however, the differentiation Ags expressed by maturing T cells are different.

Antigen-Dependent Differentiation

Activation of mature Ag-reactive T cells proceeds in a stepwise fashion through discrete stages. First, there is an encounter with Ag that leads to activation. This leads, in turn, to proliferation and differentiation. The general events of this process are outlined below.

Antigen Processing

Activation of T cell differentiation is believed to occur following presentation of immunogen by APCs. Since T cells are not activated by native Ags, this requires that Ag be internalized and processed by APCs before

TABLE 9.2 T Lymphocyte Subsets

Subset	Distinguishing Features	Role in Immunity
Regulators		
T_H cells	Class II MHC restricted; CD2, CD3, CD4	Stimulate B cells to produce antibody; promote expression of function by activated T cells
T_S cells	Class I MHC restricted; CD2, CD3, CD8	Suppress expression of immune responses
Effectors		
T_D cells	Class II MHC restricted; CD2, CD3, CD4	Promote expression of delayed hypersensitivity responses
T_C cells	Class I MHC restricted; CD2, CD3, CD8	Display cytolytic activity when stimulated

presentation. Furthermore, the resulting immunogen is presented to T cells in MHC-restricted fashion. This model limits, or restricts, recognition of Ags to those epitopes that are encountered in conjunction with particular self-MHC products. For example, T_H (CD4⁺) and T_D (CD4⁺) cells are stimulated only by foreign Ag encountered in association with class II MHC molecules, while T_C (CD8⁺) and T_S (CD8⁺) cells are predominantly stimulated by Ags associated with class I MHC Ags.

Ag is first encountered by APCs, such as Mϕs. These cells internalize the native Ag and degrade it. Subsequently, portions of the Ag become associated with MHC Ags and are expressed in the APC's surface. Two modes of processing have been identified (fig. 9.2). One mode is used for processing Ags derived from phagocytosed materials (e.g., bacteria) and leads to association of antigenic determinants with class II MHC molecules. Association between the determinants of the Ag and the MHC molecule is believed to occur in endosomes (phagosomes or related intracellular vesicles), in which catabolism of the ingested Ag occurs. The second mode is used primarily in processing Ags derived within the cell (e.g., viral Ags expressed by an

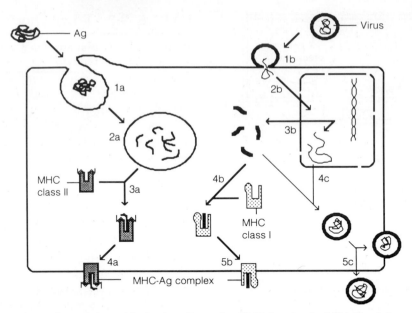

FIGURE 9.2 Antigen processing and association with class I or II MHC antigens. Either of two pathways can be followed, depending upon the nature of the Ag. Extracellular Ags are ingested (*1a*), processed (*2a*), and integrated with class II MHC molecules intracellularly (*3a*) before being expressed on the cell surface (*4a*). Proteins produced inside the cell (e.g., virus coat proteins) are integrated with class I MHC molecules (*4b*) before being expressed on the cell surface (*5b*). Other stages of viral infection are also depicted: (*1a*) viral infection; (*2a*) incorporation into host genome; (*3a*) virus reproduction; (*4c*) virus assembly; (*5c*) release of new virus. Note that in transformed cells, virus reproduction does not occur, although viral proteins are expressed.

infected cell). This leads to association of antigenic determinants with class I MHC molecules. This association is believed to occur in the endoplasmic reticulum. In either case, the MHC-Ag complex is then translocated to the APC cell surface.

Encountering Immunogen

Class I or class II MHC molecules appear to have a single binding site capable of associating with a wide variety of Ags (through their agretopes). This site exists as a cleft in the MHC molecule. In some instances, for example, with globular proteins, direct access to the agretopes of an Ag is not possible. Ag processing by APCs becomes necessary to provide conformational freedom to form secondary structures that allow exposure of the Ag's epitopes and agretopes. In these cases, it is the binding site on the MHC molecule that dictates a need for Ag processing. In contrast, other Ags apparently can associate directly with MHC molecules. However, these Ags seem to bind to the *surface* of the MHC molecule rather than within the cleft.

These Ags, known as super-Ags, include staphylococcal enterotoxins and minor lymphocyte stimulatory (Mls) gene products.

For most Ags, a composite surface unit is formed in which the self-MHC Ag stabilizes the orientation of the immunogen. This complex is presented to the T cell. TCRs, with appropriate Ag recognition specificity, will bind this composite made up of the epitope of the immunogen and the histotope of the MHC molecule. This forms a ternary complex, which is depicted in figure 9.3.

MHC Restriction

T cell activation is restricted to conditions in which Ag is presented within the context of self-MHC Ags. Ag becomes associated with either class I or class II MHC Ags through the processing mechanisms used by the APCs (see fig. 9.2). This achieves two purposes. First, it enables Ag to be modified to a form suitable for presentation to T cells. In addition, it imposes limits on which subsets of T cells can be activated by particular

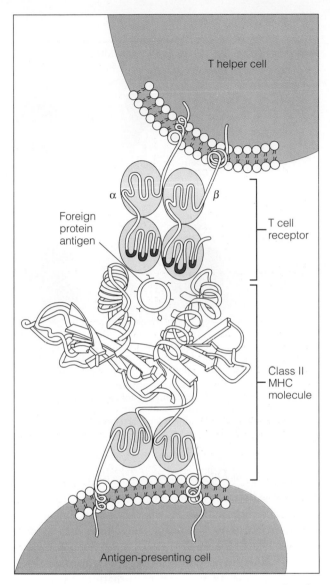

T helper cell

α β

Foreign
protein
antigen

T cell
receptor

Class II
MHC
molecule

Antigen-presenting cell

FIGURE 9.3 Ternary complex. Ag recognition occurs within the context of MHC self-Ags through the formation of a ternary recognition complex. This complex consists of (1) foreign Ag, (2) class II MHC molecule (expressed by an APC), and (3) the T cell receptor (expressed by the T_H cell). (From Sinha, A. A., Lopez, M. T., and McDevitt, H. O. Autoimmune diseases: the failure of self tolerance *Science* 248:1380, 1990. © AAAS. Reprinted by permission.)

classes of Ags. Thus, **MHC restriction** requires that two conditions be satisfied before T cell activation can occur: (1) *foreign Ags must be recognized in association with self-MHC molecules* and (2) *the class of MHC molecule must be recognized* as well.

Generally, T_C and T_S cells recognize the combination of foreign Ag and class I MHC Ags, whereas T_D and T_H cells recognize foreign Ag in association with class II MHC Ags. Two models have been proposed to account for MHC-restricted Ag recognition. The first model was a **dual recognition model.** It suggested that *two binding sites are present on the T cell membrane.* Recent evidence favors an alternative notion, an **altered-self hypothesis.** This postulates that *one receptor recognizes both the Ag and a portion of the MHC molecule,* which has been conformationally altered during the association and binding process. An associative recognition model, which would account for MHC restriction of Ag recognition, involving accessory CD4 or CD8, is depicted in figure 9.4.

According to this model, the nature of the response depends upon two factors, each of which satisfies one of the conditions of MHC restriction identified above. First, *foreign Ag must be associated with an MHC-self Ag,* either class I or class II, *before interaction with the TCR is possible.* This then enables the TCR to recognize the MHC-Ag complex. Second, the *identity of the MHC-self Ag determines the subset of T cell that is affected.* This occurs because of complementary interactions of class I MHC Ags with CD8 differentiation Ags and class II MHC Ags with CD4 differentiation Ags. Accordingly, if a foreign Ag becomes associated with a class I MHC self-Ag on an APC (fig. 9.4a), effective Ag presentation requires interaction both with the foreign Ag (in its MHC Ag) and another class I MHC Ag molecule. In this example, satisfying the dual requirement limits effective interactions to those T cells that carry CD8 differentiation Ags. Because of the nature of this interaction, **CD8$^+$** cells (T_C and T_S cells) **are class I restricted** and **CD4$^+$** cells (T_H and T_D cells) **are class II restricted.**

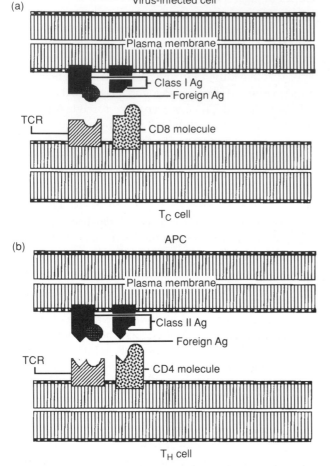

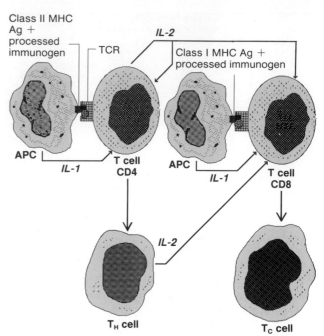

FIGURE 9.5 Influence of cytokines in T cell activation. Activation of T cells requires at least three distinct signals. The first is the immunogen presented by the APC. The other two signals are cytokines that promote proliferation and differentiation of the activated cells. IL-1, released by the APC, is required to initiate proliferation. IL-2, released by T$_H$ cells, promotes continued proliferation and ensures clonal expansion and differentiation of the activated cells.

FIGURE 9.4 Associative recognition model. An altered-self hypothesis postulates that one TCR will recognize *both* the Ag and a portion of the MHC molecule that has been altered conformationally by Ag binding. Accessory CD8 and CD4 molecules enhance binding of class I and class II molecules of the MHC, respectively.

Activation of T Cells

Converting the resting mature T cell into an activated effector of cell-mediated immunity requires several signals (fig. 9.5). Encountering the epitope of the immunogen and histotope of the MHC Ag provides the first activating signal to the T cell. In addition, APCs release interleukin 1 (IL-1), which serves as a second signal for T cell activation. T$_H$ cells responding to these signals proliferate and secrete IL-2. This lymphokine provides a third signal. IL-2 promotes differentiation of both B and T cells. Moreover, it can act in an autocrine manner on the very T$_H$ cells that have produced it.

Proliferation and Differentiation of T Cells

The immediate consequences of antigenic stimulation of T cells that lead to clonal expansion and a cell-mediated immune response do not differ from those observed in stimulating B cells (fig. 9.6; compare with figure 4.9). Binding of the immunogen/MHC-Ag complex to the TCR causes perturbations in the cell membrane. This initiates a series of membrane and cytoplasmic events that lead to proliferation and differentiation. The actions of IL-1 and IL-2 reinforce and augment these responses.

Membrane *transduction* systems are activated (possibly by the associated CD3 complex [see below]) leading to the production of cyclic guanosine monophosphate (cGMP), diacylglycerol (DAG), and inositol triphosphate (ITP). In addition, arachidonic acid metabolism and intracellular free Ca^{2+} levels are increased. The ultimate results are DNA replication and increased transcriptional and translational activity.

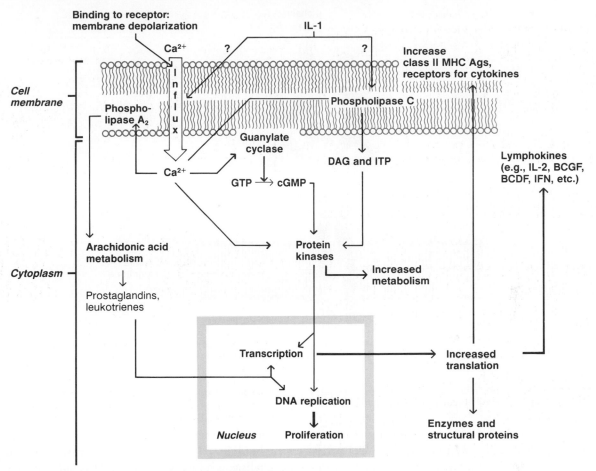

FIGURE 9.6 T cell responses to antigenic activation. Binding of Ag to appropriate TCRs triggers a series of responses. These lead to alterations in membrane function and expression of additional receptors, modifications of intracellular metabolism, and changes in gene expression. These lead to increased responsiveness to extracellular signals, proliferation, and clonal expansion. In addition, selective activities are expressed that are determined by the nature of the T cell activated, for example, cytotoxicity by T_C cells or lymphokine production and secretion by T_H cells.

Clonal expansion follows. In addition, the composition of the cell membrane changes as new surface receptors for cytokines, growth factors, and Ags are expressed. Moreover, the cells assume specific functional roles. For example, T_H cells produce and release lymphokines (e.g., ILs, growth and differentiation factors, and interferons [IFNs]). These provide helper/inducer signals for other T and B cells undergoing Ag-dependent differentiation. In yet other instances, cytotoxicity by T_C cells might be expressed. Other forms of expression are also possible; we explore them presently.

T CELL RECEPTORS FOR ANTIGEN
T Cell Receptor Structure

The TCR is a *disulfide-linked glycoprotein heterodimer.* For MHC-restricted T cell populations (approximately 98% of T cells), TCRs are composed of an acidic α chain of 45 to 55 kD and a more basic β chain of 40 to 50 kD (fig. 9.7). T cells that are not MHC restricted possess TCRs consisting of γ and δ chains (γ rather than α and δ rather than β). These T cells, which are phenotypically CD4$^-$CD8$^-$, represent only 2% of T cells.

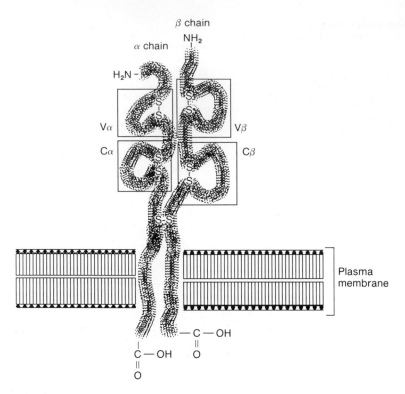

FIGURE 9.7 T cell receptor. The classical TCR is a disulfide-linked glycoprotein dimer consisting of α and β subunits that have identi-fiable internal domains. The receptor has a molecular weight of approximately 90 kD.

TCRs on CD4$^+$ and CD8$^+$ cells are sometimes referred to as $\alpha\beta$ **TCRs,** while those on CD4$^-$CD8$^-$ cells are called $\gamma\delta$ **TCRs.** Since most of our dicussions focus on $\alpha\beta$ TCRs, we will refer to them simply as TCRs and will specifically identify $\gamma\delta$ TCRs (first reported in 1986) whenever they are discussed.

TCRs of both types are noncovalently associated with **CD3,** forming a TCR/CD3 complex (fig. 9.8). CD3 consists of five subunits: δ, γ, ϵ, ζ, and η subunits (MW of 26, 21, 25, 16, and 22 kD, respectively). (Although similar nomenclature is used, note that the δ and γ chains of CD3 are different from the δ and γ chains of $\gamma\delta$ TCRs.) Two variants of CD3 are recognized. CD3 in the majority of T cells (80% of cells with $\alpha\beta$ TCRs) has a subunit composition of δ, γ, ϵ, ζ, and ζ (ζ-ζCD3). CD3s found in the remaining 20% of T cells display a subunit composition of δ, γ, ϵ, ζ, and η (ζ-ηCD3).

The intimate association between the TCR and CD3 is believed to lead to activation of intracel-lular signal transduction pathways by CD3 following Ag binding to the TCR's Ag-recognition site. Positive signaling, leading to T cell activation, occurs when TCRs are complexed to ζ-ζCD3s. In contrast, ζ-ηCD3s appear to be involved in negative signaling, that is, T cell activation does not occur following Ag binding. The significance of coupling TCRs to positive and negative transduction regulators is unclear; nevertheless, possible involvement in tolerance induction (see chapter 10) and programmed cell death have been suggested.

Recognition of foreign Ag leading to T cell activation involves three distinct molecules: TCRs, CD3, and either CD4 or CD8. Mature T cells express *Ag-specific TCRs,* which vary in primary structure. This variability in amino acid sequence is an integral part of the TCR's ability to discriminate among diverse foreign Ags. The amino acid sequence of *CD3 molecules,* however, seems to be identical, regardless of TCR specificity. CD3 molecules do not recognize Ags.

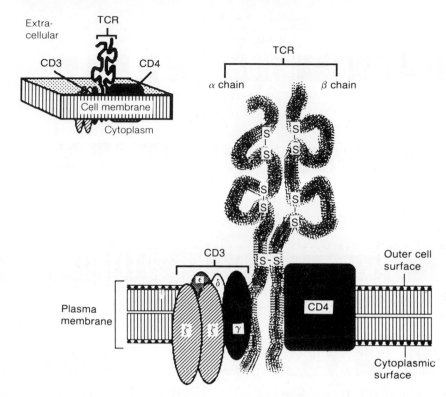

FIGURE 9.8 T cell Ag recognition complex. The T cell Ag recognition complex is composed of the TCR, CD3, and CD4 (or CD8). Depicted here is the complex as it might appear in a mature T_H cell. The TCR consists of α and β chains. It is associated with a CD4 Ag and also with the ζ-ζ form of CD3. Note that the β chain of the TCR is associated with CD4 while the α chain is associated with the γ subunit of CD3. (Adapted from Schwartz, R. H. A cell culture model for T lymphocyte clonal anergy. *Science* **248**:1348, 1990.)

However, they may be responsible for receptor conformation or transduction of the activation signal into the cell. This is suggested by the different effects of the two types of CD3s encountered in T cells. *Accessory CD4 or CD8 molecules* are also required for initial T cell activation (see fig. 9.4), which can be blocked by monoclonal antibodies (MAbs) specific for these differentiation Ags. Since CD8 and CD4 molecules do not undergo DNA rearrangments, they may serve as receptors for the constant region of class I or II MHC Ags, respectively. This question, however, has not been resolved. The apparent conservatism in amino acid sequences of CD3, CD4, and CD8 molecules reflects their association with molecules that are themselves conserved and widely expressed.

In addition to TCRs, T cells possess **CD2/E (erythrocyte) receptors** that bind to sheep red blood cells. The role of CD2 Ags in T cell function and homeostasis is not clear, although involvement in T cell MHC-unrestricted activation (not Ag specific) has been reported. Triggering of CD2 receptors (for example with MAb) has induced some cells with inherent lytic activity to express selective, but not Ag-specific, cytotoxic activity.

Generation of T Cell Receptor Diversity

Several TCR genes have been cloned and sequenced. They were found to be **members of the Ig superfamily** and thus phylogenetically related to Ig and MHC genes. The gene arrangement encoding the α, β, γ, and δ chains of the two TCRs is very similar to that of Igs, and the same nomenclature is used. Chains possess an amino-terminal variable (V) domain and a carboxy-terminal constant (C) domain. Rearrangement of DNA during Ag-independent differentiation of T cells, from their origin in the bone marrow to

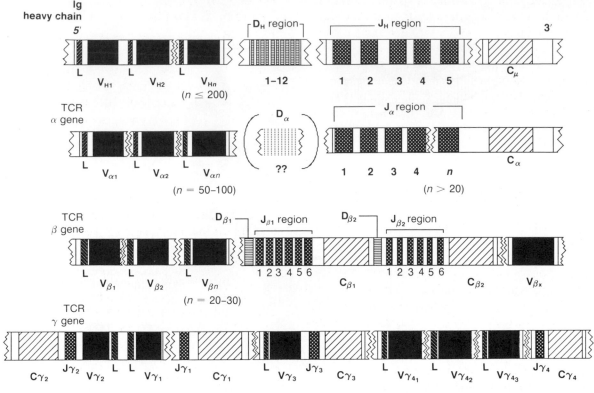

FIGURE 9.9 TCR gene organization. Subunits of the TCR are produced through assembly of gene segments in a manner that resembles the production of Igs. The organization of these gene segments bears striking parallels to the gene segment organization for Igs (as depicted by the diagram of the Ig heavy chain gene). The two primary TCR gene families, α and β, are organized similarly, and the nomenclature used for the Ig genes has been adopted. In addition, a less universally encountered member of the TCR family exists (TCR, γ gene). The organization of the segments of this gene differs somewhat from the α and β genes.

maturity in the thymus, may be analogous to Ig genes. A comparison between Ig heavy (H) chain and TCR α, β, and γ genes is provided in figure 9.9. The α gene family may consist of perhaps 50 to 100 variable (V) gene segments, 20 joining (J) segments, and a single constant (C) gene. Human α genes are located on chromosome 14, as are Ig H chain genes. There may be 20 to 30 V gene segments in the β chain gene family, upstream of two clusters consisting of one D segment and six J segments followed by a single C segment. The γ and δ gene families appear to be composed of several subfamilies, each with V, J, and C gene segments. The four TCR gene families are organized similarly to Ig light (L) and H gene chain gene families. However, the number of J gene segments encoding the αβ TCR appear to be larger than those for the Ig genes

(12 J_β and over 20 J_α). (See chapter 5 for further discussion of Ab structure and Ab gene rearrangments.)

Mechanisms for the generation of TCR diversity may be similar to those responsible for B cell receptor diversity (chapter 5). Accordingly, multiple gene segments may be transmitted in germline DNA, which are somatically rearranged during differentiation in the thymus. As with combinatorial joining of Ig gene segments, junctional site variation occurs. Further diversity is derived from the random combination of α and β chains, similar to Ig H and L chain associations. However, somatic mutation does not appear to play a significant role. Each member, or clone, comprising the repertoire of diverse T cells so generated expresses only one kind of Ag receptor, forming a unique binding site or idiotype. The idiotype is a collection of antigenic determinants or idiotopes associated with the V regions of the α and β chains (analogous to Ig idiotypes). As a result, a single T cell (or clone) is not pluripotent with respect to Ag binding. Despite the potential for recombination during V-J joining, $\gamma\delta$ TCRs appear to be very similar among all cells expressing them. Consequently, $\gamma\delta$ TCRs are less diverse than $\alpha\beta$ TCRs. As a result, it has been suggested that $\gamma\delta$ TCRs might respond to only the more common antigenic determinants in contrast to $\alpha\beta$ TCRs, which respond to unique determinants.

CYTOTOXIC T LYMPHOCYTES

T_C cells display Ag specificity and are usually detectable in the body only after they multiply following exposure to Ag. If, for example, lymphocytes are cultured with cells displaying foreign Ags, some of the lymphocytes (Ag-specific T_C cells) will reproduce and become capable of lysing cells bearing foreign determinants. They become cytotoxic to stimulator cells that carry nonself surface Ags. Stimulator cells include virally infected cells, malignant cells, histoincompatible cells, or any self-cell that may have an altered membrane or carry a membrane-attached new Ag.

MHC-Restricted Cytotoxic T Lymphocytes

Extensive studies suggest that recognition of Ag by most T_C cell populations is MHC restricted (chapter 7, Histocompatibility Systems). Most of these are restricted to class I molecules and express CD8 differentiation Ags (see fig. 9.4a). However, a subset appears to exhibit class II restriction and is CD4$^+$, characteristic of T_H cells (fig. 9.4b). Both sets recognize Ag by means of TCRs ($\alpha\beta$ TCR/CD3 complex).

Non-MHC-Restricted Cytotoxic T Lymphocytes

As noted above, some unique populations of T cells may not be MHC restricted. These were first recognized by their ability to lyse a broad spectrum of tumor cell targets, bearing different MHC Ags. A tumor Ag was recognized by clone-specific cytotoxic cells through TCRs ($\gamma\delta$ TCR); however, association with a self-Ag of the MHC was not required for lysis. These non-MHC-restricted cells are CD4$^-$ and CD8$^-$.

Mechanism of Lysis by Cytotoxic T Lymphocytes

The immune response to foreign Ags, displayed on a stimulator (or target) cell, is characterized by the generation of T cells that are cytotoxic to that target cell (i.e., T_C cells). Development of T_C cells may require assistance from T_H cells (CD4$^+$) that recognize both the Ag and class II MHC molecules on the stimulator cells. Development of T_C cells that is assisted in this fashion proceeds in two steps, as depicted in figure 9.10. During the first stage of the response, T_H cells are activated; they proliferate, and then produce IL-2 and possibly other soluble factors that promote the generation of T_C cells. In the second stage, T_C cells (CD8$^+$) respond to the foreign Ag and class I MHC Ags on the stimulator cells, which is enhanced by the soluble factors derived from T_H cells.

Alternatively, a distinct subset of T lymphocytes, designated $T\gamma$, may become cytotoxic following conferral of Ag specificity by Abs. These $T\gamma$ cells possess $\gamma\delta$ TCR/CD3 and Fc receptors (FcRs). Thus, they can mediate Ab-dependent cellular cytotoxicity (ADCC, fig. 9.11) as well as Ag-specific cytotoxicity mediated by $\gamma\delta$ TCRs.

The Lytic Process

The cytotoxic response of T_C cells to target cells is accomplished through three consecutive stages: (1) specific binding to membrane receptors (TCR/CD3 or FcR) of the T_C cell, (2) rearrangements of cytoplasmic granules with the subsequent release of cytolysins, and (3) calcium-dependent lysis of the target cell. Subsequently, the T_C cells can detach from the target cell and repeat this process with another. The events of the lytic process are the same as those already described for NK cells (see chapter 8).

DELAYED-TYPE HYPERSENSITIVITY LYMPHOCYTES

The generation of T_D cells provides a second Ag-specific cell-mediated mechanism of resistance to infection, fundamentally distinct from direct cytolysis by

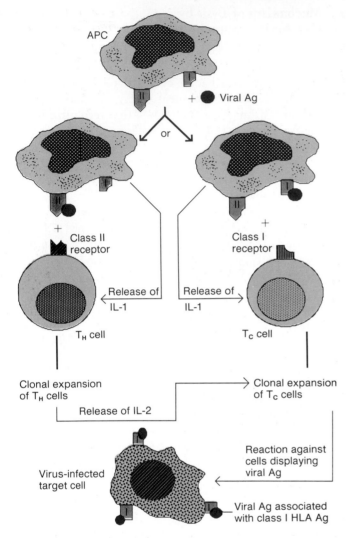

FIGURE 9.10 Development of T_C cells. In the first stage of T_C cell development, T_H cells are activated. They then proliferate and produce IL-2 (*left panel*). During the second stage, T_C cells respond to foreign Ag and class I MHC molecules. This is enhanced by T_H cell products, for example, IL-2 (*right panel*).

T_C cells. (The possible pathological consequences of DTH and T cell measurements are discussed in chapter 13, Hypersensitivity). T_D cells are intimately involved in host defense against viruses, bacteria, fungi, protozoa, and other infectious agents that may replicate intracellularly. DTH responses may also occur whenever the body encounters histoincompatible cells, or self-cells, which have been altered or transformed so

that they are no longer recognized as self. T_D cells are capable of recruiting leukocytes from various parts of the body to an active engagement site that they have recognized as nonself, and "putting them to work" defending the host.

The relative ability of T_D cells to protect the body is due principally to their capacity to produce and release lymphokines. These released products can recruit, activate, and regulate nonspecific effector cells, potentially capable of combating infectious agents. T cells (CD4+) that are active in DTH reactions are quite different from T_C cells (CD8+) involved in lytic reactions. They are not specific killer cells. Rather, they recruit potential killers, such as $M\phi$s, and control their activity.

Delayed-Type Hypersensitivity

The immune response to proteins of the "tubercle" bacillus, observed by Robert Koch in 1880, has served as a general model for DTH. Koch observed that filtrates, taken from cultures of microorganisms that cause tuberculosis, elicited a delayed-type inflammatory reaction in tubercular animals. In addition, he showed that purified Ag (tuberculin), when injected into the skin of a sensitized or immune individual, produced gradual reddening (erythema) and swelling. The reaction reached a peak within 24 to 72 hours. The response was characterized by the accumulation of inflammatory cells localized about the smallest veins. The invasive inflammatory cells found were lymphocytes, monocytes, $M\phi$s, and basophils. The time required for induction of DTH was approximately the same as for induction of Abs after exposure to Ag (a few days). Abs, however, were excluded from a role in the DTH reaction. Attempts to transfer DTH with serum from sensitized individuals regularly met with failure.

We have since discovered that the lymphocytes primarily responsible for DTH are T cells expressing CD4 differentiation Ags. Although these cells are designated T_D cells, they may be identical to one type of helper T_H cell (Type I) and thus capable of mediating both helper activity and DTH reactions. $M\phi$s (or dendritic cells) are also required for the DTH reaction. $M\phi$s present specific foreign Ag to the T_D cell in association with class II molecules of the MHC. In

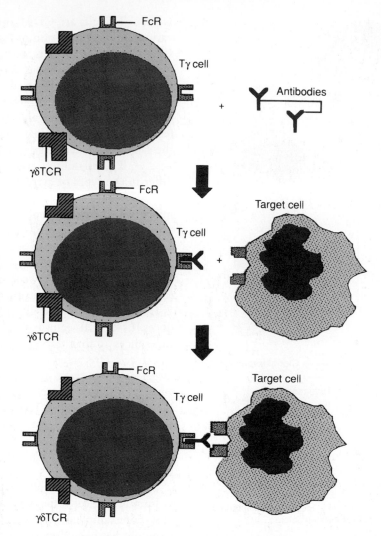

FIGURE 9.11 Conferral of Ag specificity to Tγ cells, leading to ADCC. A distinct, small subset of T lymphocytes, designated Tγ, can become cytotoxic following conferral of Ag specificity. Although lacking receptors for Ag, they can bind antibodies (cytophilic) to their FcRs. These Tγ cells can now display Ag specificity for target cell Ag that is associated with the specificity of the bound antibody. Subsequently, Tγ cells will lyse the target cells to which they bind. These cells can also exhibit TCR-directed lytic activity, as well as ADCC.

addition, they release IL-1, which promotes development of T_D cells. Ag-activated T_H cells, displaying class II MHC restriction, may also contribute to T_D cell generation. This is accomplished through the release of several lymphokines, including IL-2 (fig. 9.12).

Specific reactions with Ag cause T_D clones to release lymphokines. These may modify the immune response so that host resistance to infection is enhanced. A Mφ chemotactic factor (MCF), for example, can attract Mφs and monocytes to the area where the T_D cells have encountered Ag. A migration- inhibiting factor (MIF) may then help to keep the recruited cells in the area. At this point, a Mφ-activating factor (MAF) may be released to activate local Mφs and monocytes. In response to MAF, these cells undergo physiological changes through which their phagocytic, pinocytic, and killing capabilities are enhanced. Therefore, through the production and release of lymphokines,

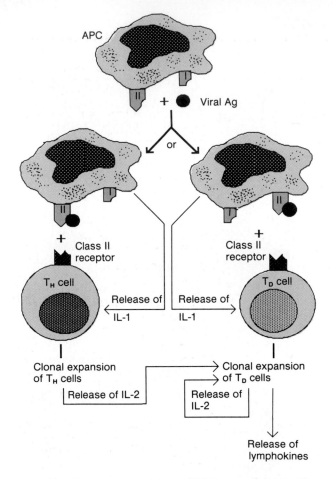

FIGURE 9.12 Generation of MHC-restricted T_D cells. Ag-activated T_H cells, displaying class II MHC restriction, contribute to T_D cell proliferation by releasing IL-2. T_D cells response to foreign Ag is also MHC restricted, by class II MHC molecules.

T_D cells can mount a rather formidable defense against invasive cells recognized as nonself.

HELPER T LYMPHOCYTES

Certain other T lymphocytes are not directly cytotoxic; however, they can profoundly affect the cytotoxic activity of other cells. These are known as helper (T_H), inducer (T_I), or helper/inducer ($T_{H/I}$) cells. As the name suggests, $T_{H/I}$ cells play primary roles in inducing or helping other cells express their functional potential.

T_H cells are CD4$^+$ and, therefore, their activation upon presentation of Ag by APCs is MHC restricted (class II). This activation, and the clonal expansion that follows, is Ag specific. Upon activation, these cells are induced to produce and secrete bioactive substances (cytokines) that potentiate proliferation, differentiation, and expression of specific effector cells that have also been specifically activated by the same (or related) Ags.

T_H cell subsets are presumed to exist. These differ in the types of cytokines that they produce and the target cells on which they act (see table 9.3). In mice, two distinct subsets have been identified. However, in humans clear discrimination of T_H cells into definable subsets has yet to be achieved. Murine T_H cells are designated T_{H1} and T_{H2}. Both produce IL-3 and granulocyte-monocyte–colony-stimulating factor (GM-CSF). They differ in that T_{H1} also produces IL-2, IFN-γ, and lymphotoxin (LTX), whereas T_{H2} produces IL-4 and IL-5 instead. The consequence of these differences is that different populations of activated target cells are acted upon (or helped). Among the target cells for these cytokines are hemopoietic precursors (GM-CSF), activated B cells (IL-2, IL-4, IL-5, IFN-γ, LTX), activated T_C cells (IL-2, IL-4, IL-5, IFN-γ,), lymphokine-activated killer (LAK) cells (IL-2, IFN-γ, LTX), Mϕs (IL-2, IL-4, IFN-γ, LTX), granulocytes (IL-4, IL-5, IFN-γ,) and fibroblasts (IFN-γ, LTX).

Certain of the effects of T_H cell participation in immunological responses have already been examined. For example, their influence on humoral immune responses has been discussed in chapter 5. In addition, T_H cell effects on nonspecific cell-mediated immune responses have been discussed in chapter 8, while influences on specific cell-mediated responses have been outlined above.

SUPPRESSOR T LYMPHOCYTES

In addition to T cells that exert positive influence on the expression of immune responses, there are other subpopulations of T cells that have a negative affect on immune expression. These populations are known as

TABLE 9.3 Selected Cytokines and Their Functions

Cytokine	Synonyms	Sources	Representative Functions
Interleukins			
IL-1	Lymphocyte-activating factor Mitogenic protein Helper peak-1	Mϕs, monocytes	Promotes differentiation and expression of both B and T lymphocytes; promotes growth and expression of many cell types (e.g., NK cells, osteoclasts, fibroblasts)
IL-2	T cell growth factor	T$_{H1}$ cells, LGLs	Stimulates T-cell growth; costimulates differentiation of B-cells; stimulates LAK expression
IL-3	Mast cell growth factor	T$_{H1}$, T$_{H2}$ cells	Stimulates growth of mast cells; stimulates growth of multipotential hemopoietic cells
IL-4	B cell stimulatory factor 1 B cell growth factor T cell growth factor 2 Mast cell growth factor 2 IgE/IgG1-enhancing factor	T$_{H2}$ cells	Costimulates proliferation of B cells; limited stimulation of T-cell growth; acts synergistically with IL-3 on mast cells; stimulates Ia expression on B cells and Mϕs, costimulates proliferation of hemopoietic progenitor cells
Il-5	T cell replacing factor B cell growth factor II IgA-enhancing factor Eosinophil differentiation factor	T$_{H2}$, T$_D$ cells	Stimulates Ab response *in vitro*; costimulates B-cell growth; enhances IgA production by activated B-cells; enhances eosinophil differentiation
IL-6	IFN-β2 B cell–stimulating factor 2 Hepatocyte-stimulating factor	Mϕs, monocytes	Stimulates growth and differentiation of B cells; promotes Ab production; stimulates production of acute-phase proteins by liver
IL-7	Pre-B cell growth factor Thymocyte growth factor	Bone marrow stromal cells	Stimulates B and T cell proliferation
IL-8	Neutrophil-activating protein Neutrophil chemotactic factor T cell chemotactic factor	Mononuclear cells, endothelial cells, skin fibroblasts	Stimulates chemotaxis of neutrophils and T cells
IL-9	T cell growth factor III T cell growth factor P-40 Mast cell growth–enhancing activity	Activated T cells	Stimulates proliferation of some IL-3 dependent myeloid cells; stimulates proliferation of BFU-Es; stimulates proliferation of mast cells and functional expression by mast cells
IL-10	Cytokine synthesis inhibitory factor	T$_{H2}$ cells	Inhibits production of IFN-γ and other cytokines by T$_{H1}$ cells

TABLE 9.3 *Continued*

Cytokine	Synonyms	Sources	Representative Functions
Interferons			
IFN-α	Leukocyte-derived IFN, Type I IFN	Leukocytes	Inhibits viral replication
IFN-β	Fibroblast-derived IFN, Type I IFN	Fibroblasts, epithelial cells, Mϕs	Inhibits viral replication; inhibits proliferation of other cell types
IFN-γ	Type II IFN, immune IFN	T_{H1}, T_D cells, NK cells	Inhibits replication of viruses; inhibits IL-4 effects on B cells; induces Mϕ Ia expression
Other Cytokines			
TNF	TNF-α, cachectin	Mϕs, T and B cells, LGLs	Acts as a cytotoxin for tumor cells; activates granulocytes; stimulates fibroblasts; induces acute-phase proteins; has antiviral/antiparasite activity
LTX	TNF-β	T_H/T_D cells	Acts as a cytotoxin for tumor cells; stimulates B cell proliferation; shares most functions of TNF-α
GM-CSF	–	T_H/T_D cells	Stimulates growth of mixed colonies of granulocytes and Mϕs derived from bone marrow progenitor cells

BFU-E, burst-forming unit–erythroid; GM-CSF, granulocyte-monocyte–colony-stimulating factor, Ia, mouse immune response gene antigen; LAK, lymphokine-activated killer cell; LGL, large granular lymphocyte; LTX, lymphotoxin; NK, natural killer; TNF, tumor necrosis factor.

Sources: Mosmann, T. R., and Coffman, R. L. *Immunology Today*. **8**:223, 1987; Marx, J. L. *Science* **239**:25, 1988; Kelso, A. *Current Opinions in Immunology* **2**:215, 1989; Jacob, C. O. *Current Opinions in Immunology* **2**:249, 1989; Moore, K. W., Vieira, P., Fiorentino, D. F., et al. *Science* **248**:1230 (1990).

T_S cells and are phenotypically CD8$^+$. T_S cells are activated in an Ag-specific manner that is MHC restricted (class I). Just as activated T_H cells exert their influence through **positive immune response modifiers** called *lymphokines,* activated T_S cells exert their influence through **negative immune response modifiers** designated as *T suppressor factors (TSFs)*. The effect of these TSFs is *induction of specific immune suppression.* This means that suppression is induced in response to particular Ags and is focused on blocking immune responses against Ags presented at the same time. This is in contrast to immune tolerance, which represents a persistent state of immunological nonresponsiveness to particular Ags (see chapter 10).

Three T_S cell subsets can be functionally discriminated: T_{S1} cells block activation of T_H and B cells. Consequently, they mediate Ag-specific suppression of cell-mediated and humoral immune responses. T_{S2} cells produce idiotype-specific suppression of humoral immune responses. This is achieved by suppressing only B cells that are activated by the same Ag that activated the T_{S2} cells. T_{S3} cells inactivate T_D cells, thereby interfering with Ag-specific DTH responses.

The role of T_S cells in humoral immune responses has been outlined in chapter 5. Mechanisms of immunological suppression and immune tolerance is explored in greater detail in the following chapter.

CYTOKINES AS IMMUNE RESPONSE MODIFIERS

There are numerous **cytokines.** They are *biologically active substances released by specific cells that elicit particular responses from other cells upon which they act.* The major cytokines are glycoproteins produced by lymphocytes (lymphokines) and Mφs (monokines), which are instrumental in orchestrating cellular activities during humoral and cell-mediated (nonspecific and specific) immune responses.

The cytokines modulating humoral immune responses, inflammatory reactions, and certain cell-mediated immune responses are well-studied. However, those participating in the DTH reaction are not as well-characterized. In the DTH reaction, specific clones of T_D cells produce lymphokines following activation with Ags. On the other hand, T cell mitogens, such as phytohemagglutinin (PHA) and concanavalin A (Con A), stimulate clones of T_D cells of any specificity to replicate and produce lymphokines. PHA (derived from the red kidney bean) and Con A (derived from the Jack bean) are lectins that bind to certain sugar residues of T cell membrane glycoproteins.

There is evidence that many cytokines are pleiotropic, that is, they can have *multiple effects on the same or different cell types.* T cell hybridomas, derived from the fusion of T cells with lymphoma cells, are being used extensively to study lymphokine production by T cells. Several have been cloned and are being produced in commercial laboratories employing recombinant DNA techniques. These commercial undertakings have clinical applications as their objectives. Cytokines that appear especially prominent as modulators of the immune response include the ILs and IFNs.

During other forms of cell-mediated immune responses, lymphokines are also produced. These are generated not only by T_D and T_H lymphocytes (CD4+), but by T_C and T_S cell subsets (CD8+) as well. In addition, B cells produce lymphokines during humoral responses. In fact, all cells involved in immune responses might, under appropriate conditions, secrete cytokines. In general, cytokines released during immune responses *regulate the growth, mobility, and differentiation of lymphocytes.* They might exert similar influence over other leukocytes and even nonwhite blood cells. In many instances, their functions are overlapping. They qualify as hormones by the broadest definition. Cytokines modify the immune response by providing signals, often in conjunction with Ags, to maximize host-defense mechanisms. As such they have captured research interest relative to their nature and

possible employment to enhance host resistance to infectious agents and tumors.

This section considers three of the most studied of the immune response modifiers: IL-1, IL-2, and IFNs. These and other important cytokines are listed in table 9.3 along with several synonyms and functions. You should note that many of the synonyms reflect functions ascribed to the particular cytokine. This often relates to characterization of a functional property of the cytokine before isolation and chemical identification has been achieved. This table does not include all known cytokines.

Interleukin 1

Source of Interleukin 1

When Mφs and monocytes are appropriately stimulated, they secrete increasing amounts of a regulatory glycoprotein, known as IL-1. A number of other nucleated cells of the body may also be capable of producing low levels of IL-1. These include dendritic cells, Langerhans' cells, endothelial cells, epithelial cells, neutrophils, B lymphocytes, and large granular lymphocytes (LGLs). Mφs can be stimulated to produce IL-1 by MHC-restricted contact with activated lymphocytes (as seen in the cytotoxic and DTH reactions). However, all cell types capable of producing IL-1 can be stimulated by a variety of T and B lymphokines, mitogens, and adjuvants, as well as by latex or silica particles.

Function of Interleukin 1

IL-1 may exist in two distinct, low molecular weight (about 15 to 18 kD) protein forms. Both forms (IL-1α and IL-1β) have been cloned (human and murine). In either form, IL-1 promotes lymphocyte differentiation and stimulates T cell functions. This includes increasing T cell production of lymphokines: IL-2, IL-3, IL-4, IL-5, IFN-γ, and chemotactic factors. During cytotoxic and DTH responses, IL-1 promotes both proliferation and differentiation responses of T_C or T_D lymphocytes. T cell activation requires not only contact with the MHC-Ag complex (on the APC), but IL-1 as well. IL-1 also promotes the production of IL-2

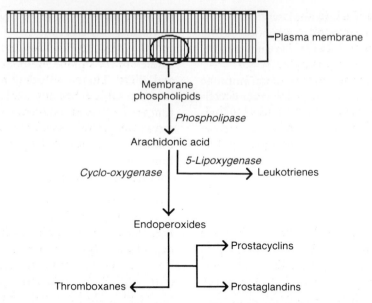

Membrane
phospholipids

Phospholipase

Arachidonic acid

Cyclo-oxygenase   *5-Lipoxygenase* ──→ Leukotrienes

Endoperoxides

──→ Prostacyclins

Thromboxanes ←──   ──→ Prostaglandins

FIGURE 9.13 Formation of leukotrienes and prostaglandins from arachidonic acid. IL-1 induces metabolism of arachidonic acid from membrane phospholipids. In turn, arachidonic acid can be metabolized into several products with potent vasoactive properties. For example, leukotrienes or prostacyclins (potent vasodilators) can be produced. Prostacyclins can be further metabolized to prostaglandins (aliphatic acids that regulate inflammatory reactions, increase vascular permeability, and stimulate smooth muscle) or thromboxanes (promote platelet aggregation, cell-to-cell interactions, and mitogenesis).

by T_H cells, and the expression of IL-2 receptors (IL-2Rs). Thus, T_H cells may serve as an IL-1 target and, later, as both an IL-2 target and producer. Moreover, this monokine promotes proliferation, differentiation, and the Ab-producing functions of B cells and expression of their membrane Ig receptors.

It has become increasingly evident that IL-1 promotes the growth and activity of a variety of cell types. In fact, this influence extends beyond lymphocytes. Monocytes/Mϕs and neutrophils, for example, are chemotactically mobilized and activated by IL-1. NK cells, liver cells, neurons, muscle cells, osteoclasts, osteoblasts, epithelial cells, endothelial cells, synovial cells, and fibroblasts may all be stimulated by IL-1 during inflammatory responses. During an inflammatory response, IL-1 can act as an endogenous pyrogen responsible for fever production. It can bring about changes in plasma levels of metals and acute-phase proteins. IL-1 can also produce an influx of leukocytes to the inflammatory site. Recent evidence suggests that certain of these effects ascribed to IL-1 might actually be produced by IL-6 (formerly known as IFN-β2).

Among the specific actions of IL-1 on cells expressing IL-1 receptors is an increase in arachidonic acid metabolism. Arachidonic acid is an unsaturated fatty acid derived from phospholipids in cell membranes. Leukotrienes and prostaglandins (PGs) are important inflammatory metabolites that are formed from arachidonic acid (fig. 9.13). These products share responsibility, with other mediators (e.g., bradykinin and histamine), for manifestations of the inflammatory response (see chapter 8).

It has become clear that IL-1 can increase activity of many cell types that are directly, or indirectly, involved in homeostatic mechanisms, and inflammation in particular. Unfortunately IL-1 can also contribute to the immunopathological conditions associated with certain autoimmune diseases, such as rheumatoid arthritis (RA). RA is characterized by active inflammation of the synovial lining of involved joints, by marked destruction of collagen, and by bone resorption. IL-1 has been found in the synovial joints of individuals afflicted with RA. It may activate synovial cells causing them to produce collagenase, with subsequent collagen destruction. It also might promote bone resorption by activating osteoclasts. Only a few substances are known to inhibit IL-1 production, at pharmacological doses. For example, steroid hormones and certain immunosuppressive drugs (e.g., cyclosporine) are inhibitory. In addition, certain antiinflammatory agents neutralize the effects of IL-1, for example aspirin, indomethacin, and ibuprofen inhibit cyclo-oxygenase, an enzyme leading to the formation of PGs.

Interleukin 2
Source of Interleukin 2

This lymphokine has been isolated and its gene has been cloned. IL-2 activity appears confined to a single protein. Human T_H cells, bearing the CD4 phenotype, produce, secrete, and respond to IL-2. Other T cell subsets and certain LGL subsets may produce IL-2 when stimulated with mitogens. Resting T cells do not produce IL-2. However, when these cells are activated, IL-2 production begins within minutes and is detectable, extracellularly, several hours later. IL-1 and a variety of neurohormones, and surface-active compounds, can enhance IL-2 production. Very low levels of IL-2 may be produced in several diseases where T cell activity is depressed. Among these disease states are lupus erythematosus, certain cancers, acquired immune deficiency syndrome (AIDS), and primary immune deficiency diseases. T_S cells and some immunosuppressive agents, such as steroid hormones, cyclosporine and PGs, can inhibit IL-2 production.

Interleukin 2 Molecules and Receptors

IL-2 is a single glycoprotein with a molecular weight of 15 kD, which is encoded by a single gene. The gene has been cloned, and recombinant IL-2 is produced by several commercial laboratories. The protein binds to specific receptors on activated T and B lymphocytes and LGLs. IL-2 is not species specific, and thus any cell with IL-2Rs may be stimulated.

All subsets of peripheral T lymphocytes, B lymphocytes, Mϕs, and LGLs can develop IL-2Rs and respond to IL-2. Studies using MAbs against Tac, which is specific for IL-2Rs, have shown that resting lymphocytes do not express IL-2Rs on their membranes.

However, they acquire both high- and low-affinity membrane receptors for IL-2 several hours following activation by Ag and IL-2 (see highlight 9.1). Moreover, these receptors can be expressed for perhaps 10 days. Furthermore, cells can be reactivated and IL-2Rs expressed again. Receptors from cells activated in this manner have been isolated. These receptors are glycoproteins (MW 55 kD) that are encoded by a single gene. These genes, also, have been cloned.

Function of Interleukin 2

Basically, IL-2 stimulates the growth and clonal expansion of specific T cells, and promotes their cellular functions. In this regard, IL-2 promotes the production of other lymphokines, such as IFN-γ, additional ILs, colony-stimulating factor, and LTX by T_H/T_D cells. It promotes enhanced cytotoxicity by T_C cells. In addition, IL-2 has been shown to stimulate clonal expansion of B cells and increased Ab formation. IL-2 can induce Mϕs to become more cytotoxic.

Evidently, triggering of IL-2Rs leads to cell division and gene expression. IL-2 binding to its receptor activates an enzyme within the cell, protein kinase C. Activated protein kinase C becomes mobilized and moves to the cell membrane. Here it phosphorylates the IL-2R, permitting the IL-2/receptor complex to be internalized. In turn, this leads to gene expression and DNA replication. However, the manner in which the internalized complex participates in intracellular signaling is not clear.

Practical or Potential Use of Recombinant Interleukin 2

IL-2 has been used as an immune response modifier in humans in attempts to correct immune deficiencies and inhibit cancer growth and metastasis. Certain cell-mediated immune deficiencies, where there is hypo production of IL-2, may be ameliorated by the addition of IL-2. However, administration of tolerable doses of IL-2 to individuals with AIDS has had no detectable beneficial effects. On the other hand, IL-2 has displayed some promising effects in inhibiting tumor growth and metastasis. Since many toxic effects were noted among individuals receiving high doses of IL-2, an alternative therapeutic approach was developed. Rosenberg and co-workers used recombinant IL-2 to

IL-2 Receptors and Expression of Cytotoxicity

Activated lymphocytes display IL-2 receptors that are detectable with monoclonal antibody against Tac Ag. Nevertheless, unstimulated lymphocytes, which do not respond to anti-Tac antibody, can respond to IL-2. Recent studies have provided an answer to this apparent enigma and, in the process, have provided additional insight into the role of IL-2 receptors in mediating activation of cytotoxic lymphocyte populations.

Activated lymphocytes possess two categories of IL-2 receptors, detectable by the anti-Tac antibody, that differ in their affinity for IL-2. One receptor has a high affinity for IL-2 (K_d = 10 pM), while the other has a low affinity (K_d = 10 nM). Both contain a 55 kD membrane glycoprotein, IL-2Rα. Both receptors apparently are absent from unactivated lymphocytes. However, Michael Sharon's laboratory reported the existence of another membrane glycoprotein that could bind IL-2 (IL-2Rβ) but that was not detectable by anti-Tac antibody. This 70 kD molecule is believed to associate with IL-2Rα to produce the high-affinity IL-2 receptor of activated cells. Moreover, IL-2Rβ was able to bind and internalize IL-2.

Siegel and associates expanded on these findings and have suggested a role for this IL-2 receptor molecule. They isolated NK cells from a population of LGLs. Exposing these cells to IL-2 (1 nM) produced a five- to 20-fold increase in proliferative rate and a three- to five-fold increase in lymphokine-activated killing. After separation of cells that bound anti-Tac antibody, the remaining cells still displayed 100% of the stimulated lymphokine-activated killer (LAK) activity and over 60% of the stimulated proliferation. These cells expressed IL-2Rβ but *no* IL-2Rα.

Characterization of functional properties of IL-2Rβ revealed half-maximal stimulation of LAK activity and proliferation by the isolated LGLs in the 0.1 to 1.0 nM range of IL-2 concentrations. In addition, they found that anti-Tac antibodies had no effect on early stimulation but blocked late (over 16 hours) effects of IL-2 stimulation. This indicates a dependence upon IL-2Rα for later expression. Moreover, increasing IL-2 concentrations were more effective in augmenting responses during the early stages than in later stages. This shows a change in receptor affinity for IL-2 (low to high) with time after stimulation.

From these results, IL-2Rβ seems to be a low-affinity receptor that mediates early events to IL-2 exposure. These events include

1. increased NK activity,
2. increased proliferation,
3. increased LAK activity, and
4. induction of high-affinity IL-2 receptors (IL-2Rα).

The significance of IL-2Rβ to lymphocyte activation, and expression of cellular cytotoxicity, remains unclear. Nevertheless, Siegel et al. offer the following suggestions. On the one hand, IL-2Rβ, expressed on LGLs, might provide a means of recruiting cytotoxic cells that are not Ag-specific, at sites of Ag-specific immune responses. On the other, IL-2Rβ on resting T lymphocytes could serve as a means of rapidly expressing high-affinity IL-2 receptors (IL-2Rα) after Ag-specific induction, while limiting their nonspecific recruitment.

Siegel, J. P., Sharon, M., Smith, P. L., et al. The IL-2 receptor β chain; role in mediating signals for LAK, NK, and proliferative activities. *Science* **238**:75, 1987.

activate fresh lymphoid cells, taken from cancer patients, which were then infused back into the individual. The procedure was first established in a murine system. Lymphocytes (LAK cells) that have been stimulated, *in vitro,* with IL-2, become capable of lysing any modified cell (such as a cancer cell) but not normal cells.

LAK cells have been administered, along with IL-2, in clinical trials to individuals with a variety of tumors. Tumor regression was observed in some cases. All participants in the study had well-advanced cancers that were not responsive to conventional therapeutic measures. Repeated administration of massive numbers of

LAK cells, augmented with maximally tolerated doses of IL-2, appear to be required for success. Although toxicity problems remain to be solved, the use of an immune response modifier to activate autologous lymphocytes appears exciting and promising.

Interferons

Several proteins interfere with viral replication. These proteins, which are produced in response to specific stimuli, are known as IFNs. IFN is produced early in an infection, before Abs and effector T cells are produced. IFN was first described in 1957 by Isaacs and Lindenmann. Since that time, we have learned that there are several IFNs. The different forms of IFN have been purified and their genes have been cloned. Once these proteins were isolated and characterized, their activities were intensely examined. It soon became clear that antigenically distinct IFNs also serve as regulatory peptides, or immune response modifiers, which promote host-defense mechanisms. For example, one type of IFN is principally antiviral, while another is primarily immunoregulatory. Using recombinant DNA technology, IFNs have been produced by several biotechnology companies for use in research and for possible clinical applications.

Types of Interferons

IFN synthesis can be stimulated by infection with viruses, bacteria, or protozoa, and by a variety of chemicals and specific Ags. IFN-α is produced by lymphocytes and other leukocytes that have been stimulated by viruses and infectious agents and by activated NK cells. Nearly a dozen different proteins that exhibit IFN-α activity have been purified. IFN-β, on the other hand, is formed by virus-stimulated fibroblasts, epithelial cells, and Mϕs. IFN-β displays 30% to 35% sequence identity with the IFN-α family, and these families are referred to as Type I IFNs. A second type (Type II), known as IFN-γ, or immune IFN, is produced by Ag- (or mitogen-) activated T cells and by activated NK cells. All IFNs are relatively small proteins, with MW ranging from 20 to 25 kD. Type I IFNs are characteristically less stable than Type II IFNs in acidic environments.

Functions of Interferons

All IFNs inhibit replication of most viruses. It is now known that IFNs can also inhibit the growth of a wide range of cell types, with each type of cell expressing a different sensitivity to the cytokine. Moreover, IFNs can also inhibit or stimulate cell differentiation, depending upon the cell type affected and the concentration of IFN used.

Some of the more interesting activities of IFNs revolve around their role as immune response modifiers. They can act on all cells involved in the body's response to Ag. For example, IFNs (especially IFN-γ) function as MAFs and MIFs (which are not themselves IFNs). Mϕs are considerably more bactericidal and tumoricidal following activation by IFN. Activated Mϕs can synthesize and secrete increased quantities of enzymes that degrade target proteins. IFNs can augment expression of FcRs on Mϕs (and other leukocytes). These cells are then more capable of engulfing immune complexes and of exhibiting ADCC against infectious agents or target cancer cells. IFNs also augment the expression of MHC class II (and class I) molecules on Mϕs, enhancing their ability to present Ag. In addition, IFNs can enhance membrane expression and secretion of IL-I by the APCs.

IFN-γ may enhance the immune response by increasing T_H cell function or decreasing T_S cell function. IFN-γ can also promote increased expression of IL-2Rs on T cells, thereby indirectly promoting T cell proliferation. Moreover, IFNs can stimulate increased expression of class I and II molecules of the MHC on lymphocytes (as noted above for Mϕs) and other APCs. On the other hand, IFNs can suppress both humoral and cell-mediated immunity. Whether IFNs enhance or suppress immunity apparently depends on the concentration of IFN employed, and the time of administration. If, for example, IFN is administered to an experimental animal before Ag is given, the immune response may be considerably lower than normal. However, if IFN is given after primary immunization with the Ag, the response may be greater than normal. It has been suggested that differences in membrane receptor expression, before or after contact with Ag, might account, in part, for the reduced or enhanced T_S cell activity observed in these studies.

All IFNs promote the activity of NK cells. NK cells are spontaneously cytotoxic to virus-infected cells and certain tumor cells. These LGLs become considerably more cytotoxic to target cells following stimulation by IFN. They become metabolically more active, and they produce larger quantities of lytic enzymes.

IFNs probably inhibit viral replication and modify immune responses indirectly, chiefly by altering the metabolism of the cells they affect. These cells have receptors for the different IFNs. Following binding of IFN, an IFN-receptor complex forms and is endocytosed into the cell. This process then leads to the active transcription of specific genes, normally silent, followed by the synthesis and secretion of new regulatory proteins. These new proteins, in turn, determine the nature of subsequent gene expression by the cells in which they appear. Thus, antiviral proteins, like the IFNs, might act by inducing the formation of new regulatory proteins that selectively inhibit the synthesis of critical viral proteins. The ultimate consequence of this action is the suppression, or inhibition, of virus production.

S U M M A R Y

1. All fine, antigen-specific cell-mediated responses involve T lymphocytes and their subsets, which are identifiable by cluster determinant (CD) differentiation antigens. T cells can engage in primary and secondary cell-mediated immune responses. Primary responses involve naive T cells, while secondary responses depend upon memory cells. [p. 229]

2. T cells undergo antigen-independent differentiation into discrete mature T cell subsets under the influence of the thymus. In addition, thymic education, leading to MHC-restricted antigen-responsiveness, occurs. [p. 230]

3. Antigen-dependent differentiation requires presentation of processed antigen by antigen-presenting cells. Processed antigen must be recognized in the context of self–major histocompatibility antigens, a phenomenon known as MHC restriction. [pp. 231–235]

4. Two forms of T cell receptors exist. Foreign antigen is recognized in MHC-restricted fashion by one form of T cell receptor, which is a clone-specific heterodimer consisting of α and β subunits associated with CD3 molecules. The alternate form of T cell receptor is comprised of γ and δ chains. This receptor appears to be suited to non-MHC-restricted recognition of conserved antigens. [pp. 235–237]

5. T cell receptor diversity is derived from DNA rearrangements that occur during antigen-independent differentiation of T cells. [pp. 237–239]

6. Cytotoxic T cells (CD8) can respond to foreign antigen on a target cell, if antigen is associated with self-MHC class I molecules. A usual consequence of this interaction is lysis of the target cell. [p. 239]

7. Delayed-type hypersensitivity T cells (CD4) are activated in a similar manner. A consequence of this interaction is the release of lymphokines that recruit and regulate cells displaying another form of host resistance. [pp. 239–240]

8. Delayed-type hypersensitivity is an inflammatory response that may follow presentation of antigen to sensitized individuals. If the Ag is given intradermally, the ensuing erthyema and swelling peak at 24 to 72 hours. Specific T lymphocytes, and nonspecific monocytes, macrophages, and basophils serve as the inflammatory cells. [pp. 240–242]

9. Helper T cells (CD4) are activated in an antigen-specific fashion to produce a variety of cytokines that potentiate, in a positive manner, expression of immune responses. [p. 242]

10. Suppressor T cells (CD8), when activated, produce suppressor factors that act to negatively regulate antigen-specific immune responses. [pp. 242–244]

11. Prominent immune response modifiers involved with cell-mediated immune responses include interleukin 1, interleukin 2, and the interferons α, β, and γ. [pp. 244–245]

12. Interleukin 1 is secreted by appropriately stimulated macrophages/monocytes and other antigen-presenting cells. This low molecular

weight glycoprotein enhances the function of lymphocytes and other cell types. Interleukin 1 is an important monokine in host defense against infection and malignancy. [pp. 245–247]

13. Interleukin 2 is produced and secreted chiefly by T_H lymphocytes and stimulates the growth of antigen-activated T cells. Accordingly, it can promote replication of T_C and T_D cells. It can also augment lytic reactions of natural killer or lymphokine-activated killer cells. [pp. 247–249]

14. Interferons are immune response modifiers with several diverse functions, including inhibiting reproduction of viruses, somatic cells, and tumor cells. They can also regulate cellular activity, producing enhanced or depressed immunity, depending on the concentration of interferon used and the time of its administration in relation to primary immunization. [pp. 249–250]

READINGS

Allen, P. M. Antigen processing at the molecular level. *Immunology Today* **8**:270, 1987.

Allison, J. P., and Havran, W. L. The immunobiology of T cells with invariant $\gamma\delta$ antigen receptors. *Annual Review of Immunology.* **9**:679, 1991.

Asklenase, P. W., and Van Lovern, H. Delayed type hypersensitivity; activation of mast cells by antigen-specific T cell factors initiates the cascade of cellular interactions. *Immunology Today* **4**:259, 1983.

Boylston, A. W. The T-cell antigen receptor gamma chain and its accomplices. *Immunology Today* **8**:144, 1987.

Brodsky, F. M., and Guagliardi, L. The cell biology of antigen processing and presentation. *Annual Review of Immunology.* **9**:707, 1991.

Cairo, M. S. (ed.). Lymphocytes and lymphokines in health and disease. *Journal of Pediatrics* **118**:S1, 1991.

Danska, J. S. The T cell receptor: structure, molecular diversity, and somatic localization. *Current Opinions in Immunology* **2**:81, 1989.

Dembic, Z., von Boehmer, H., and Steinmetz, M. The role of the T-cell receptor α and β genes in MHC-restricted antigen recognition. *Immunology Today* **7**:308, 1986.

Ding-Eyoung, J., and Liu, C. How do cytotoxic T lymphocytes avoid self-lysis? *Immunology Today* **9**:14, 1988.

Dower, S., and Urdal, D. The interleukin I receptor. *Immunology Today* **8**:46, 1987.

Frank, S. J., Niklinska, B. B., Orloff, D. G., et al. Structural mutations of the T cell receptor ζ chain and its role in T cell activation. *Science* **249**:174, 1990.

Grey, H. M., Sette, A., and Buus, S. How T cells see antigen. *Scientific American* **25**(5):56, 1989.

Harding, C. V., and Unanue, E. R. Cellular mechanisms of antigen processing and the function of class I and II major histocompatibility complex molecules. *Cell Regulation* **1**:499, 1990.

Janeway, C. A., Jr., Jones, B., and Hayday, A. Specificity and function of T cells bearing $\gamma\delta$ receptors. *Immunology Today* **9**:73, 1988.

Kelso, A. Cytokines: structure, function, and synthesis. *Current Opinions in Immunology* **2**:215, 1989.

Lanier, L., and Phillips, J. Evidence for three types of human cytotoxic lymphocyte. *Immunology Today* **7**:132, 1987.

Lydyard, P. M., and Fanger, M. W. Characteristics and functions of Fc receptors on human lymphocytes. *Immunology* **47**:1, 1982.

Marrack, P., and Kappler, J. The T cell receptor. *Science* **238**:1073, 1987.

Mosmann, T. R., and Coffman, R. L. Two types of mouse helper T-cell clone: implications for immune regulation. *Immunology Today* **8**:223, 1987.

Otten, G. Antigen processing and presentation. *Current Opinion in Immunology* **2**:204, 1989.

Robb, R. Interleukin-2: the molecule and its function. *Immunology Today* **5**:203, 1984.

Rocklin, R. E., Bendtzen, K., and Greineder, D. Mediators of immunity: lymphokines and monokines. *Advances in Immunology* **29**:55, 1980.

Shaw, S. Characterization of human leukocyte differentiation antigens. *Immunology Today* **8**:1, 1987.

Smith, K. The two chain structure of high affinity IL-2 receptors. *Immunology Today* **8**:11, 1987.

Unanue, E. R., and Allen, P. M. The basis for the immunomodulatory role of macrophages and other accessory cells. *Science* **236**:551, 1987.

Unanue, E. R., and Cerottini. Antigen presentation. *FASEB Journal* **3**:2496, 1989.

van Eijk, W. T-cell differentiation is influenced by thymic microenvironements. *Annual Review of Immunology.* **9**:591, 1991.

Von Boehmer, H. and Kisielow, P. How the immune system learns about self. *Scientific American* **265(4):**74, 1991.

Weaver, C. T., and Unanue, E. R. The costimulatory function of antigen-presenting cells. *Immunology Today* **11**:49, 1990.

Young, L. H. Y., Liu, C.-C., Joag, S., et al. How lymphocytes kill. *Annual Review of Medicine* **41**:45, 1990.

CHAPTER **10**   # Immune Tolerance and Suppression

OVERVIEW

Encounter with antigen can trigger defensive reactions characterized as humoral and cell-mediated immune responses. However, circumstances exist in which antigen does not lead to expression of an immune response. This can be the result of establishment of a nonresponsive state in which the source of antigen is tolerated by the immune system. Alternatively, this might be the result of active suppression of an immune response to encountered antigen.

CONCEPTS

1. The immune system of mature individuals can discriminate between self and nonself. Important corollaries of this ability are the persistence of a state on immunological nonresponsiveness to self-antigens (tolerance) and the expression of immune responses against nonself antigens.

2. Tolerance arising to self-antigens occurs during the course of development through at least two mechanisms affecting antigen recognition and activation. Tolerance to nonself antigens can be induced through similar mechanisms.

3. Immune responses to recognized antigens can be suppressed or inhibited. This is brought about by mechanisms that also participate in down-regulating expressed immune responses.

T he normal, healthy individual displays a variety of strategies for maintaining internal balance and equilibrium. This is accomplished, in part, through the activities of the nervous and endocrine systems. They modulate a broad range of physiological activities including metabolism, electrolyte and fluid balance, and body temperature. Other strategies are focused on maintaining personal integrity. This involves activities of the immune system that are called into play in response to foreign substances (e.g., invading organisms, spores, toxins), products of cellular and tissue damage, or aberrant expression of native tissues.

The preceding chapters have described the major components of the immune system and the genetic basis for immunological expression. In addition, interactions between products of immune response and foreign agents have been outlined. These earlier chapters have identified the means through which components of the immune system participate in expressing immune responses to encountered. Here we continue our exploration of immune system function; however, in this chapter, emphasis is focused on limiting or preventing immunological responses.

■ ■ ■ ■ ■ ■ ■ ■ ■

REGULATION OF IMMUNE RESPONSES

The relative ability of each individual to respond to the antigenic universe is inherited to a large extent. However, numerous environmental factors (e.g., such as diet, disease, and life-style) can influence our immune capacity. Homeostatic mechanisms control the size, nature, and duration of ongoing humoral and cell-mediated immune responses. Lymphocytes that are specifically activated by Ag proliferate and differentiate to become Ab-forming cells, effector T cells, or memory B and T cells. However, lymphocytes neither reproduce in uncontrolled fashion nor continuously produce increasing quantities of Abs or lymphokines. A decline in functional expression follows primary and secondary immune responses. Hence, specific immune responses must be down-regulated in some fashion.

Several mechanisms operate to modulate immunological expression. *Positive regulators* of immunological expression include Ag (in native form or processed) and cytokines (e.g., ILs, IFNs, BCGF/BCDF) from macrophages ($M\phi$s) and T_H cells. In addition, complement components and immune complexes can stimulate immune responses. *Negative regulators* include formed Abs, immune complexes, suppressor factors (from T_S cells), and Ig idiotype networks (Abs against Abs). Changes in neural and endocrine status also can modulate immunological expression in either positive or negative fashion.

The preceding discussion assumed recognition and response to foreign Ags. However, there are circumstances in which Ag is encountered, yet an immune response does not occur. For example, why does the immune system normally not become activated by encounters with self-Ags? Is the immune system incapable of recognizing these Ags? Are immune responses to these Ags actively blocked or suppressed?

Two explanations are offered for immunological nonresponsiveness to exposure to Ags. These are immune tolerance and immune suppression. Both are similar in the results achieved; namely, that an immune response is not expressed. However, they differ in the means through which this is accomplished. **Tolerance** refers to a *state of nonresponsiveness to specific Ags.* Failure to express an immune response is selectively focused on particular Ags to which the individual is said to be tolerant. This tolerance is expected to occur whenever this Ag is encountered. Responses to other Ags, even if presented at the same time, are unaffected. **Suppression** represents a *state of active inhibition* or suppression of immunological responsiveness. Suppression applies to specific instances of Ag encounter. The nature of the Ag is not central to its expression. On the one hand, this means that suppression of an immune response following exposure to an Ag might occur at one time but not at another. On the other hand, it means that immune suppression might cause down-regulation of immune responses to all Ags presented at the same time. The major features of immune tolerance and immune suppression are compared in table 10.1.

TABLE 10.1 Features of Tolerance and Suppression

Category	Tolerance	Suppression
Operational characteristics	Failure to display activation	Active inhibition
Ag specificity	Highly specific	Nonspecific
Response to repeated encounter with same Ag	Nonresponsiveness following all encounters	Variable; might not be inhibited following subsequent encounter
Response to simultaneous encounter with unrelated Ags	Normal expression of humoral and/or cell-mediated immune responses	Response to all other Ags might be inhibited

TABLE 10.2 Mechanisms for Inducing Tolerance

Mechanism	Description
Clonal deletion	T and B cell clones expressing receptors that recognize self-Ag are negatively selected, leading to their elimination.
Clonal anergy	T and B cell clones expressing receptors that recognize self-Ag are preserved, but cannot be activated following subsequent encounter with self-Ag.
Suppression	T and B cell clones expressing receptors that recognize self-Ag are preserved and actively prevented from responding to Ag.

IMMUNOLOGICAL TOLERANCE

Two forms of tolerance can be recognized: natural tolerance and acquired tolerance. **Natural tolerance** is believed to account for an individual normally not mounting an immune response against *self-Ags*. Natural tolerance *arises during development,* when the immune system is being formed and maturing (see chapter 20, Development of Immunity). **Acquired tolerance,** in comparison, arises when a *foreign potential immunogen* induces a specific, active state of unresponsiveness to itself. Specific unresponsiveness is acquired following recognition of the tolerogen by the immune system. Acquired tolerance presumably arises *after the immune system has achieved functional competence.* Acquired tolerance is of special interest for two reasons. On the one hand, from the standpoint of protection, the presence of epitopes that might be tolerogenic can compromise the body's ability to resist infectious/parasitic agents. On the other hand, induction of specific tolerance would be an asset in the case of allografts, allergens, or autoimmune responses.

Natural Tolerance

Natural tolerance *arises during the course of* embryonic and fetal *development in conjunction with maturation of the immune system.* However, in some animal species, significant maturation of the immune system continues through the neonatal period. Accordingly, natural tolerance, acquired at this time, can be referred to as neonatal tolerance.

During embryonic and fetal development, numerous cell and tissue interactions occur. Among these are interactions between the developing lymphocytes and the stromal tissues of their respective hemopoietic microenvironments. In addition, developing lymphocytes acquire the ability to recognize Ags through expression of membrane-bound or surface Igs (mIgs [or B cells]) and T cell receptors (TCRs) (see chapters 5, 9, and 20 for further discussions). This provides opportunities for interaction with Ags as well. However, during embryonic and fetal development, the only Ags available are self-Ags. It is believed that these *early encounters with self-Ags are instrumental in acquiring the ability to discriminate between self and nonself.* Associated with acquisition of this ability is the display of (1) tolerance to self-Ags and (2) immunological activation to foreign Ags.

Mechanisms for Inducing T Cell Tolerance

Tolerance can arise through three possible mechanisms (table 10.2). In all instances, there is a selective lack of response to Ag. However, the manner in which the unresponsive state arises differs among the several mechanisms. For example, cells possessing receptors with suitable specificity for the Ag might be eliminated. This mechanism is known as **clonal deletion.**

Alternatively, cells with appropriate Ag recognition specificity might remain but they might be unable to become fully activated. This is referred to as **clonal anergy.** On the other hand, Ag recognition might be capable of causing activation; however, expression of an immune response might be inhibited or blocked through active **suppression.** Clear experimental evidence has been acquired supporting clonal deletion, and good theoretical evidence exists supporting clonal anergy as mechanisms through which natural tolerance arises. Although similar documentation of suppression as an active mechanism for the induction of neonatal tolerance is not available, this mechanism cannot be excluded as a factor in establishing natural tolerance.

Clonal Deletion and Anergy of T Cells   The most universal demonstration of tolerance is that of natural tolerance to self-Ags. This tolerance arises during development, while the immune system is acquiring functional competence. Acquisition of tolerance is the result of selection of clones expressing receptors with suitable specificity for self-Ags. This process makes use of two forms of selection: *positive selection,* leading to survival and further development of the selected cell and *negative selection,* leading to the death of the selected cells.

For T lymphocytes, these selections occur primarily in the thymus and seem to affect lymphocytes only at a particular maturational stage. As T cells mature, their surface Ags change (see chapter 20). Cells that have matured to the stage characterized by the expression of CD4$^+$8$^+$ are those susceptible to selection. Apparently, cells that are phenotypically CD4$^-$8$^-$ are not sufficiently mature, and those that are CD4$^+$8$^-$ and CD4$^-$8$^+$ have already been selected. Neither the factors that determine whether selection is positive or negative nor how such selection leads to deletion or anergy are well characterized at present. Nevertheless, models have been proposed to account for clonal deletion and clonal anergy.

Figure 10.1 provides a schematic outline of how natural tolerance might be achieved. According to this scheme, interactions with self-Ags and the thymic stroma lead to selections that can be either positive or negative. An initial interaction with MHC Ags

is postulated as a step that leads to **positive selection.** *Cells capable of recognition and interaction with self-MHC will develop further,* while cells that do not interact become destined for programmed death. A second encounter subsequently occurs. At this time, cells that interact with self-Ags (not necessarily MHC) are **negatively selected** for *clonal deletion,* whereas those that do not interact are able to develop further. Cells in this population that continue to display specificity for self-Ags become anergized.

Cells expressing TCRs with specificity for foreign Ags, rather than self-Ags, become mature, Ag-responsive T cells. These cells are believed to undergo positive selection during the first round of encounter with MHC molecules displayed by stromal cells of the thymic environment. However, during the second round of selections, based on recognition of self-Ags, these cells do not participate. Consequently, they will not be negatively selected and can give rise to mature CD4$^+$ and CD8$^+$ descendants. These cells will be available for potential activation upon subsequent encounter with foreign Ag presented in conjunction with self-MHC molecules.

Several postulates have arisen to account for the events occurring during the second round of encounters and how they lead to tolerance. These include roles for (1) the affinity of the cell's TCRs for self-Ags, (2) the time when encounters occur, and (3) the nature of the presenting cells.

One widely held hypothesis considers that the **affinity of TCRs for self-Ags** plays a role in determining whether selection is positive or negative (fig. 10.2a). According to this hypothesis, cells expressing TCRs (with $\alpha\beta$ chains) with **high affinity for self-Ags are negatively selected,** and by mechanism(s) that are as yet undefined, these cells undergo clonal deletion. Consequently, those with low affinity for self-Ags undergo postive selection and survive. In addition, cells recognizing certain minor histocompatibility gene products apparently are selected for deletion. Cells whose TCRs are specific for the minor lymphocyte stimulatory (Mls, see chapter 7) haplotype of the individual have been found to disappear during development (see below). Mls products are known as super-Ags. These Ags can activate cells through interaction only with the variable portion of the β chain of a cell's

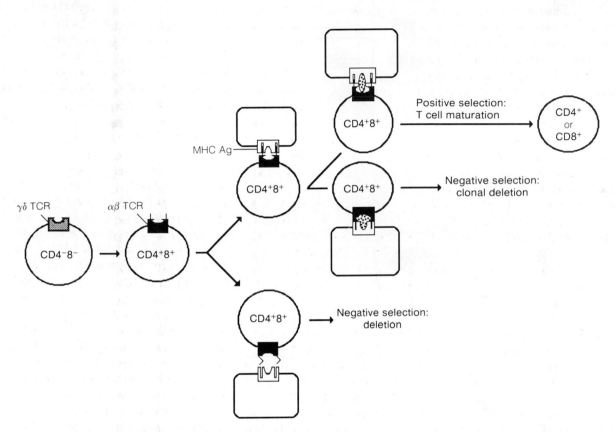

Maturation of   Engagement of   Engagement
TCR repertoire   TCR with MHC   with self-Ag

FIGURE 10.1 Clonal selection during T cell maturation. During T cell development, selection occurs that influences the composition of the TCR repertoire. This selection determines which TCRs expressed by CD4+8+ cells will persist. CD4+8+ cells that cannot interact with self-MHC Ags are negatively selected and deleted. Those cells that can interact with self-MHC Ags will survive (positive selection). A second dimension of this encounter with self-Ags determines the continued fate of CD4+8+ cells. Those that are negatively selected undergo clonal deletion. In contrast, those that are positively selected can differentiate further into mature CD4+ or CD8+ cells. (Adapted from Blackman, M., Kappler, J., and Marrack, P. The role of the T cell receptor in positive and negative selection of developing T cells. *Science* **248**:1335, 1990.)

TCRs. This activation can be demonstrated in mixed lymphocyte reactions, *in vitro,* and is believed to be a factor in negative selection of developing thymocytes.

According to a second hypothesis, the **time when interaction with self-Ag occurs** determines whether selection will lead to clonal deletion or anergy. For example, *encounters with Ag that occur early* (before 15 to 17 days, in mice) *lead to **deletion,*** whereas *those that occur later* (21 to 22 days) *lead to **anergy.*** Additional support for postulating that the maturational age of the

T cells might be important stems from the divergent responses of mature and immature T cells to monoclonal antibodies (MAbs) against CD3. Mitogenesis is stimulated in mature T cells, whereas immature T cells die.

A third hypothesis proposes that the **nature of the cells presenting self-Ags** during the encounter plays a significant role (fig. 10.2*b*). This model postulates that *encounters with self-Ag expressed by dendritic cells or M*ϕ*s leads to **deletion.*** On the other hand,

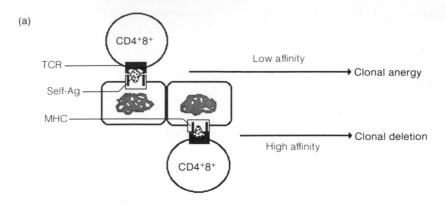

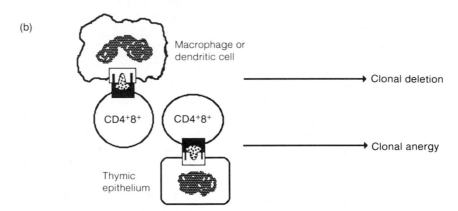

FIGURE 10.2 Means of selecting for clonal anergy or clonal deletion. Cells that are initially selected for survival because of positive interactions with self-MHC Ags undergo a second selection. Certain of these cells are subsequently negatively selected and are deleted, while others survive but are rendered nonreactive to self-Ags. Two hypotheses have been proposed to account for the criteria upon which this selection is based. These are (*a*) selection as determined by TCR affinity for self-Ags and (*b*) selection as determined by the nature of APCs. (Adapted from Ramsdell, F., and Fowlkes, B. J. Clonal deletion versus clonal anergy: the role of the thymus in inducing self tolerance. *Science* **248**:1342, 1990.)

encountering *self Ag expressed by cells of the thymic epithelium leads to* **anergy.**

A corollary to these latter two hypotheses is the proposal that a **costimulatory event** must accompany Ag recognition in order for activation to occur. This model provides a convenient *mechanism to account for anergy.* According to this hypothesis, the formation of the TCR-MHC-Ag ternary complex only predisposes to activation. The T cell involved is primed for proliferation and activation. However, another signal must be presented in conjunction with Ag presentation. Neither the nature of the costimulus nor the temporal limitations existing between presentation of Ag and the costimulus are known. Nevertheless, it appears that activation does not occur in the absence of the costimulus. Rather, the cell becomes locked in a nonresponsive state. Further exposure to Ag and even later presentation of promoting factors such as IL-2 cannot induce activation.

Immature cells might become anergized following exposure to self-Ag because they are not yet competent to recognize or respond to the costimulus. A similar encounter by a more mature cell might, therefore, involve participation of a lymphocyte that is now competent to respond to the costimulus. Using similar reasoning, we can postulate that the nature of the APC participating in the reaction determines the nature of the costimulus. In this instance, dendritic cells and Mϕs might present costimuli that are different from those of the thymic epithelium. If this costimulus is inappropriate (or ineffective), then activation cannot occur. The consequence of Ag encounter in this context is anergy.

Evidence for Clonal Deletion and Anergy Proof that clonal deletion has occurred requires that the actual loss of specific clones be demonstrated. Confirmation of clonal anergy as a mechanism through which tolerance arises requires demonstration that clones specific for particular Ags persist but cannot be fully activated. Implicating suppression in the acquisition of tolerance requires demonstration of some means of suppressing an immune response.

During the course of T cell development, diverse TCRs are expressed by different T cells. Certain of these can be discriminated by differences in which V gene region appears in the β chain of the TCR. Thus, some cells might express $V_{\beta3}$ or $V_{\beta6}$, or $V_{\beta8}$. Cells bearing TCRs with these specificities display reactivity against certain Ags. For example, $V_{\beta3}$ reacts with a product of Mls^c, while $V_{\beta6}$ and $V_{\beta8}$ react with a product of Mls^a. It has been found that mice with the Mls^c haplotype lack T cells that are $V_{\beta3}$+. Similarly, mice with the Mls^a haplotype lack T cells that are $V_{\beta6}$+ and $V_{\beta8}$+.

In other studies, transgenic mice have been constructed that express TCRs specific for the male H-Y Ag. (Transgenic mice are produced by introducing genes of interest into the nuclei of recently fertilized eggs, implanting them into a receiver mouse, and allowing them to complete development. The offspring will express these transplanted genes as well as their own.) Male transgenic mice have markedly reduced thymuses and virtually no CD4$^+$8$^+$ cells. In contrast, female transgenic mice have normal thymuses and essentially normal numbers of CD4$^+$8$^+$ cells. In addition, mice of both sexes have similar numbers of CD4$^-$8$^-$ precursors.

The results of these two types of experiments have been interpreted as showing the selective elimination of T cell clones displaying specificity for expressed self-Ag. T cells of transgenic mice of both sexes will express TCRs specific for H-Y Ags. Cells of male mice (which are phenotypically XY) express H-Y Ags, which appear as self-Ags. Consequently, when developing T cells become sufficiently mature to undergo selection within the thymus (CD4$^+$8$^+$), they will encounter this self-Ag. In contrast, female mice (which are phenotypically XX) do not express H-Y Ags, which makes H-Y Ag a nonself (or foreign) Ag. As a result, developing T cells of female transgenic mice will not encounter H-Y Ag. This evidence supports clonal deletion as a mechanism for acquisition of tolerance.

An *in vitro* model has been developed for clonal anergy as a means of acquiring tolerance. This model demonstrates a need for two signals in T cell activation. In the absence of both signals, activation does not occur. Formation of a *ternary complex between TCR, self-MHC, and Ag* represents the first signal. This interaction predisposes the T cell to activation. However, in the absence of the second (costimulatory) signal, anergy results. The nature of the costimulatory signal has not been determined. Nevertheless, it has been established that anergized cells become unresponsive to further stimulation. Two specific manifestations of the anergic state are readily identified. First, anergized cells do not undergo clonal expansion. Second, they do not produce and release IL-2. Unequivocal demonstration of clonal anergy in establishing natural tolerance has not yet been provided. However, clonal anergy has been shown to be a mechanism for establishing acquired tolerance (discussed below).

Alternatively, tolerance might arise as a result of **active suppression.** It is assumed that such suppression will be associated with the presence of suppressor substances or factors. If such factors are present, it should be possible to adoptively transfer tolerance by administration of serum or cells to a nontolerant system. This approach has failed to demonstrate the presence of suppressor factors in natural tolerance. Nonetheless, if suppression is responsible for tolerance, it is likely that the mechanism(s) by which it operates are similar to those described below.

Importance of the Thymus Two types of evidence establish the importance of the thymus in the

Clonal Selection and Immune Network: Partners in Monitoring Self-Identity

The immune system of a mature individual is known to be activated by foreign Ags and to be tolerant of self-Ags. Nevertheless, there is substantial evidence for the presence of Abs recognizing auto-Ags. The majority of these are Abs against other Abs, which are considered part of the antiidiotype network. A role for these Abs in down-regulating humoral responses is discussed elsewhere (see chapter 5). From another perspective, certain studies of neonatal rodents have revealed that "pathogen-free" mice possess similar numbers of activated lymphocytes as do normally reared mice. These cells could have been activated only by self-Ags. In addition, neonatal mice have substantial levels of IgM. Moreover, a high degree (23% to 28%) of idiotype connectively is postulated to exist among these Abs. This is believed to be a reflection of a high degree of connectivity among these Igs rather than an indication that these Igs are multireactive. The observation that the index of reactivity against self-Abs (0.30) was substantially greater than that for self-Ags (0.08) is also consistent with this interpretation. (The response to self-Abs was 3.75 times greater than the response to self-Ags, suggesting greater recognition of self-Abs than self-Ags in this experiment.)

Observations such as these have prompted some investigators to seek physiological significance for these phenomena. One result of these investigations is the proposal that the immune system expresses two functional perspectives on self-discrimination. One perspective (with which we are most familiar) presumably is expressed through immunological activation in response to foreign Ags. This is achieved through Ag-specific selection and clonal expansion. The second perspective is proposed to be expressed through an immune network that interconnects its components in affirming self-identity. This network maintains homeostatic balance and is not driven by Ag. These two immune subsystems are thought to arise sequentially and play complementary roles in monitoring self-identity.

A brief discussion of how clonal selection and the immune network are believed to interact in monitoring self-identity follows.

The **immune network** is believed to arise first. It is initially a network of interconnected Abs that are germline derived. The interconnection among the components of this network is postulated to provide a means of achieving awareness. In addition, modulating the dynamics of interactions that arise can influence the

acquisition of natural tolerance. First, T cells in nude mice do not undergo clonal deletion. This mutant strain of mouse lacks the thymus gland. They lack an environment in which normal T cell maturation can occur. Consequently, they display incomplete development of thymic-dependent immunity. In addition, T cell clones ordinarily absent in normal mature mice persist in nude mice displaying the same Ags. Second, transplantation of thymic anlagen (embryonic rudiments) to neonatal mice leads to the acquisition of tolerance to donor Ags. In these latter experiments (schematically outlined in fig. 10.3), the implanted thymus an-

lagen become populated by hemopoietic cells from the host. Subsequently, skin grafts from either host mice (BALB/c) or mice from the thymus donor strain (C3H) are tolerated. In contrast, skin grafts from other strains of mice are promptly rejected.

Although these experiments are not equivalent, their results bear on the same point. On the one hand, in the absence of the thymus gland, clonal deletion (a process shown to produce tolerance) does not occur. On the other hand, the presence of a thymus provides an environment in which tolerance can be acquired. In this instance, tolerance is simultaneously in-functional status of the components of this network. For example, low levels of ligand interaction are postulated to correlate with the resting state. In contrast, high levels of ligand interaction are believed to be associated with proliferation but no functional expression, while intermediate levels of ligand interaction are believed to lead to proliferation and functional expression.

Naturally activated lymphocytes are believed to be the mainstay of this network. The connectivity existing within the network presumably is responsible for the steady-state activity of the immune system. In addition, the activities of components of this network might be important during development. For example, the immune network might be instrumental to self-assertion and the expression of tolerance.

Clonal selection requires Ag-specific identification and activation. This process, therefore, is Ag driven. In contrast to the immune network, cells whose activation is Ag driven are thought not to be part of an interconnected network. Rather, they are believed to participate in acutely expansive reactions to external Ags (clonal expansion). These are cells that presumably have arisen outside the immune network and are specialized for reaction against nonself Ags. Therefore, they would play major roles in humoral and cell-mediated immune responses.

Thus, according to this hypothesis, immune network and clonal selection represent two complementary aspects of immunological expression. On the one hand, a cohort of naturally activated cells are interconnected into a network that operates to maintain steady-state *affirmation of self*. And, on the other hand, there also exists a constellation of noninterconnected Ag-driven cells that can be *activated against intrusion of nonself*. Confirmation of this intriguing hypothesis must await the results of future investigations.

Coutinho, A. Beyond clonal selection and network. *Immunological Reviews* **110**:63, 1989.

Jerne, N. K. The natural selection theory of antibody formation. *Proceedings of the National Academy of Sciences* (USA) **41**:848, 1955.

———. Towards a network theory of the immune system. *Annals of Immunology.* (Institut Pasteur) **124C**: 373, 1974.

duced both to host and donor tissues. This latter experiment also demonstrates acquired tolerance to Ags of C3H mice by BALB/c mice.

Induction of B Cell Tolerance

The same mechanisms through which tolerance involving T cells arose can function to induce tolerance involving B cells. However, differences in the manner through which each mechanism will be expressed are not unlikely. For example, clonal deletion of B cells will not require interaction with the thymic stroma, as was the case for T cells. In addition, clonal anergy might be achieved through deletion of T cell clones, thereby depriving B cells of appropriate T cell help. Certain of these parallels and differences are summarized in table 10.3.

B cell tolerance appears to be achieved through a combination of central and peripheral mechanisms. The **central mechanism** for tolerance induction proceeds in a manner similar to that for achieving T cell tolerance. For example, these events *occur during Ag-independent B cell differentiation*. In addition, they occur in the central hemopoietic microenvironment for B cell

TABLE 10.3 Induction of Tolerance in T and B Cells

Mechanism	T cells	B cells
Clonal deletion	Centrally mediated Affects cells with high-affinity Ag receptors; occurs early; induced by interaction with dendritic cells or Mφs (?)	Affects cells with high-affinity Ag receptors occurs early (?)
Clonal anergy	Occurs in periphery; occurs later in ontogeny; induced by interaction with thymic stroma (?); entails failure to (1) clonally expand and (2) produce IL-2	Occurs in periphery; occurs later in ontogeny consequence of failure to get T cell help (?); entails rapid down-regulation of IgM

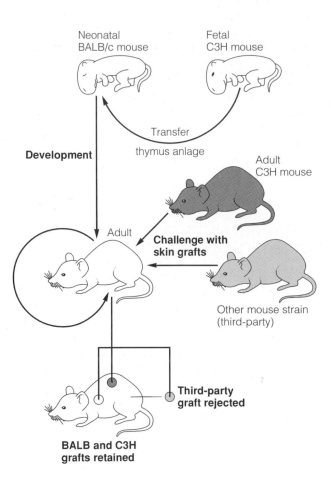

FIGURE 10.3 Tolerance induction through thymus transplantation. Embryonic or fetal thymic anlagen are transplanted to a neonatal host of a different strain (e.g., C3H to BALB/c). After the host matures, adults are challenged with skin grafts. Grafts are taken from strains of mice that are either the same as the host (BALB/c), the same as the original donor (C3H), or different from each (third-party). Grafts expressing Ags similar to those encountered within the thymic environment during development are retained (tolerated), others are rejected.

Labels in figure: Neonatal BALB/c mouse; Fetal C3H mouse; Transfer thymus anlage; **Development**; Adult C3H mouse; Adult; **Challenge with skin grafts**; Other mouse strain (third-party); **Third-party graft rejected**; **BALB and C3H grafts retained**

conditioning, namely the bursa of Fabricius (birds) or red bone marrow (mammals). Through this mechanism, B cells displaying mIg with high affinity for multivalent self-Ag apparently are selected for clonal deletion. The Ag receptors displayed by these cells

are presumed to represent preimmune mIgs arising through V-D-J recombination during Ag-independent differentiation of B cells.

In contrast, the **peripheral mechanism** seems to lead to clonal anergy. This mechanism, which occurs in secondary lymphoid tissues, appears to be one *acting on mature B cells.* One objective of clonal anergy might be censoring B cell responses to Ag encounters. B cell receptors might develop increased affinity for self-Ags as a result of hypermutation following exposure to Ag. Tolerance of these Ags requires that encounters not lead to B cell activation. Preventing presentation of T cell help might contribute to aborted activation following Ag binding. However, recent studies have observed that surface IgM is rapidly down-regulated in cells displaying tolerance. This might serve to reduce continued stimulation of B cells, thereby decreasing the likelihood that activation will result.

Acquired Tolerance

In addition to natural tolerance to self-Ags, which arises during the course of normal development, tolerance to otherwise foreign Ags can be induced. This form of tolerance is called acquired tolerance. This form of tolerance can be induced artificially (e.g., by a scientist or clinician). Acquired tolerance usually is demonstrated later in development or in mature individuals.

Inducing Tolerance to Nonself Antigens

Either T cells or B cells can become specifically unresponsive to foreign Ags. Mature T cells appear to be more susceptible to tolerization than B cells. However, immature B cells are very susceptible to tolerization. Moreover, the duration of T cell tolerance is usually longer than that of B cell tolerance. This might be related to the lifespans of these cells, since B cells are generally not as long-lived as T cells. Furthermore, the effect of Ag on the separate arms of the immune response can be variable. For example, in infectious and parasitic diseases, the host might be exposed to a constellation of foreign Ags, in differing concentrations. These Ags might be presented acutely or chronically and act either as immunogens (inducing an immune response) or tolerogens (inducing unresponsiveness). Accordingly, cell-mediated responses might be quite pronounced to an Ag, while a humoral response is lacking, or vice versa. On the other hand, both arms of the immune response might become tolerized or activated.

The means through which acquired tolerance is established appears to be dependent upon the age of the individual being tolerized. Efforts to induce tolerance in immature animals can lead to deletion of cells expressing receptors specific for the Ag. Alternatively, in mature animals, cells capable of recognizing the Ag might persist but be incapable of responding. This was illustrated in studies using mice with differing Mls haplotypes. Mice with the Mls-1^b haplotype contain T cells that are V$_{\beta 6}^+$. Following injection of cells from mice with the Mls-1^a haplotype (against which V$_{\beta 6}^+$ cells react) into neonatal Mls-1^b mice, V$_{\beta 6}^+$ cells cannot be found. This suggests that clonal deletion has occurred during maturation. On the other hand, if similar cells are injected into adult Mls-1^b mice, V$_{\beta 6}^+$ cells remain. No deletion occurs. However, these cells fail to proliferate, do not secrete IL-2, and do not respond to exogenous IL-2 following exposure to Mls-1^a cells in culture. Thus, *tolerance in the adult mice appears to be achieved by* **anergy.**

Manifestations of acquired tolerance are less universal than natural tolerance. Tolerance might occur in some individuals but not others or might exist under some circumstances but not others. In these instances, tolerance is displayed to specific nonself Ags. Any of the above-mentioned mechanisms might be responsible for this tolerance. For example, clonal deletion, or exhaustion, might occur as a result of continuous Ag stimulation. Low doses of aggregate-free Ag might stimulate T$_S$ cells, which then act to block T or B cell maturation. Alternatively, Ag might be converted to monomeric form, which is capable of blocking lymphocyte receptors, which can lead to anergy.

Tolerogens

An Ag that is recognized by the immune system, and induces a state of specific unresponsiveness, is called a **tolerogen.** However, a tolerogen, under different circumstances, can serve as an immunogen and stimulate an immune response. Tolerogens possess several characteristic features, summarized in table 10.4. For example, the quantity and mode of administration of an Ag can determine whether it will induce tolerance or elicit an immune response. Generally, high doses of Ag (high zone tolerance) tolerize B cells, while minute doses (low zone tolerance) tolerize T cells. In contrast, intermediate doses might be immunogenic. Precisely how this is accomplished is not clear. In addition, aggregate-free forms of Ag are much more tolerogenic than aggregated forms. Furthermore, intravenous injection of an Ag is more likely to promote induction of tolerance, while subcutaneous administration of the same Ag will evoke Ab production. The ability to induce tolerance also seems to be affected by the relationship between the foreign Ag and counterpart self-Ags. In particular, tolerance appears most easily induced by Ags that are closely related phylogenetically to the host's Ags. However, the tolerized state is not necessarily permanent. For acquired tolerance to be maintained, the tolerogen must persist or be repeatedly given. This appears to create a state of continuous tolerogen presence, which mimics the natural case with self-tolerance. This might be necessary because of the continued emergence of new B and T cell replacements, derived from pluripotent stem cells. Some of

TABLE 10.4 Features of Tolerogens

1. Ag can be *tolerogenic* or *immunogenic*
   Tolerogenic at high and low doses
   Immunogenic at intermediate doses

2. Ag can tolerize B or T cells
   B cells at high doses (high zone tolerance)
   T cells at low doses (low zone tolerance)

3. Aggregate-free Ag is more tolerogenic than aggregated Ag

4. Phylogenetic proximity to Ags of host favors tolerance

5. Persistent or repeated presentation is required to maintain tolerance

these might have Ag recognition receptors (TCRS or mIgs) similar to those on cells currently in a tolerant state.

Breaking Tolerance

The state of tolerance to some Ags can be broken. For acquired tolerance, this can be achieved by inoculating Ag containing epitopes present in the tolerogen but also possessing additional, unique carrier epitopes. With this method, tolerance is broken by the "new" carrier epitopes. These might engage T_H cells that were previously unavailable. B cells with receptors for the shared determinants might now be triggered to produce Ab.

Breaking natural tolerance also is possible. In these cases, the individuals display reactivity against self-Ags. The major manifestation of this occurs in autoimmune diseases. What is responsible for this breakdown of tolerance is not known in many cases. However, autoimmune responses have been observed following infections and trauma. Selected autoimmune diseases, and postulated mechanisms through which they might arise, are explored further in chapter 16.

In summary, acquired specific immunological tolerance is an active process. It involves the production of tolerant cells that cannot respond to an immunogen or are held in check by suppressor cells.

IMMUNOLOGICAL SUPPRESSION

Immune suppression pertains to the inhibition of an immune response that is being activated (or is activated). **Suppression** of an ongoing immune response represents *down-regulation of a physiologically active process*. This form of down-regulation of humoral and cell-mediated immune responses has already been reviewed (see chapters 5 and 9). However, immune suppression can also function to *block expression of an immune response* shortly after activation occurs. Since activation is not blocked, this mechanism of immunological modulation contrasts with anergy.

Physiological Immune Suppression

Several physiological means of down-regulating immune responses exist. Certain of these are humoral and one is cellular. The humoral factors that down-regulate immunological expression include (1) formed Abs, (2) immune complexes, and (3) antiidiotype Abs. Down-regulation is also achieved through T_S cells.

Humoral Suppressors

Down-regulation, or suppression, of immune responses can be achieved through **blocking access to Ag receptors.** This can occur when formed Abs bind to circulating Ag. This reduces the concentration of antigenic signal available for binding to mIg. Consequently, continued stimulation of lymphocytes bearing receptors for that Ag ceases. Continued activation of B cells can also be prevented by immune complexes. When Ab is present at low Ab:Ag ratio, complexes can form that block activation of T_H cells. This block prevents production of lymphokines required for continued expression of the immune response.

Alternatively, **antiidiotype Abs** can suppress, or inhibit, immune responses. In contrast to the above-mentioned mechanisms that interfere with Ag recognition or activation, antiidiotype Abs *interact with the product of an immune response*. These Abs recognize and react with the primary Abs. Consequently, they decrease the Ab response and limit reaction with the Ag. (See chapters 5 and 9 for further discussion of these mechanisms.)

T Suppressor Cells

T and B cell activity also can be down-regulated by T_S cells. While T_H cells are required to provide positive signals promoting the expression of immune responses, **T_S cells provide negative signals.** These

TABLE 10.5 T Suppressor Cell Subpopulations

Subpopulation	Actions on Immune Response
T_{S1}	Causes Ag-specific suppression of cellular and humoral immune responses; blocks activation of T_H or B cells
T_{S2}	Causes idiotype-specific suppression of humoral immune responses; blocks activation of B cells
T_{S3}	Causes Ag-specific suppression of delayed-type hypersensitivity responses; inactivates T_D cells

signals limit, or inhibit, the development of Ab-producing cells and of T effector cells. In addition, T_S cells can also prevent suppression (inactivation). Those T_S cells that prevent the inactivation of T_H cells are called **contrasuppressor T cells.**

Several different T_S cells and suppressor circuits have been described (table 10.5). Some T_S cells are Ag specific, targeting T_H and B cells (T_{S1}) or T_D cells (T_{S3}). These subpopulations of T_S cells might play a role in acquired tolerance. Other T_S cells are idiotype-specific (T_{S2}), acting on B cells. Ag-specific T_{S1} cells (phenotypically CD8$^+$) can bind directly to Ag on T_H and B cells. In addition, T_S cells might carry antiidiotypic determinants that can bind directly to B cells bearing the complementary idiotype. If this occurs, activation of B cells is blocked. T_{S3} cells can bind directly to T_D cells causing their inactivation. *T_S cells are believed to release suppressor factors that promote most of the functions.* These substances are possible counterparts to the cytokines produced by $T_{H/I}$ cells, T_D cells, and Mϕs.

Artificial Immune Suppression

Under certain circumstances, an immunological response might be deemed undesirable. In these cases, we seek to prevent its induction or suppress further expression. For example, we might choose to control immunological expressiveness to prevent graft rejection, control autoimmune responses, or prevent allergic reactions. Several methods of nonspecific, or relatively nonspecific, suppression of immunological activity have been developed (table 10.6). These include physical agents (irradiation), antisera, and drugs.

However, there is a negative side to this control. Since immune surveillance is compromised, prolonged immune suppression places the recipient at increased risk of contracting infectious/parasitic diseases or developing cancer.

Total lymphoid irradiation has been used to prolong transplant survival and control certain autoimmune conditions. Using a series of sublethal doses of radiation, accessible lymphoid tissue is irradiated while other parts of the body, especially the bone marrow, are protected by lead shielding. This can reduce the number of T cells that would otherwise attack histoincompatible cells. Moreover, appropriate manipulation of radiation dosage can favor expression of T_S cells. $T_{H/I}$ cells are apparently more radiosensitive than T_S cells. Irradiation can thus be used to selectively deplete $T_{H/I}$ cells. Consequently, specific T_S cells may be produced preferentially on exposure to Ag.

A variety of antisera have been produced, some with broad specificity and others with extremely narrow specificity. For example, heterologous Abs against human lymphocytes have been produced in numerous animal species (horses, goats, sheep, or rabbits). These Abs have been used to suppress allograft rejection. Antilymphocyte serum (ALS), engendered against all populations of lymphocytes, exerts a more pronounced inhibitory effect on cell-mediated responses than on humoral responses. It is not clear how ALS effects suppression. Nevertheless, it has been suggested that target cells might be destroyed or become coated with Ab, thereby blocking Ag binding by steric hindrance. Monoclonal anti-T and anti-B lymphocyte Igs have also been produced. These have been used to experimentally inhibit T cell activity or Ab formation. However, there is a complication associated with the use of antisera. The recipient might mount a response against the foreign substances (e.g., ALS), which can lead to serum sickness and serious allergic responses.

In addition, several types of drugs have been used to induce nonspecific immune suppression. In general, these agents interfere either with the proliferation or maturation of activated lymphocytes. For example, corticosteroid hormones and cyclosporine (Cs) impair maturation of activated cells by suppressing production of ILs. Corticosteroids (e.g., cortisone, produced by the adrenal glands) serve more as

TABLE 10.6 Means of Inducing Nonspecific Immune Suppression

Category	Examples	Mode of Action
Physical	Irradiation	Causes nonselective cellular and tissue damage
Antisera	Heterologous Abs; antilymphocyte serum; monoclonal anti-T and anti-B cell Abs	Have variable specificity; Ab binds to cells and impairs Ag-binding for activation or leads to cytolysis
Drugs	Corticosteroids (e.g., cortisone)	Can cause lysis of immature lymphocytes; impair production of IL-1 and IL-2
	Antimetabolites (e.g., azathioprine)	Interfere with RNA and DNA synthesis; block proliferation of activated lymphocytes
	Alkylating agents (e.g., cyclophosphamide)	Intercalate in DNA; impair proliferation of activated cells
	Cyclosporine	Suppresses IL-2 production; blocks activation of resting lymphocytes

antiinflammatory agents than as inhibitors of immunity. They can inhibit production of IL-1 and IL-2. However, steroids must be used cautiously because of the many dangerous side effects seen with prolonged use, which include hypertension, bone necrosis, cataracts, and mental disturbances. In contrast, Cs is a fungal metabolite. It has been widely used as an immunosuppressant in organ transplantation to prolong autograft survival. Although not Ag specific, Cs causes immune suppression by inhibiting the production of IL-2. In addition, Cs has been shown to generate specific T_S cells when provided in association with Ag *in vitro*. However, Cs can have considerable adverse side effects affecting the liver and kidney.

Other drugs produce immune suppression by interfering with proliferation. This is accomplished by interfering with new RNA and DNA synthesis (azathioprine) or by intercalating in the DNA causing crosslinking (cyclophosphamide [Cy]). Azathioprine (a purine analogue) is an antimetabolite capable of depressing both humoral and cell-mediated responses. It is most effective if given one day following Ag injection. Unfortunately, azathioprine can be hepatotoxic. Cy is an alkylating agent. Its selectivity is related to the metabolic activity of the cell; it is not Ag specific. Its immunosuppressive effect derives from its preferential action on proliferating cells (e.g., activated lymphocytes). Cy inhibits humoral responses more effectively than cell-mediated responses.

These means of nonspecifically suppressing immunological responses are most frequently invoked in circumstances where immunological reactions are considered unnecessary or undesirable. Hypersensitivity, autoimmunity, and transplantation are the most common situations in which these agents would be used. Further discussion of immune suppression within the context of these conditions can be found in relevant later chapters (chapters 13, 16, and 19).

S U M M A R Y

1. Immune responses are subject to negative regulation leading to antigen-specific (tolerance) or nonspecific nonresponsiveness. [p. 254]
2. Tolerance represents a state of immunological nonresponsiveness to specific antigens. Tolerance can either be natural or acquired. [p. 255]
3. Natural tolerance usually arises during development and is reflected in immunological nonresponsiveness to self-antigens [p. 255]

4. Tolerance can be achieved through three mechanisms: (a) clonal deletion, (b) clonal anergy, and (c) suppression. [pp. 255–256]

5. Clonal deletion and anergy are the primary means of establishing natural T cell tolerance. These are achieved through positive and negative selection events that are dependent upon (a) lymphocyte maturational stage, (b) receptor affinity, (c) interactions with the thymic stroma. [pp. 256–261]

6. B cell tolerance seems to be established through similar mechanisms. [pp. 261–262]

7. Acquired tolerance is typically tolerance to foreign antigens. It can be induced by a tolerogen recognized by the immune system. Any antigen can serve as a tolerogen if presented in nonimmunogenic form. Acquired tolerance arises through mechanisms similar to those for natural tolerance, but might require active maintenance. [pp. 262–264]

8. Immune suppression can be physiological or induced. Physiological immune suppression is a manifestation of normal down-regulation of immune responses and might participate in the expression of tolerance. Physiological immune suppressors include antibodies, immune complexes, and suppressor cells. Induced immune suppression is used to prevent allograft rejection, or allergic reactions and control autoimmune responses. Means of inducing immune suppression include lymphoid irradiation, antisera, and drugs (e.g., corticosteroids, alkylating agents, antimetabolites). [pp. 264–266]

R E A D I N G S

Blackman, M., Kappler, J., and Marrack, P. The role of the T cell receptor in positive and negative selection of developing T cells. *Science* **248**:1335, 1990.

Cohen, I., and Cooke, A. Natural autoantibodies might prevent autoimmune disease. *Immunology Today* **7**:363, 1986.

Festenstein, H., Kumura, S., Biasi, G. Mls and tolerance. *Immunological Reviews* **107**:29, 1989.

Fry, A. M., Jones, L. A., Kruisbeek, A. M., et al. Thymic requirement for clonal deletion during T cell development. *Science* **246**:1044, 1989.

Goodnow, C. C., Adelstein, S., and Basten, A. The need for central and peripheral tolerance in the B cell repertoire. *Science* **248**:1373, 1990.

Gorczynski, R. M., Macrae, S., and Till, J. E. Analysis of mechanisms of maintenance of neonatally induced tolerance to foreign alloantigens. *Scandanavian Journal of Immunology* **7**:453, 1978.

Herman, A., Kappler, J. W., Marrack, P., et al. Superantigens: mechanisms of T-cell stimulation and role in immune responses. *Annual Review of Immunology* **9**:745, 1991.

Lehner, T. Antigen presenting, contrasuppressor human T cells. *Immunology Today* **7**:87, 1986.

MacDonald, H. R. Mechanisms of immunological tolerance. *Science* **246**:982, 1989.

Nossal, G. I. V. Immunological tolerance: collaboration between antigens and lymphokines. *Science* **245**:147, 1990.

Ramsdell, F., and Fowlkes, B. J. Clonal deletion versus clonal anergy: the role of the thymus in inducing self tolerance. *Science* **248**:1342, 1990.

Ramsdell, F., Lentz, T., and Fowlkes, B. J. A nondeletional mechanism of thymic self tolerance. *Science* **246**:1038, 1989.

Roser, B. J. Cellular mechanisms in neonatal and adult tolerance. *Immunological Reviews* **107**:179, 1989.

Salaün, J., Bandeira, A., Khazaal, I., et al. Thymic epithelium tolerizes for histocompatibility antigens. *Science* **247**:1471, 1990.

Schreiber, S. L. Chemistry and biology of immunophilins and their immunosuppressive ligands. *Science* **251**:283, 1991.

Schwartz, R. H. A cell culture model for T lymphocyte clonal anergy. *Science* **248**:1349, 1990.

Sprent, J., Gao, E.-K., and Webb, S. R. T cell reactivity to MHC molecules: immunity versus tolerance. *Science* **248**:1357, 1990.

von Boehmer, H., and Kisielow, P. Self-nonself discrimination by T cells. *Science* **248**:1369, 1990.

Immunity and Disease

This section is comprised of three units, each with a different perspective. The section begins by examining diseases in which the immune system is called upon to respond to pathogenic organisms (unit 4). The focus of unit 5 then shifts, concentrating on the immune system itself as damaging and defective immune responses are considered. This section concludes with a discussion of two special topic areas: cancer and transplantation (unit 6). Within this section, background about the sources of disease (microbial and parasitic pathogens and cancer) is provided before a discussion of the role of the immune system is undertaken.

4 Infectious Diseases and Immunity

Pathogens and the immune responses that they evoke are explored in this unit. The nature of pathogens, their life-styles, and the means through which they infect a host and cause disease are examined in chapter 11, Agents of Infectious Disease. Following this basic foundation (or review) of disease-causing organisms, chapter 12, Immunity to Infectious Diseases, explores the interactions between pathogens (microbial or animal) and the host immune system. This unit thus acquaints the reader with (1) microbial pathogens and parasites and (2) ways in which functioning of the immune system might be distorted by infections. In addition, their role in causing disease and their interactions with host-defense systems are explored.

11 Agents of Infectious Disease

OVERVIEW

Human societies throughout the world are imperiled by the real and potential agents of infectious disease with which we coexist. This chapter examines representative microparasites and macroparasites responsible for infectious disease. In addition, it explores the broad spectrum of mechanisms for invasion of and survival in the host that these organisms already possess (and are developing). The nature of the constant battle being waged between the body's immune system and invasive viruses, bacteria, fungi, protozoa, and helminths is described in chapter 12, Immunity to Infectious Disease.

CONCEPTS

1. All infectious diseases are caused by parasites that live in or on a host organism and at its expense. This "expense" is related to the parasite's ability to cause disease (virulence), which can range from small to great, or life threatening.

2. Microparasites are pathogenic microorganisms (including viruses, bacteria, fungi, and protozoa) that multiply in the host and cause infections. In contrast, macroparasites (parasitic worms or helminths) generally do not multiply in their hosts. Technically, they cause infestations, but these are commonly referred to as infections.

3. Microparasites and macroparasites can enter the body through various routes. Once within the host, their mechanisms for survival contribute to entrenchment and to the expression of virulence.

4. Viruses, bacteria, and fungi can reproduce and propagate directly in a single host. However, parasitic protozoa and helminths might require one or more intermediate hosts to complete their life cycles.

e share this planet with a variety of other organisms. Many present no threat to us as direct sources of disease. These organisms are non-pathogenic. Some organisms, however, can cause disease and are pathogenic. All pathogenic organisms that can cause infectious diseases are parasites. Many forms of disease arise as the result of unfavorable interactions between a parasite and the host that it infects or infests.

Parasites are grouped on the basis of shared characteristics. These characteristics include size, mode of infection, and type of host. For example, **microparasites** (including viruses, bacteria, fungi, and protozoa) are pathogenic microorganisms that exhibit high rates of reproduction in their hosts. In contrast, **macroparasites** (helminths and arthropods) generally do not reproduce on or within the definitive host. Consequently, they require one or more intermediate hosts in order to complete their life cycles.

Parasites *survive at the host's expense* and return nothing of benefit to the host. However, there are related organisms (e.g., the natural flora of the body) that also *survive in a host but usually do not harm their hosts.* These organisms are considered **commensal.** Thus, the major differentiating feature between parasites and commensal organisms is their impact on the host. However, the situation is not always clear-cut. Some organisms can be either parasitic or commensal, depending upon the host's state of health.

Simplistically, the pathogenic process can be divided into two major phases. The first phase involves *entry of the parasite into the host environment.* The second phase encompasses *all of the events associated with the infection or infestation itself.* Both phases can injure the host and contribute to the pathogenesis of the infectious disease. This chapter examines aspects of the pathogenic process displayed by representative microparasites and macroparasites that infect human hosts.

■　　■　　■　　■　　■　　■　　■　　■　　■

MICROPARASITIC VIRUSES, BACTERIA, AND FUNGI

From birth, and during each subsequent minute of our lives, we confront an environment often teeming with potentially hazardous infectious agents. Yet most of us probably give this very little thought because of the sense of complacency created by the apparent ability of modern medicine to control formerly life-threatening infections (e.g., smallpox and measles). However, the recent emergence of the acquired immune deficiency syndrome (AIDS) pandemic (see chapter 15, Acquired Immune Deficiency Syndrome, for further discussion) has heightened general awareness of and concern about infectious agents.

The human immunodeficiency virus (HIV), implicated as the causative agent of AIDS, has captured worldwide attention. However, this is not an isolated illustration. For example, at a recent conference on emerging viruses, Nobel Laureate Joshua Lederberg voiced his concern about potential emerging viruses and the threat of serious infectious disease. He anticipates further viral catastrophies associated with the AIDS epidemic. Although most threatening viruses might have natural animal (rodents, birds, pigs) hosts, some investigators believe that certain of these could subsequently emerge as human parasites. They might arrive unchanged genetically or modified only slightly as a result of subtle mutations. However, what enables a virus to spread from animals to humans is still unknown. Nevertheless, it is postulated that there is a vast reservoir of viruses in nature that pose a potential threat for future infectious diseases.

Viruses are not the only microparasites posing such a threat. In May of 1990, muppeteer Jim Henson succumbed to a particularly virulent strain of group A streptococci. These organisms cause a newly recognized toxic-shock like syndrome that apparently can be fatal to otherwise healthy people within hours of the onset of symptoms. The reason that this bacterium, which causes strep throat, impetigo, scarlet and rheumatic fevers, "suddenly" produces an acute, fatal disease is not known.

Although much is known about regulators of bacterial toxicity, they are still incompletely understood. Moreover, treatment of bacterial infections often is complicated by the rapid emergence of drug-resistant strains. Because of the widespread use of antibiotics, most strains of bacteria have become resistant to at least one antibiotic. Moreover, harmless bacteria can serve as reservoirs for resistant genes, which can be transferred to virulent strains within an individual. The

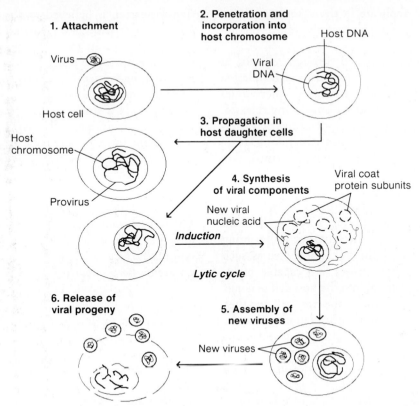

1. Attachment

2. Penetration and incorporation into host chromosome

Virus

Host cell

Host DNA

Viral DNA

Host chromosome

Provirus

3. Propagation in host daughter cells

4. Synthesis of viral components

Viral coat protein subunits

New viral nucleic acid

Induction

Lytic cycle

6. Release of viral progeny

5. Assembly of new viruses

New viruses

FIGURE 11.1 Life cycle of transforming viruses. Certain viruses do not destroy the host cell after penetration but rather incorporate their genes into the host cell's chromosomes (*step 2*). This provirus can then be passed on to future generations of cells as part of their genetic makeup (*step 3*). However, following an appropriate triggering event, a lytic cycle (*steps 4 to 6*) can be induced. This causes release of the provirus from the host cell's chromosome. Thus freed, the genetic information can now be used to produce new viral particles. The release of these new virions leads to the destruction of the host cell.

potential for emergence of highly virulent, drug-resistant bacteria is worrisome to knowledgeable observers.

The foregoing discussion identified the threat posed by microparasites. The following section examines the nature of representative viruses, bacteria, and fungi responsible for infectious diseases. In addition, this section explores interactions between these parasites and their hosts.

Microbial Life Cycles

Viruses are composed of a protein coat and an inner nucleic acid core of either DNA or RNA. Since they *have no independent means of metabolism or reproduction,* viruses can reproduce only in host cells that provide the energy, synthetic machinery, and precursors for synthesis of viral proteins and nucleic acids. Consequently, viruses are obligate parasites. Nevertheless, animal viruses have devised several means of reproduction for ensuring their propagation. Among the more common means of reproduction are the lytic cycle and cellular transformation.

During viral replication involving a **lytic cycle,** the host cell is actively invaded and taken over. The virus then uses the host cell's machinery to produce new infectious virions. This reproductive cycle involves five stages: (1) attachment to host cell receptors, (2) penetration and uncoating, (3) synthesis of viral components, (4) assembly of viral components, and (5) release of progeny viruses. The way these tasks are accomplished depends on the type of virus and on the type of cell infected. The general scheme of viral replication presented in figure 11.1 is typical of many human viruses that replicate in the cytoplasm; however, certain viruses replicate similarly, but in the nucleus.

Viruses can be released through *cell lysis,* as outlined above. In addition, viruses also can be released by *budding* from the cell membrane. Still other viruses can spread by *cell-to-cell contact* without being released. Mammalian lytic viruses can cause infections of the respiratory tract (e.g., flu by influenza virus), lungs (e.g., viral pneumonia by respiratory syncytial virus), skin (e.g., measles by a paramyxovirus), liver (e.g., hepatitis by hepatitis A, B, or C viruses), or urogenital system (e.g., herpes by herpes simplex virus type 2).

Some viruses on entering a host cell do not undergo a replicative cycle directly, but rather bring about **transformation** of the cell. These viruses, such as RNA or DNA tumor viruses, are capable of inserting their genetic material into the host cell genome. Transforming viruses can infect the host cell and then repress their own replication while integrating into the host chromosome. Once the viral DNA is integrated into the cellular DNA, it is called a provirus, and becomes a physical part of the host chromosome. Tumor viruses can remain latent within the cells that they infect. The genome of DNA viruses, in whole or in part, can be incorporated directly into the host's genome; whereas the genome of RNA viruses must first be converted to DNA, with the assistance of reverse transcriptase, before physical incorporation is possible.

In the integrated state, the provirus can be replicated with the host chromosome. All daughter cells possess the integrated provirus. Most of these cells continue to divide, showing no evidence of viral infection. However, an occasional transformed cell can undergo activation or *induction,* the onset of the productive (lytic) cycle and cell destruction. Induction may be spontaneous or triggered by external factors. Exposure to ultraviolet light or agents that interfere with DNA replication are among the external factors that can induce the lytic cycle. Like the parent virus, a virus produced following induction transforms the next cell it infects.

In certain circumstances the virus-infected cell does not actively produce viruses. Instead, this cell might undergo neoplastic transformation. This kind of transformation is believed to be one means through which cancer arises (see chapter 17).

In contrast to viruses, some microorganisms, such as **bacteria,** do *possess independent metabolic and reproductive capabilities.* These unicellular prokaryotic microorganisms are about 10 to 20 times larger than viruses. Only a small number of the many different species of bacteria cause disease. Nevertheless, they are responsible for a broad range of afflictions. For example, they cause infections of the respiratory tract (e.g., septic sore throat ["strep" throat] caused by *Streptococcus pyogenes*), lungs (e.g., tuberculosis by *Mycobacterium tuberculosis*), skin (e.g., boils and impetigo by *Staphylococcus aureus*), digestive tract (e.g., food poisoning by *Salmonella enteritidis*), urogenital system (e.g., syphilis by *Treponema pallidum*), and joints (e.g., Lyme disease by *Borrelia burgdorferi*).

These extracellular parasites reproduce by *binary fission.* Consequently, they have an incredibly short generation time, as short as 20 minutes (as compared with 12 hours required by our most prolific epithelial cells to complete mitosis). Although 100 times smaller than the mammalian host cells, they can easily outstrip our more sophisticated cells in the competition for nutrients with their exponential growth. These simplistic organisms possess a protective cell wall, but lack prominent internal cellular organelles and contain only a single circular piece of DNA. Moreover, some bacteria have additional outer structures: capsules, pili, or flagella. Despite their simplicity, bacteria can be formidable invaders since they have the ability to produce toxins that can easily cripple the functioning of our more complex cells and tissues. For example, the newly recognized toxin produced by group A streptococci that is responsible for toxic-shock like syndrome can be rapidly fatal.

There are also **atypical bacteria,** which are *intracellular parasites.* These include rickettsiae, chlamydiae, and mycoplasmas. These organisms either lack cell walls or have very poor cell walls. *Rickettsiae* are small gram-negative, pleomorphic, rodlike bacteria that require living host cells for propagation. They can cause Rocky Mountain spotted fever (*Rickettsia rickettsii*) and typhus (*R. typhi*). They require an assistant, a vector, in order to infect a prospective host. For example,

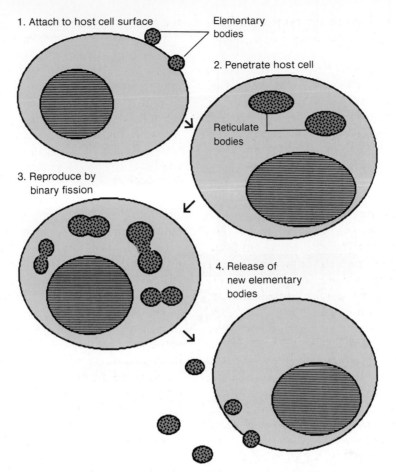

1. Attach to host cell surface

Elementary bodies

2. Penetrate host cell

Reticulate bodies

3. Reproduce by binary fission

4. Release of new elementary bodies

FIGURE 11.2 Reproductive cycle of *Chlamydia.* Elementary bodies attach to the host cell surface. After gaining entry, they enlarge to become reticulate bodies. Following several rounds of reproduction by binary fission, the newly formed elementary bodies are released to seek new cells to infect.

Rocky Mountain spotted fever is transmitted by the bite of an infected wood tick (vector), whereas transmission of typhus is achieved through the feces of infected rat fleas (vector). Once inside a human cell, the nutritionally rich cytoplasm provides this microbe with material needed for growth.

Chlamydiae are another group of intracellular parasites. Chlamydiae possess an unusual mode of reproduction. Unlike reproduction by binary fission, in which one parent cell produces two daughters of equal size, chlamydiae go through a unique developmental cycle: (l) outside a host, the organism exists as a spore-like cell called the elementary body; (2) upon entering a cell, the elementary body develops intracellularly into a larger reticulate body, which multiplies by binary fission; and (3) the progeny reticulate bodies reorganize into new elementary bodies, which are released from the host cell, completing the infection cycle (fig. 11.2). One of the most prevalent sexually transmitted diseases is caused by *Chlamydia trachomatis,* which plays a critical role in pelvic inflammatory disease. This infection can cause neonatal infections, sterility, and trachoma (which can lead to blindness). The only other species of chlamydia, *C. psittaci,* can cause psittacosis, a form of human pneumonia.

Mycoplasmas are another group of bacteria that lack a cell wall. The lack of a rigid, protective cell wall has several consequences, including an unusual,

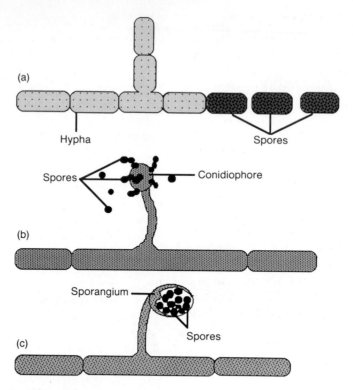

(a)

Hypha

Spores

Spores

Conidiophore

(b)

Sporangium

Spores

(c)

FIGURE 11.3 Reproduction of molds. Molds can reproduce by forming spores in several ways, for example, by budding spores from their hyphae (*a*) or from a conidiophore (*b*). Alternatively, special- ized spore sacs, called sporangia, can be formed in which spores de- velop (*c*).

changing shape (pleomorphism), and a resistance to antibiotics that inhibit cell wall biosynthesis. How- ever, mycoplasmas have triple-layered plasma mem- branes, which confer some rigidity and protection. Pathogens in this group are responsible for myco- plasmal pneumonia (*Mycoplasma pneumoniae*) and gen- itourinary tract infections like nongonococcal urethritis.

Mycology is the study of the eukaryotes known as fungi. This group includes *molds* and *yeasts*. Molds are usually larger than bacteria and produce vis- ible reproductive structures located on hyphae (as seen in bread mold). The reproductive structures at the end of the hyphae, for example, produce spores, which are capable of generating a new colony of mold (fig. 11.3). Unlike molds, which grow in colonies, yeast cells usu- ally grow as large single cells and reproduce either by the asexual process of budding or the sexual process of sporulation.

Compared with bacteria and viruses, fungal diseases are much less common in humans. Diseases caused by fungi are referred to as *mycoses* and are clas- sified according to the primary tissue affinity of the pathogen. For example, systemic mycoses (e.g., his- toplasmosis caused by *Histoplasma capsulatum*) affect the internal organs and may spread throughout the host, whereas cutaneous mycoses (e.g., athlete's foot caused by *Tinea pedis*) are limited to the skin, hair, and nails. Opportunistic mycoses afflict persons with compro- mised immune resistance (e.g., candidosis in AIDS).

HOST-PARASITE RELATIONSHIPS

Whether the pathogen is a virus, bacterium, or fungus, a well-adapted parasite obtains its essentials from the host without permanently crippling it. Most patho- gens, therefore, cause only minor disturbances in body function, and only rarely produce fatal complications.

For example, chickenpox is a highly contagious viral disease (caused by varicella-zoster virus), with symptoms including the characteristic maculopapular lesions (small, elevated regions that are discolored relative to their background) on the skin. The virus is usually disseminated to the skin and mucous membrane, where it erupts into "chickenpox" lesions, producing only mild disease. However, on occasion, the virus can enter the liver, lungs, or nervous tissue. Here it can produce fatal varicellar lesions.

Many *parasites achieve a balance with the host* that ensures the survival, growth, and propagation of both parasite and host. Thus, the relationship between parasite and host is determined by characteristics of both the parasite and the host. There is a continual struggle between forces that the parasite employs to become established in the host and the various host mechanisms that oppose these processes. Susceptibility to infections is a function both of the host's disposition to disease and of microparasite factors.

The outcome of exposure to microparasites depends upon a dynamic balance between the ability of the host to resist disease and the ability of the invader to cause disease. There are many factors that influence the balance of this host-parasite relationship. Our general health, nutrition, life-style, hormonal status, age, history of exposure to Ags, and genetic background (e.g., immune response genes in chapters 4 and 7) all bear on the status of our defense capability. The parasite brings to this balance attributes like infectivity, invasiveness, pathogenicity, and toxigenicity.

ENTRY OF MICROPARASITES INTO THE BODY

The first step to an infection is the *entrance of the parasite into the host.* The most frequent portals of entry into the body are the respiratory tract, gastrointestinal (GI) tract, urogenital tract, and breaks in the skin. Most parasites are directly ingested, inhaled, or acquired by direct contact, while others can actively invade intact mucous membranes or be injected by the bite of an arthropod vector, animal, or needle. The pathogen next must *evade or overcome three lines of host resistance* that normally confine microparasite growth to body sur-

faces: (1) surface and mechanical defenses; (2) phagocytic, cytotoxic, and inflammatory defenses; and (3) specific immune responses. Each plays an important role in preventing internal microbial colonization (explored further in chapter 12).

Skin and Mucous Membranes

The epithelial layer of the skin forms a physical barrier that tends to be impermeable to bacteria. This occurs because of the unusual structure of the outermost epithelial layer, which is composed of dead keratinized cells. We have a specialized epithelial lining in our respiratory and GI tracts to minimize infection, the mucous membrane. The mucous membrane is composed of specialized epithelial cells, which secrete a sticky substance called mucus. This secretion traps dust. In the respiratory tract, there are also ciliated cells, which move the dust-laden mucus up and out of the respiratory tract, enabling it to be swallowed and destroyed in the stomach's highly acidic environment. Should a pathogen survive, it usually cannot penetrate the mucous membrane lining the entire GI tract. Moreover, if it escapes the respiratory mucociliary escalator, it would be met by phagocytes lining the alveolar sacs of the lungs.

Nevertheless, microparasites have developed strategies to circumvent these defenses. The influenza viruses have hemagglutinins on their surfaces, which can react with cell-surface receptors on the specialized epithelial cells. Through these substances they gain entry into cells. Tubercle bacilli are resistant to phagocytosis and thus might escape macrophagic attack in the alveoli of the lung. The predisposition of the host is also important. For example, nicotine from cigarettes can paralyze the mucociliary escalator. This impairment can leave cigarette smokers more susceptible to low-grade bacterial infections which, in turn, can lead to chronic bronchitis.

The possibility of infection by way of the intestinal tract is reduced by at least four factors. First is the physical barrier produced by the mucous-producing epithelial cells. Second, secretory IgA Abs, produced here, may protect the immune individual against infection. Third, the highly acidic environment of the stomach may hydrolyze microbial invaders. Last, the already established normal flora, such

TABLE 11.1 Some Methods of Microbial Attachment to Host Cell Surfaces

Mechanism of Attachment	Microorganism	Attachment Site or Tissue	Disease
Capsid protein reacts with specific receptor	Poliovirus Adenovirus	Susceptible cells/tissues	Poliomyelitis Conjunctivitis
Attaches to carbohydrate polymer	*Neisseria gonorrhoeae*	Urethral epithelium	Gonorrhea
Interacts with neuraminic acid:			
by hemagglutinin	Influenza virus	Respiratory epithelium	Influenza
by specialized projection from bacterial surface	*Mycoplasma pneumoniae*	Respiratory epithelium	Atypical pneumonia
Interacts with mannose:			
by pili	*Escherichia coli*	Urinary tract epithelium	Urinary tract infection
by bacterial adhesin	*Salmonella typhi*	Intestinal epithelium	Enteric fever
by fimbrial components	*Escherichia coli*	Intestinal epithelium	Diarrhea
Binds to glycosyltransferase	*Streptococcus mutans*	Teeth	Caries
Binds to sialic acid:			
by unknown means	*Chlamydia*	Conjunctiva; urethral epithelium	Conjunctivitis; urethritis
by means of lipoteichoic acid	*Streptococcus pyogenes*	Pharyngeal epithelium	Sore throat
by means of pili (?)	*Shigella flexneri*	Intestinal epithelium	Dysentery

Source: Modified from Mims, C. A. *The Pathogenesis of Infectious Disease.* Academic Press, London, 1987.

as *Escherichia coli,* serves to inhibit invasion and repopulation by pathogenic microparasites.

Normal microbial flora can be a two-edged sword, however. Usually they are harmless commensals, living in harmony with the host rather than to its detriment. If the balance is upset, as in a lowering of resistance, the commensals may cause opportunistic infections. The normal microbial inhabitants of the mouth and throat include bacteria and yeasts. One of these organisms is the yeast, *Candida albicans.* This yeast is usually found in low concentrations in the mouth. However, if the immune system is deficient, as in AIDS, the yeast can cause oral and vaginal thrush. Thrush is an opportunistic infection, which occurs when *C. albicans* penetrates the oral epithelium and grows uncontrolled. Occasionally, these infections can become systemic and cause life-threatening visceral lesions.

There are microparasites, however, that can directly surmount the formidable obstacles of the mucous epithelium, acidic pH, IgA, and microbial flora.

For example, *Vibrio cholerae,* the causative agent of cholera, can hide in food pockets. They then attach and penetrate the GI tract by binding to specific receptors on the surface of intestinal epithelial cells. *Vibrio* can also produce a cholera toxin that can bind to epithelial cell receptors and trigger pathological changes. Table 11.1 summarizes examples of specific attachments of microparasites to host cells.

Urogenital Tract

The kidney produces sterile urine, which travels down the ureter to the bladder and out the urethral opening. Although the urethral tube has a normal microbial population, invading microorganisms usually do not gain access to the bladder. Much of this is the result of frequent flushing of the urinary tract by the sterile urine. Nevertheless, if pathogens have a mechanism for attaching to epithelial cells lining the tract, even frequent flushing might not evacuate them. On the other hand, urine itself can serve as an excellent culture medium, once inoculated by bacteria. Bladder infections that can result are generally more of a problem in females than in males because of anatomical differences in the urogenital tracts.

An interesting relationship exists between microbial flora in the vagina. Two colonies of microbes exist in relative harmony: *Lactobacillus* (a bacterium) and *Candida* (a fungus). Both normally colonize the vagina and keep each other's growth in check. Both are able to use the glycogen present in the vagina. The lactobacilli produce lactic acid, which lowers the pH, thereby inhibiting the growth of *Candida.* On the other hand, *Candida* inhibits the growth of lactobacilli by limiting the food supply. The prior establishment of this flora creates a barrier to invasion, yet any upset in this balance can lead to disease. This happens most frequently after the administration of broad-spectrum antibiotics used to treat other infections. This destroys the lactobacilli, releasing *Candida* from growth restraints. The result is a vaginal yeast infection. The less acidic environment that results also leaves the individual open to invasion by other microbial pathogens. Despite this barrier of normal microbial flora, certain pathogens have developed strategies to overcome this obstacle. A number of bacteria and viruses, for example, gonococci and herpes simplex, can attach to the surfaces of urethral epithelial cells and establish colonies of disease-producing cells.

Conjunctiva

Unlike the dead layer of epithelium covering the skin, the eye is composed of living tissues, which are continually being assaulted by microbe-laden dust. This is especially true of the conjunctiva, the moist outermost covering of the eye. What protects this layer from pathogenic assault is the tearing mechanism. Whenever dust hits the eye, we blink. The tears produced can mechanically wash away the particles, and a hydrolytic enzyme, lysozyme, destroys most viruses and bacteria. However, some microparasites have a special ability to attach to the conjunctival surface, for example, chlamydiae (trachoma blindness). This is the exception, however, and most pathogens only enter whenever there are breaches in the normal defense mechanisms of the eye.

EVENTS FOLLOWING INITIAL INFECTION BY MICROPARASITES

From the portal of entry, the parasite may spread directly through the tissues or proceed via the lymphatic system to the bloodstream. In this manner, microparasites can systemically spread to all parts of the body. Most organisms have "preferred" target tissues, and the biochemical environment of these tissues ultimately determines the susceptibility, or resistance, of a host to a particular parasite.

Pathogenicity of an organism refers to its *ability to cause disease,* whereas **virulence** refers to the *capacity to produce disease,* and is a measure of the degree of pathogenicity. Virulence is a function of microparasite invasiveness and toxigenicity and is measured with reference to a particular host. These factors come into play after the entry of the parasite into the host. The ability of a microparasite to cause an infectious disease can be expressed by the following formula:

$$\text{Infectious disease} = \frac{V \times D}{RS}$$

where V refers to the virulence, D to the number of pathogens or dosage, which is inversely proportional to the RS, or resistant state of the host. Thus, a disease would be most infectious if the number of virulence factors and dosage were high, and the resistance of the host was low.

The Spread of Microparasites Through the Body

There are several infections that are usually confined to the epithelial surfaces of the body. Abscesses produced by *S. aureus* provide one illustration. In this instance, an extracellular microorganism multiplies on the epithelial surface at the site of entry. This produces a spreading infection in the epithelium that is shed directly to the exterior. On the other hand, viruses can enter across epithelial surfaces and subsequently spread systematically through the body, as with measles virus. This parasite can infect the respiratory tract, spread systemically through the body, and then be shed to the exterior.

TABLE 11.2 Means Used by Bacteria to Escape Phagocytosis

Organism	Mechanism or Agent Used	Action on Phagocyte
Clostridium perfringens	θ toxin Capsule	Inhibits chemotaxis Resists phagocytosis
Mycobacterium leprae	Leaves phagolysosome by unknown means	Resists phagocytosis
Mycobacterium tuberculosis	Cell wall component	Resists killing and digestion
Pseudomonas aeruginosa	Exotoxin A	Kills phagocytes
Salmonella typhi	Vi Ag	Resists phagocytosis
Staphylococci	Cell wall mucopeptide Leukocidin-induced lysosomal discharge within phagocytes	Resist lysosomal destruction Kill phagocytes
Streptococci	M substance Streptolysin Streptolysin-induced intracellular release of lysosomal enzymes	Resist phagocytosis Inhibit chemotaxis of neutrophils Kill phagocytes

Source: Modified from Mims, C. A. *The Pathogenesis of Infectious Disease.* Academic Press, London, 1987.

After crossing the epithelial cell layer, the pathogen must penetrate the subepithelial tissue, where it encounters the lymphatic filtration system and phagocytic cells that have migrated to the tissues by way of the bloodstream. In addition, in order to successfully continue its invasion, a pathogen must be able to resist the defenses that are involved in the inflammatory response. Numerous means of accomplishing this have evolved. For example, *S. typhi* can circumvent the destructive consequences of phagocytosis since it can actually multiply in the macrophages that have ingested them. Certain strains of *S. aureus* can produce a mucopeptide that suppresses early events of inflammation. In contrast, bacteria with capsules (e.g., pneumococci) are not engulfed by phagocytes, unless Ab is present. Moreover, some microbes produce factors, called agressins, that damage the defense reactions of the host. *S. aureus* is able to produce a toxin, leukocidin, that can kill the phagocyte by inducing lysosomal discharge into the cell cytoplasm. Another strategy, exhibited by *M. leprae,* evades lysis in the phagolysosome by escaping from the phagosome and entering the cytoplasm at an early stage after endocytosis. On the other hand, certain viruses, like herpes simplex, are able to regularly multiply in macrophages. Table 11.2 summarizes antiphagocytic strategies used by microparasites.

Once beyond the physical barriers and inflammatory effectors, microparasites can be spread via the lymph, blood, cerebrospinal fluid, body cavities, or nerves, to any site where the pathogen can find a suitable environment to colonize.

MECHANISMS OF CELL AND TISSUE DAMAGE
Virulence Factors that Can Establish Infection

To establish infection, most microparasites must first *attach to the host tissue cells.* The ways in which this is accomplished are varied. Certain gram-negative bacteria possess pili. These are tubular proteinaceous appendages extending from the cell surface of bacteria. Long hairlike pili can attach to the mucous epithelial surface lining the intestinal, urinary, or genital tracts. Alternatively, secretory substances, called adhesins, can be used to achieve adherence. The causative agent of whooping cough, *Bordetella pertussis,* employs this mechanism. These bacterial proteins seem to mediate attachment by binding to respiratory cilia and to the bacterial surface, creating an adherence bridge. In addition, *B. pertussis* adhesins can bind to the surfaces of other pathogens, such as pneumococci. Thus, the adherence system of the primary pathogen could con-

Artificial Hearts and Joints: You Can't Fool Mother Nature

ith the advent of the Jarvik-7 artificial heart, artificial joint, and other prosthetic devices, many advances have been made in replacing biological body parts with artificial, man-made body parts. However, unexpected complications have arisen. One of these is a phenomenon called **biomaterial-centered infection.** The biomaterials used in artificial devices do not create as smooth a surface as living tissues. This provides a focus for bacterial adhesion. Bacteria are able to seek out the irregularities of the biomaterial surface, adhere to them, and colonize the surface. Pathogens that easily adhere to biomaterial surfaces include *S. aureus, S. epidermidis, P. aeruginosa, Pseudomonas, Streptococcus,* and *Proteus* species.

In addition, there seems to be poor **tissue integration** of biomaterial surfaces. For a transplant to be successful, the tissue cells must form a bond with the biomaterial surface that is comparable to the bond formed between adjacent cells in a tissue. This process is currently a slow one at best. Yet it can and must happen in order for the artificial organ to become compatible with the body's tissues.

These two phenomena, of microbial adhesion and tissue integration of biomaterials, interact as the two forces compete with one another for the surface of the artificial organ. If the rapidly dividing bacteria colonize first, the implant is doomed; but if the tissue cells integrate with the biomaterial surface first, it is rigorously defended by host defenses, and bacterial colonization is prevented. Understanding how to tip the balance in favor of tissue integration will prevent the catastrophic infections that doom so many artificial organ transplants.

Interactions of both biomaterials and tissue cells are controlled by specific receptors and other membrane molecules interacting with the surface. Bacterial colonization and tissue integration seem to be based on similar molecular mechanisms. Antiadhesive films have not met with much success. It is thought that the best strategy for decreasing bacterial colonization is to develop an adhesive for biomaterial that would encourage rapid eukaryotic colonization and integration. Along with the use of prophylactic antibiotic therapy, the race for the biomaterial surface may eventually be consistently won by the tissues.

Gristina, A. G. Biomaterial-centered infection: microbial adhesion versus tissue integration. *Science* **237**:1588, 1987.

tribute to secondary pneumonias during whooping cough. Other means of establishing a foothold include penetrating the mucous layer itself. The influenza virus can release neuraminidase from its capsid. This enzyme can dissolve the neuraminic acid of mucus. Viral attachment to the cell membrane can be easily accomplished once the integrity of the mucous layer is compromised.

Virulence Factors that Promote Pathogen Survival

Once the microbe has invaded, it has to *establish itself in the body and evade host defenses.* Survival can be promoted if the pathogens have mechanisms that protect them from phagocytosis. Beta-hemolytic streptococci have surface "M" proteins, which resist phagocytosis and digestion. *S. aureus* can release coagulase, an enzyme that triggers the clotting of plasma. These bacteria protect themselves from attacking phagocytes by cloaking themselves in an impenetrable wall of clotted fibrin. Another strategy involves the manufacture of enzymes that can hydrolyze host tissues, enabling the pathogen to move and easily renew its nutrient source. Use of these enzymes, or spreading factors, can be seen in the dissemination of *Clostridium perfringens* in gas gangrene. This pathogen releases collagenase, which destroys the collagen matrix of skin, cartilage, and bone. As the physical barriers collapse, the microparasite is able to invade tissues and multiply rapidly.

Viruses also contribute to bacterial survival in the host. This is typified by the lysogenic viruses. Some lysogenic cells acquire new properties through a process called *lysogenic conversion. Corynebacterium diphtheriae* is a gram-positive rod that can be infected by a lysogenic bacteriophage (bacterial virus). Once the phage genome is established in the bacterial chromosome, a powerful exotoxin can be produced that causes diphtheria in humans. The diphtheria toxin, which inhibits protein synthesis in tissue cells, causes cellular necrosis. This also increases the availability of nutrients to the exploding population of corynebacteria, which is now firmly established in the host.

Virulence Factors that Promote Host Injury

Once within the host, many microbial pathogens have the ability to multiply within host tissues and spread from the original site of infection. Often the host tissue is damaged by virulence factors released by the microparasites during this process. Gram-negative (denoting the presence of a lipid-rich cell wall) pathogens are able to release endotoxins when lysed. **Endotoxins** are *derived from the lipid portion of the cell wall's lipopolysaccharide layer.* Endotoxins are able to mediate a number of physiological events in the body including fever, pain, diarrhea, hemorrhage, and even circulatory collapse.

Gram-positive (denoting the presence of a lipid-poor cell wall) bacteria can produce **exotoxins.** These are *proteins released from living pathogens* that can act as virulence factors and promote the pathogenesis of a number of bacterial diseases. Fibrinolysin, a virulence factor produced by *S. pyogenes,* can dissolve fibrin clots, thereby promoting the spread of the pathogen. Hemolysins are produced by *S. aureus.* They destroy nutrient-rich erythrocytes, promoting the growth of the microbe. However, with the elimination of oxygen-carrying red blood cells, the host can develop anemia. The botulinum toxin produced by *C. botulinum* is a neurotoxin that can cause flaccid paralysis and fatal food poisoning. Table 11.3 summarizes some factors that can increase microbial virulence.

Many fungi, also, can produce powerful toxins. *Aspergillus flavus,* a contaminant of ground nuts, produces a powerful aflatoxin that can cause liver cancer in animals. *Claviceps purpurea* is a rust fungus that grows on rye and produces an ergot toxin. After contaminated grain is ingested, muscle spasms and restricted blood flow can occur in humans. The action of ergotamine can cause systemic necrosis of tissues. This begins in the extremities and spreads to the internal organs. The toxin can also act as a powerful hallucinogen, producing a state of euphoria, while the toxin is killing the person.

Certain viruses can inflict direct damage to host tissues. The rhinoviruses, for example, may infect epithelial cells in the upper respiratory tract during a cold. As a consequence of infection, cells fall off the mucosal surface, exposing areas of underlying tissue. This exposed area is now susceptible to secondary infection by bacteria.

Summary of Damage to Host by Pathogenic Microorganisms

Production of virulence factors can enable the microparasite to overwhelm the host-defense network at numerous points. Some pathogens possess surface components that can attach to the host cells, enabling them to easily invade the tissues and circumvent the first line of defense. These include our skin, mucous membranes, and antimicrobial secretions as found in our tears and stomach acids. Other pathogens produce toxins that can kill the phagocytic cells released to the tissues during inflammation. This enables the infectious agents to circumvent the body's second line of defense, inflammation and phagocytosis. Portals of exit can be established by toxins that are released, triggering diarrhea or coughing spasms, thereby discharging the pathogens to infect new hosts. Spreading factors can remove physical barriers to microparasite dispersal throughout the body. Unfortunately, the body's third, and most effective, line of defense, the specific immune response, might never be given a chance to be effectively expressed. Since it often takes 10 to 14 days to establish clinical expression of disease to initial (first) infections, the rapidly expanding populations of microparasites could overwhelm the body long before a specific immune response could address the pathogen. Thus, many infections are a race against time to eliminate the virulent pathogen before it elim-

TABLE 11.3 Factors That Can Increase Microbial Virulence

Effect on Virulence	Factors	Mechanism of Action	Organisms Using This Mechanism
Establish infection	Pili	Facilitate attachment to target tissues	*Neisseria gonorrhoeae*; *Escherichia coli*
	Capsule	Facilitates attachment	*Cryptococcus neoformans*; *Streptococcus pneumoniae*; *Klebsiella pneumoniae*
	Neuraminidase	Facilitates attachment	Influenza virus
Resist host defense; survive in host	Capsule	Resists phagocytosis	*Cryptococcus neoformans*; *Streptococcus pneumoniae*; *Klebsiella pneumoniae*
	Coagulase Leukocidins	Walls off site of infection Kill phagocytes	*Staphylococcus aureus*
Spread from site of infection	Collagenase	Dissolves collagen in connective tissues	
	Lecithinase	Destroys cell membranes	*Clostridium perfringens*; *Streptococcus pyogenes*
	Hyaluronidase	Dissolves matrix of connective tissues	
	Fibrinolysin	Dissolves fibrin clots	
Damage host	Exotoxins (e.g., cholera, diphtheria, and botulinum toxins; aflatoxin and ergot)	Interfere with physiological processes	*Corynebacterium diphtheriae*; *Clostridium tetani*; *Clostridium botulinum*; *Staphylococcus aureus*; *Vibrio cholerae*; *Aspergillus flavus*; *Claviceps purpurea*
	Endotoxins	Release endogenous pyrogens; cause vascular collapse, shock, death	Most gram-negative pathogens

Source: Modified from McKane, L., and Kandel, J. *Microbiology: Essentials and Applications.* McGraw-Hill, New York, 1985.

inates the host. Table 11.4 lists certain pathogenic microparasites of viral, bacterial, and fungal origin that are responsible for disease in humans.

MICROPARASITIC PROTOZOA

Our understanding of infections caused by protistans (single-celled eukaryotes) and animal parasites has lagged far behind our understanding of infections caused by viruses and bacteria. For example, in contrast to viral and bacterial diseases, we are still not able to successfully immunize individuals against diseases caused by protistans and animal parasites (except in isolated instances). Yet, each year, billions of people throughout the world are infected by protistans and

animal parasites and millions die as a result. The public health impact is obviously enormous. These diseases perhaps have not received as much attention as they might. Several factors might contribute to this situation. Among these reasons are the facts that (1) these diseases are endemic primarily in less developed countries, where multiple infections are common and (2) the organisms responsible have complex life cycles involving multiple hosts. However, the scientific and medical communities recently have begun to focus greater attention on these intriguing parasites.

Parasitic protistans, chiefly protozoa, are typically larger than bacteria. Their life cycles often *involve differentiation through several morphological and antigenically distinct stages.* The vast majority of protozoan

TABLE 11.4 Representative Microbial Pathogens Afflicting Humans

Group	Pathogens	Diseases
Viruses		
DNA viruses	Hepatitis B virus	Infectious hepatitis
	Herpes simplex virus	Herpes infections
RNA viruses	Paramyxovirus	Influenza
Atypical Bacteria		
Mycoplasmas	*Mycoplasma pneumoniae*	Atypical pneumonia
Rickettsiae	*Rickettsia burneti*	Q fever; typhus
Chlamydiae	*Chlamydia psittaci*	Psittacosis
	Chlamydia trachomatis	Trachoma
Bacteria		
Cocci (gram positive)	*Staphylococcus aureus*	Boils; septicemia; food poisoning; toxic shock syndrome
	Streptococcus pyogenes	Tonsilitis; scarlet fever; erysipelas; food poisoning; toxic-shock like syndrome
Cocci (gram negative)	*Neisseria gonorrhoeae*	Gonorrhea
Bacilli (gram positive)	Clostridia	Tetanus; botulism; gangrene
	Corynebacterium diphtheriae	Diphtheria
Bacilli (gram negative)	*Bordetella pertussis*	Whooping cough
	Escherichia coli	Urinary tract infections; infantile gastroenteritis
	Hemophilus influenzae	Pneumonia; meningitis
	Proteus spp.	Urinary tract and wound infections
	Salmonella spp.	Enteric fever; food poisoning
	Shigella spp.	Bacillary dysentery
Bacilli (acid-fast)	*Mycobacterium tuberculosis*	Tuberculosis
	Mycobacterium leprae	Leprosy
Miscellaneous	*Treponema pallidum*	Syphilis
	Borrelia burgdorferi	Lyme disease
	Vibrio cholerae	Cholera
Fungi	*Candida albicans*	Thrush; dermatitis
	Histoplasma capsulatum	Histoplasmosis

Source: Mims, C. A. *The Pathogenesis of Infectious Disease.* Academic Press, London, 1987.

TABLE 11.5 Representative Parasitic Protozoa

Classification	Taxonomic Features	Characteristics of Parasitism	Examples
Subphylum Sarcodina	Have ameboid morphology	Contain parasites of human gastrointestinal tract (order Amoebida) and neural tissues (order Schizopyrenida); transmission does not involve passage through intermediate host that acts as vector	Amebic dysentery caused by *Entamoeba histolytica;* Meningoencephalitis caused by *Naegleria fowleri*
Subphylum Mastigophora	Are pear-shaped to elongate; have one or more flagella for locomotion	Contain parasites of digestive or genital tracts which do not require intermediate vector (orders Diplomonadida and Trichomonadida); Parasites affecting wide range of tissues that use insects as vectors and intermediate hosts (order Kinetoplastida)	*Giardia lamblia* infects duodenum and jejunum, *Trichomonas vaginalis* affects genital tract; Sleeping sickness and Chagas' disease are caused by trypanosomes; a broad range of disorders result from *Leishmania*
Phylum Ciliophora	Are ciliated protozoa	Only one human pathogen; these parasites have sexual phase in their life cycle (in contrast to preceding forms); they do not require vector	*Balantidium coli* produces intestinal ulcers similar to those of amebiasis
Phylum Apicomplexa (Sporozoa)	Lack locomotor structures; produce large numbers of spores after conjugation; usually intracellular at some stage of life cycle	Infect several different organs; employ numerous mammalian species as intermediate hosts (subclass Coccidia, family Sarcocystidae); Affect blood and other tissues, employ insects as vectors and intermediate hosts (Coccidia, family Plasmodidae); rarely afflict humans but are serious veterinary problem (subclass Piroplasmia)	*Toxoplasma gondii*, which causes toxoplasmosis; Malaria caused by *Plasmodium vivax, Plasmodium falciparum, Plasmodium ovale, Plasmodium malariae;* Babesiosis (similar to malaria) caused by *Babesia microtus*

diseases occur in tropical and developing countries. A sampling of parasitic protozoa, and the diseases that they cause, are outlined in table 11.5. Some of the more important parasites are highlighted in this chapter.

Amebas

There is only one species of ameba that is pathogenic to humans, *Entamoeba histolytica.* This intestinal parasite is very cosmopolitan, afflicting about 40 million individuals throughout the world. Transmission of amebiasis from host to host is by a fecal-oral route that involves contaminated food or liquids. As might be expected, incidence of amebiasis is highest in areas where sanitation is poor and hygienic standards are low.

E. histolytica passes through distinct morphological stages as it progresses through its life cycle (fig. 11.4). An extremely resistant cyst represents the form that is usually ingested and initiates infection of a new host. The mature cyst releases four actively motile trophozoites. These organisms feed mainly on bacteria in the gut, principally in the large intestine (ileum). However, they can also invade tissues and feed on phagocytes and erythrocytes. The microparasites can migrate through the bloodstream to other organs or tissues. Moreover, they can encyst and be passed through the feces to infect yet another host.

Within the afflicted host, *E. histolytica* can invade the intestinal epithelium where they can cause local ulcerations. Extensive ulceration can lead to secondary infections as opportunistic intestinal bacteria take advantage of the compromised host. The host might also exhibit abdominal tenderness, dysentery,

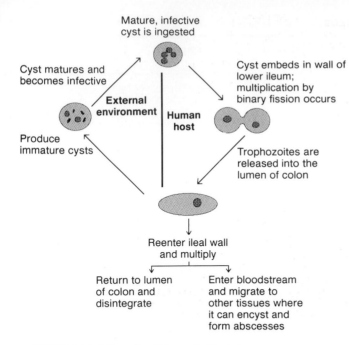

Mature, infective
cyst is ingested

Cyst matures and
becomes infective

**External
environment**

**Human
host**

Cyst embeds in wall of
lower ileum;
multiplication by
binary fission occurs

Produce
immature cysts

Trophozoites are
released into the
lumen of colon

Reenter ileal wall
and multiply

Return to lumen
of colon and
disintegrate

Enter bloodstream
and migrate to
other tissues where
it can encyst and
form abscesses

FIGURE 11.4 Life cycle of *Entamoeba histolytica.*

dehydration, loss of appetite, and weight loss. In certain instances, abscesses in the liver, lungs, brain, and other organs can develop.

Several strains of *E. histolytica* have been identified that can be distinguished on the basis of isoenzyme patterns of three specific enzymes. Recently, it was shown that nonpathogenic strains of the ameba can acquire pathogenic properties under appropriate culture conditions, presumably as a result of interactions with bacteria indigenous to the gut. It is believed that expression of pathogenic amebiasis, *in vivo,* is influenced by interactions between *E. histolytica* trophozoites and local intestinal bacteria. This conclusion is supported by the observation that these amebas are not pathogenic in "germ-free" experimental hosts.

Flagellates
Trichomonas

Certain related protozoa follow a life-style similar to that of *E. histolytica.* However, these organisms are flagellates, that is, they possess flagella. Moreover, some display a preference for infecting the small intestine. A representative of this type of protozoan is *Giardia*

lamblia, which causes diarrhea. Another member of this group displays a propensity for infecting the mucosa of the genital tract. This organism, *Trichomonas vaginalis,* may cause inflammation of the vagina in females. In infected males, the prostate gland, seminal vesicles, and urethra are common sites of inflammation. In contrast to *E. histolytica,* these flagellates have a consistent, distinctive morphology—they are pear-shaped. A further distinction between *Trichomonas* and the intestinal parasites is that the fecal-oral route of transmission is abandoned, and a genital means of transmission is adopted in its place.

Trypanosomes

Trypanosomes are slender organisms possessing an undulating membrane and a single, whiplike flagellum that extends anteriorly (fig. 11.5). They are two to three times the size of human erythrocytes. As flagellates, trypanosomes belong to the same subphylum as *Giardia* and *Trichomonas;* however, they belong to a different order. Transmission of the previous organisms did not require an intermediate host or carrier. In contrast, *trypanosomiasis generally is transmitted with the assistance of an intermediate host.* Trypanosomes are transmitted from host to host through insect bites. Two important trypanosomiases, sleeping sickness in the Old World and Chagas' disease in the New World, are briefly reviewed as illustrations.

Trypanosomes are responsible for a disease endemic to tropical Africa known as sleeping sickness. This disease afflicts perhaps 35 million people, primarily living in rural areas. Sleeping sickness is caused by *Trypanosoma gambiense* or *T. rhodesiense.* The protozoa are transmitted from one host to the next by a vector, or carrier, that is related to the common housefly. This vector is the tsetse fly.

Upon taking a blood meal from an infected person, the tsetse fly might ingest several trypanosomes. These develop, divide, and populate the fly's salivary glands. Here they mature into infective trypanosomes. When this fly bites another human, infective trypanosomes can be introduced. Skin lesions, or chancres, might develop at the site of inoculation. Nevertheless, trypanosomes spread to the lymphatic system and bloodstream. From here, they can eventually make their way into the cerebrospinal fluid. In

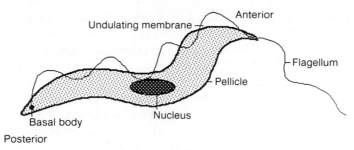

FIGURE 11.5 Trypanosome.

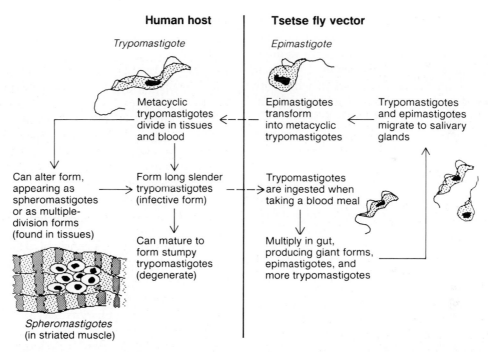

FIGURE 11.6 Life cycle of trypanosomes causing sleeping sickness. Trypanosomes pass through several stages, some of which occur in a human host, while others occur in the tsetse fly. The fly acquires the parasite when it feeds on an infected individual. In turn, it trans- mits the disease to a new host when taking a blood meal on that individual. Note that the form of the trypanosome that is infective for humans is not the stage that infects the fly, nor is the stage that infects the fly the one that normally infects a new human host.

any, or all, of these sites, the parasites can reproduce. In doing so, they release toxins and a variety of Ags. In time, immune complexes form. These complexes can damage the brain, heart, or kidneys. If untreated, sleeping sickness can cause listlessness, nausea, an inability to eat, swelling of lymph nodes, coma, and death. The life cycle of these trypanosomes is schematically outlined in figure 11.6

A particular problem that arises in trypanosomiasis is that of *antigenic variation*. During chronic trypanosomiasis, waves of parasites appear in the blood. Each wave represents antigenically distinct variants of the parasite. During this process, trypanosomes can actually switch surface glycoproteins by programmed gene rearrangements. This helps elude the host's immunological defenses (see chapter 12, Immunity to Infectious Diseases). This has complicated attempts at controlling this disease, which have been frustrating. On the one hand, treatment is unsatisfactory (in part, because of antigenic variation). On the other hand, regulating the parasite and its vector has not been economically feasible. In the case of sleeping sickness caused by *T. rhodesiense,* the problem is further exacerbated by the ability of this organism to infect wild animals and cattle upon which local populations depend for their livelihood.

Another trypanosomiasis is known as Chagas' disease. This disease is caused by *T. cruzi* and is endemic to the New World, specifically Central and South America. It is estimated that over 12 million people suffer from this disease. *T. cruzi* resembles the trypanosomes responsible for African sleeping sickness. However, it differs in two very important ways. First, it is less selective in its host. *T. cruzi* can infect dogs, rats, bats, and several other mammals. Thus, there is an almost unlimited supply of hosts in which this parasite can breed and be perpetuated. The second difference is that they are intracellular parasites.

The vector for *T. cruzi* is the triatomid bug. This is a nocturnally active insect that hides in cracks and crevices of thatched roofs and buildings by day. Although transmission from host to host is accomplished in a manner similar to the transmission of sleeping sickness, *T. cruzi* infects the hindgut of the vector rather than the salivary gland. Infection of a new host occurs when trypanosomes, deposited in the feces of the insect, make their way into the bite wound, other local skin abrasion, or conjunctiva. Once in the host, the protozoa invade cells near the site of inoculation. There they multiply and cause an inflammatory reaction. Five days later, the trypanosomes are released into the bloodstream and interstitium. They pass through the body fluids to other tissues, which now become infected. Here they can again multiply. As with sleeping sickness, toxic products and immune complexes eventually accumulate. During the acute phase of Chagas' disease, lymph nodes, liver, and spleen might be enlarged. Anemia, diarrhea, and coughing are also common symptoms. During the chronic phase, which can extend for 10 to 20 or more years, damage to the heart or digestive tract might occur. Effects on the heart can lead to congestive heart failure and death. Alternatively, accumulations of trypanosomes can distend the GI tract, creating a depository for fluid and salt accumulation because of impaired peristalsis. Blood pH

is altered; toxicity, shock, and frequently death follow. The life cycle of this trypanosome resembles that of its Old World cousins.

Treatment of this disease and management of its insect vector have not progressed substantially. Improvements in housing and sanitation conditions have not adequately been implemented or kept pace with the growing populations of Central and South America. As a result, Chagas' disease actually appears to be increasing.

Leishmania

Other flagellated protozoa are responsible for a broad range of diseases throughout much of the world. For example, *Leishmania tropica,* which causes a disease called "Oriental sore," is endemic to Africa as well as China, India, Pakistan, and several other countries in the Near and Middle East. *L. donovani* causes kala-azar, which is widespread in Africa, Iran, Iraq, southern USSR, India, and South America. In the New World, *L. braziliensis* is responsible for espundia throughout Central and South America.

Each of these disease forms has characteristic features that differ from each other. Oriental sore is a cutaneous leishmaniasis. Infected individuals display ulcerous skin lesions. These sometimes are over an inch in diameter. Espundia is somewhat related, as a mucocutaneous leishmaniasis. However, in this form, secondary lesions and gross disfigurement (e.g., extensive erosion of the nose, pharynx, larynx, and trachea) are common. On the other hand, kala-azar is a visceral leishmaniasis. This form is associated with anemia, leukopenia (reduced white blood cell levels), and weight loss. Despite their differences, all are transmitted by bites from sand flies. Moreover, in all cases the parasitic flagellate infects the host's macrophages, where they develop and multiply.

Sporozoa
Plasmodium

Over 100 million people are infected each year with malaria and over a million of these die from its effects. Malaria, a disease of the tropics and subtropics (80% of all cases occur in Africa), is the result of infection by

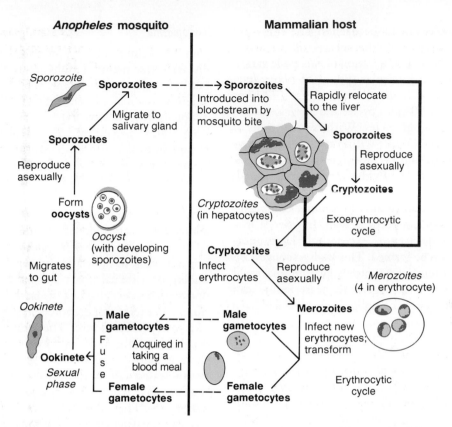

FIGURE 11.7 Life cycle of *Plasmodium*. The protozoa that cause malaria must complete their life cycles in two different hosts. This cycle contains a sexual phase that is initiated in the mammalian host (formation of gametocytes) but completed (fusion of gametocytes) in the insect host.

one of four species of parasite: *Plasmodium vivax, P. ovale, P. malariae*, and *P. falciparum*. All forms of malaria are transmitted by bites from infected female *Anopheles* mosquitoes. Male mosquitoes feed on plant juices and, therefore, are not part of the life cycle of the plasmodial parasite.

The infective life cycle of *Plasmodium* is complex and involves several maturational stages (fig. 11.7). Infection occurs when immature parasites, called sporozoites, are introduced from the mosquito's saliva into the host. Sporozoites enter the host's bloodstream and, within minutes, disappear from the peripheral blood. This disappearance actually represents a relocation of these parasites to the liver of the host. While in the liver cells, the sporozoites reproduce asexually. At this stage, the parasite is called a cryptozoite (since it is hidden from view). Within a few days, the crypto-

zoites erupt from the liver cells and reenter the bloodstream where they infect erythrocytes. Invasion of the host erythrocyte is dependent on the presence of sialic acid residues on the surface receptors. Within the erythrocytes, another round of asexual reproduction occurs. This stage varies between 48 and 72 hours, depending upon the species of infecting protozoan. However, at the end of this stage, 6 to 32 new merozoites emerge. Some merozoites enter erythrocytes and become either male or female gametocytes (sex cells). When the next *Anopheles* mosquito takes a blood meal, if these gametocytes are ingested, they can sexually unite and give rise to a new generation of sporozoites in the mosquito's salivary gland. When this occurs, the cycle is ready to be repeated.

An initial attack of malaria involves recurring chills, fever, and sweating. This often is accompanied by convulsions, nausea, and headaches. The chills and fevers are correlated with the release of successive broods of merozoites. The duration of this cycle varies, depending upon the particular species of *Plasmodium* responsible for the infection; *P. malariae* has a 72-hour cycle, *P. ovale* has a 50-hour cycle, and *P. vivax* and *P. falciparum* have 48-hour cycles. With certain forms of malaria, these cycles subside within two weeks. However, relapses occur and cycles of chills and fever invariably return. As the individual's vitality is sapped, anemia, splenomegaly (enlargement of the spleen), and debilitation become apparent. If immune complexes form, renal damage can occur as well. In cases of malaria caused by *P. falciparum,* exceedingly large numbers of parasites can be formed. This leads to congestion of capillaries. Violent GI symptoms, pneumonia, renal and cerebral (stroke) damage, and heart failure can eventually follow. These complications invariably have fatal consequences.

Attempts to deal with malaria focus on three points: (1) insect control, (2) treatment after infection, and (3) immunization against infection. Insect control is largely a matter of trying to eliminate or control breeding grounds for mosquitoes—stagnant bodies of water. Treament has characteristically been in the form of drugs, principally quinine and related compounds. This approach endeavors to focus properties of specific substances against sensitive stages of the malarial parasite's life cycle. For example, quinine and chloroquine can effectively abort the asexual erythocytic stages of *P. falciparum,* but are essentially ineffective against the gametocytic and extraerythrocytic stages. In contrast, primaquine acts against the gametocytic and extra-erythrocytic stages of most forms of malaria, but does not block the asexual erythrocytic stages. Quinine and chloroquine appear to interfere with DNA and RNA synthesis, while primaquine presumably induces hemolysis of erythrocytes deficient in glucose-6-phosphate dehydrogenase. The great diversity of Ags available because of the size of the parasites and the number of stages to their life cycles presents considerable challenge to the production of effective vaccines (see highlight 11.2 and chapter 12, Immunity to Infectious Diseases).

Toxoplasma

Another member of the Sporozoa is responsible for a disease whose manifestations are usually mild in adults but extremely severe in infants. Furthermore, it has emerged as a major opportunistic infection among individuals with AIDS or experiencing immune suppression. This organism, *Toxoplasma gondii,* causes toxoplasmosis. It can be transmitted through several routes: across the placenta from mother to fetus, by eating raw or improperly cooked meat containing encysted parasites, or by exposure to cysts in cat feces. The somewhat boat-shaped parasite seems able to infect almost any warm-blooded animal.

The life cycle of *T. gondii* (fig. 11.8) is similar, in many ways, to those already seen. In the cat, *T. gondii* undergoes a sexual phase and produces oocysts. The oocysts can infect almost any animal. Following ingestion, it can release sporozoites into the intestinal tract of a newly infected host. There they invade the intestinal epithelium and can form pseudocysts. Within these pseudocysts, endozoites are formed. These are then released and, in turn, invade other tissues where they can give rise to larger cysts. These cysts produce cystozoites. These larger cysts can be found in muscle and brain, particularly of small mammals. Cystozoites are resistant to proteolytic enzymes. This is especially advantageous since it ensures that they will be able to survive in the gut of the cat after it eats an infected mouse. The released cystozoites can then undergo an asexual phase with the eventual production of gametocytes and oocysts.

If an adult human should become infected, manifestations of toxoplasmosis might resemble infectious mononucleosis with concomitant swelling of lymph nodes, muscle pain, mild anemia, and low-grade fever. In contrast, if *T. gondii* is transmitted during pregnancy to a developing fetus, the results can be extremely serious. For example, pregnancy might be aborted or stillbirth might result. On the other hand, the infant might be born blind, mentally retarded, or displaying evidence of other damage to the central nervous system.

Plasmodium: Parasite with a Thousand Disguises

The title of this highlight might seem a bit farfetched. However, the analogy has merit. This protozoan, which is responsible for malaria, has a rather complex life cycle. Moreover, individual plasmodia can display a broad range of antigenic markers. These features, in a sense, are like different costumes that this parasite can "wear." This is an important feature in this organism's success as an animal parasite.

In order to be successful, all parasites have to simultaneously play two games rather effectively. First, the parasite *must draw its nutrients from the host*. However, it *must not endanger the host*; at least, not too soon, if it is to reproduce more of its own kind. The second game that it must play also addresses its own survival. This time, it is *survival against possible attack by the host's defenses.* Several strategies have been developed through phylogenetic history by all existing parasites (see chapter 12, Immunity to Infectious Diseases). One rather successful strategy involves frequent alteration of the parasite's appearance to the immune system.

In the case of an organism like *P. falciparum*, these "face-lifts" are expressed in the several stages of its life cycle within its mammalian host: sporozoite → cryptozoite → merozoite → gametocyte. At each stage, the appearance of the organism changes. Surface Ags, undoubtedly, have been altered as well. Thus, at each stage, it might appear that a new organism has emerged to replace the former one. In addition, the great antigenic variability that can be displayed by *P. falciparum* is further augmented by genetic recombination in the insect vector. Since different genetic forms of *P. falciparum* occur within the same host, intermixing of gametocytes becomes possible before infection of a new host.

Aspects of this genetic recombination have recently been described. Using *P. falciparum* parasites that had been cloned through mosquitoes, Walliker et al. (1987) demonstrated that Mendelian patterns of inheritance occurred. However, they also observed a high frequency of recombination of traits from the parental parasite strains. This suggested extensive genetic rearrangement after crossfertilization. Since multiple genomic forms of *P. falciparum* are common within any host, genetic rearrangement of this sort is likely to occur frequently. The results of this investigation suggest that genetic rearrangements among *P. falciparum* parasites are a major mechanism for maintaining parasite heterogeneity and for creating parasites with new genotypes. This strategy seems to ensure a continuing supply of new "costumes" for use by *P. falciparum* as it infects yet new hosts.

Cohen, S. Survival of parasites in the immunocompetent host. In *Immunology of Parasitic Infections.* Cohen, S., and Warren, K. S. (eds.). Blackwell Scientific Publications, Ltd., Oxford, 1982.
Walliker, D., Quakyi, I. A., Wellems, T. E., et al. Genetic analysis of the human malaria parasite, *Plasmodium falciparum. Science* **236**:1661, 1987.

MACROPARASITIC WORMS

Worms of one form or another make up several animal phyla. Among these are *free-living* and *commensal forms,* as well as *macroparasites.* Although there are five phyla of worms, flatworms (Platyhelminthes) and roundworms (Nematoda) are the organisms generally in mind when people are speaking about parasitic worms. These macroparasites differ from microparasites previously discussed in that they are much larger, more complex, and multicellular. In addition, they display wide geographic distribution and the occurrence of *multiple infections of the same host is common.* The total number of infections (or infestations) among humans far exceeds the world population.

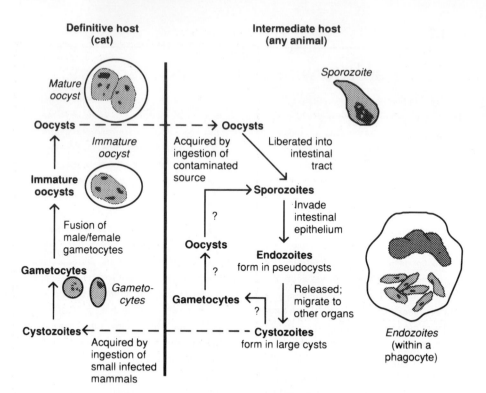

**Definitive host
(cat)**

**Intermediate host
(any animal)**

Sporozoite

*Mature
oocyst*

Oocysts - - - - - - → Oocysts

*Immature
oocyst*

Acquired by
ingestion of
contaminated
source

Liberated into
intestinal
tract

**Immature
oocysts**

↑

→ **Sporozoites**

Invade
intestinal
epithelium

Fusion of
male/female
gametocytes

?

Oocysts

Endozoites
form in pseudocysts

?

Gametocytes

*Gameto-
cytes*

Gametocytes ←

Released;
migrate to
other organs

?

Cystozoites← - - - - - - **Cystozoites**
form in large cysts

Acquired by
ingestion of
small infected
mammals

*Endozoites
(within a
phagocyte)*

FIGURE 11.8   Life cycle of *Toxoplasma.* The life cycle of *T. gondii* is very similar to that of *Plasmodium.* In this cycle, the entire sexual phase occurs in the cat. Infective oocysts can be transmitted by the cat to other organisms. The cat acquires infective cystozoites when it eats infected mice. The cycle that is depicted with question marks represents a pathway that might occur within an infected cat that leads to self-infection. Under these conditions, the cat serves as both a definitive host and an intermediate host. This cycle also occurs in cannibalistic carnivores—since they acquire infective cystozoites embedded in the tissues of infected members of their species on whom they feed. However, unlike the cat, they do not shed oocysts.

Trematodes

One of the major parasitic groups of the Platyhelminthes is the class Trematoda. This group contains parasites known as "flukes." These parasites infest the skin, mouth, gills (or lungs), digestive tract and glands, urinary bladder, or blood of their hosts. They characteristically possess suckers for attaching to their hosts. Examples of trematodes are the blood flukes, *Schistosoma mansoni, S. japonicum,* and *S. haematobium.* Trematodes are responsible for over 300 million infections throughout the world.

Schistosomes were described by Bilharz in 1852, but had apparently been known to the ancient Egyptians from evidence in their hieroglyphics. Although not frequently causing death, schistosomiasis is a debilitating disease. For example, eggs from flukes can cause pulmonary, renal, or neural damage. In addition, reactions to the eggs can cause local inflammation and fibrosis. Alternatively, cirrhosis of the liver or chronic diarrhea might result. Moreover, abdominal distension, and especially hepatomegaly (enlargement of the liver) and splenomegaly (enlargement of the spleen), can occur. Schistosomiasis constitutes a serious health problem in certain parts of the world, notably in Africa, the Middle and Far East, South America, and the Carribbean (e.g., Puerto Rico, Jamaica, Haiti, and the Dominican Republic).

The life cycles of schistosomes are complex and involve snails as intermediary hosts (fig. 11.9). In general, the sexual phase of the schistosome's life cycle occurs in the definitive host, humans, while the asexual phase takes place in an appropriate intermediate, snail,

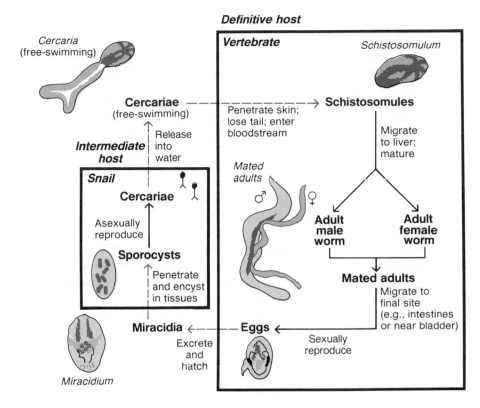

FIGURE 11.9 Life cycle of schistosomes. As with protozoan parasites, schistosomes require two different hosts in order for their life cycles to be completed. In contrast to most protozoa, schistosomes use snails as intermediate hosts. A further difference is that the adult worms exist as either male or female. Mating of two worms of opposite sex is required. Mating of these worms is unusual in that the small male worm remains tucked within the folds of the larger female worm as they migrate through the bloodstream of the host and remain mated at their final destinations.

host. Schistosomes are selective in their use of snail hosts. For example, *S. mansoni* uses large aquatic *Biomphalaria* snails, *S. japonicum* infects small amphibious *Oncomelania* snails, while *S. haematobium* selects globose *Bulinus* snails. In brief, male and female schistosomes mate and produce eggs. These eggs hatch liberating miracidia that can infect snails. The sporocysts that develop within the snail give rise, in turn, to free-swimming cercariae that can now infect a new definitive host. Following maturation into adult schistosomes, the cycle can be repeated.

The three species of schistosomes identified above differ not only with regard to the type of snail used as an intermediate host, they also differ with regard to where the adults mate and the number of cercariae produced within the snail host. For example, adult *S. mansoni* and *S. japonicum* live in small mesenteric veins in the intestines. Eggs that they produce most likely are released into the intestinal lumen and are discharged in the feces. Adult *S. haematobium,* on the other hand, live in veins close to the urinary bladder. Consequently, their eggs are probably released in the urine. In addition, *S. mansoni* sporocysts can produce and release hundreds of cercariae each day for several weeks. Sporocysts of *S. japonicum* produce only a few cercariae each day, while *S. haematobium* sporocysts release an intermediate number.

In all instances, however, the free-swimming male and female cercariae must infect a new host within a few days or they lose their infectivity. Infection is accomplished by attachment to the skin followed by enzymatic penetration. Transformation into a schistosomule, a process that can take three hours, might occur during penetration. Schistosomules, when

phase of their life cycles in dogs, wolves, and other canines. Their larval stages are completed in intermediate hosts, which include sheep, swine, cattle, and moose, as well as humans. The hydatid cysts represent the cysticercal stage of this cestode. Unlike *T. solium* and its relatives that display a propensity for taking up residence in muscle, the cysticerci of *E. granulosus* shows a distinct preference for lung, liver, spleen, kidney, heart, and brain. Passage through humans as intermediate hosts is not an obligatory part of this parasite's life cycle; however, the relationship between humans and dogs has created ample opportunity for humans to serve as accidental intermediate hosts with severe consequences.

The infective impact of the pork tapeworm on the host depends upon the number of parasites. If only a single worm has infected the host, it is quite possible that few, if any, symptoms will be manifest. However, if heavy larval infections (cysticercosis) occur, muscle pain, weakness, meningoencephalitis, and epilepsy may deveop. A potential consequence of infection by *E. granulosus* is the expression of serious anaphylactic reactions should the hydatid cysts rupture and release their toxic contents.

Nematodes

Nematodes, or roundworms, comprise the largest group of parasitic worms that infect humans. It is believed that, at some time during their lives, over half of the world's population will be infected by nematodes. In contrast to trematodes and cestodes, which are flatworms, nematodes have cylindrical bodies that are tapered at the ends. In addition, nematodes have separate sexes.

Roundworms include *Enterobius vermicularis,* known as "pinworm," and *Necator americanus,* commonly known as "hookworm." Pinworm is usually more of an annoyance than a serious threat. This worm, which infects the upper GI tract and occasionally the female genital tract, causes itching in its host. Pinworm infections are common among children. In contrast, *N. americanus* presents quite a different problem. This parasite attaches to the lining of the small intestine where it bites into blood vessels. Here it releases an anticoagulant and feeds on the host's blood. These worms can produce symptoms that include abdominal pain, iron deficiency anemia, and possibly heart failure. Moreover, in the young, they can cause growth retardation. Both *E. vermicularis* and *N. americanus* mature and mate in the digestive tract. From here, they discharge their eggs, which are expelled with the feces. However, they differ in their means of infecting a new host. *E. vermicularis* enters through the mouth, whereas *N. americanus* forcibly gains entry by burrowing through the skin.

Other roundworms that spend their adult lives in the human GI tract are *Ascaris lumbricoides* and *Trichinella spiralis*. *T. spiralis* possesses an extremely simple life cycle in that it lacks an intermediate host and matures very rapidly. The infective stage of this parasite is the cyst normally found in muscle tissue. If someone eats improperly cooked pork that is infected, the ingested cysts produce larvae within that individual's digestive tract. Within three to four days, these larvae will develop into adults. The adults mate and produce larvae, microfilariae, that bore through the intestinal wall and enter the bloodstream. These microfilariae make their way to muscle tissue where they encyst. Adult worms survive for only a few weeks, but the microfilarial cysts can remain infective for one to two years. Passage of trichinosis from one person to another does not occur (at least not in modern cultures). Nevertheless, this disease is perpetuated though ingestion of pork scraps fed to pigs (domestically) and within various cannibalistic carnivores (e.g., polar bears, foxes, hyenas, and wild pigs).

Approximately a billion people are believed to be infected by *A. lumbricoides*. This worm possesses a complex life cycle, although it too does not pass through an intermediate host (fig. 11.12). Eggs, which are capable of surviving for long periods, under adverse conditions can lie dormant in soil. Alternatively, if the soil is moist and warm, larvae develop within the eggs. Nevertheless, when the eggs (containing developed larvae) are ingested, the larvae hatch in the intestines. Subsequently, they embark on a round-trip journey to the oropharynx and back to the intestines. First, they penetrate the intestinal wall and enter the bloodstream. From here, they make their way through the heart and on to the lungs. Within the lungs, the larvae become lodged in the alveoli. Progressively, they then make their way through the bronchial passages to the

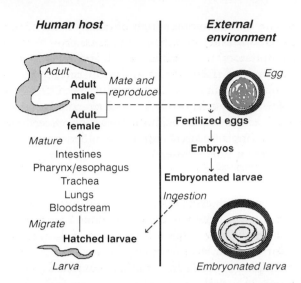

Human host

Adult

Adult male ⎤
           ⎬ Mate and reproduce
Adult female ⎦

Mature ↑
Intestines
Pharynx/esophagus
Trachea
Lungs
Bloodstream

Migrate |

Hatched larvae

Larva

External environment

Egg

↓

Fertilized eggs

↓

Embryos

↓

Embryonated larvae

Ingestion

Embryonated larva

FIGURE 11.12 Life cycle of *Ascaris lumbricoides*. This roundworm has a very complex life cycle. Only one host is used, and a portion of the life cycle is completed in the external environment. However, within the human host, these worms migrate from the intestines up through the lungs, then back to the intestines again as they mature.

trachea and into the mouth and pharynx. Once in the alimentary tract, they return to the intestines. Only now will they mature into adults and mate. Reproducing females can produce up to 200,000 eggs per day. Ascarid infections rarely persist for more than one year. If the infestation is limited, symptoms might be negligible. However, with infections produced by large numbers of worms, the lumen of the intestinal tract might become partially blocked. In addition, larvae that become permanently lodged in the lungs can lead to ascarid pneumonia, while migration of adults to unusual sites (e.g., eye, brain, spinal cord, kidneys, or heart) can present serious risks to the host.

Other roundworms have intermediate hosts that act as vectors in the transmission of disease. In one sense, this is reminiscent of the parasitic life cycles displayed by certain protozoans (e.g., trypanosomes and *Plasmodium*). These nematodes are the filaria. Unlike their cousins, discussed above, filaria do not focus on the digestive tract as the major site of infection. Rather, there is a tendency to find these worms in the blood, lymphatics, or the skin. These sites apparently serve to enhance the chances of transmission to a new host. Other features displayed by these worms are modifications in their behavior. For example, microfilariae of

Wuchereria bancrofti in Africa, India, and China are typically inactive during the day but rather active at night, while in the Eastern Pacific the cycle is reversed. The periods of activity of microfilariae coincide with peak periods of activity of their insect vectors. On the other hand, microfilariae of *Onchocerca volvulus* distribute themselves in regions of the body where the insect vectors show a preference for biting in procuring their blood meals. Thus, filarial worms appear to have developed behavioral patterns that enhance the chances of further transmission. These parasites also appear to be very host specific and tissue specific in their patterns of infection.

Arthropods

Arthropods are invertebrates that possess a hard, chitinous exoskeleton and jointed legs. The number of pairs of legs, the presence or absence of wings, and the number of body segments that they have depends upon whether we are referring to insects or arachnids. Characteristically, members of the class **Insecta** have three pairs of legs, wings, and three major body segments (head, thorax, and abdomen). Members of the class **Arachnida** (which includes spiders, scorpions, mites, ticks, and lice) have four pairs of legs, two major body segments (cephalothorax and abdomen), but lack wings. In contrast to protozoan and helminthic parasites, arthropodal parasites are **ectoparasites.**

Arthropods, as parasites, are of far greater concern to veterinary medicine. Among the more prevalent parasitic forms are fleas, lice, mites, and ticks. These organisms present a two-fold threat. First, they can serve as the parasitic organism on the infected host. Second, they often serve as vectors for other parasites, usually protozoan. Consequently, they can add a second parasite to the total infective burden imposed on the host. As primary parasites, arthropods cause local inflammatory and allergic reactions. These are brought about by the secretions that they produce and release into the skin when they bite their hosts. Infestations of human hosts by fleas, mites, and ticks are not especially common occurrences. On the other hand, infestations by lice are much more prevalent, especially where sanitation is poor and personal hygiene is neglected. In their roles as carriers of parasitic disease, they do not themselves have to parasitize the host they infect. Even though they might fall from their intended host, if they have bitten the individual and introduced infective microorganisms, protozoans, or worms, then they have played their part in infecting the host with a parasite. Among the diseases that they can induce in this manner are Rocky Mountain spotted fever and Q-fever, both of which are caused by rickettsiae; Lyme disease, caused by a spirochete; babesiosis and trypanosomiasis, which are caused by protozoa. Of these, only trypanosomiasis is not transmitted by ticks. In addition, all can occur in humans, although babesiosis tends to produce only mild symptoms.

SUMMARY

1. Viruses, bacteria, and fungi are microparasites residing on or within another living organism. These agents of infectious disease can affect any organ system of the body. [p. 272]

2. Viruses are obligate parasites that are able to attach and penetrate into cells, take over, and either utilize cellular machinery of the host to replicate new virions, remain latent within the cell, or cause transformation of the infected cell. [pp. 273–274]

3. Bacteria can multiply at a much faster rate than human host tissue, compete for foodstuff, and often produce virulence factors that can cause disease. [pp. 274–276]

4. Fungi are eukaryotic organisms that can be obligate intracellular parasites and cause disease by interfering with the normal functioning of specific host tissue cells. [p. 276]

5. Although microparasites harm the host, the most successful parasites achieve a balance with the host, which ensures the survival, growth, and propagation of both parasite and host. [pp. 276–277]

6. The relationship between parasite and host is determined by the susceptibility of the host and the pathogenicity of the parasite. [p. 277]

7. Among the microparasite's attributes are infectivity, invasiveness, pathogenicity, and toxigenicity. [p. 277]

8. The most common portals of entry of microparasites into their hosts are the respiratory, the gastrointestinal, and the urogenital tracts, breaks in the superficial mucous membranes, and the skin. [pp. 277–279]

9. From the portal of entry, the microparasite may spread directly through the tissues or proceed via the lymphatic circulation to the bloodstream, where it can be disseminated systemically. [pp. 279–280]

10. Virulence is the ability of the pathogenic organism to cause infectious disease and is usually mediated by the production of virulence factors. Virulence factors that promote pathogen survival and host injury include toxins, antiphagocytic factors, and spreading factors. [pp. 280–282]

11. How the body's defense mechanisms address viral, bacterial, and fungal invasion determines whether host-parasite interactions result in microparasite elimination or disease. [pp. 282–283]

12. Protistan microparasites (protozoa) and macroparasites (worms) cause infectious diseases that are more prevalent in less developed countries of the world. [p. 283]

13. Protozoa are unicellular organisms that can act as animal microparasites. There are several diverse forms that are distinguishable by their physical appearance and distinctive life cycles, which often include one or more intermediate hosts in addition to a definitive host. [pp. 283–285]

14. Pathogenic amebas directly infect millions of people and cause colon infections ranging from mild diarrhea to dysentery, which may be complicated by liver abscess. [pp. 285–286]

15. Flagellates include the protozoa that are responsible for African sleeping sickness and Chagas' disease (trypanosomes), kala-azar and espundia (*Leishmania*), and trichomonad infections (*Trichomonas vaginalis*). Certain flagellates make use of intermediate hosts to complete their life cycles and to ensure transmission to new definitive hosts. [pp. 286–288]

16. The Sporozoa include the microparasites responsible for the various forms of malaria and toxoplasmosis. [pp. 288–290]

17. Flukes and tapeworms (Platyhelminthes) and roundworms (Nematoda) are responsible for the majority of diseases caused by macroparasites. [p. 291]

18. Flukes, or trematodes, can infect humans and localize in the blood, liver, intestines, or lungs of their hosts. Their life cycles include intermediate (snails) and definitive hosts; however, the infective stages are capable of free-living existence for short periods. [pp. 292–294]

19. Cestodes, or tapeworms, are hermaphroditic organisms that, as adults, are essentially egg-producing machines composed of a scolex (head) and a series of reproductive segments (proglottids). They infect principally the digestive tracts of their hosts. Although intermediate and definitive hosts are included in their life cycles, both hosts are vertebrates. [pp. 294–296]

20. Nematodes, or roundworms, are a group of parasitic worms whose adult stage is dioecious. They infect a variety of organs which include blood and muscle. Their life cycles can occur with (filarial worms, *Trichinella spiralis*) or without (*Ascaris lumbricoides*) intermediate hosts. [pp. 296–297]

21. Arthropods are mostly free living; however, some are involved in parasitic relationships. Insects are not generally parasites, but often serve as intermediate hosts and vectors for several protozoan parasites (e.g., *Plasmodium vivax* and *Trypanosoma cruzi*). Arachnids serve both as vectors and intermediate hosts in the transmission of protozoan parasites. In addition, they are occasionally parasites themselves. Among the diseases they transmit are Rocky Mountain spotted fever, Q-fever, and Lyme disease. [pp. 297–298]

READINGS

Viruses, Bacteria, and Fungi

Culliton, B. Emerging viruses, emerging threat. *Science* **247**:279, 1990.

Feduchi, E., Alonso, M., and Carrascoo, L. Human gamma interferon and tumor necrosis factor exert a synergistic blockade on the replication of herpes simplex virus. *Journal of Virology* **63**:1354, 1989.

Goldfeld, A., and Maniatis, T. Coordinate viral induction of tumor necrosis factor alpha and interferon beta in human B cells and monocytes. *Proceedings of the National Academy of Science* (USA) **86**:1490, 1989.

Greenfield, L., Johnson, V. G., and Youle, R. J. Mutations in diphtheria toxin separate binding from entry and amplify immunotoxin selectivity. *Science* **238**: 536, 1987.

Jawetz, E., Melnick, J. L., and Adelberg, E. A. *Review of Medical Microbiology.* 17th ed. Lange Medical Publications, Los Altos, Calif., 1987.

Joklik, W. K. *Virology.* Appleton-Century-Crofts, Norwalk, Conn., 1985.

Mims, C. A. *The Pathogenesis of Infectious Disease.* Academic Press, Inc., New York, 1987.

Moxon, E., and Kroll, J. The role of bacterial polysaccharide capsules as virulence factors. In Jann, K., and Jann, B. (eds.). *Current Topics In Microbiology and Immunology: Bacterial Capsules.* Springer-Verlag, New York, 1990.

Notkins, A. L., and Oldstone, M. B. A. (eds.) *Concepts in Viral Pathogenesis II.* Springer-Verlag, New York, 1986.

Wright, K. Bad news bacteria. *Science* **240**:22, 1990.

Protozoa and Helminths

Andrysiak, P. M., Collins, W. E., and Campbell, G. H. Stage-specific and species-specific antigens of *Plasmodium vivax* and *Plasmodium ovale* defined by monoclonal antibodies. *Infection and Immunity* **54**:609, 1986.

Cohen, S., and Warren, K. S. (eds.). *Immunology of Parasitic Infections.* Blackwell Scientific Publications, Ltd., Oxford, 1982.

Cross, G. A. M. Cellular and genetic aspects of antigenic variation on trypanosomes. *Annual Review of Immunology.* **8:**83, 1990.

Hughes, H. Toxoplasmosis—a neglected disease. *Parasitology Today* **1:**6, 1985.

Klein, A. E. *The Parasites We Humans Harbor.* Elsevier/North Holland Publishing Co., New York, 1981.

Mahmoud, A. Parasitic protozoa and helminths: biological and immunological challenges. *Science* **246:**1015, 1989.

Russell, D., and Talamas-Rhohana, P. Leishmania and the macrophage. *Immunology Today* **10:**328, 1989.

Stavitsky, A. B. Immune regulation in schistosomiasis japonica. *Immunology Today* **8:**228, 1987.

Walliker, D., Quakyi, I. A., Wellems, T. E., et al. Genetic analysis of the human malaria parasite *Plasmodium falciparum. Science* **236:**1661, 1987.

CHAPTER 12

Immunity to Infectious Diseases

OVERVIEW

Immunity to infectious diseases involves interaction between the infectious agent, on the one hand, and the body's defenses on the other. This includes the expression of immunological function in the face of challenge by infectious agents. In addition, it depends upon, and is influenced by, the several strategies that have been evolved by these organisms for counteracting and evading the host's immunological defenses. Vaccines, to date, have had a tremendous impact on world health, and there is now promise of modern vaccines being developed against other critical and potentially devastating infectious diseases.

CONCEPTS

1. The host employs innate and acquired immunological defenses to combat invasion by infectious agents. Both humoral and cell-mediated mechanisms can be fully expressed against these invasions.

2. Which mechanisms of defense are employed may be affected by the manner in which the pathogen confronts the host. Organisms that inhabit the blood are more likely to evoke humoral immune responses, whereas those afflicting host tissues might preferentially elicit cell-mediated responses.

3. Infectious organisms have elaborated several mechanisms that enable them to elude the host's immune system. Generally these include means of evading detection or of modulating the nature of the host's response.

4. Several avenues are actively being explored to develop and improve vaccines not currently available (or less than ideal) that will effectively provide acquired immunity against pathogenic organisms.

301

I mmunity to infectious diseases refers to resistance of a host organism to pathogens or their toxic products. The kinds and numbers of pathogens (e.g., viruses, bacteria, fungi, protozoa, and helminths) encountered varies from one environment to another. A biological environment that is normally not threatening to healthy individuals may be devastating to those that are immunodeficient, and thus subject to opportunistic infections. On the other hand, the most menacing environment might contain infectious agents capable of overcoming both innate defenses and the most sophisticated acquired defense mechanisms presently known. Generally, however, the body does remarkably well in protecting us from the many possible pathogens encountered in our environment. In accomplishing this, the body's defenses are continuously responding to agents of disease.

Although all humans possess basically similar defense mechanisms, each is individually unique in being able to cope with the biological environment. Generally health, nutrition, life-style, hormone status, sex, age, history of exposure to Ags, and genetic background all influence defense capability. Those with the least effective defense systems are more likely to succumb, in whole or in part, to assault by infectious agents of disease.

This chapter considers some of the factors that contribute to innate and acquired immunity to infectious diseases. Immune effector systems that provide protection against, or are overcome by, microparasites (viruses, bacteria, fungi, and protozoa) and macroparasites (helminths) are examined. Finally, the nature of vaccines and their potential for protection against infectious agents of disease are explored.

■ ■ ■ ■ ■ ■ ■ ■ ■ ■

RESISTANCE TO VIRAL, BACTERIAL, AND FUNGAL MICROPARASITES

Viruses, bacteria, and fungi are microparasites that present acute challenges to the organisms that they infect. The *duration of the infections that they cause are usually short,* on the order of days or weeks, although more protracted or persistent infections can occur. Within this period, the mechanisms for infection elaborated by the pathogen, and the defenses of the host, are pitted against each other. Resolution of the ensuing conflict is based on responses by the host, as well as the pathogen. These responses can lead to eradication/control of the pathogen or, rarely, death of the host.

Innate Immunity

Innate host defenses against microparasites are relatively **nonspecific** (table 12.1). They *include physical and anatomical barriers.* In addition, the potential host employs cellular and biochemical defenses. The cellular defense is provided by antagonistic indigenous flora (bacteria) and a variety of cells that either directly phagocytize free viruses and bacteria or destroy virus-infected cells, while the biochemical factors include antiviral and antibacterial substances.

In order for viruses and bacteria to become established in a host, they must first pass through or across **anatomical barriers** designed to protect the body from invasion. In order to infect a host, microparasites must circumvent these barriers. The most frequent routes of entry are the mouth (e.g., eating contaminated food), the respiratory tract (e.g., airborne droplets and dust), and the urogenital tract (by direct contact). The intact skin normally bars penetration by most microparasites. In addition, it discourages microparasites from colonizing by perspiration and sebaceous secretions with an acidic pH. The ciliated mucous membranes of the respiratory tract also present a barrier against microbial attachment and invasion. The ciliated cells of this epithelium can sweep particles containing pathogens to the pharynx where they then are moved to the gastrointestinal (GI) tract. The GI tract has several additional defenses against microparasitic invasion. First, the mucous membrane lining the GI tract makes attachment and entry difficult. In addition, viruses and bacteria can be destroyed by the hydrochloric acid present in the stomach. Moreover, other digestive secretions (e.g., saliva, which contains numerous hydrolytic enzymes, and the digestive enzymes of the stomach and small intestine) can have devastating effects on ingested viruses and bacteria. Furthermore, the normal bacterial flora of the large intestine (colon) tend to discourage viral invasion and

TABLE 12.1 Innate Defenses Against Microparasites

Category	Nature of Defense	Examples
Anatomical barrier	Provides physical barrier against direct penetration by virus or bacterium	Skin; mucous epithelium of respiratory, GI, and urogenital tracts
Cellular defense	Creates nonpermissiveness (passive)	Genetic incompatibility with infecting virus
	Displays phagocytosis (active)	Mφs; granulocytes
	Provides cytotoxicity (active)	Phagocytes; NK cells
Biochemical factors	Exert antimicrobial action	Lysozyme; IFNs
	Augment cellular defense	IFNs; ILs

bacterial colonization. For example, many coliforms can release antibiotic materials or serve as active competitors for nutrients.

Microparasitic invaders that penetrate the physical barriers are next confronted by nonspecific **cellular defenses.** Certain of these defenses are somewhat passive while the majority are active. For example, passive defense is offered to viruses that gain entry to a host only to encounter cells that are genetically nonpermissive. The cells are simply not susceptible to the intracellular infection by these viruses. Active cellular defense against microparasitic invaders is provided by *phagocytes* (macrophages [Mφs] and granulocytes) and by a subpopulation of lymphocytes known as *natural killer (NK) cells* (see chapter 8, Effectors of Nonspecific Cellular Immunity). For example, bacteria that have successfully gained access to body tissues and fluids can be confronted by phagocytic cells, which continually survey the body for foreign invading cells. Usually this is accompanied by an acute inflammatory response. Upon reaching the site of inflammation (where the bacteria are located), the phagocytes (e.g., polymorphonuclear neutrophils [PMNs]) can engulf, kill, and digest the bacteria. On the other hand, viral invasion might be countered by NK cells. Residing in the peripheral lymphoid organs, NK cells recognize virus-infected cells, bind to them, and subsequently lyse them. NK cytotoxic activity can be widespread since it is neither virus specific nor MHC restricted. Fungi are likely to be confronted by PMNs, Mφs, and NK cells.

The activity of *cellular defenses can be augmented and amplified by the participation of biochemical factors.* These factors include substances that can act directly on the invading microparasites and substances that act on the phagoctyes and NK cells to increase their effectiveness. Two substances, for example, that act against pathogens are lysozyme and interferon (IFN; see chapter 9). Both are directed against viruses. Lysozyme is an antimicrobial enzyme, which is present in many locations of the body, including the surface of the skin, tears, and nasal passages. It acts by chemically degrading the virus particles and bacteria. IFNs are host-coded proteins that are produced whenever viruses have escaped chemical destruction or phagocytosis, have invaded permissive host cells, and have initiated a lytic cycle (see also chapter 9, Effectors of Specific Cellular Immunity). Within hours after viral invasion, the levels of IFN-α (produced by leukocytes) and IFN-β (synthesized predominantly in fibroblasts) rise rapidly in infected tissues. IFN might act directly on virus-infected cells inhibiting virus production, on Mφs stimulating phagocytosis, or on NK cells activating cytotoxicity. In addition, exposure of noninfected host cells to IFN can provide protection against viral infection. Since IFN is relatively species specific (but not viral specific) once induced, it is capable of inhibiting the lytic cycle of the virus that stimulated its production. Moreover, it may inhibit any antigenic variants of the virus that might develop. However, induction of IFN using synthetic substances or administration of recombinant IFN prevents only certain viral infections. Thus, not all viral infections are equally sensitive to control by IFN alone. Potentiation of the actions of phagocytes and NK cells is achieved through cytokines, which include the IFNs (α, β, γ), interleukin 2 (IL-2), and tumor necrosis factor (TNF).

Innate immunity is critical to resisting microparasites; however, age also appears to play a role. Many viruses and bacteria produce mild or no disease in mature animals, while they produce severe disease in neonates and the aged. For example, studies with herpes simplex virus show an age-dependent variation in pathogenicity. This appears to be correlated with increased or decreased capability of Mϕs to effectively respond to the virus. In general, Mϕs and PMNs can collectively exert significant activity against microparasites in an immunocompetent host. Free viruses and bacteria are readily taken up and destroyed by phagocytes, especially when they are activated by lymphokines like IFN.

Acquired Immunity

In contrast to innate immunity, acquired immunity is **specific.** It is directed against a particular agent. Acquired immunity can be actively acquired, arising after exposure to an infective agent, or passively acquired by transfer of Abs against a particular infective agent.

Upon entering the body, bacteria, free virions, or virus-infected cells might be recognized by Mϕs, granulocytes, and NK cells as foreign. These cellular components of innate immunity do not distinguish one microparasite Ag from another, or even one microparasite from another. Nevertheless, they possess a recognition system that permits them to act spontaneously whenever they encounter free microparasites or parasitized cells. However, meaningful specific resistance to infection can only be acquired following exposure to specific Ags. While early nonspecific defenses are active, microparasitic Ags are being recognized specifically by Ag-reactive lymphocytes. These cells subsequently produce specific Abs and clones of specific T effector cells.

Acquired *specific immunity against viruses* is induced by viral Ags. Ags from different viruses, or even a single virus, exhibit varying degrees of immunogenicity. These can induce both specific humoral and specific cell-mediated immune responses. Viruses are antigenic mixtures, the complexity of which is determined largely by the number of virus-encoded proteins. The viral Ags that appear to be most immunogenic are the viral glycoproteins that are expressed on the surface of infected cells and on the surface of virus particles. Most Ags are dependent on T cell help for the induction of an Ab response by B cells (fig. 12.1), although some polymeric Ags are T independent and can activate B cells directly.

The mechanisms by which specific Abs and specific T cells might complement and enhance our innate *defenses against toxigenic and/or invasive pathogenic bacteria* are multifold. In this regard, responses can lead to the formation of antitoxin Abs that neutralize distinct poisonous substances produced by bacteria, for example, tetanus toxin responsible for tetanus (spasms of skeletal muscles) and botulinum toxin responsible for a fatal type of food poisoning. Unfortunately, our natural defenses are largely ineffective against these bacterial toxins, although there are basic polypeptides in serum that provide some protection. On the other hand, if the disease-causing agent is a bacterial cell, specific Abs also can be produced. These Abs can provide immunological protection in several ways. For example, they can bind to pathogenic bacteria and, in the presence of complement, cause bacterial cell lysis. The binding of specific Abs to bacteria can enhance opsonization of the cells by phagocytes. Abs can also agglutinate bacteria, permitting their clearance from tissues more rapidly. Specific T cells also contribute to the recruitment of phagocytes and the activation of Mϕs for more effective engulfment and destruction of bacteria.

Humoral Defenses Against Viruses

Humoral responses protect the host against viruses in several ways (table 12.2). One important antiviral mechanism is *virus neutralization.* Neutralizing Abs can be induced by whole viruses, single proteins, or small peptides. Induced neutralizing Abs, as well as passively transferred neutralizing Abs, have the ability to protect the host from virus infection. Since Abs cannot normally enter intact cells, they are ineffective against latent endogenous viruses or viruses that are spread from one cell to another through intracellular bridges. IgG, IgM, IgA (and probably IgE) might be capable of

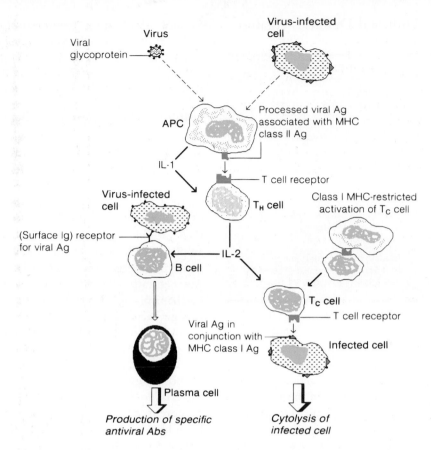

FIGURE 12.1 Stimulation of T-dependent immune responses to viral Ags. Viral Ags, whether on a virus or expressed by virus-infected cells, can provoke T-dependent immune responses. Processing and presentation of Ag to T_H cells by APCs leads to their activation. This is promoted with the aid of IL-1 produced by APCs. In turn, acti-vated T_H cells release IL-2, which promotes the proliferation (clonal expansion) of T_C cells and B cells that have specific receptors for the same viral Ags. This then leads to cytolysis of virus-infected cells or the production of specific Abs against viral Ags.

specifically neutralizing free virions that are spread from one cell to another by other means. IgM and IgG are the major classes of Ab responsible for virus neutralization in serum. IgA neutralizes virus on mucosal surfaces, where it prevents virus binding to the mucosa. In contrast to IgG, IgA does not recruit phagocytic cells or complement. IgE usually binds to mast cells and, with Ag, can cause the release of inflammatory mediators. IgE is probably made in response to virus Ags, but it is not clear whether its actions account for any of the clinical complications produced by virus infection. In addition, some Abs might cover viral coat proteins that normally interact with cell receptors. This type of binding would prevent viral attachment and penetration of host cells. Recently, monoclonal neutralizing-Abs have been used to map functional epitopes of infectious agents or synthetic peptides. This has enabled protective epitopes to be distinguished from those that are resistant to neutralization. Variation by viruses of neutralization-sensitive epitopes can lead to persistent infection.

Complexing of viruses with IgG can also produce viral aggregates, forming readily phagocytized complexes. *Complement* can enhance the neutralization of viruses by Ab. This is achieved by increasing the size of the virus-Ab complex and by producing and incorporating C3b into complexes that can then bind to C3b receptors on phagocytic cells. Abs and complement thus

TABLE 12.2 Humoral Defenses Against Viruses

Mechanism	Means of Expression
Neutralization	Binding of Ig to virus, blocking spread of virus to other cells (e.g., interference with binding or inhibition of penetration of host target cell)
Opsonization	Formation of viral aggregates and incorporation of C3b, leading to enhanced engulfment by phagocytes
Complement-mediated lysis	Direct lysis of virus by Ab and complement; cytolysis by means of properdin pathway
ADCC	Binding of Ab-coated infected cell to FcRs of nonspecific effector cell, leading to cytolysis

can act as opsonins by coating extracellular viruses, thereby permitting the particles to be more effectively phagocytosed. Ab and complement can also directly lyse enveloped viruses. In addition, complement alone can inactivate certain viruses directly in the absence of Ab. In a retrovirus infection, one of the viral proteins can act as a receptor for Clq. In Sindbis virus infections, the alternative complement pathway is activated, leading to inactivation of the virus, independent of Ab. Furthermore, infected cells displaying viral Ags on their surfaces can be lysed by specific Abs capable of fixing complement. Although lysis is by the classical complement pathway, it is dependent on the activation of the alternate pathway, which is required to amplify the signal to significantly damage the cell membrane.

Another important humoral defense mechanism involves coating of virus-infected cells with Ab, thereby marking them for destruction by nonspecific cytotoxic cells, mainly killer (K) and NK cells by *Ab-dependent cellular cytotoxicity (ADCC)*. K and NK cells possess Fc receptors (FcRs) that can bind to the exposed Fc region of the membrane-attached Ab. The amount of bound IgG required to trigger ADCC reactions is much less than that required to provoke a complement-dependent Ab-mediated lysis.

Not all Ab-mediated reactions specific for viral Ags are helpful, however. Antigenic modulation is an example of a harmful repercussion. Ab can react with cells carrying viral Ags to effect their removal from the cell surface. Since these antigenically modulated cells cannot be recognized as infected, they might escape destruction by specific cytotoxic T (T_C) cells.

Humoral Defenses Against Bacteria

Several humoral immune mechanisms are set in motion when bacteria invade the body. Specific B cells are activated to clone and differentiate into Ab-producing plasma cells. The Abs can then bind to the foreign cell surface and activate (1) phagocytes, (2) NK cells, and (3) the complement cascade. Alternatively, some Abs (IgA) inhibit attachment to host cell surfaces: for example, Ab to fimbriae and capsules can block attachment of bacteria to the host cell membrane. Yet other Abs neutralize the actions of bacterial toxins. These mechanisms contribute to the concerted elimination of foreign bacteria from the body and reduce or prevent the expression of clinical symptoms of disease.

Virulence of many pathogenic bacteria is related, in part, to their ability to escape phagocytosis. It has been suggested that the cell surfaces of nonvirulent bacteria do not readily absorb water. Consequently, they are more susceptible to phagocytosis than are virulent bacteria which have hydrophilic surfaces. In addition, some strains of virulent bacteria secrete antiphagocytic materials. The humoral immune response enhances both the mechanism and the specificity of the phagocytic response. Abs directed against surface Ags of bacteria might neutralize antiphagocytic substances or bind directly to the capsule or cell wall of the nonencapsulated forms. Specifically bound Ab can then bind and activate complement. Through this specific interaction, bacteria become opsonized and can be more readily phagocytosed. Ultimately, almost all pathogenic bacteria are controlled by phagocytes, which can be activated by a variety of microparasitic products including endotoxins, muramyl dipeptides, and carbohydrate polymers.

Some Abs can induce complement-dependent lysis of gram-negative bacteria, which are responsible for diseases such as gonorrhea (*Neisseria gonorrhoeae*), dysentery (*Shigella dysenteriae*), and cholera (*Vibrio cholerae*). Gram-negative endotoxins can also activate the alternative complement pathway, causing lysis of bacteria in the absence of Abs. As such, this mechanism represents a component of innate immunity.

In contrast, secretory IgA serves in many instances to protect epithelial surfaces from microbial invasion. IgA does not fix complement, lyse cells, or enhance phagocytosis. However, it seems to prevent binding of invasive and noninvasive bacteria to host cell membranes. Some bacteria have evolved the ability to resist IgA blocking. These bacteria produce enzymes that are capable of degrading IgA.

A variety of bacterial toxins can be neutralized by Abs that exhibit antitoxin activity. In these instances, protection from disease rests almost exclusively with the presence of these neutralizing Abs. In the case of tetanus, pathogenicity comes less from the bacteria, *Clostridium tetani,* than from the toxin it produces. The tetanus toxin is a potent spasmogen, which produces the symptoms associated with the disease. Neutralization of the toxin is essential to preventing the exotoxin from reaching its target cells. Abs can also neutralize bacterial products that inhibit phagocytosis (e.g., M-proteins) or promote their penetration into tissues (e.g., hyaluronidase produced by *C. perfringens*).

Humoral Defenses Against Fungi

Fungi are not usually very invasive pathogens in the normal human host. Humoral reactions against fungi are **nonspecific** and, to a certain extent, nonimmunological. These defenses occur in the form of serum agglutinins (causing clumping), serum inhibitors of fungal growth, and opsonins. Opsonins, in fact, play a more prominent role by interfacing with phagocytes in nonspecific cell-mediated immune responses. Furthermore, specific Ab production does not appear to be significantly stimulated in response to most fungal infections.

Cell-Mediated Responses Against Viruses

Virus-infected cells displaying new surface Ags can stimulate the formation of specific T_C and **delayed-type hypersensitivity (T_D) lymphocytes.** There is ample evidence to support a critical role for T lymphocytes in the control of viral infections. *Cytolysis* of virus-infected cells by T_C cells has been demonstrated in both acute and persistent virus infections. Humans who are immunodeficient, with respect to cell-mediated immunity, appear to be considerably more vulnerable to virus diseases than those deficient in humoral immunity. T effector cells recognize specific viral Ags in association with self-Ags of the MHC, displayed on the virus-infected cell. T_C cells, therefore, must possess receptors for both viral Ag and self class I Ag of the MHC for it to interact with and destroy the virus-infected cell. T_D cells are also MHC restricted. After interaction with the Ag, T_D and T_C clones are expanded and become part of the resulting adaptive immunity. Consequently, large numbers of virus-specific cells, including T memory cells, are acquired following clinical (and subclinical) exposure to viral infections and following immunization with viral vaccines.

Clones of T_D and **T helper (T_H)** cells, which emerge in response to viral Ags, can produce a host of lymphokines that recruit and regulate both specific and nonspecific effector cells. For example, sensitized T_D cells produce lymphokines that are responsible for the recruitment and activation of Mϕs. **Mϕs** play a major role in the response to delayed-type hypersensitivity reactions and, once activated, show increased phagocytic activity and an enhanced ability to kill virus-infected cells. Although spontaneous nonspecific cytotoxicity, mediated by NK cells, is a component of innate immunity, NK activity also can be enhanced during T cell responses to viral Ags. This occurs as a result of the formation and release of immune response modifiers like IL-2 and IFN-γ. Specifically generated Abs, resulting from a humoral response, can also promote nonspecific cell-mediated activity in the form of ADCC reactions from K cells, which results in a cell-to-cell contact killing of infected cells.

Activation of T_H cells also leads to an augmentation of Ag-specific humoral responses against the viruses or virus-infected cells. This is accomplished through the action of cytokines, including ILs, IFNs, and TNFs.

Cell-Mediated Responses Against Bacteria

T lymphocytes play a crucial role in the host response to bacteria, especially in those that are capable of replicating within host cells, such as phagocytes. During the induction of immunity against bacteria, **Mϕs** not only engulf bacteria, they also process and present Ag to specific clones of T cells that are capable of responding to Ag. Ag-activated T cells can interact with mononuclear phagocytes to enhance cellular resistance to bacterial infection. Lymphokines, such as Mϕ-activating factor (MAF) and chemotactic factor (CTF), that are produced by T_D cells increase Mϕ efficiency in engulfing and killing bacteria. In addition, activated Mϕs spread out more extensively, exhibit more surface receptors, and are biochemically more active than unstimulated phagocytes. For example, there is increased lysosomal enzyme activity inside and outside the Mϕ at the tissue site. Although these phagocytes are induced by specifically activated T_D cells, they can act nonspecifically against potential target bacteria. Thus, animals infected by one type of bacterium might become more resistant against a second unrelated species because of the activated Mϕs present. Activated Mϕs, derived from a specific cell-mediated response, can complement a humoral response. In this instance, Ab-coated bacteria can be selectively destroyed. This occurs in granulomatous leprosy and tuberculosis, two infections produced by mycobacteria (*Mycobacterium leprae* and *M. tuberculosis,* respectively).

Protection against intracellular bacteria can also be provided through target cell lysis by T_C cells. For example, Kaplan and colleagues found that local application of recombinant IL-2 to skin lesions of individuals with leprosy induced a marked influx of CD4+ and CD8+ cells. This was followed by destruction of local tissue Mϕs. Killing of Mϕs primed with mycobacterial Ags was predominantly a function of class II MHC-restricted CD4+ T cells (presumably T_C cells). However, CD8+ T cells and NK cells might also have participated. Destruction of host cells, which harbor bacteria that they are unable to eliminate, is a significant mechanism for host protection.

Although T cells usually respond to Ag-specific activation, *broad T cell activation* can occur. For example, polyclonal Ags (e.g., mitogens like concanavalin A and phytohemagglutinin) can stimulate almost all T cells. Some bacterial toxins can apparently behave somewhat like mitogens. On the other hand, some Ags are broadly conserved, and are comprised of some epitopes that are shared by a variety of microparasites (and often self-components). T cells with specificity for these shared determinants have the potential to recognize a whole spectrum of infectious agents. For example, toxic shock syndrome toxin, produced by *Staphylococcus aureus,* stimulates most, but not all, human T lymphocytes. Thus, this toxin acts as polyclonal T cell activator or "super-Ag." Super-Ags are not only found in the *staphylococci,* but in certain other bacteria as well. Broad T cell activation can contribute to pathogenicity by promoting secretion of high levels of TNF. Although TNF contributes to normal immune response to Ag at physiologic levels, it might exhibit harmful effects as a mediator of circulatory collapse and widespread tissue necrosis at higher levels.

Cell-Mediated Responses Against Fungi

Immune responses against fungi appear to be principally cell mediated. This is suggested by the high incidence with which granulomatous reactions occur in association with fungal infections. In addition, delayed-type hypersensitivity reactions are common in mycoses. In these reactions, T_D (CD4+) **cells** and activated **Mϕs** clearly play significant roles. Moreover, recent studies with an animal model for histoplasmosis suggest a role of T cells that are reactive to fungal Ags. For example, mice treated with monoclonal Ab (MAb) against L3T4 (equivalent to CD4+) cells did not not clear *Histoplasma capsulatum* from their spleens as well as control animals did. Presumably, T cells that are reactive to *H. capsulatum* produce IFN-γ, which, in turn, activates Mϕs to restrict the intracellular growth of the yeast cells. In general, the immune responses against fungi are similar to those induced by mycobacteria.

HOW MICROPARASITES OVERCOME THE BODY'S DEFENSES

Acquired host defense against a particular virus or bacterium depends upon the development of T and B memory cells and quantities of Abs that can recognize and interact with specific viral or bacterial Ags. In order to successfully infect a previously immunized host, a microbial pathogen must either escape detection by the host's immune system or in some way incapacitate it. Several mechanisms have been devised by viruses and bacteria to achieve these objectives (table 12.3).

Fungal Infections in AIDS: Taking Advantage of a Weak Host

Most fungi, the yeasts and molds, found in nature are usually *harmless opportunistic* flora in immunocompetent individuals. When fungal infections (mycoses) occur, such as athlete's foot or thrush, it is usually more of a nuisance than a serious pathological event. In those instances when fungi cause serious infections, it is usually associated with depressed immune reactivity, in particular, depression of delayed-type hypersensitivity. It is, therefore, not surprising that individuals with AIDS (where T_H function is impaired) are candidates for certain serious mycoses.

The most common fungal infections encountered in AIDS patients are caused by the yeast *Candida albicans*. Although candidoses can produce painful oral thrush and extend to the esophagus, they rarely become systemic and are not usually fatal. On the other hand, cryptococcoses (caused by the yeast *Cryptococcus*) can arise in the respiratory tract and spread to the brain. There they can cause a severe meningitis, which is very resistant to chemotherapy and is often fatal. A third class of fungal infection frequently seen in AIDS patients is histoplasmosis, caused by *Histoplasma*. This fungus enters the body by way of the respiratory tract and can rapidly spread to the liver, spleen, GI tract, and brain. *Histoplasma* organisms can usually be kept in abeyance with the antibiotic amphotericin B. However, chronic use of this antibiotic can produce debilitating side effects. Thus,

treatment of AIDS patients with fungal disease is difficult. In addition, treatment with antibiotics controls certain opportunistic mycoses only temporarily; they do not prevent the development of other AIDS-related illnesses.

These mycoses ordinarily are prevented by active cell-mediated mechanisms mediated by nonspecific effectors (e.g., macrophages and NK cells) and T_D cells. In AIDS, amplification of these defenses is prevented. The primary targets of the AIDS virus (human immunodeficiency virus-I, HIV-I) are T cells expressing CD4 Ag. These are mostly T_H and T_D cells. Viral infection of T_D cells directly impairs response against fungi. In addition, viral infection of T_H cells removes the usual means for amplifying immune responses, the production of IL-2 and other lymphokines. As a consequence, immunological defenses against fungi become limited to the nonspecific cellular immune responses. These are further compromised by being deprived of amplification signals normally provided by Ag-specific T_H and T_D cells.

Although many of the mycoses are not life threatening, unless disseminated systemically, the sudden appearance or worsening of fungal infections in individuals with AIDS is often seen as a sign of rapidly declining immune competence. Thus, the course of a fungal infection can be used as a barometer for this unrelenting progressive disease.

Wetherbee, R. E. Infections in AIDS. *Laboratory Medicine* **17**:679, 1986.

TABLE 12.3 Means of Escaping Immunological Destruction Used by Microparasites

Category	Mechanism	Description
Evasion	Antigenic drift	Alters antigenic nature of microorganism
	Antigenic modulation	Modifies or masks Ag expression on infected cell
Immune suppression	Cellular immunity	Cripples specific effector cells (e.g., T_H cells or Mϕs); stimulates T_S cells
	Humoral immunity	Destroys Igs
Subversion	Ag-related damage	Causes immune-complex formation
	Autoimmunity	Induces Ab formation against host tissues

Survival of a pathogenic microorganism can be achieved by duping the immune system into believing that no defense is needed. Alternatively, a slower and less aggressive response results if the immune system can be made to accept the invading organism as a newcomer. If the microparasite entering the body has changed antigenically from the initial immunizing Ag, it may not be recognized and might thereby escape from T cell and Ab attack. One class of strategy is **evasion.** Viruses and bacteria display antigenic drift, or variation. Through this mechanism viruses, or bacteria, modify their exposed antigenic determinants over the course of time. This can give rise to new, or variant, strains of pathogenic microbes. These newly evolved strains might be able to parasitize the presumably immune host. The constantly changing strains of influenza virus provide excellent examples of this mechanism in action. A related stratagem employed by viruses is known as *antigenic modulation.* When executed, this mechanism leads to the removal of surface Ags from the infected cells. This enables the infected cells to escape destruction, since they are no longer recognized as foreign, or defective. Binding of Ab to measles virus glycoproteins that are located on the surface of infected cells can modulate the expression of viral proteins. This can lead to shedding of virus Ag-Ab complexes from the cell surface and depression of intracellular synthesis of specific viral proteins.

An alternative means of prolonging survival in the host is to **reduce the host's response.** This can be accomplished in several ways. For example, viruses might destroy primary or secondary lymphoid tissues, causing *immune suppression.* Particular immune cells (e.g., T_H cells) might be destroyed, thereby crippling the immune response. This is the mechanism used by Epstein-Barr virus (EBV), measles virus, and HIV-1, which gives rise to acquired immune deficiency syndrome (AIDS). Viruses can also promote the formation and release of immunosuppressive proteins that might alter the membranes of cells of the immune system. Certain reoviruses produce a gene product, a specific viral capsid protein (σ-l), which is capable of inducing the expression of suppressor T (T_S) cells, which then might play a role in allowing the virus to overcome the body's defenses. In addition, some bacteria (e.g., coliform bacteria, staphylococci, mycobacteria, vib-rios, and treponemes) are capable of secreting factors that *suppress phagocytosis.* Other bacteria produce enzymes that cleave Ig molecules such as IgA. Furthermore, fungi employ immunosuppressive mechanisms as well. For example, intravenous injection of cryptococcal Ags induced Ag-specific T_S cells, which inhibited cell-mediated immune responses in a murine model.

A third method used by microparasites involves a **subversion of the host's immune responses.** Response to certain viruses (e.g., hepatitis B virus) can *produce circulating immune complexes,* which are capable of damaging host tissues. In mice, chronic infection by lymphocytic choriomeningitis virus can lead to the formation of circulating immune complexes of virus and antiviral Ab. In turn, this produces an inflammatory reaction, immune-complex glomerulonephritis, with ensuing kidney damage. Moreover, viruses and bacteria can cause further debilitation by stimulating destructive autoimmune reactions. For example, certain reovirus infections are responsible for the development of auto-Abs that react with Ags in the anterior pituitary gland and pancreas, causing endocrine disorders. Although these reactions might arise as natural consequences of microbial infection, they, nevertheless, interfere with eradication of the infectious agent and cause damage to host tissues.

RESISTANCE TO PROTISTAN AND ANIMAL PARASITES

While viruses, bacteria, and fungi produce acute disease states, protozoan and animal parasites **produce chronic disease states.** Rather than measuring the time of infection in days or weeks, these parasitic infections may extend for months or even years. Thus, interactions between the infectious agent and the immune system are likely to differ from those involving bacteria, viruses, and fungi. Since protozoan and animal parasites usually establish long-term relationships with their hosts, *damage to the host must be limited and the host's defenses must be eluded.* Successful parasites accomplish both of these objectives.

There is a broad spectrum of effects associated with protistan and animal parasitic infection (table 12.4; fig. 12.2). Some of these are directly associated with

TABLE 12.4 Pathological Consequences of Infection by Protistan and Animal Parasites

Pathological Feature	Method of Expression	Examples
Mechanical tissue damage or destruction	Physical obstruction of anatomical sites, with loss of function	Obstruction of intestinal lumen by worms (e.g., *Ascaris*)
Loss of essential nutrients	Competition by parasite, leading to host deprivation	Depletion of vitamin B$_{12}$ by tapeworms (e.g., *Diphyllobothrium latum*)
Tissue damage (direct)	Release of proteolytic enzyme that digests host tissues	Actions of protozoa invading host tissues (e.g., *Entamoeba histolytica*)
Tissue damage (indirect)	Reactions to parasites and their excretions that evoke immunological reactions with secondary damage to host tissues	Inflammatory and granulomatous responses to *Leishmania;* formation of immune complexes with Ags of *Schistosoma*
Secondary infections	Irritative actions of parasite attachment, allowing opportunistic infection by bacteria	

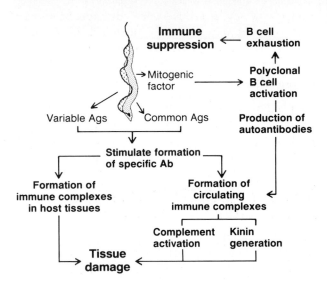

FIGURE 12.2 Some effects on a host of confrontation by animal parasites. Animal parasites (e.g., trypanosomes) can produce pathological changes in their hosts. Two important effects are tissue damage and immune suppression. Both effects can be generated as a consequence of immune responses to parasite Ags or parasite products (e.g., mitogenic factors).

the parasites or their products. Others are consequences of reactions on the part of the host that the parasites provoke. The nature and extent of these pathological effects is determined by the parasite's habits (its site and mode of infection) and the parasitic load (number of invading parasites and progeny).

Innate Defenses

Natural, or innate, mechanisms of resistance to protistan and animal parasites, whether they are protozoan (unicellular) or metazoan (multicellular), are *similar,* in principle, *to those employed against viruses, bacteria, and fungi.* Some are nonimmunological, while others comprise part of the host's immunological defense (table 12.5). The nonimmunological factors might present a **physical barrier** or create an **inhospitable environment** that discourages invasion by certain parasites, for example, the presence of sickle cell trait or absence of Duffy Ag. Individuals possessing sickle cell trait (the heterozygous occurrence of alleles for sickle cell anemia, hemoglobin S [HbS]) display a reduced susceptibility to malaria. In these individuals, Hb tends to more readily deform and crystallize. This causes mechanical distortion that can destroy intracellular malarial parasites. In contrast, the Duffy Ag is believed to be a molecule necessary for parasite attachment to host cells. Its absence, therefore, reduces the incidence of successful association between an infecting parasite and host cells. However, these defenses are not effective against all parasites, nor are they effective in all instances against particular parasites. For example, the skin provides a barrier that is effective against bacterial penetration; however, many successful protistan and animal parasites have developed means of defeating this barrier. For example, malarial

TABLE 12.5 Host Defenses Against Protistan and Animal Parasites

Defense	Mode of Expression
Nonimmunological	
Mechanical barrier	Physical impediment to parasitic entry (e.g., skin)
Genetic status	Presence of factor (e.g., HbS) or absence of trait (e.g., Duffy Ag) that creates conditions unfavorable for infection or parasite survival
Filtration	Action of spleen in monitoring erythrocytes, leading to preferential elimination of those harboring intracellular parasites
Immunological	
Nonspecific	Defensive responses triggered by parasites, leading to their cytotoxic removal
Cellular	Reactions involving participation of phagocytes (Mϕs and granulocytes) or NK cells
Humoral	Ab-independent complement activation
Specific	Defensive responses triggered against specific parasite Ags, leading to elimination of parasites and acquired immunity
Cellular	T_C-, T_D-mediated cytotoxicity; T_H stimulation of humoral responses
Humoral	Specific Ab against parasite Ags

parasites use an insect vector, while schistosomes have evolved mechanisms for actively penetrating the skin.

Other host defenses are more active. These include several nonspecific and specific responses to parasites. The **nonspecific immunological defenses** are similar to those employed against bacteria, viruses, and fungi. This includes direct cellular responses by *Mϕs and granulocytes (neutrophils, eosinophils, basophils) and NK cells.* In addition, a humoral component is provided through the *alternate complement pathway,* which is Ab independent.

These defenses, on occasion, may be frustrated by particular parasites. For example, certain protozoan parasites, such as *Leishmania,* actually infect Mϕs. They are completely dependent upon Mϕs, where they thrive in the phagolysosomes. However, this does not mean that a potential mammalian host is defenseless against infection by *Leishmania.* Although this parasite specifically infects Mϕs, not all Mϕs are equally susceptible to attack. Nonstimulated Mϕs are more likely to fall victim to leishmanial parasites, whereas Mϕs activated by lymphokines display increased resistance.

Acquired Immunity

An infected host will mount **specific** responses against invading protistan and animal parasites. The response can be *antiparasite, antidisease, or both.* For example, an effective response might provide protection against the parasite itself or against parasite toxins that cause disease. These responses are triggered by exposure to specific parasite Ags. Since parasites usually cause chronic infections, there is often persistent Ag stimulation due to circulating Ags and immune complexes. B and T cell activation occurs giving rise to **Abs** and **effector T cells** directed against particular parasite Ags. Moreover, **memory B** and **T cells** are produced. They are *responsible for specific, acquired immunity.* Unfortunately, acquired immunity is largely ineffective in protecting the host against recurrent infection by most parasites, for reasons to be explored below. This is not always the case, however. For example, immunity to amebiasis and toxoplasmosis after recovery seems fairly complete. One study of individuals cured of amebiasis found a reinfection rate of only 0.29% in 1,021 cases over a five-year period. Moreover, an immunity of sorts is sometimes derived as a result of an ongoing infection. In schistosomiasis, the presence of surviving adults in a host can protect against reinfection. However, this may be a consequence of adaptive mechanisms employed by the schistosomes rather than effective immunity on the part of the infected host.

Stimulation of specific responses is highly variable. Extracellular parasites (and the extracellular stages of parasite life cycles) are more likely to be encountered by cells of the immune system. These would be expected, therefore, to provoke cell-mediated and humoral immunological attack. They are also more likely to encounter Ab than intracellular parasites, since Ab does not enter cells directly (although it may be pinocytosed). On the other hand, intracellular parasites may provoke, and be subject to, cell-mediated immunity by antigenic modification of host cells. In contrast, parasites that lack a tissue stage may escape detection by the host's immune system. These organisms might not stimulate any response whatsoever, despite their ability to produce copious amounts of foreign Ag.

Humoral Responses to Protistan and Animal Parasites

Protistan and animal parasites stimulate the production of Abs, especially IgG, IgM, and IgE. Infection by protozoan parasites is associated with increased production of IgG and IgM, predominantly. However, intestinal protozoan parasites (e.g., *Entamoeba* and *Giardia*) might induce production of IgA. In contrast, helminthic parasites stimulate the production of IgE much more strongly than other Ig classes.

The **Abs** produced may provide protection through several mechanisms (table 12.6). For example, binding of Ab to the surfaces of protozoan parasites can *block invasion of host cells.* Alternatively, Ab binding to parasite surfaces might *opsonize the parasites, cause their agglutination, or mark them for ADCC.* All of these mechanisms are readily displayed against blood parasites (e.g., trypanosomes, toxoplasmas, and plasmodia). For example, Abs against merozoites of *Plasmodium* are able to block penetration into host erythrocytes. In addition, agglutination of blood parasites, when it occurs,

TABLE 12.6 Humoral Defenses Against Protistan and Animal Parasites

Physical interference	Binds to parasite surface, blocking attachment to host cells (used against protozoa)
	Obstructs oral or genital orifices; deprives parasites of nutrients or impairs reproduction (used against helminths)
Agglutination	Increases clearance of parasites from blood (used against protozoa)
Opsonization	Increases phagocytosis of parasites coated with Ab and complement (used against protozoa)
Cytotoxicity	Enhances complement-mediated cytolysis (used against protozoa)
	Promotes ADCC (used against protozoa and helminths)
Neutralization	Binds to toxins or enzymes, preventing them from damaging host tissues (used against protozoan and helminthic products)

is frequently accomplished by IgM. Abs also contribute to ADCC and complement-mediated lysis of protozoa (e.g., trypanosomes) and certain helminths (e.g., *Trichinella, Filaria,* and *Schistosoma*). Through their FcRs and complement receptors, cytotoxic cells such as Mφs, neutrophils, and eosinophils adhere to worms coated with Ab. Schistosome larvae can be damaged and killed by degranulating eosinophils that adhere to the IgG-coated worms. The increased number of eosinophils (eosinophilia) in worm infections appears to be T cell dependent.

In addition, Abs have been found to interfere with the functioning of worms in somewhat unexpected ways. Abs can impair feeding and reproduction of worms by blocking particular orifices (oral and genital). This limits the extent of the infection by either destroying the worms (through starvation) or curtailing their ability to reproduce. Moreover, Abs provide protection by binding to and neutralizing products of parasites. These products include toxins and enzymes released by the parasites that are potentially harmful to the host organism. Since these toxic products contribute to the manifested infectious disease, neutralizing Abs may prevent disease even though the parasites are not eliminated.

Some protozoan Ags are T independent and, at appropriate concentrations, are mitogenic. The Ags can induce nonspecific polyclonal activation of B and T cells. Not only are these responses ineffective at counteracting the parasite responsible, they can be actually harmful to the host. B cell exhaustion and production of auto-Abs are among the consequences of nonspecific polyclonal B cell activation. Polyclonal activation of T cells might produce autoreactive T_C cells or lead to immune suppression (by activation of T_S cells). Helminthic parasites, through their promotion of IgE production, can induce Type I hypersensitivity reactions (anaphylaxis [see chapter 13, Hypersensitivity]). Moreover, IgE-mediated reactions can induce physical expulsion of helminths from the gut through these reactions. Specifically, sensitized mast cells that are coated with IgE, in response to Ags from parasitic worms, can be induced to release vasoactive amines. These substances increase vascular permeability which, in turn, increases fluid flow into the lumen of the gut. In addition, these same substances can trigger vigorous spasmodic contraction of the smooth muscle of the digestive tract. The combination of increased lubrication and sudden, violent contraction is occasionally sufficient to dislodge infecting nematodes, which can then be expelled from the host.

Cell-Mediated Responses to Protistan and Animal Parasites

Dependence upon cell-mediated immune responses for counteracting protozoan infections can be demonstrated using nude (athymic) mice. These animals display a reduced capacity to control trypanosome and malaria infections. The type of T cells involved, and the nature of their participation in protection, appears to differ with the nature of the infection.

Recently, it was shown that T_C cells are important for protection against protozoa, although it is not clear how they mediate this protection. For ex-

ample, T_C cells from mice immunized against *Toxoplasma* have been shown to be capable of directly lysing these parasites. These cells might also control toxoplasmosis by the production of lymphokines which subsequently activate Mϕs. T_C cells are also important in resistance to leishmaniasis and malaria. In addition, T_H and T_D cells play central roles through their recruitment and activation of nonspecific cytotoxic cells (phagocytes and NK cells) and by augmentation of humoral responses. For example, cytokine-activated Mϕs display much more active and efficient responses to several blood parasites, including trypanosomes, leishmanias, toxoplasmas, and plasmodia. Moreover, evidence has emerged that suggests that some genes responsible for defense against animal parasites segregate independently of the MHC; that is, they are not part of the MHC, but lie outside it. Furthermore, these appear to be genes that regulate expression of Mϕ/monocyte responses. For example, certain of these genes encode enzymes involved in cell killing (e.g., superoxide dismutase and peroxidase).

On the other hand, cell-mediated immune *responses to helminths probably are induced more by their secretions and excretions* than by surface Ags. As with protozoan parasites, T_C cells may be less pivotal to host defense than T_H and T_D cells. Nevertheless, there is evidence of direct T_C cytotoxicity directed against the migrating larvae of some helminths. In addition, helminths are more likely to produce inflammatory reactions. This arises from two sources. On the one hand, release of IL-1 by activated Mϕs can induce the liver to produce acute-phase proteins. Certain of these proteins (e.g., C-reactive protein) can stimulate complement with the subsequent release of vasoactive products. These increase vascular permeability locally and promote the influx of additional effector cells. On the other hand, inflammatory responses are provoked through the action of IgE on basophils and mast cells. This prompts release of vasoactive substances that similarly alter vascular permeability, and induce further leukocyte immigration. However, this second mechanism can also produce other symptoms of anaphylaxis.

In the case of helminthic infections, eosinophils are perhaps the most significant effector cells that are attracted to the site of inflammation. They are

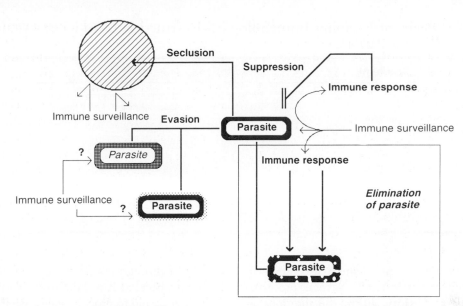

FIGURE 12.3 Interactions between animal parasites and host immune surveillance systems. Parasites can interact with the immune surveillance systems of their hosts in ways that ensure their survival. These include *anatomical seclusion* that reduces or prevents their detection, *evasion* by presenting Ags that confuse the immune surveillance mechanisms about their true identity (e.g., antigenic variation, Ag masking, or by *suppression* of immune responses). However, when these strategems fail, *elimination* of the parasite is likely to occur.

drawn to this area by chemotactic factors derived from worm Ags or from IgE-activated mast cells. Eosinophils can attach to IgE-coated worms through their FcRs. Their subsequent degranulation releases products that are toxic to the parasites. The elevated plasma IgE levels accompanied by eosinophilia, characteristic of helminthic infections, appear to be regulated by T cells. This is supported by the absence of these features following helminthic infection of mice that are depleted of T cells. In addition, recent evidence shows that the T_{H2} cell products, IL-4 and IL-5, can regulate respectively IgE and eosinophil production.

Further consequences of inflammatory reactions to parasitic infections give rise to the formation of fibrous tissue or granulomas. These are not restricted to worms, but rather can arise during the eradication of any protozoan or metazoan parasite that infects host tissues. For example, in response to *Leishmania* or to schistosome eggs, phagocytes endeavor to isolate, or wall off, the parasite. The lymphokines released during the inflammatory reaction stimulate not only Mϕs but also local fibroblasts. This leads to the deposition of extracellular fibrous materials in the affected area. Although this response does not restore normal tissue integrity, it reflects successful elimination of the parasite from that area.

HOW PROTISTAN AND ANIMAL PARASITES ELUDE IMMUNOLOGICAL ATTACK

Protistan and animal parasites must effectively evade or thwart a host's defenses if they are to survive, and thrive, at the host's expense (fig. 12.3). In chapter 11, we reviewed several characteristics and life-styles of animal parasites. In the foregoing discussion, we identified the ways in which the host responds to the presence of detected parasites. What, then, are the means that protistan and animal parasites use to limit these responses and better ensure their survival? Protistan and animal parasites make use of the similar basic devices that serve viruses, bacteria, and fungi well (table 12.7). This includes evasion, suppression, and subversion. However, to these, protistan and animal parasites add a personal touch—anatomical seclusion.

The first approach against immunological attack is to remain hidden. Protistan and animal parasites attempt to accomplish this in two principal ways.

TABLE 12.7 Means of Escaping Immunological Destruction Used by Protistan and Animal Parasites

Category	Mechanism	Description
Seclusion	Inaccessible parasite	Parasite enters host cells or anatomical site that removes it from exposure to immune surveillance
Evasion	Antigenic variation	Antigenic identity of parasite is altered
	Antigenic masking	Host proteins are attached to parasite's surface to mask it
Suppression	Cellular immunity	Specific effector cells (e.g., Mφs) are crippled; T_s cells are stimulated
	Humoral immunity	Ags are shed (leading to Ab depletion; immune-complex formation); destruction of Igs, polyclonal expansion, and B cell exhaustion
Subversion	Autoimmunity	Ab formation is induced against host tissues

One way is to seek an anatomical site that is removed from immunological surveillance. Several protozoa seek **anatomical seclusion** within the interiors of cells. For *Plasmodium* these are erythrocytes, while *Leishmania* prefer Mφs. Toxoplasmas are less selective in the cells that they infect. In addition, they are believed to be able to affect nonphagocytic cells by some undefined mechanism that compels these cells to engulf them. With their intracellular habitat they avoid the effects of Ab. Many (e.g., *Leishmania*) have also learned to avoid intracellular killing by oxygen metabolites and lysosomal enzymes. Helminths, which are multicellular, cannot infect individual cells. They nevertheless achieve anatomical seclusion by encystment (e.g., *T. spiralis*) or by taking up residence in the lumina of ducts (e.g., *Fasciola hepatica* in the bile duct) or of major organs (e.g., *Taenia* spp. in the intestinal lumen).

Alternatively, parasites seek to **evade detection** by confusing or duping the host's immune system. The primary means of evading specific recognition are *antigenic variation* and *Ag masking*. Some parasites, like trypanosomes and plasmodia, exploit antigenic variation very successfully. Trypanosomes can change the antigenic nature of their surface coats. By presenting novel Ags throughout their lives, these protozoa thus confront the immune system as "new" infective agents repeatedly. This mechanism is used by Old World (African) trypanosomes, which have been shown to display more than 100 antigenic coats, but does not seem to be exploited by New World (American) trypanosomes, such as *T. cruzi*. Plasmodia, on the other

hand, pass through several discrete development stages, each with peculiar Ags. Moreover, plasmodia recently have been found to produce stage-specific classes of ribosomes; however, the significance of this variation to infectivity and parasite survival is obscure. Certain helminths also modify their surface Ags. For example, *Trichinella* undergoes five molts during its migration, changing its surface identity at each molt. As a result, each new stage of the life cycle is perceived by the host as a new infective challenge. Consequently, these strategies prevent the host's Ag-specific defenses against Ags that were seen earlier from being called into play against the parasites.

In contrast to undergoing antigenic variation, some parasites (e.g., trypanosomes and schistosomes) *adsorb host proteins* to their surfaces. These proteins confer on the parasite a bizarre pseudo-self-identity that masks their true antigenic nature and enables them to evade immunological attack. In addition, certain other parasites retain a surface coating, or glycocalyx, that blocks direct exposure of its surface Ags. This device is used by members of the genus *Fasciola*. In yet other instances, the surface Ags are shed by the parasite into the circulation, causing immune complexes to form as they remove Abs.

Evasion is not always possible or successful. Most parasites, therefore, have alternative means of counteracting immunological attack. These include depressing, or suppressing, the host's normal defenses or diverting them into responses that reduce their direct impact on the parasites. **Immune suppression** can be induced by several parasites (e.g., trypanosomes, plasmodia, and trichinella). For example, certain blood parasites achieve immune suppression through polyclonal expansion. This leads to two very important results: (1) production of large amounts of low-affinity Ab and (2) eventual clonal exhaustion. Both are responsible for decreased efficiency of humoral immunity. Similar T cell clonal exhaustion can be induced with a diminution of the cellular immune response. In addition, persistent circulating Ags associated with chronic malaria and trypanosome infections can produce Ag overload, leading to Mϕ dysfunction. Dysfunctional Mϕs might display reduced phagocytic capability and monokine production, might not process Ag properly, or might release prostaglandins (which suppress some inflammatory reactions). Alternatively, trypanosomes have been reported to be capable of producing suppressing factors that might act directly against cells of immunological defense. Moreover, suppression is also accomplished by degradative cleavage of Abs or by complement resistance or inactivation. Nonspecific immune suppression is a general feature of microparasite and macroparasite infections.

Protistan and animal parasites also derive some benefit by **diverting, or subverting, the host's normal responses.** This is accomplished, in part, through the production of auto-Abs and autoreactive T$_C$ clones that might inadvertently arise during polyclonal activation. Other damage to the infected host sometimes occurs as a consequence of immune responses against parasites. This characteristically arises from the formation of immune complexes that might become lodged in organs. These complexes are formed by parasite Ags and Igs (usually IgM, but occasionally IgG). Complement is sometimes associated with these complexes as well. In addition, in trypanosomiasis, complexes can form between the trypanosomes themselves and antitrypanosome Abs or between trypanosome DNA and anti-DNA Abs. These complexes can affect the kidney and systemic blood vessels, causing glomerulonephritis and vasculitis.

IMMUNIZATION WITH VACCINES

Vaccines contain naturally occurring components or secretions of pathogens as Ags used to stimulate humoral and/or cell-mediated immunity. Ags in **vaccines** can be (1) *inactivated whole organisms,* (2) *harmless organisms,* (3) *isolated structural components or products of organisms,* (4) *synthetic Ags,* or (5) *Abs that serve as Ag mimics.* Vaccination is a form of prophylaxis that has clearly exerted a profound influence on world health. To date, active immunization with vaccines has been effectively employed against numerous infectious diseases caused by microparasites, for example, cholera, diphtheria, hepatitis, influenza, Japanese encephalitis, measles, mumps, polio, tuberculosis, typhoid fever, smallpox, and yellow fever. Nevertheless, immunological prevention of many, often alarming, infectious diseases (e.g., AIDS) is lacking and for many others (e.g., rabies) is less than ideal. In contrast, successful immunoprophylaxis against protistan microparasites and animal macroparasites has yet to be achieved. No effective vaccines are available for infectious diseases caused by parasitic protozoa or helminths. However, many new vaccines are being developed and a number of the older vaccines are being improved (table 12.8).

Characteristics of Good Vaccines

Vaccines should display several features if they are to be effective. For example, a vaccine should activate Ag processing and the production of ILs by Ag-presenting cells. In addition, a high yield of diverse memory T and B cells should be produced by vaccination. Moreover, stimulating Ags within the vaccine should persist in lymphoid tissues to promote continued production of Abs and effector cells, which are short-lived. Last, the vaccine should not cause adverse reactions.

Clearly, any potential vaccine *must contain epitopes capable of eliciting an immune response* if it is to confer immunity. Moreover, a vaccine should provide a variety of epitopes in order to stimulate expansion of several lymphocyte clones, each responding to a different epitope. This is important since individual variations in the nature of immune response genes and of MHC molecules expressed will cause members of a population to respond differently (or not at all) to any particular epitope. For example, synthetic peptides containing several epitopes reognizable to both B and T cells can be highly immunogenic in their free form. However, vaccines containing peptides possessing only a single epitope recognizable by each class of lymphocyte might not be effective for all members of a pop-

TABLE 12.8 Representative Diseases for Which Vaccines Are Being Developed Or Improved

Infection	Vaccines Being	
	Developed	Improved
Viral		
AIDS	+ +	
Cytomegalovirus infections	+ +	
Hepatitis (types A and C)	+ +	
Herpes (caused by herpes simplex 2)	+ +	
Influenza (types A and B)		+ +
Poliomyelitis		+ +
Rabies		+ +
Bacterial		
Cholera		+ +
Leprosy	+ +	
Meningitis (meningococcus type A/C)		+ +
(meningococcus type B)	+ +	
Pertussis		+ +
Pneumonia (streptococcal)		+ +
Streptococcal infections (caused by group A and B streptococci)	+ +	
Tuberculosis		+ +
Protozoan		
Chlamydiasis	+ +	
Gonorrhea	+ +	
Leishmaniasis	+ +	
Malaria	+ +	
Trypanosomiasis	+ +	
Yellow fever		+ +
Helminthic		
Filariasis	+ +	
Schistosomiasis	+ +	

Source: Robbins, A. Progress towards vaccines we need and do not have. *Lancet* **335**:1436, 1990.

with epitopes recognized by B cells in order to ensure broad activation following vaccination.

Production of *immunity by vaccination should be long lasting*. This persistence can be achieved by the generation of long-lived memory cells. In addition, retention of epitopes from the vaccine by lymphoid tissues can provide continued activation of short-lived effector cells.

Amino acid sequences within so-called foreign Ags might be quite similar to self–protein Ags. Thus, epitopes might be presented to T and B cells that lead to the production of auto-Abs. This complication occasionally arises after vaccination.

Classical Methods of Vaccine Production
Vaccines Using Whole Organisms

Interest in controlling infectious diseases probably emerged before written records were kept. However, systematic efforts to control infectious diseases date back to the eighteenth century, to the introduction of vaccination. Initially, vaccines made use of fully potent, live "organisms." This was the case with Jenner's use of vaccinia (cowpox) virus to induce immunity to a related strain, variola (smallpox) virus. The term vaccine originated at this time, when reference was made to the vaccinia virus used to immunize humans. Greater specificity and greater safety were achieved when attenuated live organisms or killed (inactivated) organisms were used to produce vaccines. For example, vaccines against measles, mumps, poliomyelitis (Sabin), and tuberculosis make use of attenuated (nonvirulent), live viruses or bacteria. On the other hand, vaccines against poliomyelitis (Salk), rabies, and cholera employ inactivated viruses or bacteria.

These earlier vaccines made use of **entire organisms.** These vaccines induced immunity by confronting the individual's immune system in essentially the same fashion as did the virulent pathogen. Thus, the immunized host's *immune system encountered a variety of epitopes* or antigenic determinants, just as if they were infected with microparasites. However, these vaccines have disadvantages. First, most of the specific Abs and effector T cells generated provide no protective function whatsoever since they are directed against Ags that are not essential for survival of the pathogen

ulation. Some immunologists believe that highly immunogenic proteins widely used in vaccines, such as tetanus toxoid, could be used as carriers to develop new vaccines for poorly immunogenic protective epitopes. Others suggest that a universal T cell epitope (capable of association with polymorphic MHC Ags) should be sought. This epitope could be complexed

or induction of disease symptoms. Second, some non-protective epitopes within the vaccines might induce immune suppression or immune enhancement. These events can lead to inappropriate responses with undesirable consequences to the host. Moreover, for vaccines using inactivated pathogens or attenuated (weakened) organisms, one must always confirm that no live organisms are present. Furthermore, with attenuated organisms, the danger of reversion to virulence is present. Handling and storage of vaccines with either inactivated or attenuated organisms create potential hazards to both the personnel involved and the environment.

Vaccines Using Isolated Antigens

Other strategies emerged that yielded vaccines that contained **specifically isolated Ags** rather than whole organisms. These vaccines use purified Ag fractions such as toxoids (chemically altered exotoxins that have lost their toxicity but retained their antigenicity). The acquired immunity displayed by individuals immunized with these vaccines is directed against the specific Ag or toxin used. For example, most individuals vaccinated with Pneumovax® (prepared from purified extracts of capsular Ags from *Streptococcus pneumoniae*) are immunized against pneumococcal pneumonia caused by any of the 14 strains of *S. pneumoniae* (all of which possess these capsular Ags). Vaccines prepared from toxoids can provide immunity against the toxic effects of *C. tetani* (tetanus) and *Corynebacterium diphtheriae* (diphtheria) exotoxins.

Modern Vaccines

These approaches have been very beneficial in preventing many important infectious diseases. However, there are diseases for which whole organism or natural product vaccines are quite unsatisfactory. Attempts to produce an improved generation of vaccines began in the 1980s. **New approaches** in the development of vaccines include (1) *construction of recombinant vectors,* (2) *synthesis of protective Ags,* and (3) the *use of internal image Abs* (antiidiotypes).

Recombinant Vaccines

Selected immunogenic proteins derived from infectious agents have been produced in large quantities using recombinant DNA methodology. Genes encoding these structural antigenic determinants have been identified, cloned, and expressed in a variety of systems. Genes that recently have been cloned and expressed in bacteria include those encoding immunogenic peptides from *V. cholerae* (B toxin subunit), herpes simplex virus (glycoprotein D), and *Plasmodium falciparum* (circumsporozoite protein). Moreover, recombinant forms of immunogenic peptides (envelope glycoproteins) of HIV have been expressed in mammalian and insect cell systems, while genes encoding immunogenic proteins of hepatitis B virus have been cloned in yeast. Proteins expressed in mammalian and yeast cells are glycosylated and resemble naturally occurring surface proteins. Recombinant DNA vaccines provide a supply of selected immunogenic peptides in quantities that might otherwise be unavailable. These recombinant products can be coupled with adjuvants and safely employed for immunization.

Recombinant Infectious Vaccines

The effectiveness of a recombinant DNA vaccine was found to be greatly enhanced by incorporation into a "live" vaccine. Live viral vectors can potentially improve immunogenicity of the expressed recombinant insert by mimicking the presentation of a pathogen's Ags through replication in the host. More importantly, however, this enhancement of immunogenicity is achieved without inducing the disease.

The value of this approach was first appreciated in the early 1980s by Paoletti and Moss, who showed that vaccinia virus (used to eradicate smallpox) could be used to express foreign Ags in laboratory animals. This virus can take up to 30 kilobases of foreign inserted DNA. In this system (fig. 12.4), foreign DNA is inserted into a recombinant vector that is then introduced into mammalian cells infected with vaccinia virus. Subsequently, a recombinant virus is produced that expresses the foreign gene. The recombinant vaccinia virus formed can replicate in the host in the same

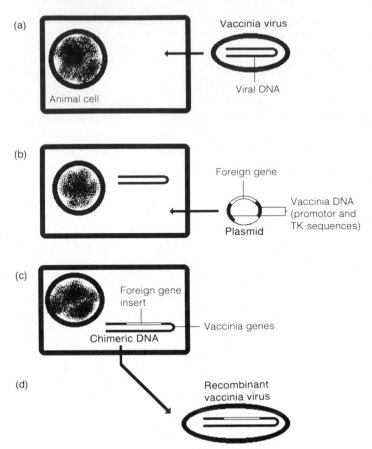

FIGURE 12.4 Construction of recombinant vaccine. Recombinant vaccines can be generated by incorporating foreign genes into vaccinia virus DNA. (*a*) Animal cells are first infected with vaccinia virus. (*b*) Subsequently, a plasmid containing the foreign gene of interest and promoter and thymidine kinase (TK) sequences from vaccinia virus is introduced. (*c*) During replication of vaccinia virus DNA, the plasmid sequences are also replicated and chimeric viral DNA containing the foreign gene is produced. (*d*) Recombinant vaccinia virus can be shed, which will express proteins encoded by the foreign gene.

way as an attenuated vaccine. Using this technique, chimeric vaccinia viruses have been constructed to express Ags from malarial parasites and from influenza, rabies, Epstein-Barr, and immune deficiency viruses.

Recombinant Viruslike Particles

Viruslike particles (VLPs) are made up of proteins of the same size and structure as viruses; however, they do not contain DNA or RNA and, therefore, are not infective. Since these particles can be engineered to include foreign proteins, they can serve as vehicles for presenting Ags to the immune system. Yeast cells possess a gene known as *Ty,* which can be fused to foreign

genes. (*Ty* is a retrotransposon, that is, a transposable genetic element capable of insertion at different sites within the genome which reproduces like an RNA virus.) Following fusion of *Ty* with foreign genes, yeast cells make hybrid proteins that become assembled into VLPs. These VLPs display Ags on their surfaces that correspond to the foreign genes. VLPs are significantly more immunogenic than globular proteins.

Kingsman and colleagues created hybrid VLPs carrying p24 protein, which forms part of the core of HIV-1. These VLPs are being used in trials as a potential new AIDS vaccine. VLP-p24 might be a useful form of immunotherapy for individuals afflicted with AIDS. Moreover, it is hoped that reagent might also

Soluble CD4 Antigen: Distracting HIV-1 Virus

T he HIV-1 virus is responsible for inducing AIDS. A primary means through which immune suppression is achieved in AIDS is through the destruction of T_H cells. These cells express CD4 Ag, which is used as a recognition ligand by gp-120 (a 120 kD envelope glycopeptide of HIV-1). This interaction between CD4 and gp-120 appears to be important to the formation of multinucleated giant cells (accomplished by cell fusion of macrophages) as well.

Chinese hamster ovary (CHO) cells were transfected with plasmids containing versions of CD4. Plasmids encoding the entire CD4 molecule directed the synthesis of CD4 that was retained by the CHO cells. Plasmids of the encoded versions of CD4 that lacked the anchoring sequence for CD4 directed the synthesis of CD4 that was shed into the culture medium. Both forms of CD4 reacted with MAbs against CD4. In addition, both forms bound isolated gp-120 with comparable affinity ($K_D = 1.3 \times 10^{-9}$ M for the intact CD4 vs. $0.72-0.83 \times 10^{-9}$ M for the truncated CD4).

Although CD4 and gp-120 displayed appropriate affinity characteristics in a binding assay, the question remained: Did secreted, recombinant CD4 have any therapeutic potential? This could be tested only by observing its ability to block infection by HIV-1. A $CD4^+$ cell line (H9 human T cells) was used for this purpose. A challenge dose of 100 $TCID_{50}$ units (50% tissue culture infective dose) of HIV-1 was presented for three days. Cells were scored after seven days in culture. When undiluted CD4 was included in the medium, infection of H9 cells by HIV-1 was reduced from $61\% - 65\%$ to $0.4\% - 1.4\%$. However, if CD4 was diluted 1:4, HIV-1 infection was reduced to only $16\% - 36\%$.

This demonstration suggests the potential for using isolated, soluble CD4 as a therapeutic tool in the management of AIDS, in the future. In addition, this might provide an approach for using naturally occurring ligands, for which pathogens display a strong affinity, as tools for reducing pathogenicity and virulence.

Smith, D. H., Byrn, R. A., Marsters, S. A., et al. Blocking of HIV-1 infectivity by a soluble, secreted form of the CD4 antigen. *Science* **238**:1704, 1987.

---

serve as a preventive vaccine. An apparent correlation exists between anti-p24 Ab levels and expression of clinical symptoms of AIDS. Individuals who are HIV-1 positive (which indicates exposure to the AIDS virus) and who possess high anti-p24 levels tend to have longer onset times for display of clinical symptoms of AIDS than do those with low anti-p24 titers. Accordingly, it is believed that boosting the anti-p24 titer with VLPs might be beneficial in delaying or preventing the expression of the clinical symptoms of AIDS.

Synthetic Vaccines

In view of the difficulties in obtaining large amounts of Ag from many important infectious agents (as seen for stages of malaria below), only genetically engineered or synthetic vaccines are being contemplated. Noninfectious vaccines can be produced by synthesis of peptides containing the primary structure of antigenic regions of an infectious agent. However, these antigenic regions might contain nonoverlapping epitopes reactive with B cells, T_H cells, and T_S cells. The coexistence of helper and suppressor determinants within an Ag could lead to nonimmunogenicity. Consequently, whenever a T_S epitope is located it can be deleted from the Ag. Nevertheless, there is the basic problem of deciding which peptides should be synthesized to elicit protective immunity, which often appears in the form of neutralizing Ab, specific cell-mediated immunity, and immunological memory.

Epitopes that activate B cells are more often conformational, rather than linear. Consequently, factors like surface accessibility, hydrophilicity, and segmental motility (folded [high motility] versus

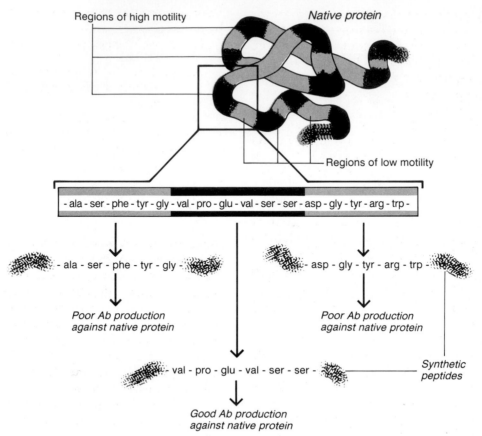

FIGURE 12.5 Antigenic potential of synthetic peptides mimicking diverse regions of globular proteins. Globular proteins possess numerous diverse epitopes. Certain of these occur at regions where the native peptide is folded (regions of high motility), while others are found in nonfolded regions (low motility). Synthetic peptides can be made that mimic these regions. Those peptides that mimic regions of high motility are most effective in generating Abs with good reactivity against the native protein. Although this figure illustrates the section of these peptides in linear fashion, it should be emphasized that mimicking the conformation of that region of the native protein is extremely important.

nonfolded [low motility] regions of a molecule) become important. In addition, three-dimensional analyses of the binding of synthetic peptides are of interest. Crumpton showed that fragments of globular proteins, corresponding to regions of the whole protein in folded conformation, often react with Abs directed against the native protein. It is believed that synthetic peptides corresponding to regions of high motility (edges of a folded chain) are most likely to stimulate the production of Abs that will react with the native protein. In contrast, synthetic peptides mimicking folded regions of low motility are not likely to give rise to Abs that will react with the native protein. These

relationships are depicted in figure 12.5. It has been suggested that synthetic peptide fragments might exist in various configurations in equilibrium. Among these diverse forms are a small number of molecules whose shape is recognized and stabilized by Ab.

A synthetic peptide of native sequence might contain epitopes that stimulate B cells and others that stimulate T cells. Nevertheless, carrier proteins have been coupled to some synthetic peptides to enhance T-dependent humoral responses. Spacing and synthesis of repeating immunodominant epitopes have also been employed. In developing a vaccine against the sporozoite stage of malaria, it was found that the protective

Ags were polypeptides that cover the surface membrane of the parasite. The species-specific dominant epitope consists of the tandem repetition (23 repeats) of four amino acids (asp-ala-asp-pro). Abs raised against this synthetic peptide (coupled with a carrier), react with the surface protein (circumsporozoite) of the parasite and neutralize its activity.

Recent field trials of a potential malaria vaccine found that the circumsporozoite vaccine tested was not immunogenic in many (about 40%) adults throughout an endemic region of Africa. Some members of the population apparently expressed MHC molecules that simply did not respond to the T cell epitopes in the vaccine. This precluded expression of a humoral response controlled by class II MHC-restricted T_H cells. The response observed in this human population supported the belief, previously based on murine studies, that immunity is under the control of immune response (Ir) genes. Moreover, these results indicate that an ideal synthetic peptide vaccine should be immunogenic in each and every member of the population to be vaccinated. This requires that the vaccine contain pathogen-specific epitopes recognizable by T and B cells of everyone being vaccinated.

Strides in this direction are already being made. Recently, epitopes recognizable by T cells have been characterized in protein Ags from a variety of viruses, bacteria, and protistan and animal parasites. Epitopes were identified by cloning pathogen-specific T cells from several of immune and nonimmune individuals. The various T cell clones generated in this manner can be used to determine *in vitro* whether a particular synthetic peptide will associate with diverse MHC molecules (Ags), which is a necessary condition for the constructed peptide to be immunogenic. In this manner, vaccines can be identified that contain peptides which will react with T (and B) cells from most members of a target population.

Idiotype Vaccines

Vaccines based on Ag mimicry by Ab are referred to as internal image, or as idiotypic, vaccines. The regulatory network envisioned by Jerne in the 1970s holds that Abs become immunogenic as their concentrations increase in response to Ag. This can produce physiological autoimmunity. The sequence following immunization with a classical Ag might occur as follows:

1. Ab (Ab-1) to foreign Ag A with a certain idiotype (Id-1) becomes immunogenic as their concentration increases.
2. Id-1 of Ab-1 gives rise to anti-Id-1 (Ab-2).
3. Ab-2 (or anti-Id-1) has antigenic determinants (or idiotopes), designated Id-2, which might resemble (internal image) and behave like epitopes of Ag A.
4. In turn, Ab-2 (or Id-2) could stimulate the formation of Ab-3 (or anti-Id-2), which is the same as Ab-1.

However, the host would be immunologically tolerant of the Fc region of these Abs. Some idiotopes might share identical amino acid sequences with the immunogenic epitopes of the classical Ag. In addition, some idiotopes might share stereochemical mimicry with the epitope. This mimicry does not require matching of primary amino acid sequences. Roitt and colleagues suggest that the similarity between idiotopes and epitopes might be an intrinsic ability to provide similar contact noncovalent bonds.

Internal image Abs or antiidiotypic vaccines have been tested in syngeneic murine systems, with or without adjuvants, against a variety of viruses (e.g., hepatitis B, rabies, and polio); bacteria (e.g., *S. pneumoniae* and *Listeria monocytogenes*); protistan (e.g., trypanosomes) and animal parasites (e.g., schistosomes). Idiotypic vaccines can be safer and more readily available than classical vaccines. In addition, they efficiently induce neutralizing Abs and specific cell-mediated immunity, which appears to be non-MHC restricted. Potentially idiotypic vaccines may be immunogenic to all members of a population, regardless of their MHC type. Furthermore, they can be substituted for polysaccharide Ags, which are nonimmunogenic in infants, and poorly immunogenic in adults. Recombinant DNA and synthetic vaccines, by comparison, are apparently not very effective in inducing immunity against carbohydrate epitopes on pathogens (e.g., *N. meningitidis* and *S. pneumoniae*). Idiotypic vaccines provide an alternative approach when the Ag in question is either difficult to isolate or unavailable. In addition, idiotypic vaccines can also substitute for a synthetic peptide when that peptide does not present the tertiary structure of the native Ag.

Antigen and Antibody Mimetics

Novel reagents, called *mimetics,* have been developed recently. Mimetics are designed to intentionally mimic particular Ags or Abs. Moreover, as specially designed reagents, the desired ligand-binding properties needed for Ag-Ab recognition can be combined with characteristics that enhance immunological benefits. For example, mimetics can be designed to (1) have little or no immunogenicity as foreign Ags (e.g., nonpeptide compounds), (2) have extended serum half-lives and potentially be active for longer periods than Igs, or (3) be able to cross the blood-brain-barrier and act where native Igs cannot penetrate.

Although not yet exploited as vaccines, the properties just cited suit mimetics for this purpose. For example, a CD4-mimetic has been developed which can bind viral recombinant gp120. This binding parallels the interaction that occurs between HIV (which produces gp120) and its target lymphocytes (which express CD4) in AIDS. Thus, CD4-mimetic has the potential for limiting or blocking the spread of AIDS in an infected individual. Another reagent, designated 87.1-mimetic, mimics the second complimentarity-determining region (CDR) of a MAb against reovirus type 3 receptor. This non-peptide, CDR-mimetic reproduces characteristics of the MAb; particularly, it binds to the reovirus receptor and suppresses concanavalin A induced mitogenesis in T cells expressing this receptor. These results suggest that other nonpeptide CDR-mimetics can be created as substitutes for other Abs. This approach might provide powerful tools for protection against infectious agents.

S U M M A R Y

1. Confrontation by potentially infective biological agents occurs on a regular basis. Defense against these agents is one function of the immune system. [p. 302]

2. Microbial pathogens (which include viruses, bacteria, and fungi) usually produce acute infections. [p. 302]

3. Innate defenses against microbial pathogens include: (a) anatomical barriers to physical entry of the pathogens, (b) nonspecific cellular defenses that seek to eradicate the intruders (e.g., natural killer cells and phagocytes), and (c) biochemical factors that augment cellular responses or directly impair successful infection by the pathogen (e.g., interferons and lysozyme). [pp. 302–304]

4. Acquired immunity is antigen specific. It is induced by specific antigens of the pathogen and is directed against particular antigenic determinants. It has the additional advantage of conferring immunological memory. [p. 304]

5. Humoral defenses against microbial pathogens lead to (a) neutralization or inteference with binding to host cells, (b) opsonization, (c) complement-mediated lysis or (d) antibody-dependent cellular cytotoxicity reactions. [pp. 304–307]

6. Specific cell-mediated responses against microbial pathogens are mediated by T_C and T_D cells. Cytolytic responses that occur can also be mediated by nonspecific killers (e.g., macrophages and natural killer cells) that are specifically recruited by T_H cells. [pp. 307–308]

7. Microbial pathogens can escape reprisal by a host's immune system by either avoiding detection (antigenic drift or modulation) or by modulating the host's immune response (e.g., immune suppression). [pp. 308–310]

8. Infections by protistan microparasites (protozoa) and animal macroparasites (helminths) are generally chronic. [p. 310]

9. Innate defenses against protistan and animal parasites are similar to those employed against microbial pathogens, namely, mechanical defense and nonspecific cellular and humoral defenses (e.g., natural killer cells and phagocytes; alternate complement pathway). [pp. 311–312]

10. Acquired immunity against protistan and animal parasites includes the production of specific antibodies, activation of specific effector T cells, and the generation of B and T memory cells. However, acquired immunity frequently does not confer protection against reinfection by protistan and animal parasites. [pp. 312–313]

11. Humoral responses against protistan and animal parasites involve IgM, IgG, and IgE. IgE is especially important against helminths. These defenses act against parasites in several ways. These include (a) physical interference (blocking attachment or obstructing orifices), (b) causing agglutination, (c) promoting more active phagocytosis (opsonization), (d) inducing cytotoxicity, and (e) neutralizing parasite products. [pp. 313–314]

12. Cell-mediated responses against protistan and animal parasites are primarily conducted by macrophages, neutrophils, eosinophils, and platelets. Their effectiveness may be enhanced by lymphokines released by antigen-activated T cells. Antigen-specific cytotoxic T cells may, nevertheless, be involved in direct lysis of some parasites. [pp. 314–315]

13. Protistan and animal parasites escape immunological destruction by (a) anatomical seclusion, (b) evasion, and (c) immune suppression. Through seclusion parasites seek to escape detection. Evasion mechanisms attempt to avoid recognition as foreign agents (antigen masking) or elude immunological memory (antigenic variation). Immunosuppressive mechanisms endeavor to diminish the efficiency of the host's response against the parasite. [pp. 315–317]

14. Vaccines are used as a means of generating immunity against infectious agents. Traditional approaches have used live, attenuated, or killed pathogens, their antigens (purified), and toxoids. Newer approaches (a) make use of recombinant DNA technology to produce analogues of the infectious vectors, (b) generate synthetic versions of antigenic epitopes, and (c) exploit antiidiotype antibodies, and (d) create mimetics of particular Ags or Abs. [pp. 317–324].

R E A D I N G S

Ada, G. Vaccines. In Paul, W. (ed.). *Fundamental Immunology.* 2d ed. Raven Press, New York, 1989.

Blackwell, J. Immunology of leishmaniasis. In Lachmann, P., Peters, D., Rosen, F., and Walport, M. (eds.). *Clinical Aspects In Immunology.* 5th ed. Blackwell Scientific Publications, Ltd., Oxford, 1990.

Bloom, B. R. Games people play: how parasites evade immune surveillance. *Nature* **279:**21, 1979.

————. New approaches to vaccine development. *Review Infectious Diseases* **11:** 460, 1989.

Cherfas, J. U.K. vaccine trial: stalking horse for the future. *Science* **249:**626, 1990.

Cohen, I., and Weiner, H. T-cell vaccination. *Immunology Today* **9:**332, 1988.

Cox, R. A. (ed.). *Immunology of the Fungal Diseases.* CRC Press, Inc., Boca Raton, Fla., 1989.

Cryz, S. J., Jr. (ed.) *Vaccines and Immunotherapy.* Plenum Press, New York, 1991.

Ettinger, H., Gillessen, D., Lahm, H., et al. Use of prior vaccinations for the development of new vaccines. *Science* **249:** 423, 1990.

Fawcett, P. T., Fawcett, L. B., Doughty, R., et al. Suppression of malaria induced autoimmunity by immunization with cryoglobulins. *Cellular Immunology* **118:**192, 1989.

Fine, P. BCG vaccination against tuberculosis and leprosy. *British Medical Bulletin* **14:**691, 1988.

Good, M., Kumar, S., and Miller, L. The real difficulties for malaria sporozoite vaccine development. *Immunology Today* **9:**351, 1988.

Good, M. F., Kumar, S., Weiss, W. R., et al. T-cell antigenic sites of the malaria circumsporozoite protein. *Blood* **74:**895, 1989.

Hiernaux, J. Idiotypic vaccines and infectious diseases. *Infection and Immunity* **56:**1407, 1988.

Hoffman, M. "Superantigens" may shed light on immune puzzle. *Science* **248:**685, 1990.

Kierszenbaum, F., Sztein, M., and Beltz, L. Decreased human IL-2 receptor expression due to a protozoan pathogen. *Immunology Today* **10:**129, 1989.

Koff, W., and Fauci, A. Human trials of AIDS vaccines: current status and future directions. *AIDS* **3**(suppl. 1):125, 1989.

Kreier, J. P., and Mortensen, R. F. *Infection, Resistance, and Immunity.* Harper & Row, New York, 1990.

Laurence, J., and Schild, G. AIDS 1989. Vaccines and immunology: overview. *AIDS* **3**(suppl. 1):119, 1989.

Mahmoud, A. A. F. Parasitic protozoa and helminths: biological and immunological challenges. *Science* **246**:1015, 1989.

Marx, J. Taming rogue immune reactions. *Science* **249**:246, 1990.

Milich, D. Synthetic T and B cell recognition sites: implications for vaccine development. *Advances in Immunology* **45**:195, 1989.

Moss, B. Vaccinia virus: a tool for research and vaccine development. *Science* **252**: 1662, 1991.

Nussenzweig, R. Parasitic disease as a cause of immunosuppression. *New England Journal of Medicine* **306**:423, 1982.

Oehen, S., Hengartner, H., and Zinkernagel, R. M. Vaccination for disease. *Science* **251**:195, 1991.

Oeltmann, T. N., and Frankel, A. E. Advances in immunotoxins. *FASEB Journal* **5**:2334, 1991.

Pink, J., and Sinigalia, F. Characterizing T-cell epitopes in vaccine candidates. *Immunology Today* **10**:408, 1989.

Playfair, J. (ed.). Immunity to infection. *Current Opinion in Immunology* **2**:345, 1990.

Playfair, J., Taverne, J., Bate, C., et al. The malaria vaccine: anti-parasite or anti-disease. *Immunology Today* **11**:25, 1990.

Saroca, R., Schwab, C., and Bosshard, H. Epitope mapping employing immobilized synthetic peptides. *Journal of Immunological Methods* **141**:245, 1991.

Saragovi, H., Fitzpatrick, D., Raktabutr, A., et al. Design and Synthesis of a mimetic from an antibody complimentarity-determining region. *Science* **253**:792, 1991.

Sher, A., James, S., Correa-Oliveira, R., et al. Schistosome vaccines: current progress and future prospects. *Parasitology* **98**:561, 1989.

Wakelin, D. *Immunity to Parasites: How Animals Control Parasite Infections.* E. J. Arnold, London, 1984.

Watson, J. D. Leprosy: understanding protective immunity. *Immunology Today* **11**:218, 1989.

Weller, P. F. The immunobiology of eosinophils. *New England Journal of Medicine* **324**:1110, 1991.

Woodrow, G., and Levine, M. M. *New Generation Vaccines: The Molecular Approach.* Marcel Dekker, New York, 1990.

World Health Assembly. Global eradication of poliomyelitis by the year 2000. Resolution WHA 41.28, 41st World Health Assembly, May 13, 1988.

Zanetti, M., Sercarz, E., and Salk, J. The immunology of the new generation vaccines. *Immunology Today* **8**:18, 1987.

Damaging and Defective Immune Responses

This unit explores the immune system under conditions in which its roles in defense and homeostasis are not properly performed. Chapter 13, Hypersensitivity, discusses mechanisms and consequences of the immune responses that are exaggerated or inappropriate to the stimulus. In chapter 14, Immune Deficiency, the general means through which the immune system might become impaired in its function are examined, as are the results of reduced immune responses. Special attention is provided in chapter 15 to acquired immune deficiency syndrome (AIDS). Last, chapter 16, Autoimmunity, explores the situations in which the immune system reacts against the individual's own cells and tissues as though they were foreign. This unit provides an overview of ways in which functioning of the immune system might be distorted. In addition, examples are presented for each of the major categories of immunological dysfunction.

13 Hypersensitivity

OVERVIEW

The four types of hypersensitivity reactions are defined according to their immune mechanisms and clinical manifestations. Ways of measuring or detecting hypersensitivity reactions are also explored.

CONCEPTS

1. Hypersensitivity reactions lead to pathological events in the body and are mediated by immune mechanisms.

2. Antibodies play an essential role in Type I, II, and III hypersensitivity reactions, whereas Type IV is mediated by antibody-independent effects of T lymphocytes upon target cells.

3. Hypersensitivity reactions are a complex network of interactions among mediators released by immune triggers.

The immune response is a powerful weapon against disease, but it sometimes goes awry. Usually the immune system protects us, to varying degrees, from invading disease-causing organisms. However, for some of us, the immune system reacts to certain foreign substances in a way that is not beneficial, and so is responsible for a diverse group of pathological states, such as atopic allergic diseases and asthma. Whenever the immune system acts excessively or inappropriately to an Ag and pathological changes occur, the person is said to be *hypersensitive.*

Historically, hypersensitivity reactions were divided originally into two classes based on the relative amount of time for an immunological response to develop in a sensitized host. **Immediate hypersensitivity** reactions develop in less than 24 hours after reexposure to an Ag, whereas **delayed hypersensivity** reactions occur within 24 to 48 hours.

In 1963, Coombs and Gell refined the classification, identifying four classes (or types). Within the category of immediate hypersensivity reactions, there are three subdivisions, namely, Type I (anaphylaxis), Type II (cytotoxic), and Type III (immune-complex-mediated) reactions, which are all Ig-dependent hypersensitivities involving B lymphocytes. Type IV is a cell-mediated or delayed hypersensitivity and is mediated by T lymphocytes.

An alternative scheme identifies five classes of hypersensitivities. Using the Coombs and Gell nomenclature, the additional category is called Type V hypersensitivity. This is known also as stimulatory, or antireceptor, hypersensitivity. This is a form of immediate hypersensitivity that is mediated by non-complement-fixing antibodies directed against receptors of the affected tissue. Kirkpatrick has recently (1987) offered the following alternative nomenclature: class 1, reagin-dependent injury (former Type I); class 2, cytotoxic reactions (former Type II); class 3, immune-complex-mediated reactions (former Type III); class 4, antireceptor Abs (the new class); and class 5, delayed hypersensitivity (former Type IV). Since the majority of manifestations of class 4 (Type V) reactions appear to be caused by auto-Abs (anti-self Abs), we have considered these under autoimmunity (chapter 16).

Consequently, the discussion of hypersensitivity in this chapter employs the traditional Coombs and Gell classification scheme.

The different types of hypersensivity reactions are compared in table 13.1. In this chapter, we explore how Ags can lead to an immune response that is detrimental to the host.

■ ■ ■ ■ ■ ■ ■ ■ ■ ■ ■

TYPE I HYPERSENSITIVITY: ANAPHYLAXIS

If an Ag is administered to a sensitized host and produces a sudden (or immediate) allergic response that is pathological in nature and mediated by IgE Abs, the reaction is termed **anaphylaxis** or antiphylaxis (as distinguished from the helpful prophylaxis). Localized anaphylaxis is exemplified by such conditions as hay fever and asthma. Systemic anaphylaxis is a shocklike condition that can occur in individuals who are intensely allergic to such things as bee venom. Both conditions are mediated by IgE and are considered *atopic* allergic disease states (from the Greek, *atop-* ["out of place"]).

An antigenic substance that can trigger the allergic state is known as an **allergen.** It can be a protein or a chemically complex low molecular weight substance. Most allergens are considered weakly immunogenic and most people do not react or respond to them adversely. However, an allergic person is often sensitive to several different allergens. In the United States, about 20% of the people develop allergic disorders during their lifetimes.

Mechanism of Ige-Mediated Hypersensitivity

The first phase in Type I immediate hypersensitivity is the sensitization stage. It starts with the first exposure to an allergen, which initiates the biosynthesis and release of humoral Ab, in this case primarily IgE. Once the reaginic Ab, IgE, is released from a plasma cell, it locates and binds to mast cells and basophils. Basophils are found in the circulation, while mast cells (or fixed

TABLE 13.1 Hypersensitivity Reactions

Type*	Alternate Name	Characteristics	Examples
Immediate			
Traditional			
Type I	Anaphylactic type	IgE binds to mast cells/basophils; allergen binds to IgE on sensitized cells, triggering release of vasoactive substances (histamine, serotonin, leukotrienes, etc.)	Allergies; anaphylactic shock due to bee sting
Type II	Cytotoxic	Ag elicits formation of Ab, which binds to target cell, causing its destruction (e.g., by complement-mediated cytolysis)	Drug/transfusion reactions; erythroblastosis fetalis
Type III	Immune complex	Ab combines with large amount of Ag, forming Ag-Ab complexes that trigger release of histamine and other mediators; damage to blood vessels occurs with inflammation and necrosis resulting	Serum sickness; lupus erythematosus
Nontraditional†			
Type V	Stimulatory antireceptor	Ab against receptor binds, causing impaired physiological responses—this is sometimes displayed as stimulation of the cell or tissue (Abs do not fix complement)	Graves' disease; myasthenia gravis; insulin-dependent diabetes mellitus
Delayed			
Type IV	Cell mediated	Ags cause proliferation of lymphoid cells: sensitized cells react to Ag by activating T_C cells or T_D cells, which release lymphokines that mediate hypersensitivity reaction; humoral Abs are *not* involved	Graft rejection; tuberculin reaction; contact sensitivity (e.g., poison ivy)

*Classification scheme described by Coombs and Gell in 1963 is used. This defined four classes (types) of hypersensitivity reactions—Types I through III being manifestations of immediate hypersensitivity, and Type IV representing delayed hypersensitivity. Type V does not exist in this scheme. However, discovery of an increasing number of diseases attributed to antireceptor Abs, some of which lead to stimulation of the affected cell, has led to creation of a fifth category.

†Manifestations of this form of hypersensitivity are considered separately under the heading of autoimmune disorders (see chapter 16, Autoimmunity).

basophils) are located in the lymphoid regions of the respiratory and gastrointestinal (GI) tract, and linings of blood vessels, including capillaries. They have large numbers of vesicles containing pharmacologically potent compounds like histamine and serotonin. Thus, from the first exposure, allergen-specific IgE is fixed to the mast cells and basophils, thereby sensitizing them. The part of the IgE molecule that binds to the surface of the mast cells and basophils is the Fc portion of the molecule. It binds to specific *FcE receptor* sites on the cell membrane, where it can remain attached for up to six weeks. The individual is now sensitized, and the stage is set for the second exposure to allergen which will result in the expression of the atopic, or allergic, reaction. After a second exposure, the allergen travels to the mast cells and basophils, where it binds to the Ag-binding site on the IgE molecule. Ag-Ab binding triggers the process of degranulation, through which the mast cell explosively discharges its pharmacologically active agents (fig. 13.1).

Mediators

The contents of the mast cell secretory vesicles include a variety of substances with similar physiological effects on inflammation (table 13.2; see also chapter 8).

Histamine is the most abundant and fastest acting of these substances. It induces smooth muscle contractions, release of mucus, vasodilation, and increases capillary permeability. All of these actions can have profound effects. For example, excessive smooth

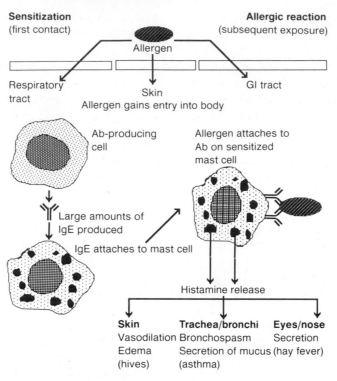

FIGURE 13.1 Type I hypersensitivity. An Ag (allergen) stimulates Ab (IgE) production, leading to the sensitization of mast cells. Subsequent exposure to this same allergen leads to activation of the sensitized cells with the release of histamine and other mediators that give rise to the symptoms of the allergic reaction.

TABLE 13.2 Mediators of Anaphylactic Reactions

Mediator*	Activities
Preformed	
ECF-A	Attracts and deactivates eosinophils; increases number of complement receptors
Histamine	Increases vascular permeability; induces smooth muscle contraction; is chemoattractant for eosinophils; stimulates prostaglandin synthesis; stimulates T_S cells
NCF-A	Attracts and deactivates neutrophils
Serotonin	Increases vascular permeability
Generated	
Bradykinin	Causes contraction of bronchioles, induces vasodilation and hypotension
Leukotrienes (SRS-A)	Increases capillary permeability; stimulates contraction of bronchioles; inhibits mitogenic response of lymphocytes
PAFs	Stimulate aggregation and lysis of platelets
Prostaglandins	Are vasodilators, bronchoconstrictors, and regulators of hemostasis
Thromboxanes	Are bronchoconstrictors

*Mediators that are present before initiation are defined as *preformed*, as opposed to mediators that are *generated* during (or as a result of) hypersensitivity reactions.

muscle contraction and release of mucus in the respiratory tract can close the air passages of the trachea and bronchi, causing asphyxiation and death by suffocation. Another target area is the uterus. Pregnant women who are severely allergic can abort the fetus during an attack from histamine release and subsequent smooth muscle contractions in the uterus. Histamine can also lead to edema in which excess fluid accumulates in the tissues. This is due to a histamine-induced increase in capillary permeability. Vasodilation through histamine release also ensures that the area will have an increased blood flow. Thus, there can be extensive loss of blood fluids into the tissues. This can lead to circulatory shock, when cells no longer are supplied with the proper levels of oxygen and glucose from the blood. Under these conditions, cells, tissues, organs, and eventually organ systems begin to fail and death can occur.

Serotonin is another substance released during mast cell degranulation that acts as a chemoeffector of smooth muscle. In addition to causing smooth muscle contraction, it also increases the respiratory rate, produces pain, depresses central nervous system activity, and further stimulates histamine release. All of these effects act as a positive feedback mechanism, which heightens the allergic symptoms brought on by the major effector, histamine.

Bradykinin is a small peptide, which also stimulates slow, sustained contraction of smooth muscle. Even though it is released in minute amounts, it is effective in enhancing capillary permeability, increased secretion from mucous glands, and leukocyte emigration from blood vessels into the tissues.

Slow-reacting substance of anaphylaxis (SRS-A) is a mixture of three **leukotrienes** (LTs), which causes edema through capillary dilation as well as smooth muscle contraction. LTs are very potent muscle spasmogens. They cause the same symptoms as histamine, serotonin, and bradykinin, but the effects are slower and longer lasting.

Platelet-activating factors (PAFs) induce the aggregation and lysis of platelets. Platelets are needed for proper blood clot formation (hemostasis). Heparin is another substance released during degranulation. It blocks the formation of thrombin, which converts fi-brinogen into fibrin in the blood. Thus, heparin also decreases blood coagulation.

Eosinophil chemotactic factor of anaphylaxis (ECF-A) and *neutrophil chemotactic factor of anaphylaxis* (NCF-A) draw eosinophilic and neutrophilic leukocytes to the inflamed site. Eosinophils and neutrophils are believed to reverse some of the deleterious effects of anaphylaxis. Accordingly, eosinophils release antihistaminelike substances, and neutrophils phagocytize (engulf) damaged cells and remove them from the area.

Prostaglandins (PGs) and *thromboxanes* are products generated by mast cells. The binding of allergen to IgE on the mast cell causes perturbations of the cell membrane, initiating enzymatic breakdown of phospholipids and the release of arachidonic acid, the precursor of PGs and thromboxanes. PGs can act as vasodilators, bronchoconstrictors, and regulators of blood coagulation; thromboxanes can cause bronchoconstriction.

Thus, histamine alone does not produce all of the symptoms associated with anaphylaxis. In fact, it is the well-tuned orchestration of several substances that interact and enhance each other's activities that is responsible for these manifestations. Consequently, whenever degranulation of a mast cell or basophil occurs, the capillaries fill with blood causing redness, and plasma leaks into the tissues causing swelling, itching, pain, and discharges—thereby accounting for the classical, cardinal signs of inflammation.

Since mast cells are located in such diverse areas of the body as the respiratory tract, GI tract, reproductive tract, and skin, exposure to allergens may lead to the development of hives, eczema, red eyes, sneezing, nasal congestion, puffiness, and itching. Smooth muscle involvement can lead to symptoms of respiratory distress (coughing, wheezing, and breathing difficulties), complications of the GI tract (nausea, vomiting, and diarrhea), or complications of the reproductive tract (severe cramping).

One of the few instances in which an IgE-mediated immediate hypersensitivity reaction is beneficial is in fighting parasitic infections. IgE can contribute significantly to the body's defense against parasitic worms and insects (see chapter 12, Immunity to Infectious Diseases). As long as the reactions are not

HIGHLIGHT 13.1

Regulation of Mast Cell Degranulation by cAMP

The release of vasoactive amines by mast cells is mediated in a stepwise fashion. The Ag-IgE complex acts as a first messenger. The complex binds to Fc receptors in the mast cell plasma membrane. This membrane receptor is linked to a membrane-bound enzyme, adenylate cyclase (AC). When activated, AC generates a second messenger molecule, cyclic adenosine monophosphate (cAMP). In turn, cAMP activates specific protein kinases (PKs) to phosphorylate proteins that are involved in the degranulation process of the mast cell, leading to the release of allergic mediator molecules. The enzyme, cyclic nucleotide phosphodiesterase (PDE), inactivates cAMP by converting cAMP to inactive AMP. In addition, binding of the Ag-IgE complex to the Fc receptor leads to perturbations of the mast cell membrane. These, in turn, are associated with increased phospholipid turnover and increased Ca^{2+} influx. The increased intracellular Ca^{2+} and phospholipid products seem to be involved in interactions of intermediate filaments with secretory vesicles and the fusion of vesicles with cell membranes. (See fig. 13.A.)

The level of cAMP appears crucial in controlling mast cell degranulation and release of secretory vesicle contents. However, *mediator release (degranulation) is greater when the intracellular levels of cAMP are low.* This creates an apparent contradiction in that stimulation of cAMP production is necessary for initiating degranulation, but maintenance of an elevated intracellular cAMP concentration seems not to be compatible with maximal degranulation.

Drawing on this information, Type I hypersensitivity reactions are treated with drugs that modulate cAMP levels, blocking release of inflammatory mediators from mast cells.

1. Stimulation of AC through other receptors causes cAMP levels to rise. Since mast cells possess α- and β-adrenergic receptors, which interact with AC, hormones such as epinephrine can stimulate cAMP production. This explains the therapeutic value of epinephrine in treating anaphylactic reactions: epinephrine stimulates AC, causing a rise in cAMP and a diminished level of histamine release.

2. An alternative means of increasing cAMP concentration is by reducing its breakdown by PDE. Anaphylaxis is occasionally controlled by theophylline, which blocks PDE, thereby reducing the destruction of cAMP. The elevated cAMP levels inhibit, or depress, degranulation.

On the other hand, the use of drugs like propranolol (which blocks β-adrenergic receptors) impairs stimulation of AC. This is associated with a failure to increase cAMP levels and an increase in histamine release. Since propranolol is a drug commonly used to treat heart disorders, such as arrhythmias and angina, severe reactions can occur if a person medicated with propranolol is having an allergic episode. The effect is the result of physiological antagonism, rather than direct competition for the same mediator system.

The modulation of degranulation, and mediator release, from mast cells can be regulated by the second messenger molecule, cAMP. It appears that a transient increase in cAMP is necessary as a trigger to subsequent degranulation, but that persistently elevated cAMP interferes with other events that actually bring about degranulation.

Austen, K. F. Tissue mast cells in immediate hypersensitivity. *Hospital Practice* **17**:98, 1982.

Buisseret, P. D. Allergy. *Scientific American* **247**:86, 1982.

Peachell, P. T., Macglashan, D. W., Jr., Lichtenstein, L. M., et al. Regulation of human basophil and lung mast cell function by cyclic adenosine monophosphate. *Journal of Immunology* **140**:571, 1988.

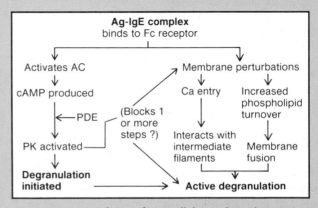

FIGURE 13.A Regulation of mast cell degranulation by cAMP.

excessive, the mast cell secretions, following binding of the parasite's Ags to surface IgE, can lead to expulsion of the parasite from the body via coughing, sneezing, vomiting, or diarrhea.

Late-Phase Reaction

When allergen binds to an IgE–mast cell complex, degranulation of vasoactive granules by the mast cell can cause immediate hypersensitivity reactions, such as anaphylaxis, within minutes. However, many allergic persons can experience a type of backlash reaction several hours after the initial event. For example, after being challenged by bee venom, the site of injection will become immediately swollen and red, a typical wheal and flare reaction. This reaction might subside within an hour. However, hours later, the site can become reinflamed, and remain so for the next 24 hours. This late-phase reaction is not entirely understood, but histological studies have shown differences in the early versus late reactions. Mast cells and basophils are present in the early reactions; however, in the late-phase reaction, the site becomes infiltrated by mononuclear cells, neutrophils, and eosinophils. The latter cells can express histamine receptors and are perhaps drawn to the site by the chemotactic property of histamine. Once there, these effector cells can reestablish an acute inflammatory response, thus prolonging allergic injury.

The late-phase reaction might be important in explaining the previously puzzling phenomenon of delayed symptoms in persons with allergic asthma or allergic rhinitis. Alerting people to subsequent reactions after the initial event should enable earlier intervention and help to minimize tissue injury. Interestingly, antihistamines are not effective in blocking late-phase reactions; however, pretreatment with blockers of histamine receptors inhibits the development of this type of reaction.

Measurement of Type I Hypersensitivity

If a person is suspected to be allergic to a particular substance, a skin or scratch test can be performed. In this clinical test, a small dose of allergen is injected under the skin. In less than 30 minutes, the results can be read. If an individual is allergic, there will be a **wheal**

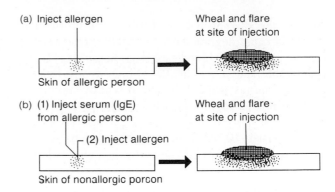

FIGURE 13.2 Demonstration of Type I hypersensitivity. (*a*) The wheal and flare response can be induced in a sensitized person by injecting a small quantity of the allergen into the skin. (*b*) The Prausnitz-Küstner test demonstrates the presence of serum IgE against an Ag. In this test, serum believed to contain specific IgE is injected into the skin of a nonallergic person. A wheal and flare response occurs after the allergen is administered.

and flare response at the injection site, which is now blanched, swollen, and itchy. Since the injection site is small, it is possible to test for hundreds of substances on a person's back (fig. 13.2). The wheal and flare response can be used to determine the specific substance to which the atopic patient is sensitive. Intense reactions to such tests are interpreted as being the allergens responsible for the immediate difficulties of the person.

In 1921, Prausnitz and Küstner used blood serum to passively transfer allergic reactivity (IgE) from an allergic patient to the skin of a normal individual. As was formerly demonstrated, subsequent to the injection of serum IgE, inoculation of the allergen to that site will evoke a wheal and flare reaction in the nonallergic person (fig. 13.2). The **Prausnitz-Küstner (P-K) procedure** can be used to test people for life-threatening allergens such as bee venom. Individuals who are extremely sensitive to an allergen can undergo this indirect mode of testing to determine if their serum contains the specific IgE to the allergen, without having to come into direct contact with the allergen.

Another assay, similar to the P-K procedure, is **passive cutaneous anaphylaxis (PCA)**. This test is used to assay IgE in experimental animals, where it measures local anaphylaxis *in vivo*. In this procedure, test serum is injected intradermally, and 48 hours later the test animal is challenged with allergen and Evans blue dye, injected intravenously. If IgE is present in the serum, the allergen will bind to the IgE on the mast cell and cause degranulation and the release of vaso-active amines. The blood capillaries in the area become permeable and allow the Evans blue dye to leak out into the dermis of the skin. The area of dye in the skin can be related to the quantity of IgE present in the serum.

In 1910, while investigating anaphylactic reactions, Schultz and Dale demonstrated separately that sensitized strips of smooth muscle can contract *in vitro* following exposure to allergen. This *in vitro* tissue model of anaphylaxis is still used for experimental studies and is called the **Schultz-Dale test.** Smooth muscle strips can be passively sensitized by bathing them in serum from a hypersensitive animal. The actual test is performed by adding the Ag and observing subsequent contractions.

There are also two radioactive *in vitro* tests for quantifying specific IgE concentrations: the **radioallergosorbent test** (**RAST**) and the **radioimmunosorbent test** (**RIST**). In the RAST, purified allergen extract is absorbed onto paper disks. The serum of a patient suspected of containing IgE is incubated with the disk. Radioactively labeled rabbit anti-IgE is then added. The disk is incubated, washed, and then tested for radioactive content. If the person is sensitive to the allergen, the disk will be radioactive. This positive reaction results from binding of the radioactive anti-IgE to the complex formed between the individual's IgE Abs and the allergen in the disk (fig. 13.3). The RIST, on the other hand, is a radioimmunoassay (RIA) (see chapter 4) in which serum IgE competes with radiolabeled IgE for binding to allergen. Allergen is bound to a solid-phase carrier, and is incubated with a known quantity of labeled IgE and an aliquot of serum to be tested. Maximal binding of labeled IgE to allergen occurs when the assay is performed using serum samples containing no IgE. The presence of endogenous IgE in serum samples causes competitive displacement of labeled IgE from allergen. Consequently, progressively lower levels of radioactivity are encountered with increasing IgE concentrations in the serum samples being evaluated. These tests are used for individuals who are thought to be extremely sensitive to the al-

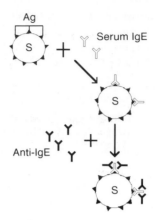

FIGURE 13.3 Radioallergosorbent test. Sorbent (S) coated with Ag is incubated with serum, allowing attachment of Ab. Radioactively labeled anti-IgE Ab is then added. When the Ag-coated S is recovered, radioactivity is found only if IgE reacted with the Ag. Failure to detect radioactivity with the S at the end of the assay indicates that IgE specific for the Ag was absent.

lergen being tested, or when the reliability of skin tests is questionable because of drug exposure, disease, or the individual's age.

Systemic Anaphylaxis

Systemic anaphylaxis is an *acute IgE-mediated reaction* affecting a variety of organ systems, including the skin (urticaria), the respiratory tract (bronchospasm and laryngeal edema), and the cardiovascular system (hypotension). Within five minutes after exposure to an allergen, clinical manifestation can begin. The systemic release of mast cell mediators induces generalized smooth muscle contraction, hypotension, edema, and irregular heart rate (arrhythmia). Unless counteracted (e.g., by epinephrine) death can occur within an hour from strangulation (narrowing of the air passages by bronchospasms), fluid accumulation in the respiratory tract (laryngeal edema), shock (hypotension), or cardiac arrhythmias (e.g., fibrillation).

Atopic Disease States and Treatment

Atopic allergy refers to a category of *chronic human allergy states,* which include hay fever, asthma, hives, and food allergies. The mechanisms through which these

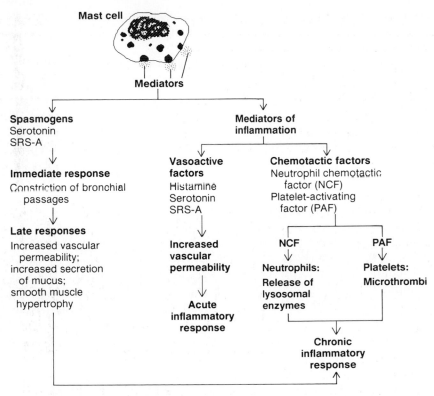

FIGURE 13.4 Inflammatory response in the asthmatic lung. Sensitized mast cells release mediators that are spasmogens and mediators of inflammation. Repeated activation of these pathways ultimately leads to manifestations of chronic inflammation.

are expressed are essentially the same as those involved in systemic anaphylaxis. Atopic responses are likely to arise when allergen is localized or absorbed slowly, in contrast to systemic anaphylaxis, which is more likely to occur if large quantities of allergen are quickly distributed throughout the body.

Allergic Rhinitis

In early spring, when the pollen count begins to climb, about 10% of the people in the United States start sneezing, wheezing, coughing, and reach for their handkerchiefs and antihistamines. Hay fever, or allergic rhinitis, is an IgE-mediated allergic reaction that affects the upper respiratory tract. It gives rise to symptoms such as nasal congestion, sinus headache, runny nose, watery eyes, itching, and sneezing. There are two types of hay fever: seasonal and chronic. Seasonal hay fever is generally caused by pollens: tree pollen in spring, grass pollen in summer, and weed pollen in autumn. Nonseasonal hay fever can be chronic unless the source (which can include such culprits as animal dander, dust, or other types of fine particles suspended in air) is removed. If the allergen cannot be removed, treatment of the symptoms can be accomplished by drugs. Antihistamines appear to be the pharmacological agents of choice for allergic rhinitis since histamine seems to be the major mediator of these allergies.

Allergic Asthma

Asthma is a more severe form of respiratory allergy that produces contraction of the trachea and bronchi (fig. 13.4). Asthma attacks can be brought on by airborne allergens. In addition, attacks can be precipitated by asthma-producing foods such as milk, milk products, eggs, meat, fish, or cereal. In fact, a person can even become sensitive to the normal microbial flora of the upper respiratory tract and become a victim of endogenous asthma attacks.

In allergic asthma reactions, constriction of the smooth muscles brings about a progressive closure of the airways. The subsequent inability to fill the lungs with air can cause serious complications. It is interesting that antihistamines do nothing to alleviate these symptoms. Antihistamines are ineffective in reversing the smooth muscle contraction because the main mediators are serotonin and SRS-A. Thus, drugs that act to reverse the muscle spasms, such as epinephrine (adrenaline), are used and are dispensed as atomizers for quick delivery. In addition, corticosteroids and cromolyn sodium have proved beneficial in treating allergic asthma attacks. These appear to act by affecting basophil and mast cell functions. Cortisone, a corticosteroid, can interfere with reaccumulation of histamine by mast cells following their degranulation. On the other hand cromolyn sodium appears to prevent degranulation (and histamine release) by stabilizing the granule and lysosomal membranes. Other therapeutic interventions include methotrexate, which modulates T cell function (e.g., possibly increasing the numbers of T_S cells), and diethylcarbamazine, which impairs the activity of LTs (especially LT-4), which can stimulate and augment inflammatory responses.

Atopic Dermatitis (Urticaria)

Allergic skin eruptions can come from such varied sources as foods, drugs, chemicals, and clothing materials. The skin condition can express itself as wheals (whitish swellings), hives (red lesions), or even eczema (scaly sores). Avoidance of the food, chemical, or material is the easiest treatment, although urticaria usually responds to antihistamines if avoidance is not possible.

Gastrointestinal Allergy

Allergies to food can cause a wide range of GI disturbances, including diarrhea, nausea, vomiting, and cramps. This type of allergy can be triggered by a wide range of foods from citrus fruits and eggs to milk and chocolate. In the severe form, the person starts to choke as the offending food is being chewed. The allergen–IgE–mast cell reaction can be so rapid that swallowing and breathing can become difficult before the first bite enters the stomach. An easy "cure" for food allergies is to avoid the food unless it is a common ingredient of prepared foods, such as eggs or flour.

Desensitization Therapy

Another approach in the treatment of allergic disease is desensitization, a procedure that attempts to modify a person's reaction to an allergen. This is accomplished by actually injecting the person with the offending allergen. Injections of an extremely small dose of allergen are started, and over a long period of time (months) it is progressively increased to a higher dose, until the person no longer reacts to the naturally occuring allergen. In this way, it is possible to "cure" the patient and permanently abolish the allergic reaction. (Note that this is induction of tolerance to the allergen.) However, there are no guarantees with this therapy. In fact, some individuals, after years of this type of allergy immunotherapy, may still be allergic, while others, although apparently "cured," may have a sudden relapse and be required to undergo treatment from the beginning. (This is equivalent to breaking tolerance.) (See chapter 10 for further discussion of tolerance.)

Densensitization seems most successful with ragweed pollen and insect venom. Although clinically effective, the precise mechanism of immunotherapy is still unknown. It is known, however, that serum IgG Abs can rise during allergy therapy. One possible explanation for this phenomenon is that large aggregates of polymerized allergen (e.g., pollen extracts treated with glutaraldehyde) present few exposed epitopes with which to stimulate sensitized mast cells. However, following degranulation of the mast cells that are activated, these aggregates are degraded, exposing several of the hidden epitopes. These exposed epitopes, in turn, stimulate the production of IgG Abs. These IgG Abs are called *"blocking"* Abs because they are able to bind to the allergen in the bloodstream before they reach the IgE–mast cell complex and thus block degranulation. The production of blocking Ab is referred to as hyposensitization since most subclasses of IgG cannot bind to mast cells themselves (IgG4 being an exception) and can remove the allergen from circulation. Thus, a person's allergic symptoms can steadily decrease as the levels of blocking IgG Ab rise during therapy (fig. 13.5).

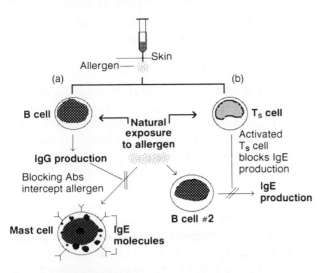

FIGURE 13.5 Treatment of Type I hypersensitivity by immunization. By means of inoculation with an allergen, immunity can be induced either by (a) the production of "blocking Ab" or (b) the activation of T_S cells.

An alternate theory states that this type of immunotherapy stimulates the expression of T_S cells. This is supported by the observation that, in some patients, the allergen injections produce a lowering of IgE Ab production. This could be brought about when the immune system responds by stimulating formation of T_S lymphocytes that induce a partial state of tolerance for the allergen. In this way, T_S cells would block B cell activation and the subsequent production of IgE; thus, as the levels of IgE drop, so would the symptoms. Why some people respond to allergy therapy by producing IgG-blocking Abs and others by T cell tolerance via suppressor cells, while others do not respond at all, are questions yet to be answered (fig. 13.5).

TYPE II HYPERSENSITIVITY: CYTOTOXIC REACTION

Type II is an **IgG-complement-mediated hypersensitivity** in which cell damage is brought about by complement fixation and lysis of the foreign antigenic cell. Thus, the damage in cytotoxic reactions is brought about by serum complement, which has been activated on a tissue cell Ag-Ab complex. In addition, there may be further cell damage by Ab-dependent cells of the immune system, such as phagocytic leukocytes. Harmful cytotoxic reactions include transfusion reactions to incompatible blood and erythroblastosis fetalis.

Mechanisms of Antibody-Dependent Cytotoxic Hypersensitivity

Type II cytotoxic reactions involve the combination of IgG or IgM serum Abs with foreign antigenic determinants on a cell membrane. Alternatively, a free foreign Ag or hapten may be adsorbed onto a cell membrane, which subsequently combines with Ab. Cytotoxic reactions can be induced, which are directed against cells displaying this configuration of Igs bound to Ags on their surfaces (fig. 13.6).

Certain of these cytotoxic reactions are complement dependent. Once IgG Abs become membrane bound, complement can be activated. Activation of the classical complement pathway leads to the lysis of the cell through generation of a membrane attack complex (fig. 13.6a). Alternatively, activation of the complement cascade can lead to the formation of C3a and C5a fragments. Since these fragments are chemotactic for phagocytic cells, they can focus a phagocytic response against the target cell (fig. 13.6b). In addition, these fragments have anaphylatoxic activity, causing histamine release and ensuing inflammation. (See chapter 6, Complement and its Role in Immune Responses, for additional details.)

In addition to the complement-dependent cytotoxic reactions outlined above, Ab-dependent cellular cytotoxicity (ADCC) reactions can be induced (fig. 13.6c). In these cases, IgG or IgM interacts with Fc receptors of natural killer (NK) cells initiating the ADCC response. These ADCC reactions can damage normal tissues. For example, auto-Abs binding to acetylcholine receptors in myasthenia gravis can induce ADCC reactions directed against normal skeletal muscle.

An example of immunohematologic disease is drug-induced immune hemolytic anemia. In this situation, a drug, such as the antibiotic penicillin, can bind to the membrane of an erythrocyte and form an antigenic complex with the surface of the blood cell. This can bring about the production of Abs, which can bind to the drug–cell membrane complex. Thus, the drug

Regulating IgE Synthesis

I mmunologically, there are strains of mice known as responders and nonresponders. A responder strain produces an elevated immune response, such as a high Ab titer, to a specific Ag; low responders or nonresponders display little or no immune reaction to the same Ag. Such strains of mice are helpful as experimental models in determining regulatory factors involved in immune responsiveness. For example, for studies of IgE production, the BDF-1 and SJL strains can be used.

When challenged with Ag, the inbred strain BDF-1 produces a high level of IgE, whereas strain SJL produces little or no IgE. Upon examination of the spleen cells, two soluble factors can be isolated from T cells: (1) an IgE-potentiating factor from BDF-1 splenic cells producing IgE and (2) an IgE-suppressive factor from splenic cells from SJL mice, which failed to form IgE Ab. These two factors comprise a class of molecules termed IgE-binding factors. IgE-potentiating factor is found whenever IgE is expressed, whereas IgE-suppressive factor appears whenever IgE synthesis is suppressed.

It is also possible for T cells from one strain to switch from producing IgE-potentiating factor (and high IgE levels) to producing IgE-suppressive factor (and reduced IgE levels). The switch seems to depend on which type of inducing factor is present: glycosylation-enhancing factor (GEF), derived from T_H cells, or glycosylation-inhibiting factor (GIF), released from T_S cells. T cell clones release IgE-potentiating factor in the presence of GEF, but the same cells can form IgE-suppressive factor in the presence of GIF.

There are exciting therapeutic implications associated with these factors. It should be possible to administer inducers, such as GIF, in the presence of a specific IgE, that would selectively induce the formation of IgE-suppressive factors and terminate the IgE response. It also appears that human lymphocytes produce T cell factors similar to the mouse IgE-binding factors. Thus, another clinical approach to allergy therapy might be the administration of human IgE-suppressive factors. Either treatment could provide a viable alternative to the current desensitization treatment, which is effective against only a small percent of allergens.

Huff, T. F., and Ishizaka, K. Formation of IgE-binding factors by human T cell hybridomas. *Proceedings of the National Academy of Science* (USA), 81:1514, 1984.

Ishizaka, K. Regulation of IgE synthesis. *Annual Review of Immunology* 2:159, 1984.

acts as a hapten, since it is bound to the red cell membrane, and stimulates the production of a high level of antidrug Abs. Since the Abs produced are IgG and IgM, the complement cascade can be activated and the resulting erythrocyte destruction can induce severe anemia. Individuals afflicted with this disease usually show symptoms of fever, weakness, fatigue, and jaundice. Fortunately in most cases, once the patient is taken off the drug, recovery is complete.

Blood Groups

Experiments in blood transfusions were first undertaken seriously during the seventeenth century, but were so unsuccessful that the practice was outlawed in Europe. The reason for the death of so many recipients remained mysterious until 1904, when Landsteiner discovered that the serum of some human donors clumped or agglutinated the red blood cells of other normal donors. After analyzing many blood combinations, he found that all human blood was not the same, but instead could be subdivided into groups. Blood could only be transfused safely if the blood group of the donor matched that of the recipient. Life-threatening reactions occurred whenever the serum of the recipient agglutinated the donated red blood cells.

Since that time, it has been found that there are serum IgG Abs that can react to Ags present on the red blood cells. These erythrocyte Ags, called *agglutinogens,* number over 100 and comprise some 20 blood group systems. Abs to these Ags, called *agglutinins,* can

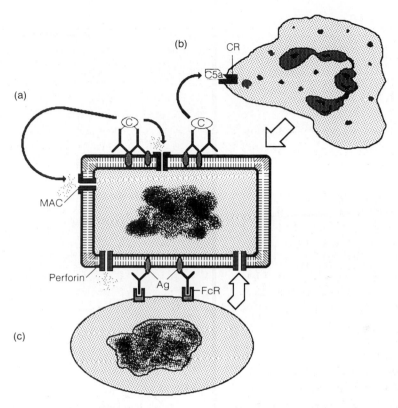

FIGURE 13.6 Mechanisms of cell destruction in Type II hypersensitivity. (*a*) Complement (C) binding to attached Abs can activate the classical complement pathway causing cytolysis through membrane attack complexes (MACs). (*b*) Generation of active intermediates from the complement pathway (e.g., C5a) can recruit phagocytes (e.g., neutrophils) through binding to their complement receptors (CRs). These cells subsequently ingest target cells. (*c*) Binding of Ab through Fc receptors (FCRs) can also stimulate NK cells to express Ab-dependent cellular cytotoxicity directed against cells displaying Ab bound to Ag.

be encountered in two clinical situations: (1) during pregnancy, if the fetus has any erythrocyte Ag that the mother's erythrocytes lack and (2) in blood transfusions, if the transfused blood is mismatched and has red cell Ags different from those of the recipient's blood. The blood group Ags that are discussed below are the ABO system and the Rh system; however, several other blood-grouping systems also exist (e.g., the Kell, Lewis, Duffy, and Kidd systems).

The ABO blood group system was discovered by Landsteiner by mixing the red cells of one set of donors with the serum of others and checking for agglutination (table 13.3). From the results, he defined the blood groups as O, A, B, and AB, which was based on the distribution of two serum agglutinins (IgG) and two agglutinogens (Ags) on the erythrocyte surface.

TABLE 13.3 Blood Typing Based on Agglutination

Blood Type	Agglutination Reaction to	
	Anti-A Serum	**Anti-B Serum**
O	−	−
A	+	−
B	−	+
AB	+	+

+ denotes that agglutination occurs, − that it does not.

The agglutinins are known as anti-A and anti-B Abs. The agglutinogens are Ag A and Ag B. If a person has blood type 0, the erythrocytes lack agglutinogens but

TABLE 13.4 ABO Blood Group System

Genotype	Blood Group Phenotype	Antigens on Erythrocytes (*agglutinogens*)	Serum Antibodies (*agglutinins*)
AA or AO	A	A	Anti-B
BB or BO	B	B	Anti-A
AB	AB	A and B	None
OO	O	None	Anti-A and anti-B

Configuration of terminal sugars in the antigenic groups for each blood type:

Blood type O
—*N*–acetylgalactosamine—[D]–galactose—*N*–acetylglucosamine—[D]–galactose

[L]–fucose

Blood type A
—*N*–acetylgalactosamine—[D]–galactose—*N*–acetylglucosamine—[D]–galactose-***N*–acetylgalactosamine**

[L]–fucose

Blood type B
—*N*–acetylgalactosamine—[D]–galactose—*N*–acetylglucosamine—[D]–galactose-**[D]–galactose**

[L]–fucose

Blood type AB
—*N*–acetylgalactosamine—[D]–galactose—*N*–acetylglucosamine—[D]–galactose-***N*–acetylgalactosamine**

[L]–fucose

—*N*–actylgalactosamine—[D]–galactose—*N*–acetylglucosamine—[D]–galactose-**[D]–galactose**

[L]–fucose

agglutinins anti-A and anti-B are found in the serum. Blood type A indicates the presence of agglutinogen A and agglutinin anti-B, whereas blood type B contains agglutinogen B and agglutinin anti-A. On the other hand, a person having type AB blood has both A and B Ags on the red cell surface and no serum agglutinins against the AB Ags. Table 13.4 summarizes the characteristics of the ABO blood group system.

Abs to the Ags of the ABO system occur in the plasma of people lacking the Ag, even though they have neither had a blood transfusion nor been pregnant. These anti-A and anti-B IgG Abs had developed during childhood from exposure to colon bacteria, which normally inhabit the lower GI tract. These bacterial Ags bear a strong resemblance to the A and B erythrocyte Ags, and hence the Abs formed against the antigenic determinants on the surface of the bacterial cells can effectively crossreact to any foreign blood cells that may enter the body during the person's lifetime.

The Ags of the ABO blood groups are inherited characteristics. The AB genes are inherited in a codominant manner since a person with an A/B genotype has both A and B Ags on the surface of the red blood cells. On the other hand, O is recessive to either A or B. Thus, a person whose genetic makeup is A/O is blood type A. If an individual had a maternal B gene and a paternal O gene passed on, the person would have blood type B. However the A/O and B/O individuals would be phenotypically indistinguishable from A/A or B/B genotypes, respectively. Accordingly, A/O or A/A both would result in blood type A, and B/O or B/B would give blood type B. The fact that an A/O person may pass the O gene on to an offspring is the basis of paternity exclusion testing. Paternity is ex-

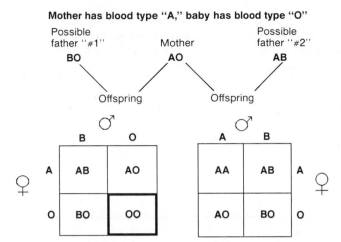

Mother has blood type "A," baby has blood type "O"

Possible father "#1"   Mother   Possible father "#2"

BO   AO   AB

Offspring   Offspring

♂   ♂

	B	O
A	AB	AO
O	BO	**OO**

	A	B
A	AA	AB
O	AO	BO

FIGURE 13.7 Paternity exclusion testing. Knowing the blood types of the mother, the baby, and the suspected father(s), the **probability of paternity** can be determined. Note that this testing can determine that someone is *not* the father or that he *might be* the father.

cluded if the child has a blood type Ag that both the supposed father and the mother lacked or if the child does not have an Ag that the father must have passed on to the offspring (fig. 13.7).

The other blood group that is discussed is the Rh factor, or D Ag. This Ag can also be found on the surface of human erythrocytes. It was named Rh since a similar Ag was detected in serum produced in rabbits immunized with rhesus monkey red blood cells. Approximately 85% of the population possess this Rh(D) Ag and are said to be Rh⁺. Persons who do not have the Rh factor on their red blood cells are Rh⁻. The plasma of Rh⁻ persons does not contain agglutinins against the Rh factor, but such Abs can develop if blood transfusions of Rh⁺ blood are given to these people. Such incompatible blood transfusions, if continued, would lead to serious transfusion reactions. The Rh factor is also an inherited trait, and each person has two of these gene complexes, one inherited from each parent. Furthermore, one or the other is passed on to an offspring. The genetics of the Rh system is most important in determining fetal-maternal compatibility. As discussed later in the chapter, if there is an Rh incompatibility, hemolytic disease of the newborn might arise. Since the Rh⁺ allele is dominant to Rh⁻, a person who is heterozygous (Rh⁺/Rh⁻) for the trait

has Rh⁺ blood, as does the homozygous dominant individual (Rh⁺/Rh⁺). The only way one can have Rh⁻ blood is to be homozygous recessive (Rh⁻/Rh⁻) and have both recessive alleles in the pair.

Transfusion Reactions

If a person whose blood belongs to one group receives a blood transfusion from a donor of another group, a hemolytic transfusion reaction is likely to occur. This occurs because the serum of the recipient may agglutinate the cells of the donor, or the serum of the donor may agglutinate the cells of the recipient. Reactions to transfusion of mismatched blood are associated with such physiological pathologies as agglutination of red cells in the blood circulation, hemolysis of erythrocytes, and liberation of free hemoglobin from the lysed red blood cells into the plasma. A rise in free hemoglobin levels can cause secondary complications such as jaundice, fever, and failure of kidney function. An adverse reaction is actually much more likely to occur if the recipient's serum agglutinated the donor's cells, than vice versa, since the donor's serum becomes considerably more diluted in the circulation of the recipient. This effect tends to minimize the agglutinating capacity of the donor's serum.

If we consider only the ABO blood group system, a person with blood type O can theoretically be considered a universal donor since there are no A or B Ags on the erythrocyte surface, which could react with anti-A or anti-B agglutinins in the serum of the recipient. Conversely, a person with blood type AB can theoretically be considered a universal recipient since both the A and B agglutinogens are already present as surface Ags.

The perception of "universal donor" or "universal recipient" is somewhat misleading. On the one hand, this perception ignores the presence of other blood group systems and the reactions that they might induce. On the other hand, this relationship applies only to washed erythrocytes. Washed erythrocytes from a type O individual would lack A or B agglutinogens, and thus should not elicit a response from individuals whose blood types are O, A, B, or AB. By similar reasoning, an individual with type AB blood could receive washed erythrocytes from individuals of any blood type, since they would not possess agglutinins in their plasma against either A or B agglutinogens. Neither whole blood nor plasma could be used, however, since the donor might possess agglutinins that could react against the recipient's erythrocytes. For example, a person with type O blood would possess anti-A and anti-B agglutinins that could react with erythrocytes in recipients with blood types A, B, or AB. Consequently, unless there is an emergency, blood transfusions always make use of type-specific blood (i.e., type A recipients receive type A blood, type B get type B, and so on).

In general, it is safe to transfuse whole blood if it can be demonstrated that the recipient and the donor have the same major and minor blood groups. This requires that serum from a candidate for transfusion be screened for atypical Abs to erythrocyte Ags, and that a potential donor's erythrocytes be crossmatched for their compatibility with the recipient's serum. In the absence of careful screening, incompatible transfusion can occur. This was more common in the past than it is today. The clinical consequence of an incompatible transfusion can range from subclinical symptoms to death, depending upon the Ab concentration, the nature of the Ag, and the immune system's ability to stimulate hemolysis.

Transfusion reactions are divided into three main types. The first, called major hemolytic reaction, occurs when there is a sudden and massive destruction of the transfused blood. Death of the patient may occur from systemic shock brought about by massive erythrocyte destruction and kidney failure consequent to a filtering overload from the excess of red cell debris. The lysis of erythrocytes is mediated by binding of circulating agglutinins to surface agglutinogens and the resultant activation of complement. Activation of the complement cascade will destroy the red cells and produce a severe drop in the hematocrit.

Minor hemolytic reactions occur when the rate of red cell destruction is less rapid. The results might only be anemia due to a lowered red blood cell count brought on by IgG-complement-mediated destruction. The transfused blood can be removed by the spleen, and the liver can metabolize the released hemoglobin; however, the person will appear jaundiced.

Fortunately, treatment is simple; we need only to find compatible blood for another transfusion.

Delayed transfusion reaction takes place when the proper blood group Abs are absent in the serum. This sometimes occurs if the agglutinins are not renewed and therefore do not persist in the serum. Thus, at the time of testing, there was no sign of incompatibility, even though the patient had been previously sensitized. An anamnestic (memory) response is elicited when the blood is transfused and the concentration of Ab rises rapidly within five to ten days posttransfusion. This results in the complement-mediated destruction of the transfused blood. The reaction, however, is not usually serious, as long as the person is retransfused with type-specific blood.

Rh Incompatability

If an Rh⁻ woman and Rh⁺ man have children, the children will probably be Rh⁺ since the Rh⁺ allele (gene) is dominant. (If the male is homozygous [Rh⁺/Rh⁺], all offspring will be Rh⁺, but if he is heterozygous [Rh⁺/Rh⁻], there is a 50% chance that each child will be Rh⁺.) If the fetus is either homozygous dominant or heterozygous, the erythrocytes will possess the Rh factor, and hence the fetus will be Rh⁺. Normally the fetal-maternal circulation does not mix but small hemorrhages can occur, especially during the last trimester when the fetus is relatively large. If this happens, there is an intermingling of fetal and maternal blood. In this situation, the Rh⁺ blood cells of the fetus would cross the protective placental barrier and enter the blood circulation of the mother. The antigenic Rh⁺ red cells of the fetus would then trigger the production of anti-Rh Ab by the mother's immune system. The maternal Ab produced is IgG, which is able to cross the placental barrier and enter the fetal circulation. Once the anti-Rh Abs have bound to the fetal Rh⁺ erythrocytes, complement is activated and fetal red cells are destroyed. As a consequence, the baby may be born with a disease state called erythroblastosis fetalis or hemolytic disease of the newborn (fig. 13.8). The disease is manifested in the fetus before it is born or within the first few days of neonatal life. The clinical symptoms include severe anemia, jaudice, edema, and enlargement of the infant's spleen and liver. The measures used

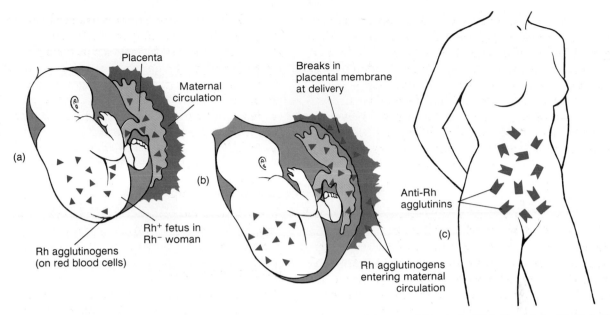

Placenta

Maternal circulation

Breaks in placental membrane at delivery

(a)

(b)

(c)

Rh⁺ fetus in Rh⁻ woman

Rh agglutinogens (on red blood cells)

Rh agglutinogens entering maternal circulation

Anti-Rh agglutinins

FIGURE 13.8 Hemolytic disease of the newborn. If blood from an Rh⁺ fetus spills into the bloodstream of an Rh⁻ mother, she will make Abs against the Rh agglutinogens. These anti-Rh agglutinins can cross the placenta and cause hemolytic disease in a subsequent pregnancy if the second fetus is also Rh⁺. (From John W. Hole, Jr., *Human Anatomy and Physiology,* 4th ed. Copyright © 1987 Wm. C. Brown Publishers, Dubuque, Iowa. All Rights Reserved. Reprinted by permission.)

in treating erythroblastosis fetalis will depend upon the severity of the symptoms. In extreme cases, total blood transfusion might be performed in order to save the baby from death due to shock.

This disease is not common with the first pregnancy since the extent of hemorrhage is usually slight and the concentration of fetal Rh factor is too low to induce maternal Ab formation. But the large amount of bleeding that occurs during delivery of the baby often ensures that the Rh⁺ cells of the infant will enter the mother's circulation and hence stimulate Ab formation. In fact, Abs formed against Rh⁺ fetal cells begin to appear about 6 weeks later. Once that happens, this disease can occur in subsequent pregnancies.

Several means exist for evaluating hemolytic disease of the newborn. For example, maternal blood can be examined for the presence of circulating Abs against fetal blood Ags. Alternatively, fetal cord blood can be tested for the presence of anti-Rh(D) Abs or Abs against other blood Ags circulating in the fetal blood.

Erythroblastosis fetalis can be prevented by passive immunization of the Rh⁻ mother with Abs against Rh⁺ blood. Designated Rh Ig, or RhoGAM ™,

and comprised of human γ-globulin containing anti-Rh Ab, its mode of action is to cancel out the antigenic effect of the fetal Rh⁺ cells that might enter the circulation. Thus, any of the baby's Rh⁺ erythrocytes that might enter the mother's bloodstream at birth are rapidly destroyed by the Rh Igs, and once removed cannot stimulate the mother's immune system. With the generation of anti-Rh Abs effectively blocked, the immunological basis for this hemolytic disease has been eliminated for any subsequent child. Rh Ig is routinely administered both during pregnancy and at the time of birth to prevent Rh immunization of the mother.

TYPE III HYPERSENSITIVITY: IMMUNE-COMPLEX DEPOSITION

If an Ag is not cellbound but rather is small and soluble, the body can encounter severe difficulties if it is repeatedly exposed to that Ag. Ag-Ab complexes might form under these conditions and can lead to Type III hypersensitivity reactions or **immune-complex syndromes.** Some of these reactions are relatively mild and self-limiting, such as the Arthus reaction, while

TABLE 13.5 Consequences of Complement Activation in Type III Hypersensitivity Reactions

Event	Role of Complement	Consequences
Release of lysosomal enzymes	Immune complexes	Proteolytic and hydrolytic enzymes can cause damage to healthy local tissues
Cytolysis	C5–9 cause rupture of cell membrane	Discharge of intracellular contents can lead to further stimulation of inflammatory responses with damage to local tissues
Chemotaxis	C3a and C5a	Lymphocytes and phagocytes can be attracted to site, thereby prolonging inflammatory response
Histamine release	C3a and C5a	Histamine discharge by basophils/mast cells and platelets can prolong inflammatory response and cause damage to blood vessel walls

others can lead to fatal organ system complications, as occurs in systemic lupus erythematosus (SLE).

In order to understand how these complexes form, one must review the physical consequences of Ag-Ab combinations (see chapter 4). The combination of Ag-Ab can cause the formation of a secondary precipitating complex if the concentrations of Ag and Ab are in the same proportion. Thus, if Abs combine with soluble Ags under appropriate conditions, complexes might form that can precipitate out of solution. This precipitation reaction is maximal when the amount of Ab equals that of Ag and is called the zone of equivalence.

Monocytes/macrophages (Mϕs) are very efficient at binding and removing large, precipitating Ag-Ab complexes. They can also remove the smaller complexes made in Ab excess, but are relatively inefficient at removing immune complexes formed in Ag excess. Polymorphonuclear neutrophils (PMNs) also remove large Ag-Ab complexes but are very inefficient at clearing smaller, soluble ones. Thus, if a physiological situation arises that mimics Ag excess, immune complexes are not cleared and their persistence can trigger an acute inflammatory response, which is classified as a Type III hypersensitivity reaction.

Mechanism of Immune-Complex Deposition

The stage is set for an immune-complex reaction whenever the combination of Ab with a large dose of Ag produces Ag-Ab complexes that cannot be effi-

ciently removed by phagocytosis. The resulting Ag-Ab complexes can then trigger the activation of serum complement, platelets, and phagocytes, all of which can set into motion events that result in tissue damage.

Usually the role of complement is to protect the host afflicted by infection. Its main function is to destroy foreign cells by lysing the plasma membrane. It also induces phagocytic PMNs to engulf and kill the harmful invaders. However, in Type III hypersensitivity, the immune complexes formed will interact with and activate the complement system. As a result, fragments C3a and C5a, which are created, can cause healthy body cells to be damaged and killed (necrosis). The C3a and C5a fragments are anaphylatoxic since they bind to plasma membrane receptor sites on basophils and mast cells, causing histamine release (inflammatory response). The C5a fragment can also attract various cells of the immune system, such as PMNs. These PMNs can respond by releasing their degradative lysosomal enzymes into the extracellular fluid, damaging the host cells in the vicinity of the reaction. The lysis of the host cells is also mediated when C5–C9 becomes activated and binds to any cells near immune complexes. Thus, in Type III hypersensitivity reactions, one level of damage is actually caused by serum complement that has been activated on a free Ag-Ab complex (table 13.5).

On another level, the generation of immune complexes can lead to blood clotting (thrombosis) and hemorrhaging. Both of these reactions involve platelets. Immune complexes can bind to receptors on the platelet membrane, causing the release of stored vasoactive amines. These chemicals lead to increased vascular permeability and damage to small blood vessels. The actual binding of the complexes to the platelets also causes platelet aggregation, which leads to thrombosis.

The generation of C5a causes infiltration of the affected area by PMNs and is a crucial step in the production of the next pathogenic level in Type III hypersensitivity. The binding of immune complexes to neutrophils can lead to the release of lysosomal enzymes whose degradative character produces tissue damage. Phagocytosis need not occur before these lysosomal enzymes are released. The cells retain their viability and can release additional degradative enzymes at a later time.

Generally, the degree of damage generated depends upon the ratio of the concentration of soluble Ag to that of Ab. For example, if a situation is created where there are equal amounts of Ag and Ab (or slightly into the Ab or Ag excess zones), the Ag-Ab complexes precipitate at the site of Ag injection and create a localized and mild Type III hypersensitivity, as in the Arthus reaction. In contrast, if there is a large Ag excess, the Ag-Ab complexes become soluble and circulate, causing more serious systemic reactions (serum sickness) or eventual deposition in organs (e.g., kidneys) joints, and skin (autoimmune disorders).

Local Deposition—Arthus Reaction

Every year there seems to be an influenza (flu) epidemic somewhere in the world, and every year millions of people receive the newest flu virus vaccine in an attempt to escape the disease. The vaccination is usually a series of two injections, the second (booster) usually given about six weeks after the initial injection. For most of us, the booster shot is as painless as the first, but for some, receiving the booster leads to a very painful, local inflammatory response at the site of the injection. The affected area becomes red, hot, swollen, and is painful to touch. This is due to an Arthus reaction. It is caused by a higher Ab titer to the influenza Ags in these individuals than the rest of the population. Accordingly, when they receive the booster (Ag),

in the wake of high Ab titers, the high Ag-Ab levels result in the formation of local, precipitating immune complexes.

Within several hours after injection, an acute inflammatory reaction develops. The immune aggregates complex in the tissue area and will fix complement. The resulting complement fragment, C5a, will attract phagocytic neutrophils, and the binding of the Ag-Ab complexes will cause them to release lyosomal enzymes. These degradative enzymes will cause tissue damage to neighboring cells, including the destructive inflammation of small blood vessels (vasculitis), which can lead to minor hemorrhaging. However, it must also be noted that while the lysosomal enzymes that are released can damage tissue, they will also degrade most of the immune complexes and, thereby, limit the course of inflammation.

The anaphylatoxin activity of C3a and C5a will trigger histamine release from local basophils and mast cells. Histamine will dilate capillary beds near the site of injection and produce swelling, as plasma leaks into the tissue area. Erythema (redness) is also due to histamine, as vasodilation increases the blood flow to the region. Histamine is also released from platelets when Ag-Ab complexes bind to membrane receptors, which then leads to platelet aggregation and eventually blood clotting. Figure 13.9 summarizes the local changes brought about during an Arthus response.

Fortunately, within a short time (12 to 24 hours), the PMNs are replaced by Mφs, which are able to successfully phagocytize and degrade the remaining immune complexes. Eosinophils also infiltrate at this time and release an antihistaminelike substance. The inflammatory response subsides and is totally resolved within a few days.

Generalized Deposition—Serum Sickness

During World War II, soldiers with bacterial infections were often treated by repeated injections of antiserum prepared in horses. Within a few weeks, the recipients often developed such symptoms as swollen lymph nodes, high fever, body rash, sore joints, and renal involvement. This syndrome was named serum sickness and is another form of Type III hypersensitivity. It was due to an immune response to horse Ags,

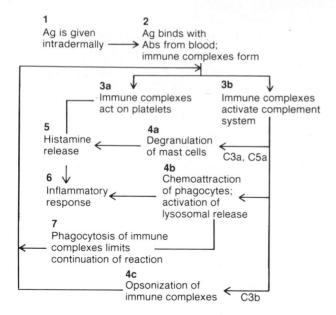

1
Ag is given
intradermally $\longrightarrow$

2
Ag binds with
Abs from blood;
immune complexes form

3a
Immune complexes
act on platelets

3b
Immune complexes
activate complement
system

5
Histamine
release $\longleftarrow$

4a
Degranulation
of mast cells

C3a, C5a

6
Inflammatory
response $\longleftarrow$

4b
Chemoattraction
of phagocytes;
activation of
lysosomal release

7
Phagocytosis of immune
complexes limits
continuation of reaction

4c
Opsonization of
immune complexes $\longleftarrow$ C3b

FIGURE 13.9 Arthus reaction. Intradermal administration of an Ag can initiate a cascade, leading to an inflammatory response. This response would be self-perpetuating, except for the stimulation of phagocytosis of immune complexes that is induced. This removes the initiating trigger and limits the extent of the inflammatory response.

and this practice has been discontinued; however, the same syndrome is now encountered in allergic reactions to certain drugs. No matter what the precipitating cause, they all result from the deposition of soluble Ag-Ab complexes formed as a result of Ag excess.

These soluble immune complexes can circulate and be subsequently deposited in various sites throughout the body, for example, in the joints. The Ag-Ab aggregates can fix complement and release C3a and C5a, which lead to degranulation of basophils and the release of histamine and PAF. These vasoactive chemicals bring about vascular changes, such as increased capillary permeability, that allow the immune complexes to localize in vessel walls. Once deposited in vessel walls, they can further fix complement with the release of chemotactic factors (CTFs). The area then becomes infiltrated with phagocytic PMNs. The accumulated PMNs ingest the Ag-Ab complexes and release lysosomal enzymes. These degradative enzymes cause systemic necrosis of the blood vessel walls. Ad-

jacent cells can also be damaged as the lysosomal enzymes diffuse out into the tissue area. Edema (swelling) is another physiological effect of the increased vascular permeability produced by histamine. In fact, this is the actual cause of the swelling of the eyes, face, and joints that occurs in this syndrome. Moreover, localized clotting also occurs. This is the result of the release of basophil-derived PAF, thus setting the events of blood clot formation into motion (table 13.6). The kidneys might also become affected if the capillaries comprising the nephron's glomeruli become involved through the deposition of immune complexes. In such instances, significant inflammatory lesions might develop (glomerulonephritis) and renal failure might result.

Initially, the circulating immune complexes are in Ag excess and produce inflammatory lesions, but as Ab production rises, the immune complexes increase in size as the zone of equivalence is reached. These larger immune complexes are more easily phagocytized and cleared by the cells of the reticuloendothelial (mononuclear-phagocytic) system of the liver and spleen. Once all immune complexes are removed from the circulation, the serum Ab titer rises and the symptoms are usually resolved within a week of developing symptoms.

In both serum sickness and the Arthus reaction, if the Ag cannot be avoided, the symptoms can be controlled by treatment with antihistamines, epinephrine, corticosteroids, and aspirin. These substances act as antiinflammatory agents.

Detection of Immune Complexes

There are many tests for the detection of circulating immune complexes in individuals with suspected immune-complex disorders. The fact that several tests are used to detect circulating complexes suggests that no single test is adequate for all situations. This is not surprising because of the dynamic nature of the processes involved in the formation of immune complexes at different stages of Ag access. To complicate matters, the identity of the Ag is often unknown and, thus, specific detection of the Ag is not always possible. Where the identity of the Ag is known, as in antigenic drug sensitivity, immune complexes are generally detected

TABLE 13.6 Reactions in Serum Sickness

Early Reactions	Late Reactions
Ag and Ab combine to form complexes	Ag-Ab complexes are deposited in blood vessel walls
Ag-Ab complexes activate complement, and trigger release of histamine from basophils and platelets	Ag-Ab complexes activate complement, stimulate platelets to form microthrombi, and attract neutrophils and stimulate release of their lysosomal enzymes
Vascular permeability is increased; inflammatory response is initiated	Blood vessel wall sustains damage

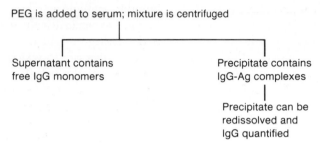

(a) **Polyethylene glycol assay**

PEG is added to serum; mixture is centrifuged

Supernatant contains free IgG monomers

Precipitate contains IgG-Ag complexes

Precipitate can be redissolved and IgG quantified

(b) **Platelet aggregation test**

Immune complexes are mixed with platelet suspension

Platelet aggregation is induced

(c) **C1q binding test**

C1q is linked to inert solid-phase support

Serum containing immune complexes is added

Complexes bind to C1q

Amount of complex is determined using radioactively labeled anti-IgG Ab

FIGURE 13.10 Assays for immune complexes.

by (1) their physical characteristics, (2) their tendency to adhere to cell membranes, or (3) their property of interaction with certain components of the complement system (fig. 13.10).

In the first category of tests (based on physical characteristics), tissue samples may be taken and examined by *immunofluorescence* for the presence of Ig and complement. We can also use the ability of polyethylene glycol (PEG) to precipitate the high molecular weight immune complexes. In this test, a serum sample is added to buffer containing PEG. If there are Ag-Ab complexes, they will be selectively precipitated by PEG and monitored by laser nephelometry.

In the second category (the ability to adhere to cell membranes), we can detect complexes in serum via the *platelet aggregation test*. This test exploits the fact that Ag-Ab complexes interact with membrane surfaces of blood platelets and produce aggregation. The presence of clumps of platelets is a positive test indicating that immune complexes are present in the serum.

Clumps can be detected either visually, with a microscope, or electronically, by changes in turbidity measured with a platelet aggregometer.

In the assay, C1q is bound to an inert support (e.g., bound to the sides of a test tube) and is exposed to a serum sample to be tested. If immune complexes are present, they will bind to the C1q. Following incubation, serum is removed and a second incubation is performed with radiolabeled anti-IgG Abs. The amount of radioactivity remaining after this second incubation correlates with the concentration of immune complexes in the serum sample.

Immune complexes have a higher molecular weight than free Ab and have a propensity for precipitation. This has provided a basis for a novel therapeutic procedure called plasmapheresis. Individuals with certain immune-complex disorders can be treated by this technique to remove Ag-Ab complexes from their serum. This test is performed with an automatic, continuous-flow, cell separator that physically removes the large, proteinaceous complexed Abs and returns the cleared plasma to the individual.

Immune-Complex Disorders

The development of immune complexes is associated with a number of pathological states in humans. Many of these diseases appear to be autoimmune in nature and are covered in chapter 16, Autoimmunity. Among these disorders are SLE, in which the immune complex consists of DNA/anti-DNA complexes, and rheumatoid arthritis, in which the normal Ig is complexed to an auto-Ag called the rheumatoid factor.

In general, all immune-complex disorders have certain pathogenic mechanisms in common. IgG and IgM are the Abs most often involved in these syndromes. However, the formation of the complexes themselves depends upon many factors that affect the ratio of Ag and Ab concentrations (Ag excess, equivalence, or Ab excess). Physiological changes in the tissues and blood greatly affect the formation and deposition of these complexes.

Once the immune complexes are formed, the complement system becomes activated. With the generation of C3a, C5a, and $\overline{C567}$, inflammation and chemotaxis might result. Since immune complexes also bind to platelet membranes, release of vasoactive amines might occur, leading to increased vascular permeability and possibly damage to small blood vessels. As a result, immune complexes could leave the circulation, precipitating in the basement membrane (basal lamina) lining of the organs.

The final stage occurs when the PMNs arrive on the scene. The infiltration by these phagocytic leukocytes is crucial to the ensuing tissue damage. Engulfment of immune complexes causes these cells to release lysosomal enzymes to the interstitial fluid. These potent hydrolytic enzymes not only destroy the immune complexes, but also produce substantial damage to normal cellular structures. Consequently, tissue damage might occur that, in more serious instances, gives rise to widespread necrosis and severely compromises the integrity of the affected organ and supporting organ systems. The most pathological clinical feature of immune-complex disorders is usually the result of lysosomal damage to tissues in the organ system that is directly affected.

Acute Poststreptococcal Glomerulonephritis

Kidney failure can be a sequel to a severe streptococcal infection. If a commonplace "strep" throat is not treated, the mass of free streptococcal Ags in circulation can increase to the point of forming soluble Ag-Ab complexes in Ag excess. If these immune complexes subsequently deposit on the glomerular basal lamina of the kidney, an acute inflammatory response can occur. Most people who develop this complication recover and respond to antiinflammatory drugs, but a few do not respond to treatment and ultimately develop chronic renal failure, which can lead to death.

Lepromatous Leprosy

In patients with lepromatous leprosy, there is a widespread, systemic invasion by the bacterium, *Mycobacterium leprae.* The mass infiltration of these bacilli into tissues can produce a high titer of antigenic fragments. Ag-Ab complexes can then form, causing an Arthus-type immune-complex reaction in the skin. This is characterized clinically by the presence of hundreds of sore, red skin lesions occurring over the entire body. Another complication of lepromatous leprosy is the deposition of immune complexes in the joints and kidneys, leading to arthritis and kidney malfunctions.

Secondary Syphilis

This sexually transmitted disease is caused by the spirochete, *Treponema pallidum*. Usually, this disease is diagnosed and treated in the primary stage, while the parasite is infectious and produces sores or chancres at the site of the infection. If the infection is not treated with antibiotics, the disease can progress to the secondary stage within a few months. In secondary syphilis, antitreponemal Abs complex with soluble treponemal Ags and these immune complexes can be detected in the serum. If these complexes lodge in the glomeruli, kidney disease will result from complement-mediated kidney damage. These same immune complexes can also lodge in the joints, and the attracted PMNs can release tissue-destroying lysosomal enzymes causing arthritislike symptoms. Afflicted persons can actually develop sores covering the entire surface of the body as immune complexes deposit in capillary beds beneath the skin and initiate local inflammatory responses. Depending upon where the immune complexes form, other organ systems can become involved during this Type III hypersensitivity inflammatory reaction. Syphilis can still be easily treated with antibiotics at this time, and the disease does not become life-threatening until years later, when tertiary syphilis develops and the stage is set for a cell-mediated Type IV hypersensitivity reaction.

TYPE IV HYPERSENSITIVITY: DELAYED OR CELL MEDIATED

The term **delayed hypersensitivity** was first coined by Koch in the late nineteenth century from his studies on immunity to tuberculosis. He was performing research with guinea pigs that had been previously exposed to the causative agent of tuberculosis, the tubercle bacillus, *M. tuberculosis*. He reexposed the guinea pigs to a heat-killed preparation of tubercle bacilli by injecting a sample under the skin. After a delay of 24 to 48 hours, there appeared at the site of injection an acute inflammatory response. The area was red, hard, and swollen. This delayed reaction was so pronounced and reproducible that it became a standard diagnostic procedure with a number of bacterial, fungal, plant, and protozoan Ags. To this day, skin testing with tuberculin extracts is used as a way of testing for prior (or current) exposure to tuberculosis.

What we now know is that delayed-type hypersensitivity (DTH) or Type IV hypersensitivity is the clinically observable outcome of a cell-mediated immune reaction in the tissues of a sensitized individual. Cell-mediated immunity refers to the immune responses of T lymphocytes and Mϕs, rather than the B lymphocytes and Abs. The major points of difference between delayed and immediate-type hypersensitivity are the time course, histology, transference, and specificity of the reactions (table 13.7). The Type IV delayed, cell-mediated reaction is so named because it appears 24 to 48 hours after the presensitized host encounters the Ag. It is characterized by redness (erythema) and formation of a hard lump (induration) in the affected region. The erythema is due to the increased blood flow to the damaged area, and the induration is a consequence of accumulated Mϕs and lymphocytes. The T lymphocytes and Mϕs are activated by the foreign, cell-bound Ags and the reaction can cause severe tissue destruction.

Mechanism of Cell-Mediated Immunity

Mechanistically, DTH reactions involve the activation of T cells by Ags that are typically cell bound. The activated T lymphocytes will produce clones (populations of cells derived from a single precursor) of T_D (CD4$^+$) and T_C (CD8$^+$) lymphocytes.

The cell-bound Ag is recognized by specific receptors located on the membrane of the T lymphocytes. In the initial recognition step, a Mϕ, which has previously engulfed the foreign cell, "presents" the Ag to specific T lymphocytes that can recognize the foreign Ags of its cell surface. These T cells will clone, and two subsets of T cells, T_D and T_C, will be created, thus establishing a Type IV reaction.

Upon reacting with Ag, the T_D cells secrete lymphokines (table 13.8). These are glycoproteins, which exert a regulatory effect chiefly on Mϕs. The lymphokines themselves are neither Ag binding nor Ag specific, but instead are substances that can attract

TABLE 13.7 Comparison of Hypersensitivity Reactions

Characteristic	Hypersensitivity Reaction			
	Immediate			Delayed
	Type I	Type II	Type III	Type IV
Approximate time to develop clinical signs	30 min	5–12 hours	3–8 hours	24–48 hours
Reaction mediators	IgE, histamine, SRS-A, etc.	IgG, IgM, complement	IgG, IgM, complement; eosinophils, neutrophils; lysosomal enzymes	T cells, Mϕs; lymphokines
Reaction to intradermal injections	Wheal and flare	–	Erythema/edema	Erythema/induration
Passive transfer with serum from sensitized donor	Yes	Yes	Yes	No
Examples	Asthma, food/insect allergies; anaphylaxis	Transfusion reaction; drug-induced allergies; hemolytic disease of the newborn	Arthus reaction; serum sickness	Graft rejection; contact dermatitis; tumor immunity

TABLE 13.8 Representative Lymphokines and Their Actions

Lymphokine	Designation	Actions
Chemotactic factor	CTF	Stimulates chemotaxis of Mϕs
Interleukin 2	IL-2	Stimulates clonal expansion and maturation of T and B cells and NK cells
Macrophage-stimulating factor	MSF	Stimulates Mϕ migration to site of Ag
Macrophage-activating factor	MAF	Restricts Mϕ movement and increases phagocytic activity
Migration-inhibiting factor	MIF	Inhibits migration of Mϕs
Interferon (gamma)	IFN-γ	Stimulates NK activity

and activate Mϕs to the area in the body where the Ag is located. Thus, the T effector cells need not leave the lymphoid area, but can operate and regulate from afar via their lymphokines. The lymphokines include CTF, which attracts Mϕs; migration- inhibiting factor (MIF), which impedes their movement from the site of infection; Mϕ-stimulating factor (MSF), which enhances Mϕ migration to the Ag area; and Mϕ-activating factor (MAF), which keeps them at the site of infec-

tion and causes them to actively phagocytize and destroy foreign cells at the site of infection.

Mϕs are nonspecific effectors of inflammation. Some of these activated Mϕs release their degradative lysosomal enzymes into the tissue where the Ag is located and thus effect a localized inflammatory response. This can lead to necrosis and fibrosis in the host tissue as well as destruction of the infecting agents or cells. Since the killing is nonspecific, a secondary

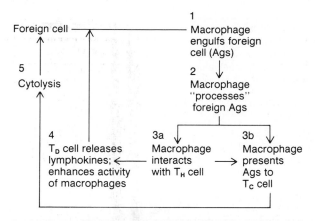

```
                                    1
Foreign cell ──────┬──────→   Macrophage
             │     │          engulfs foreign
             │     │          cell (Ags)
       ↑     │     │             2
   5   │     │     │          Macrophage   ↓
Cytolysis    │     │          "processes"
             │     │          foreign Ags
       ↑     │     │
       │     │     │
   4   │         3a  ↓           3b  ↓
 T_D cell releases  Macrophage     Macrophage
 lymphokines;  ←──  interacts   →  presents
 enhances activity  with T_H cell  Ags to
 of macrophages                    T_C cell
       │                               │
       └───────────────────────────────┘
```

FIGURE 13.11 Cell-mediated immune mechanisms. Cell-mediated mechanisms of an immune response can involve production and activation of cytotoxic lymphocytes, with subsequent lysis of the foreign cells or the stimulation of lymphokine release, leading to increased phagocytic destruction of the foreign cells.

infectious agent (such as a pathogenic bacterium) can also be killed via $M\phi$ phagocytosis (fig. 13.11).

A second subset of T cells, T_C or cytotoxic T lymphocytes, is also generated in cell-mediated immunity. These T cells can recognize and specifically react with Ags on target foreign cells and cause their lysis. Specific receptors on the surface of these cytotoxic T cells allow for cell-to-cell binding. Once this has occurred, the T_C cell is able to kill the antigenic cell by lysis. Since this killing is Ag specific, innocent host "bystander" cells are not damaged. The T_C cell itself is left unharmed and can repeat this cytotoxic process, killing dozens of target cells during its lifetime. The mechanism of the T_C cell's "lethal one-way hit" needs clarification; however, there is a clear difference between complement-mediated lysis and T_C cell lysis. Cells lysed by Ab and complement slowly leak out their cytoplasmic contents, but cells lysed by cytotoxic T cells explode. The aftermath of cytotoxic T cell destruction is cellular debris rather than a ghost cell remnant as occurs through complement lysis.

Since the Type IV hypersensitivity reaction is mediated by T cells and $M\phi$s rather than Ab and complement, immunity cannot be passively transferred to a nonsensitized individual by serum or γ-globulin injections. Nevertheless, an individual could acquire this sensitivity through a blood transfusion containing the activated T lymphocytes. Thus, the slow time course

of delayed hypersensitivity is due to the relatively slow cell division, mobilization, and migration of T lymphocytes and $M\phi$s to the Ag, as compared with the more rapid synthesis, diffusion, and delivery of soluble, noncellular Abs and complement that occurs during immediate hypersensitivity reactions.

If multiple doses of Ag are given over time to a hypersensitive individual, these Type IV inflammatory lesions can progress from acute to chronic causing local ulceration, necrosis, and fibrous scarring (granuloma).

Measurement of Cell-Mediated Immunity

There are a number of tests that can measure the efficiency of cellular immune function to a certain Ag in an individual. These fall into four basic categories: (1) delayed hypersensitivity skin tests, (2) lymphocyte activation, (3) assays for T lymphocytes, and (4) T cell function. One representative test from each category is discussed in this section in order to introduce the principles, applications, and interpretations of these assays to cellular immune function (fig. 13.12).

In **delayed hypersensitivity skin testing,** the Ag to be tested is injected into the skin and the reaction interpreted two to three days later. The *tuberculin skin test* (*Mantoux test*) provides an example of this type of testing. It is used to establish previous (or current) exposure to tubercle bacilli. A positive inflammatory lesion at the injection site confirms exposure but must be documented by a chest x-ray. The x-ray data would be the only way that we could distinguish between a previous exposure and a currently active infection of tuberculosis in an individual.

Lymphocyte activation refers to an *in vitro* test that scores for actively cloning, Ag-stimulated T lymphocytes. Lymphocyte activation is commonly used to assess cellular immunity in individuals with immune deficiency, autoimmunity, infectious diseases, and cancer. In the lymphocyte culture technique, purified lymphocytes are cultured in media containing substances called mitogens. Mitogens are plant or bacterial-derived chemicals that have the ability to stimulate lymphocyte division (blastogenesis). A radioactively labeled precursor of DNA is then added since DNA synthesis is very active during blastogenesis. The mixture is incubated and the radioactivity

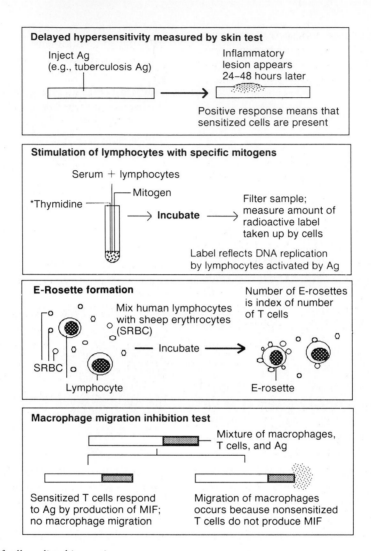

Delayed hypersensitivity measured by skin test

Inject Ag
(e.g., tuberculosis Ag)

Inflammatory
lesion appears
24–48 hours later

Positive response means that
sensitized cells are present

Stimulation of lymphocytes with specific mitogens

Serum + lymphocytes

*Thymidine —— Mitogen

→ **Incubate** →

Filter sample;
measure amount of
radioactive label
taken up by cells

Label reflects DNA replication
by lymphocytes activated by Ag

E-Rosette formation

Mix human lymphocytes
with sheep erythrocytes
(SRBC)

Number of E-rosettes
is index of number
of T cells

SRBC

Lymphocyte

—— Incubate ——→

E-rosette

Macrophage migration inhibition test

Mixture of macrophages,
T cells, and Ag

Sensitized T cells respond
to Ag by production of MIF;
no macrophage migration

Migration of macrophages
occurs because nonsensitized
T cells do not produce MIF

FIGURE 13.12 Evaluation of cell-mediated immunity.

incorporated into lymphocytes is then measured. If a person has a very large number of active lymphocytes, blastogenesis will be stimulated by the mitogen, and the amount of radioactive DNA will be high. However, the amount of DNA synthesis is decreased in someone with depressed levels of reactive lymphocytes, and the resulting stimulation index is lower than normal.

In the **assays for human T lymphocytes,** we can get information about the number of T cells in an individual. This information can be used diagnos-

tically to assess immune deficiency disorders (e.g., acquired immune deficiency syndrome [AIDS]), certain infectious diseases, and cancer. However, these tests give no specific information about the functional capacity of these cells. One of these tests, the E-rosette test, measures the number of T lymphocytes by exploiting the unusual fact that human T cells can bind sheep erythrocytes. The lymphocytes are larger in size than the erythrocytes, and so a flowerlike rosette is formed, with the T cell as the flower's center and the sheep erythrocytes as the petals. This marker is termed

E(rythrocyte) rosette and is a widely used means of identifying and quantifying human T lymphocytes. The role of this test is being superceded by the use of the fluorescence-activated cell sorter (see chapter 4 for further description).

One **T cell function** that can be tested is the *ability to produce lymphokines* upon reexposure to a specific Ag. One lymphokine that is produced by a reactive T cell is MIF, which inhibits the normal migration of Mφs. In the *Mφ migration inhibition test,* lymphocytes, isolated from a patient, are packed into capillary tubes containing macrophages. These capillary tubes were previously coated with the specific Ag to be tested. If the lymphocyte population had previous memory of being exposed to the Ag, the T cells will release MIF and the Mφs will not emigrate from the capillary tube. Thus, whenever migration is inhibited, the lymphocytes in that tube are sensitive to that Ag and can functionally respond and produce the lymphokine, MIF.

Type IV Disease States
Contact Dermatitis: Poison Ivy

Allergic contact dermatitis is a cell-mediated allergic reaction that occurs when certain chemicals come in contact with and bind to skin cell components. For example, in poison ivy, the oily substance coating the underside of the leaves contains chemicals called catechols. When the catechols come in contact with skin, they can be easily absorbed and then bind to high molecular weight skin proteins. The initial steps of sensitization appear to involve Ag processing via the Langerhans' cells of the epidermis. This triggers a sequence of events, leading to the clonal expansion of specific T lymphocytes. Thus, in seven to ten days, there is a T cell response and memory cells are formed. There is usually no ensuing poison ivy rash upon first contact since the catechol-bound protein complexes have been sloughed off. However, once sensitized, if a person is reexposed to the poison ivy catechols, the same carrier (skin protein)-hapten (catechol) conjugate is formed and recognized. T memory cells are rapidly (one to two days) converted to activated T cells, which produce lymphokines and mediate Mφ-induced inflammation. This produces severe blistering of the skin accompanied by severe itching. T_C cells are also involved in

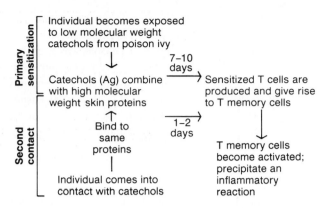

FIGURE 13.13 Events of contact dermatitis to poison ivy.

and cause the destruction of all epidermal cells associated with the catechol–skin protein complex (fig. 13.13).

Treatment for such a condition includes washing with brown soap (Fels-Naptha) to remove the oily catechol complexes from the skin and weeping blisters, the topical use of antiinflammatory (containing hydrocortisone) cream to control the itching. In severe cases, systemic corticosteroids are employed to reduce the inflammation.

Tertiary Syphilis

Syphilis is a sexually transmitted disease that can progress through three distinct phases. The causative agent is the spirochete *T. pallidum,* which is sensitive to the antibiotic pencillin. The first stage of syphilis is characterized by the formation of a chancre (ulcerous lesion) at the site of infection. This primary syphilitic stage lasts approximately two weeks, whereupon the chancre heals and the person appears to be asymptomatic. However, if left untreated, secondary syphilis follows months later and is characterized by infectious skin rashes, swollen glands, and general malaise. If syphilis still remains untreated, tertiary syphilis is expressed years after the primary infection. In this stage, unusual skin lesions, called gummas, are formed on the body. These lesions arise as a result of cell-mediated immunity to circulating *T. pallidum* Ags. The lesions are due to tissue destruction by T cells and Mφs at sites of infection in the body.

Unfortunately, the skin is not the sole organ involved at this stage. Type IV hypersensitivity reactions can also occur in the brain, kidney, liver, bone, and blood vessels. This can lead to brain degeneration, kidney and liver dysfunctions, bone deformation, and circulatory system disintegration. Death usually ensues from a chronic tertiary syphilitic infection because of cell, tissue, and organ system damage brought on by cell-mediated allergic reactions.

Leprosy

Leprosy, or Hansen's disease, is caused by the acid-fast bacillus, *M. leprae.* This bacterium has a propensity for attacking human skin and nerve cells. Leprosy is a disease that is characterized by the development of multiple lesions of the skin accompanied by numbness. There are three forms of leprosy: (1) the relatively benign tuberculoid leprosy, which results in skin discoloration; (2) an intermediate form called borderline, which includes anesthetic (loss of sensation) skin lesions; and (3) severe lepromatous leprosy, which can include systemic organ involvement.

The form the disease takes depends very much on the cell-mediated response following infection. The later the cell-mediated immune response develops, the longer the parasite can reproduce inside human host cells and the more severe the infection. For example, in tuberculoid leprosy, there is a strong cell-mediated response that inhibits the growth of the bacilli, while there is little evidence of cell-mediated immunity in the severe, life-threatening, lepromatous leprosy.

In leprosy, we might also observe the phenomena of reversal and downgrading reactions. These "reactions" are characteristic of borderline forms of leprosy and represent abrupt shifts in cell-mediated immunity. Formerly benign skin lesions suddenly become sore and tender. There is a concomitant decline in the number of circulating lymphocytes (downgrading reaction), and the skin lesions can spread and involve surrounding nerve cells (reversal reaction). This cell-mediated hypersensitivity reaction can lead to extensive skin and nerve damage. Thus, the destruction of tissue cells that occurs in leprosy is largely due to an attack by T lymphocytes and activated Mϕs on infected host cells.

These immunological complications can be very severe and require treatment with antiinflammatory agents such as corticosteroids, which can depress the immune response. A sulfa-derived antibacterial drug, dapsone, is usually the chemotherapeutic agent of choice in treating leprosy.

SUMMARY

1. The immune system sometimes goes awry and malfunctions, or overreacts, causing a disease state called hypersensitivity. Four classes of hypersensitivity reactions are characteristically identified, and occasionally a fifth is included. [p. 330]
2. Type I hypersensitivity or anaphylaxis consists of two stages: sensitization and atopic reaction. (a) In sensitization, the antigen (allergen) stimulates the production of IgE antibody, which binds to mast cells and basophils. (b) In the atopic reaction, a second exposure to allergen leads to antigen binding to IgE-bound mast cells and basophils. This stimulates the release of mediators, such as histamine. [pp. 330–331]
3. Histamine causes the contraction of smooth muscles, dilation of blood vessels, increased capillary permeability, and the release of mucus. The ensuing inflammatory response can lead to contraction of air passages and loss of blood fluids, resulting in asphyxiation and shock. [pp. 331–335]
4. Antihistamines and epinephrine are the drugs of choice in treating certain Type I hypersensitivity reactions by neutralizing histamine and serotonin, respectively. Since numerous cell mediators are released during an allergic reaction, one drug cannot alleviate all symptoms of an allergy, which can take many forms (e.g., food, respiratory, skin). [pp. 333–335]
5. Type I hypersensitivity to certain allergens can be measured by skin tests (wheal and flare, Prausnitz-Küstner tests) or *in vitro* testing (radioallergosorbent test). [pp. 335–336]

6. Hay fever, asthma, eczema, hives, and food allergies are all forms of Type I reactions. These conditions are due to different types and locations of cell mediators. [pp. 336–338]

7. Desensitization to an allergen can be accomplished by injecting varying doses of the offending allergen over a long period of time. This treatment might lead to the production of blocking antibodies (IgG or IgA), the activation of suppressor T cells, or both. The former inactivates the antigen before it can bind to IgE, and the latter suppresses synthesis of IgE. [pp. 338–339]

8. Type II hypersensitivity or cytotoxic reaction is an IgG-complement-mediated hypersensitivity. Cell damage is caused by complement-mediated or antibody-dependent cytolysis of the foreign antigenic cell to which antibody is bound. [p. 339]

9. A further complication arises in Type II reactions since the activation of the complement cascade leads to the formation of C3a and C5a fragments. Their ensuing chemotactic and anaphylatoxic activity leads to phagocytosis and histamine release, respectively. [pp. 339–340]

10. Harmful cytotoxic reactions include blood transfusion reactions, drug-induced hemolytic anemia, and erythroblastosis fetalis. [p. 340]

11. In 1904 Landsteiner discovered the ABO blood group system, which provided the basis for successful blood transfusions. Erythrocytes can have type A, B, or A and B antigens (agglutinogens) on their surfaces. If blood is mismatched, circulating antibodies (agglutinins) can bind to foreign erythrocytes, causing agglutination and complement-induced lysis. [pp. 340–344]

12. Another blood group, Rh(D), also must be considered in blood transfusions. Rh incompatibility is more of a problem during pregnancy when the mother is Rh⁻ and the fetus is Rh⁺. This can lead to the disease erythroblastosis fetalis if the mother becomes sensitized to the fetus' Rh⁺ antigens. Once

sensitized, the maternal immune system can produce cytotoxic immunoglobulins that are able to cross the placenta and attack the erythrocytes of the fetus. [pp. 343–345]

13. In Type III hypersensitivity (immune-complex deposition), repeated exposure to a small, soluble antigen can cause the formation of antigen-antibody complexes that can activate complement. [pp. 345–346]

14. C3a and C5a fragments can be generated and be chemotactic for phagocytes, which can then release harmful lysosomal enzymes. These fragments are also anaphylatoxic and can cause mast cells and basophils to release histamine, producing an inflammatory response. [pp. 346–347]

15. Repeated subcutaneous injections of antigen can lead to antibody excess and local deposition of immune complexes, called the Arthus reaction. This causes local inflammation and minor tissue damage at the site of injection. [p. 347]

16. Repeated injection of antigen can cause serum sickness, a condition due to antigen excess and the formation of circulating antigen-antibody complexes. The resulting activated complement components can damage the vascular bed and cause leakage of complexes into tissue regions, such as joints and kidneys, where tissue damage can occur. [pp. 347–348]

17. Immune complexes can be detected by a variety of clinical tests such as the polyethylene glycol assay, complement-binding tests, and immunofluorescence. [pp. 348–350]

18. There are many types of immune-complex disorders including acute poststreptococcal glomerulonephritis, lepromatous leprosy, and secondary syphilis. Tissue damage in all of these disease states is mediated by antigen-antibody complexes and complement activation. [pp. 350–351]

19. Treatment of certain immune-complex syndromes can be accomplished by plasmapheresis, which removes harmful complexes from the plasma before they are deposited and damage organ tissues. [p. 350]

20. In Type IV hypersensitivity or cell-mediated reactions, foreign cell-bound antigens activate T lymphocytes and macrophages to produce a cell-mediated response. [p. 351]

21. Activated T_D cells produce soluble lymphokines, which can attract attacking macrophages to the site of infection where they can bind, phagocytize, and destroy the foreign cells. [pp. 351–353]

22. T_C cells are also produced, which can bind to and destroy foreign cells on contact. [p. 353]

23. Type IV cell-mediated immunity can be measured by delayed hypersensitivity skin testing, lymphocyte activation tests, E-rosette assay, or MIF tests. These tests measure different aspects of cellular immune function to antigens. [pp. 353–355]

24. Type IV disease states include contact dermatitis, borderline leprosy, and tertiary syphilis. Allergic contact dermatitis is a cell-mediated reaction to certain chemicals that contact and bind to the skin. Damage in Type IV disease states is mediated by T cells and macrophages. [pp. 355–356]

R E A D I N G S

Austen, K. F. Systemic anaphylaxis in the human being. *New England Journal of Medicine* **291**:661, 1974.

Beall, G. N. Asthma: New ideas about an old disease. *Annals of Internal Medicine* **78**:405, 1973.

Buisseret, P. D. Allergy. *Scientific American* **247**:86, 1982.

Conrad, D. H., FcεRII/CD23: the low affinity receptor for IgE. *Annual Review of Immunology* **8**:623, 1990.

Fathman, C., and Fitch, F. *Isolation, Characterization and Utilization of T-lymphocyte Clones.* Academic Press, Inc., Orlando, Fla., 1982.

Fearon, D. T. Cellular receptors for fragments of the third component of complement. *Immunology Today* **5**:105, 1984.

Gleich, G. J. The late phase of the immunoglobulin E-mediated reaction. *Journal of Allergy and Clinical Immunology* **70**:160, 1982.

Gottlieb, A. R., Mazicaz, G. A., Tamaki, N., et al. The effect of dialyzable products from human leukocyte extracts in cutaneous delayed hypersensitivity responses. *Journal of Immunology* **124**:885, 1980.

Haeney, M. *Introduction to Clinical Immunology.* Butterworth Publishers, Stoneham, Mass., 1985.

Herberman, R. B. Natural killer cells. *Hospital Practice* **17**:93, 1982.

Holborow, E., and Reeves, W. *Immunology in Medicine,* Grune & Stratton, Inc., Orlando, Fla., 1983.

Hollingsworth, H. M., Giansiracusa, D. F., and Upchurch, K. S. Anaphylaxis. *Journal of Intensive Care Medicine* **6**:55, 1991.

Insalaco, S. J. Massive transfusion. *Laboratory Medicine* **15**:325, 1984.

Ishizaka, T., White, J. R., and Saito, H. Activation of basophils and mast cells for mediator release. *International Archives of Allergy and Applied Immunology* **82**:327, 1987.

Karenblat, P. E., and Wedner, H. J. *Allergy:Theory and Practice.* Grune & Stratton, Inc., Orlando, Fla., 1984.

Landsteiner, K., and Levine, P. On the inheritance of agglutinogens of human blood demonstrable by immune agglutinins. *Journal of Experimental Medicine* **48**:431, 1928.

Lockey, R. F., and Bukantz, S. C. (eds.). *Principles of Immunology and Allergy.* W. B. Saunders Co., Philadelphia, 1987.

Milgrom, F., Abeyounis, C. J., and Albini, B. *Antibodies: Protective, Destructive and Regulatory Role.* S. Karger, Publishers, Basel, 1985.

O'Hehir, R. E., Garman, R. D., Greenstein, J. L., et al. The specificity and regulation of T-cell responsiveness to allergens. *Annual Review of Immunology* **9**:67, 1991.

Oppenheim, J., and Landy, M. *Interleukins, Lymphokines and Cytokines.* Academic Press, Inc., Orlando, Fla., 1983.

Ptak, W., Rozycka, D., Askenase, P. W., et al. Role of antigen-presenting cells in the development and persistence of contact hypersensivity. *Journal of Experimental Medicine* **151**:362, 1980.

Theofilopoulos, A. N., and Dixon, F. J. The biology and detection of immune complexes. *Advances in Immunology* **28**:89, 1979.

Turgeon, M. L. *Fundamentals of Immunohematology.* Lea and Febiger, Philadelphia, 1989.

Wilson, C. B., and Dixon, F. J. Immunopathology and glomerulonephritis. *Annual Review of Medicine* **25**:83, 1974.

he compo
teract wit
work tha
against a constan
protozoa, tumors.
the potential for
sists of an innate
quired arm (B cell
mediated] immu
pendently or in

Deficien
can be **inherite**
quired. In gene
dividual with im
the role that the
system plays. Fo
encounter viral
whereas B cell
bacterial infecti

Treatm
many avenues,
In the sections t
orders that are d
entire spectrum
netic, developm
netic, developm
psychological.

■ ■ ■

TABLE 14

Disorder
Reticular dysgenesis
CID
A-T
Wiskott-Aldric syndrome
ADA deficien

Consequently, the child suffers from severe, recurrent infections throughout life. This disease results from failure of stem cells to differentiate into lymphocytes. (These could be processed later by the secondary lymphoid organs into B and T cells.) Although the individual has phagocytes (neutrophils and monocytes) to combat infections, if they are overwhelmed, there is no backup system in the form of lymphocytes to call upon. Prophylactic antibiotic therapy can help, but the child is still very vulnerable to infection and, unless placed in a sterile "bubble," the child will usually succumb to an infection within the first few years of life. If a close tissue match can be made, the most effective treatment is bone marrow transplantation. When successful, the individual's immune system becomes functional through this therapy.

Ataxia Telangiectasia

A partial CID is ataxia telangiectasia (A-T). (Ataxia refers to uncoordinated muscle movements, and telangiectasia refers to the vascular dilation that frequently occurs in this disorder.) In contrast to the previously mentioned disorders, in A-T the developmental defect *occurs prior to stem cell maturation,* and the lesion affects the embryonic mesoderm. Hence, A-T is a *multisystem defect,* involving the vascular, endocrine, nervous, and immune systems. There is evidence of both bone marrow and thymic lesions in A-T. This disorder is progressive. Mental capacity, immune status, and other physiological conditions deteriorate with time. Severe infections begin to occur during the first year of life, and may be either viral (T cell) or bacterial (B cell). Interestingly, Ab levels and T lymphocyte populations are only slightly decreased initially, but their depression becomes more severe with time. Persons afflicted with A-T rarely survive past puberty, due to physiological complications.

Wiskott-Aldrich Syndrome

Another partial CID is Wiskott-Aldrich syndrome, which is an X-linked recessive syndrome. It is characterized by three cardinal symptoms: bleeding, recurrent infections, and eczema. The bleeding is due to reduced platelet output (thrombocytopenia); recurrent bacterial, viral, and fungal infections from abnormal-

ities in cell-mediated (thymic hypoplasia) and Ab-mediated (lymphoid hyperplasia) immunity; and allergy-related eczema from elevated IgE levels. There is also evidence of *decreased functional reactivity of lymphocytes, monocytes, and platelets.* The *Ig pattern is aberrant* in that IgM levels are low but IgA and IgE levels are elevated. Males with Wiskott-Aldrich syndrome are also prone to malignancies, perhaps due to decreased immune surveillance. Treatment of the disorder might involve the prophylatic use of antibiotics and administration of intravenous immune serum globulin preparations. Successful bone marrow transplantation has resulted in correcting both the platelet and immunological abnormalities.

Enzyme Deficiency

Certain types of immune deficiency disorders arise as a consequence of reduced enzymatic activity. One interesting example of a CID has a genetically inherited enzyme deficiency disorder. The enzyme that is deficient in this disorder is adenosine deaminase (ADA), which is essential in nucleic acid metabolism. This defect means that adenosine accumulates in the lymphocytes and exerts a suppressive effect on the functioning of T cells, especially the T_H cells. Suppression of the T_H cells interferes with Ab production, as well as cell-mediated immunity. Consequently, the person with this deficiency has depressed humoral and cellular immune responses. The most successful way to treat this type of CID is transplantation of stem cells from fetal bone marrow or liver. This can lead to the subsequent restoration of full immunological function.

Two experimental procedures for treating CID are currently under investigation. One procedure involves *gene replacement* to compensate for ADA deficiency. In this procedure, leukocytes from an individual with CID are grown in cell culture with nonpathogenic retroviruses (e.g., vaccinia virus) containing a functional human ADA gene. Cells that become infected by the virus incorporate and can express the ADA gene. When returned to the person, these cells can compensate for ADA deficiency so long as the cells survive. The second procedure *replaces functional ADA* itself by linking it to polyethylene glycol (PEG). Since the ADA-PEG complex retains biological activity, it also can compensate for ADA deficiency in individuals with CID. However, replacement of ADA is only short-term since it is determined by the half-life of the ADA-PEG complex in the circulation. Consequently, repeated administration of ADA-PEG is needed. This second approach has already been used in treating a few children with CID. It appears to be a reasonable, albeit temporary, strategy in cases where bone marrow transplantation is not possible.

ANTIBODY (B CELL) IMMUNE DEFICIENCY DISORDERS
Hypogammaglobulinemias

There are several types of B cell defects which are referred to as hypogammaglobulinemias. These disorders are so named because they are characterized by a *severe reduction in the plasma proteins known as γ-globulins.*

This class of immune deficiency includes inherited and developmental disorders. For example, in X-linked infantile hypogammaglobulinemia (Bruton's disease), male infants suffer from severe, chronic bacterial infections after placental Abs or Abs from breast-feeding have been degraded. In this syndrome, the *B cell presursors are believed to be absent or arrested* at a pre-B cell stage of differentiation. This is suggested by the absence, or deficiency, of all five classes of serum Igs. Infants with this disorder respond well to antibiotic treatment for bacterial infections and seem able to handle viral infections relatively well. Administration of γ-globulin is the mainstay of such therapy. Even with these therapies, it is rare that children afflicted with this disease reach puberty; in fact, many develop chronic lung disease and die of respiratory complications.

Acquired hypogammaglobulinemia differs from congenital hypogammaglobulinemia in three important ways. First, the person with this deficiency has B lymphocytes and low (not absent) Ab titers. Second, the onset of the disease usually occurs after puberty. Third, there is some abnormality in T lymphocyte function. These include possible decreases in T_H function and increased numbers of T_S cells. The cardinal sign of this disorder is recurrent pyogenic infections caused by gram-positive pathogenic bacteria. Onset of these infections can occur at any age. Although the numbers of B cells appear to be normal, the

levels of all classes of Abs are abnormally depressed. What triggers this disorder remains unknown, but T cells appear to be involved. The treatment of acquired hypogammaglobulinemia is identical to that of infantile hypogammaglobulinemia, which includes γ-globulin replacement therapy and prophylactic antibiotic treatments.

Dysgammaglobulinemia

There is also a class of syndromes that include a *deficiency in only one type* of Ab class. This type of disorder is called a dysgammaglobulinemia, reflecting a disturbance of the "normal" γ-globulin fraction. One example of this class of disorder is a selective IgA deficiency. The cause of this disorder is unknown and this disease can strike at any age. The numbers of IgA-producing B cells are usually normal. The defect appears to be in the production of T_S cells specific for the secretory Ab, IgA. The most frequent symptoms are recurrent bacterial lung infections, such as lobar pneumonia. Other complications include increased incidence of allergies, gastrointestinal disease, autoimmune disease, and increased risk of developing cancer. Without the protective function of IgA present in the mucosal linings, the body is more open to pathogenic agents, which can produce these complications. Unlike the more generalized hypogammaglobulinemias, people suffering from selective IgA deficiency should not be treated with γ-globulin therapy. Since they are capable of forming normal amounts of Ab of other Ig classes, they may recognize injected IgA as foreign and form anti-IgA Abs, which could trigger an immune-complex syndrome. Broad-spectrum antibiotics are used to prevent bacterial infections, but there is, as yet, no means by which the deficient IgA can be replaced safely.

CELLULAR (T CELL) IMMUNE DEFICIENCY DISORDERS

Individuals with defects in T cell function have more severe and resistant infections than those with Ab deficiency disorders. Rarely do individuals with cellular immune deficiency disorders survive to puberty. Disorders in T cell immunity are also often associated with

TABLE 14.2 Characteristics of B and T Cell Disorders

Disorder	Organ Affected	Cell Type Affected	Consequence	Treatment
X-linked infantile hypogamma-globulinemia	Bursa equivalent	B cell	Increased bacterial infections	Antibiotics; γ-globulin
Acquired hypogamma-globulinemia	Unknown	B cell (T cell)	Increased infection by gram-positive bacteria	Antibiotics; γ-globulin
Selective IgA deficiency	Unknown	B cell	Increased bacterial infections	Antibiotics only
DiGeorge syndrome	Thymus	T cell	Increased bacterial, viral, and yeast infections	Antibiotics; calcium and hormone therapy
Nezelof's syndrome	Thymus	T cell	Increased bacterial, viral, and protozoan infections	Antibiotics; γ-globulin; thymus transplants; transfer factor

abnormalities of B cell immunity in view of the close link between T_H function and the expression of Ab production by B cells. Cellular immune deficiency disorders are most often associated with viral, fungal, and protozoan infections, rather than with bacterial infections. In most cases of primary defects in cellular immunity, Ab production is secondarily depressed, but the Abs produced are functional and can protect the person from some bacterial pathogens. Other pathologies associated with this class of immune deficiency disorder include growth failure, susceptibility to graft-versus-host reactions, fatal infections with live (attenuated) viral vaccines, and increased risk of malignancy. Table 14.2 describes the major similarities and differences between B and T cell disorders.

DiGeorge Syndrome

In *congenital thymic aplasia,* or DiGeorge syndrome, the person is born with little or no thymus gland. In addition, the parathyroids, endocrine glands near the thymus, are also absent. The functions of both organs are essential for survival—the thymus for the formation of competent T cells to carry out cellular immune functions, and the parathyroids for the production of the hormone, parathormone, which regulates calcium levels in the blood.

The thymus and parathyroid glands are absent as a result of interference with normal embryonic development during the first trimester of pregnancy. In addition to the absence of these glands, persons with DiGeorge syndrome also display abnormal facial features. The first signs of this disorder appear immediately after birth and are manifest as heart problems so severe that the baby can die of congestive heart failure within days of birth. This is usually a consequence of impaired calcium regulation caused by the absence of the parathyroid glands. This yields a condition called hypocalcemia (low blood calcium levels). Since the heart is very sensitive to calcium levels, an imbalance in either direction can be life threatening. If left untreated, the baby might die of cardiac arrest before passive maternal immunity ceases and problems with cell-mediated immunity due to thymic aplasia commence. Injections of calcium and parathormone can correct the hypocalcemia and the resulting cardiac problems. However, individuals who survive this immediate neonatal period develop recurrent and chronic infections including pneumonia, diarrhea, and yeast infections.

Examination of the white blood cells reveals a lymphocytopenia with *T cell numbers being markedly reduced.* B cells are present, but Ab levels, although very low, are functional. These Abs are primarily maternally transferred IgG type. If a diagnosis of DiGeorge syndrome is made soon after birth, the baby can be given a fetal thymus transplant that can permanently restore T cell immunity. Thus, the key to prolonged survival is the proper and prompt diagnosis and treatment of the disease soon after birth.

Nezelof's Syndrome

In contrast to DiGeorge syndrome, Nezelof's syndrome is a T cell deficiency disorder that results in *abnormal Ig synthesis.* Persons with this disease are susceptible to recurrent fungal, viral, protozoan, and bacterial illnesses, and are usually diagnosed around two to three years of age. While the cause for this disorder is unknown, findings show a marked decrease in T (but not B) cells, which reflects the abnormalities in thymus architecture in which the number of thymocytes is reduced. Although the *levels of B cells and Abs appear normal, humoral immunity is abnormal.* There usually is no Ab response following specific immunization, and much of the circulating Abs in these individuals are not specific for any known Ag.

In order to improve the person's prognosis, aggressive treatment of infections is necessary. In addition, continuous antibiotic treatment and monthly γ-globulin administration is required. Thymus transplantation and administration of thymic factors can restore cellular immunity and partial humoral immunity. Transfer factor therapy has been utilized with questionable success, on occasion. Transfer factor is a soluble extract derived from immune T cells and has been implicated in T cell differentiation, activation, and expression.

MURINE MODELS FOR B AND T CELL IMMUNE DEFICIENCY DISORDERS

Several animal models have been developed to study immune deficiency disorders. Three specific murine models are outlined briefly.

The **athymic,** or **nude (Nu/Nu), mouse** represents a mutant strain of mouse which serves as a model *congenital T cell immune deficiency disorder.* The nude mouse arises as an autosomal recessive mutant that displays failure of hair growth (hence the name "nude") and arrested development of the thymus gland (see highlight 2.1). In nude mice, the thymus is present as a rudimentary structure, if it is present at all. Consequently, these animals are unable to properly support Ag-independent differentiation of T cells.

A T cell population can be identified in nude mice by the presence of Thy-1 Ag. However, these cells fail to express Ag-specific T cell receptors (TCRs) characteristic of mature T lymphocytes. In particular, T cells of nude mice display TCRs expressing the γδ gene sequences rather than αβ normally encountered in mature Ag-responsive T cells. This observation suggests a role for the thymus gland in determining the repertoire of TCRs in mature, functional T cells. This model is used to study influences of the thymic environment on (1) Ag-independent differentiation of T cells, (2) determination of the repertoire of TCRs, and (3) induction of neonatal tolerance.

A second murine model is associated with a partial B cell defect. Since this model *B cell immune deficiency disorder* is associated with a mutation to a member of an X-linked gene family, it has been designated as an **X-linked immune deficiency (*xid*).** The gene affected appears to be an X-linked lymphocyte regulatory (XLR) gene. The XLR gene is selectively expressed in both B and T lymphocytes and encodes a filamentlike protein that possesses certain properties of a nuclear regulatory protein. In *xid* mice, this gene apparently is not transcribed. However, it is not yet clear how this mutation is associated with the impaired B cell function associated with this immune deficiency.

A third murine model produces a **severe combined immune deficiency (*scid*).** The defect responsible for this mutation is focused to a site designated *scid,* which maps on chromosome 16. The *scid* mouse serves as a model *T and B cell immune deficiency disorder* arising from defective B and T cell differentiation. In particular, this mutant displays abnormal recombinase activity. As a result, defects arise in joining disparate gene regions contributing to the repertoires of Ag receptors (surface Igs or TCRs). For example, V-D-J recombination during Ig production by B cells appears to be impaired in *scid* mice. This is seen as an inability to properly join the cleaved ends of V region gene segments. Consequently, there is impaired production of fully functional lymphocytes. The *scid* mutation provides a model for exploring the mechanisms of gene rearrangement (recombination) responsible for producing the diversity of Ag-specific receptors displayed by mature lymphocytes.

These, and other, model systems provide powerful tools for characterizing the altered functional status of T or B cells (or both) encountered in immune deficiency states. In addition, these models enable genes that influence immune expression to be identified, characterized, and their roles in immunity defined. Furthermore, in conjunction with advances in cellular and molecular biology pertaining to gene therapy, the possibility arises that immune deficient states might, someday, be partially or fully corrected by therapeutic intervention.

PHAGOCYTE DYSFUNCTION DISEASES

Phagocytic disorders fall into two categories: extrinsic and intrinsic. Included in the extrinsic phagocytic disorders are suppression of phagocytic cell number by immunosuppressive agents, interference with phagocytic function by corticosteroids, and suppression of circulating neutrophils by auto-Abs directed against the phagocyte's surface Ags. Intrinsic phagocytic disorders include various inherited enzyme deficiencies within the metabolic pathway involved in microbial killing during phagocytosis. Included among these enzyme disorders are chronic granulomatous disease and Chédiak-Higashi syndrome. Characteristic of these disease states is a susceptibility to bacterial and fungal, but not viral or protozoan, infections.

Chronic Granulomatous Disease

Chronic granulomatous disease involves a phagocytic *dysfunction in certain enzymes involved in bacterial killing.* The enzyme most often affected is NADPH oxidase. As a result of these enzyme deficiencies, the metabolism of neutrophils and monocytes/macrophages is abnormal, with a consequent decrease in intracellular killing of certain bacteria and fungi.

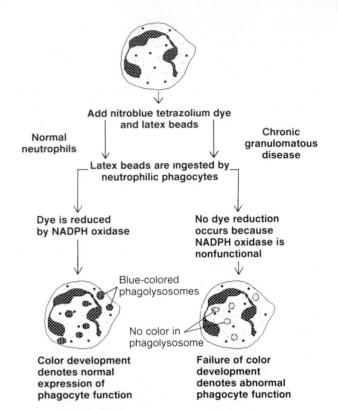

FIGURE 14.1 Nitroblue tetrazolium test of phagocyte function in diagnosing chronic granulomatous disease.

The disease is usually diagnosed before two years of age, when the child shows susceptibility to infection, such as multiple abscess formation by organisms of low disease-causing ability. The most common form of this disease is an X-linked disorder, affecting only male offspring. Phagocyte function tests can be performed, such as the quantitative nitroblue tetrazolium test. Normal phagocytes exposed to this dye will develop blue precipitates in their cytoplasm as enzymes, like NADPH oxidase, reduce the colorless precursor to a blue-colored dye. Neutrophils from a person with chronic granulomatous disease will not form the blue precipitate because of the dysfunction or absence of these enzymes (fig. 14.1). The long-term survival of individuals with this disorder depends on early diagnosis, followed by prophylactic antibiotic and antifungal treatment and white blood cell infusion therapy.

Chédiak-Higashi Syndrome

Another inherited disorder affecting phagocyte function is Chédiak-Higashi syndrome. It affects both males and females and its symptoms include albinism, central nervous system abnormalities, and recurrent bacterial infections by a wide variety of organisms. The phagocytic killing *defect is due to fragile lysosomal membranes,* which do not degranulate properly leading to delayed killing times. At times the lysosomes burst and cause local tissue damage in the area of infection. This multisymptom disease of unknown cause can also adversely affect the activities of NK and T_C cells. The only treatment against infecting organisms is specific antibiotic therapy. The prognosis is poor because of increasing susceptibility to infection and progressive neurological deterioration. Few individuals with Chédiak-Higashi syndrome survive to puberty.

Deficient Expression of Leukocyte Adhesion Molecules

Clinical symptoms similar to those arising from defects in phagocyte killing can arise by other means. For example, impaired mobility and ingestion of granulocytes also can be associated with increased susceptibility to infectious agents. In certain of these instances, the defect seems to be associated with expression of leukocyte cell adhesion molecules (Leu-CAMs) found on the surfaces of lymphocytes, phagocytic leukocytes, and hemopoietic cells (see chapter 8). Because of the broad expression of Leu-CAMs among leukocytes, impaired functional expression by both phagoctyes and lymphocytes can be observed. For example, granulocytes from individuals with this genetic lesion display reduced adhesion and adhesion-dependent function. This can lead to reduced margination and extravasation of granulocytes into inflammatory sites (whether induced by wounding or infection). Impaired lymphocyte function can be associated with (1) abnormal migration to lymphoid organs leading to hypoplasia in these organs, (2) poor adhesion between B and T cells resulting in decreased T cell help, and (3) diminished cytotoxicity.

Decreased expression of Leu-CAMs can lead to deficiencies in expression of both Ag-specific and nonspecific immune responses. Treatment of individuals with this type of disorder includes prophylactic administration of antibiotic and antifungal agents. Bone marrow transplantation also has been used in some instances. The recent production of a complementary DNA clone for a human Leu-CAM β chain might lead to the correction of this defect by gene insertion at some future date.

COMPLEMENT IMMUNE DEFICIENCY DISORDERS

A variety of complement deficiencies have been associated with increased susceptibility to infection (table 14.3). Complement factors are involved in (1) phagocytosis; (2) Ab killing of bacteria; (3) lysis of viruses, virus-infected cells, and tumor cells; (4) histamine release (anaphylatoxin) by mast cells and basophils; and (5) chemotaxis of phagocytic neutrophils and monocytes. Most disease states are inherited by both males and females (autosomal), and usually are associated with the complete absence of one or another proteinaceous complement component. This implies that the lesion is at the level of the DNA structural gene for that product. The diseases that are associated with complement disorders can be divided into three groups based on common symptoms. These include disorders affecting (1) components C1, C2, and C4; (2) C3; and (3) C5–C9.

C1–C4 Deficiencies

Deficiencies in C1, C2, and C4 are associated with increased susceptibility to bacterial infections, as well as dramatic increases in immune-complex autoimmune diseases, such as systemic lupus erythematosus (SLE). This association is probably due to failure of complement-mediated phagocytosis to clear immune complexes. Treatment is directed toward control of infection by chemotherapy and toward the specific symptoms of the autoimmune disease. Complement replacement therapy is not suggested for persons with autoimmune disorders as it might produce an increase in immune complexes, worsening the SLE symptoms.

The absence of the C3 complement component is associated with increased susceptibility to bacterial infections, which can be life threatening. Among

TABLE 14.3 Characteristics of Phagocyte and Complement Deficiency Diseases

Disorder	Cell Type Affected	Defect	Consequence
Phagocyte Defects			
Chronic granulomatous disease	Phagocytes, chiefly neutrophils	NADH oxidase deficiency	Increased bacterial infections
Chédiak-Higashi syndrome	Phagocytes, NK, and T_C cells	Defective lysosomal membrane	Increased bacterial infections
Adhesion molecule deficiency	Phagocytes, NK, and T_C cells	Deficient Leu-CAM expression	Increased bacterial infections
Complement Deficiencies			
C1, C2, or C4		Structural gene deficiency	Increased bacterial infections; autoimmune disease
C3		Deficiency in C3 inactivator	Increased bacterial infections
C5, C6, C7, or C8		Structural gene deficiency	Increased infections by *Neisseria*; immune-complex disorders

the common problems encountered are septicemia, pneumonia, and meningitis. The decrease in serum C3 levels is usually a result of a deficiency of C3b inactivator. As a consequence, C3 is not easily conserved and its levels are rapidly depleted. Antibiotic therapy is used to control the infections, but the prognosis is poor since the primary defect remains.

C5–C9 Deficiencies

Persons with deficiencies in C5–C8 can be asymptomatic for years and then develop infections caused by *Neisseria* (e.g., meningitis and gonorrhea). These organisms can be found in the nasopharynx, urethra, and vagina. Their spread to other sites suggests that complement-mediated lysis is the primary means of controlling the growth and distribution of these opportunistic pathogens. Immune-complex syndromes, with rheumatoidlike symptoms, are also found with C5–C8 disorders. Antibiotic therapy controls infections, but complement replacement therapy cannot be used due to the possible exacerbation of immune-complex disorders. Interestingly, there are no known diseases associated with deficiencies of C9.

NEUROIMMUNOENDOCRINOLOGY

It has long been suggested that stress might adversely affect the status of a person's immune system. Yet, until recently, evidence for such a connection was only circumstantial. Statistically, people who have recently lost a loved one and are in a state of deep grief are very susceptible to debilitating infectious diseases and even cancer. Since the immune system monitors and responds to infections and cancers, it has been assumed that there was some link between the stress being experienced and the depression of the immune system observed. However, if we argue that a link exists between stress and immune status, links between the immune, nervous, and endocrine systems must be demonstrable. Such links recently have been demonstrated on a number of fronts.

Neural and Endocrine Influences on the Immune System

Behavioral Influence on Immunological Expression

Clinically, it has been shown that mates of people dying of cancer show lymphocytopenia (reduced lymphocyte count) and depressed lymphocyte activity within months of the mate's death. In addition, persons hospitalized for severe clinical depression have suppressed lymphocyte responses. Milder forms of stress have been correlated with negative changes in cellular immunity. For instance, a study of students preparing for final exams revealed that their cellular immunity was depressed, even though they were accustomed to taking exams. Of particular note was the observation that the lymphocytes most adversely affected were T_H cells. Since this cell type is needed for the expression of both humoral and cellular immunity, impairment of function could have disastrous consequences if the person was exposed to disease-causing agents at that time.

If stress can cause immune suppression, can these effects be reversed? The answer to this question is not straightforward and appears controversial. Nevertheless, studies using behavioral interventions (e.g., relaxation techniques, meditation, and mental imagery of the immune system) and alternative therapies (from Eastern medical practices), in conjunction with traditional Western medical practices, showed enhanced survival among individuals with cancer or acquired immune deficiency syndrome.

Additional evidence for behavioral modification of immune responsiveness comes from studies with animals. In one study, investigators injected mice with a chemical (poly I:C, which stimulates interferon [IFN] production) that enhances NK activity while exposing the mice to the distinctive odor of camphor (which has no effect of the immune system). In this classical (Pavlovian) conditioning experiment, the mice soon were able to be exposed to camphor alone and to show a large increase in NK activity. In another experiment, rats were given saccharine in conjunction with the immunosuppressant, cyclophosphamide. After their conditioning, when the rats were given saccharine alone, they became sick and died. In this case, the animals were conditioned to suppress their immune response. These, and other experiments, indicate that the immune and nervous systems can interact to influence the nature of immune responses.

Another study has demonstrated a more substantive link between the nervous, endocrine, and immune systems whereby stress might be producing immune suppression through the hypothalamic-pituitary-adrenal pathway. In this pathway, stress

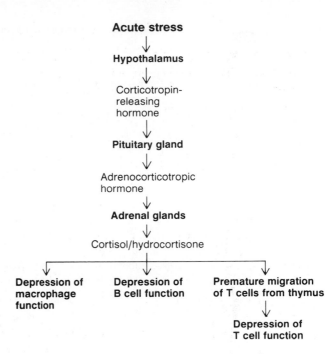

FIGURE 14.2 Interaction of nervous, endocrine, and immune systems in response to acute stress.

triggers the hypothalamus to release the hormone corticotropin-release factor (CRF), which stimulates the pituitary to secrete adrenocorticotropic hormone (ACTH). The adrenal gland responds to ACTH by releasing cortisone and other steroids, which then act as immunosuppressants (fig. 14.2).

Neuronal Influence on Immunological Expression

Anatomical studies reveal a direct neural connection between the spinal cord and immune organs. Nerve fibers from the autonomic nervous system connect to the thymus gland, which is responsible for T cell maturation. The thymus can also exert influence on the immune system by releasing hormones that could potentially reach all lymphocyte populations in the body through the vascular and lymphatic circulation (fig. 14.3a). These thymic hormones, thymosin and thymopoietin, influence the expression of both humoral and cell-mediated immunity. The importance of these hormones is seen by the positive therapeutic results obtained in studies using thymosin on patients with immune deficiency, autoimmune, and neoplastic

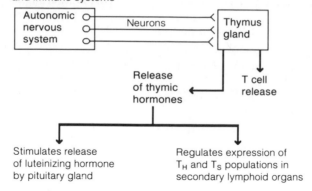

(a) Anatomical connection between nervous and immune systems

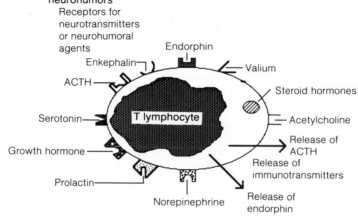

(b) Immune modulation by neurotransmitters and neurohumors

FIGURE 14.3 Illustrations of immunoneural communication.

(cancer) diseases. Thus, through the innervation of the thymus gland, there might be neural control of release of these hormones.

Other organs involved in the immune response that are innervated by the nervous system include the spleen, lymph nodes, and bone marrow. By carefully following nerve paths, neurons can be seen to branch out and synapse in lymphocyte-rich regions of these organs, especially the T cell regions. The neurotransmitters released by these neurons could act as *immune modulators* (fig. 14.3b). In fact, cell membrane receptors for the tranquilizer diazepam (Valium) have been found on T cells. This suggests a possible link between an antianxiety substance in the brain and the immune system. Other receptors found on lymphocytes include receptors for the neurotransmitters acetylcholine, norepinephrine, and the brain opiates, endorphins and enkephalins. In addition, other cells of the immune system can respond to neurotransmitters; macrophages can bind serotonin and substance P. Serotonin causes macrophage activation, whereas substance P inhibits their movement and activity.

Moreover, neurosurgical manipulation of the brain can affect the cellular composition of lymphoid organs. For example, if lesions are made in the anterior or ventromedial regions of the hypothalamus of rodents, the number of nucleated cells in the spleen and thymus is reduced. A similar effect can be achieved by

TABLE 14.4 Representative Hormonal Influences on Immunological Expression

Hormone	Effect	Function Modulated
Steroid Hormones		
Glucocorticoids	+	Ab or cytokine production, NK cell killing
Sex steroids	+/−	Lymphocyte transformation, cytotoxicity in MLC
Polypeptide Hormones		
ACTH	+/−	Ab or cytokine production, NK cytotoxicity, macrophage activation
β-endorphin	+/−	Ab production, T cell and macrophage activation
met-enkephalin	+/−	T cell activation (at low doses) T cell suppression (at high doses)
Growth hormone	+	Ab production, IL-2 modulation, macrophage activation
Oxytocin	+	T cell proliferation
Prolactin	+	IL-2 production, macrophage activation
Amino acid Derivatives		
Catecholamines	+	Mitogen-induced proliferation
Thyroxine	+	T cell activation, expression of plaque formation by B cells

+, enhancement or stimulation of function; , suppression or inhibition of function; +/−, enhancement or suppression of function depending upon assay conditions.

MLC, mixed lymphocyte culture.

making lesions in the mammillary bodies. However, the mechanism through which these manipulations of the central nervous system are able to profoundly affect cell numbers of major lymphoid organs is not known.

Endocrine Influence on Immunological Expression

Modulation of immunological expression by several hormones has been demonstrated. Table 14.4 provides a partial list of hormones that have been shown to exert positive (enhancing) or negative (suppressing) effects on various parameters of immune response. For example, the stress-induced release of ACTH, glucocorticoids (e.g., cortisol), or catecholamines (epinephrine and norepinephrine) can lead to immune suppression. This is achieved either through suppression of mitogenic stimulation of lymphocytes (catecholamines) or of functional expression of activated cells (ACTH and glucocorticoids). On the other hand, prolactin (which might also be released during stress) can enhance activation of macrophages and interleukin 2 (IL-2) production by T_H cells.

Immunological Influence on Neuroendocrine Function

Conversely, the immune system seems to be capable of influencing behavioral, neuronal, and endocrine activity. Activated cells of the immune system can release IFN and ILs, which have been shown to alter the activity of brain neurons and of endocrine tissues. One manifestation of this interaction is induced by a bacterial peptide, Factor S (muramyl peptide). Factor S is capable of stimulating the immune response and inducing fever and deep sleep. This peptide can bind to receptors found on both macrophages and neurons. Following its release by bacteria, Factor S can stimulate phagocytosis in macrophages. In addition, the macrophages also respond by releasing IL-1, which can interact with neural receptors and trigger slow-wave sleep and fever. This nervous-immune system link might have evolved as a mechanism through which the host could address infection on several levels.

Products of the immune system are also able to affect neural and neuroendocrine function in other ways. For example, lectin-activated T cells secrete a neurotrophic peptide, called neuroleukin. This lymphokine promotes the survival, in culture, of a subpopulation of embryonic spinal neurons and of sensory neurons that are insensitive to nerve growth factor. In addition, another cytokine, IL-1, can directly stimulate the release of several hormones from the pituitary gland. Among the hormones released are ACTH, thyroid-stimulating hormone, and growth hormone. Moreover, thymosin can activate the hypothalamic-pituitary-adrenal circuit, thereby causing an increase in corticosteroid levels. Thus, these "immunotransmitters" could have as profound an affect on the nervous system as the neurotransmitters have on the immune system.

Neural-immune interactions include extracellular signaling molecules such as hormones, neurotransmitters, and cytokines, which act as chemical messengers by which lymphocytes and neurons can communicate with each other. Although it is clear that the immune and nervous systems interact with one another, much remains to be learned about their mutual influences.

AGING AND THE IMMUNE SYSTEM

Every cell in the body has a biological clock. Its spring slowly unwinds as time passes. Some cells can "rewind" by cell division, making new daughter cells identical to the original mother cell. Other cells never again divide in the adult and, when death occurs, there is no replacement. As time marches on, organs, organ systems, and ultimately the whole organism become affected by this irreversible aging process, until the cellular death load becomes too great and the organism dies. This programmed decline in physiological competence seems concomitant of changes manifested in the immune system.

As people age, certain normal immune functions, including both T and B lymphocyte activities, usually decline. Since the immune system can come in contact with most of the cells, tissues, and organs within the body, alterations of immune function could affect all other systems. Moreover, associated with this aging immune system is an increased susceptibility to disease states, such as cancer and autoimmune and immune deficiency disorders. These adversely affect many organ systems and compromise the survival of the individual.

In this section, we explore age-related changes in the immune system, mechanisms responsible for the decline in immune function, and mechanisms responsible for diseases associated with aging and declining immune function. The comprehension of how the immune system ages and influences the health of the individual becomes even more important in light of the projected increase in life expectancy. By the turn of the twenty-first century, close to half the American population will be around retirement age. As it is, most elderly people die of either heart disease or cancer. In many cases, heart disease can be prevented (or its progress retarded) by appropriate life-style changes, such as proper diet, exercise, and stress reduction. But what about cancer? The chances of developing cancer increase with age. If one contributing factor is the age-related decline of the immune system's cancer surveillance function, then determining the causes of and finding the remedies for this depressed functional state could bring about dramatic decreases in the number of cancer cases among the elderly.

Morphological findings show that certain tissues and organs of the immune system decrease in both mass and function with age. In humans, the thymus gland begins to atrophy at puberty. There is also an age-related reduction in the thymic lymphatic mass, which is detected after menopause in women and at approximately age 50 in men. At that time, we can also detect age-related histological changes in other lymphatic tissues, including diminishing numbers of germinal lymphocyte centers in the lymph nodes.

By the sixth decade, there is approximately a 30% decrease in the numbers of circulating T lymphocytes, as compared with young adults. However, the numbers of B lymphocytes remain essentially the same. When functional tests are performed, the greatest change appears in the helper function of T cells, which decline dramatically with age. In addition, the serum concentration of the thymic hormone, thymosin, begins to decline after age 40. Perhaps thymic atrophy and the decline in thymic hormone levels adversely

Immunotransmitters

Immunotransmitters are chemicals released by immunocytes (lymphocytes and macrophages) that can communicate not only with the immune system but with other control systems as well. Although they are produced by immunocytes, these substances resemble neuromodulators (neurotransmitters) and hormones in several instances.

One immunotransmitter, identified by Blalock and Smith at the University of Texas, is ACTH. ACTH is a hormone released by the anterior pituitary gland, whose target organ is the adrenal cortex, where it stimulates the release of cortisone. The fact that immune cells can release ACTH suggests that the cells of the immune system might act as small endocrine-hormone factories. As these cells migrate throughout the body, they seem to possess the ability to modulate the immune response in accordance with the physiological events occurring locally.

Immunotransmitters can also communicate with the brain. Blalock and Smith have reported that lymphocytes can release the neuromodulator, β-endorphin. Endorphins are the brain's opiates and were previously thought to have been made only by the brain in response to pain. Why would lymphocytes synthesize endorphins? Perhaps during an infection, they release endorphins to overcome pain. Alternatively, they might act as sensors telling the brain that microbes are invading, enabling the brain to regulate the body's response.

The immunocytes not only mimic neurotransmitters, but their own lymphokines can influence brain function directly. Besedovsky of the Swiss Research Institute has shown that interferon can alter the neuronal discharge rate in the brain. Other chemicals of the immune system, including the thymic hormones, can also influence the central nervous system. Rats injected with thymosins show depressed brain levels of norepinephrine. Since norepinephrine can influence the hypothalamus, it may be that thymosins could themselves stimulate the hypothalamus indirectly and set into motion the hypothalamic-pituitary-adrenal reaction.

This two-way communication between the immune system and the brain could be an effective means of accelerating recovery from invading microbes. Immunotransmitters could inform the brain of the invasion. The brain could then adjust immune response through the release of modulators that bind to receptors on immunocytes, altering immunocyte expression. Pert and Ruff at the National Institute of Mental Health have shown that neuromodulators, such as endorphin, can bind to macrophages, altering their migrational activity. Perhaps the binding of endorphins could increase the numbers of macrophages arriving at the site of microbial attack, to more effectively combat infection.

Proponents of psychoneuroimmunology (PNI) feel that delineation of pathways of interaction between the brain and the immune system will clarify the link between emotions and disease. Behavioral medicine has long been the approach in the East and the ridicule of Western medicine. Perhaps as researchers further define the link between the immune system and the brain, it will be possible to meld therapies, such as behavioral modification, with traditional therapies (e.g., chemotherapy) to treat, or even prevent, disease.

Jankovic, B. D., Markovic, B. M., and Spector, N. H. (eds.). *Neuroimmune Interactions: Proceedings of the Second International Workshop on Neuroimmunomodulation. Annals of the New York Academy* (Vol. 496). New York, 1987.

affect T_H cells, consequently yielding diminished humoral and cell-mediated immunity with advancing age.

Studies of Ag-induced Ab responses show that primary, but not secondary, Ab responses decrease with age. This suggests that regulator T lymphocytes, but not necessarily B cells, are affected. Memory B lymphocytes formed in early life can function properly throughout life. Antigenic challenge usually requires the cooperation of T cells to stimulate Ab production by B cells. Accordingly, a person who had contracted pneumococcal pneumonia at age eight would be protected for life against a second invasion of *Streptococcus pneumoniae* bacteria, due to the persistence of memory B lymphocytes. However, if a person was first exposed to these bacteria at age 60, an immune response might not be mounted because of T cell defects and, consequently, the person might succumb to pneumonia.

The decline with age of normal immunological function might be secondary to changes in the cellular environment ("milieu") of the organism. The effects of changes in the physiological milieu on the expression of immune potential has been investigated by cell transfer experiments in mammals. In these experiments, old cells were transferred to young recipients and young cells to old recipients. The results indicate that old cells transferred to young recipients can be "rejuvenated," while young cells placed in old recipients will age prematurely and show reduced functional capacity. Therefore, there is a deleterious physiological milieu in the aging animal that adversely affects cells of the immune system, whatever their source. At present, we do not know what these factors are. They could be "toxic" substances of metabolic origin, or alternatively, they might be essential substances that are no longer produced by aging animals.

Evaluation of the various immune cell types in aging mammals has shown that the number of bone marrow stem cells remains relatively constant throughout life. However, the rate of B lymphocyte generation and the size of the colonies produced seem to decline with age. The accessory cell of the immune system, the macrophage, needed for Ag processing, does not seem to be affected by age. The relative numbers of this phagocyte remain constant throughout life. Furthermore, the results of studies on aging macrophages show that the activities of this cell in handling

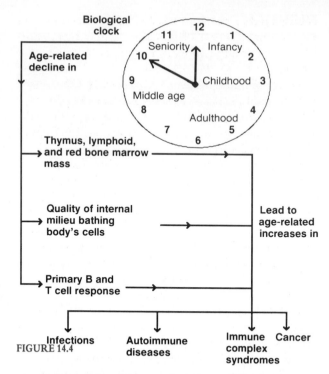

FIGURE 14.4

FIGURE 14.4 Alterations in the immune system due to aging. With advancing age (approaching 12 o'clock), several parameters of immunological status and function can decline. These, in turn, lead to increased incidence of several disorders.

Ags, initiating the immune response to that Ag, and during phagocytosis, do not diminish as a function of age.

Present evidence suggests that the decline in normal immune function that accompanies aging is due primarily to changes in the T lymphocyte component of the immune system (fig. 14.4). This is not surprising in light of the thymic changes that occur. What is happening in the aging thymus to produce aberrant T cells? One theory postulates that there are subtle error-accumulating mechanisms operating at the level of DNA which result in mutated cells. In general, aging cells begin to lose their ability to repair damage to their DNA. If this happened to differentiating T cells, disruption of normal function could easily occur, with devastating results.

As normal immune function declines with age, the incidence of infections, autoimmune and immune-complex diseases, and cancer increases. Elderly individuals tend to be more susceptible to infections and have a longer course of infection, with higher mortality, than young adults. Autoimmune disorders also increase with age. For example, among women, the incidence of autoimmune diseases, such as rheumatoid arthritis and SLE, increases after age 40. Perhaps defects in the aging thymus gland disrupt the self-tolerance mechanism through changes in the T_s population. Cancer is another disease state whose incidence increases with age. The mechanism whereby decreased immune function permits the growth of neoplasms is not, as yet, fully elucidated. One theory suggests that depression of T lymphocytes allows for a breakdown in the immunological surveillance system for neoplastic cells. Moreover, once the transformed cells start to grow, impaired T_C lymphocyte function cannot stop the growth of the tumor.

Can the events of immune senescence be prevented? There appears to be no definitive answer to this question; however, the nutritional state of the individual seems to play an important role in maintaining a healthy immune system. There seems to be a relationship between nutrition, immunity, and disease. Deficiencies in minerals (e.g., zinc) and vitamins (e.g., folic acid) seem to impair immune function. Calorie restriction and low fat intake appear to be beneficial for the continued maintenance of good immune status into advanced age. Malnutrition among the aged is a worldwide problem. We now realize that deficiencies, or excesses, of each major dietary component, (including proteins, fats, total calories, vitamins, and minerals), may profoundly affect the immune system, and the occurrence and progression of disease, and longevity.

On another front, investigators are exploring immunorestoration therapy (e.g., thymic hormone treatment) or the use of immune modulators for maintaining proper immune status. However, a word of caution is necessary. There is no magical diet or treatment. How an individual reacts to such treatments will depend on a multitude of physiological factors that, as yet, are undefined. As knowledge about normal immunological mechanisms grows, however, we can anticipate a time when a scientifically modified "immunotherapeutic" diet might be realized.

SUMMARY

1. Immune deficiencies can involve one or more of the components of the immune network and lead to an individual being more susceptible to pathological disorders. [p. 361]
2. In stem cell deficiency diseases, both humoral and cellular immunity are impaired. Lacking functional B and T lymphocytes, the individual suffers from severe, recurrent infections throughout life. [pp. 361–363]
3. Humoral immune deficiency disorders (hypogammaglobulinemias) include defects in B lymphocytes and antibody production. This leaves the individual extremely susceptible to bacterial, but not viral, infections. Specific B cell disorders include X-linked infantile hypogammaglobulinemia, acquired hypogammaglobulinemia, and dysgammaglobulinemia. [p. 363]
4. Cellular immune deficiency disorders are associated with viral, fungal, and protozoan (rather than bacterial) infections. In congenital thymic aplasia (DiGeorge syndrome), the individual is born without a thymus gland and therefore cannot produce functioning T lymphocytes. In Nezelof's syndrome, the T cell disorder leads to abnormal B cell immunity as well. Most T cell disorders respond well to thymus transplantation, which is usually successful in restoring T cell and partial B cell immunity. [pp. 363–365]
5. Several animal models have been developed to explore immune deficiencies. Three particular murine models are especially useful in this regard: (a) the nude mouse as a model for T cell immune deficiencies, (b) the *xid* mouse as a model for partial B cell immune deficiency, and (c) the *scid* mouse as a model for B and T cell immune deficiency. [pp. 365–366]
6. Phagocytic dysfunction diseases can be either extrinsic (acquired) or intrinsic (inherited). Extrinsic disorders include impaired phagocytic activity due to drugs or other external agents,

while intrinsic disorders pertain to inherited enzyme deficiencies, which affect bacterial killing by phagocytes. In chronic granulomatous disease, the enzyme NADPH oxidase is lacking, and in Chédiak-Higashi syndrome, improper degranulation of lysosomes with phagosomes causes delayed killing of bacteria. Other disorders arise because of deficiencies in expression of adhesion molecules, which are associated with impaired migration and ingestion. Individuals with malfunctioning phagocytes are more prone to bacterial infections and the associated complications. [pp. 366–367]

7. Complement deficiency disorders are associated with increased susceptibility to infection. Disorders are grouped into three categories: (a) deficiencies in C1, C2, and C4, which include problems dealing with bacterial infections, and immune-complex disorders; (b) C3 disorder, which affects the ability to fight foreign bacteria; and (c) C5–C8 disorders with ensuing problems in controlling the levels of pathogenic *Neisseria.* [pp. 367–368]

8. Neuroimmunoendocrinology is a field that explores the relationship between the nervous, endocrine, and immune systems. For example, stress may produce immune suppression through the hypothalamic-pituitary-adrenal pathway, by means of cortisone. Anatomical studies show neural connections between the nervous system and immune organs like the thymus gland and spleen. T lymphocytes have been shown to have membrane receptors for neurological agents (e.g., tranquilizers). Conversely, T cell products, such as interleukins and interferon, have been shown to alter neuronal activity in the brain and hormone release from endocrine glands. Thus, there is evidence to support the notion that the immune, endocrine, and nervous systems interact and mutually affect each other's activity. [pp. 368–372]

9. The aging of the immune system is seen in individuals as a decline in many immune functions. The inability to fight infections and a high incidence of cancer and immune-complex disorders increase with age and can be related to such changes as the atrophy of the thymus gland (T cell, cell-mediated immunity) and the decrease in red bone marrow (B cell, humoral immunity). [pp. 372–375]

READINGS

Anderson, D. C., and Springer, T. A. Leukocyte adhesion deficiency: an inherited defect in the MAC-1, LFA-1 and p150,95 glycoproteins. *Annual Review of Medicine* **38**:175, 1987.

Ansell, J. D., and Bancroft, G. J. The biology of the SCID mutation. *Immunology Today* **10**:322, 1989.

Baskin, Y. The way we act. *Science 85* **6**:94, 1985.

Bercza, I. Immunoregulation by neuroendocrine factors. *Developmental and Comparative Immunology* **13**:329, 1989.

Bosma, M. J., and Carroll, A. M. The SCID mouse mutant: definition, characterization, and potential uses. *Annual Review of Immunology* **9**:323, 1991.

Bosma, M. J., Freid, M., Custer, R. P., et al. Evidence of functional lymphocytes in some (leaky) *scid* mice. *Journal of Experimental Medicine* **167**:1016, 1988.

Ferrari, G., Rossini, S., Giavazzi, R., et al. An in vivo model of somatic cell gene therapy for human severe combined immunodeficiency. *Science* **251**:1363, 1991.

Hanahan, D. Transgenic mice as probes into complex systems. *Science* **246**:1265, 1989.

Hartman, D. P., Holaday, J. W., and Bernton, E. W. Inhibition of lymphocyte proliferation by antibodies to prolactin. *FASEB Journal* **3**:2194, 1989.

Khansari, D. N., Murgo, A. J., and Faith, R. E. Effects of stress on the immune system. *Immunology Today* **11**:170, 1990.

Marx, J. L. The immune system "belongs in the body." *Science* **227**:1190, 1985.

Murasko, D. M., and Goonewardene, I. M. T-cell function in aging: mechanisms of decline. *Annual Review of Gerontology and Geriatrics* **10**:71, 1990.

Schultz, L. D., and Sidman, C. L. Genetically determined murine models of immunodeficiency. *Annual Review of Medicine* **5**:367, 1987.

Siegel, J. N., Turner, C. A., Klinman, D. M., et al. Sequence analysis and expression of an X-linked lymphocyte-regulated gene family XLR. *Journal of Experimental Medicine* **166**:1702, 1987.

Su, T.-P., London, E. D., and Jaffe, J. H. Steroid binding at s receptors suggests a link between endocrine, nervous, and immune systems. *Science* **240**:219, 1988.

Verma, I. M. Gene therapy. *Scientific American* **263**(5):68, 1990.

Yoshikai, Y., Matsuzaki, G., Takeda, Y., et al. Functional T cell receptor delta chain gene messages in athymic nude mice. *European Journal of Immunology* **18**:1039, 1988.

15 Acquired Immune Deficiency Syndrome

OVERVIEW

In acquired immune deficiency syndrome (AIDS), human immunodeficiency virus (HIV) infects CD4+ cells, especially T_H lymphocytes, and impairs their function leading to a complete breakdown in immune responsiveness. AIDS is characterized by a variety of clinical symptoms that reflect conditions ranging from opportunistic infections to cancer, to which the infected individual becomes increasingly susceptible.

CONCEPTS

1. The etiologic agent of AIDS is HIV-1, a retrovirus that can be transmitted among adults by sexual intercourse or administration of contaminated blood products and during the perinatal period from the mother to her fetus or newborn infant.

2. AIDS compromises the immune system of the infected individual, rendering the person more susceptible to opportunistic viral and fungal infections and cancers like Kaposi's sarcoma.

3. Ligand-specific binding of HIV to CD4 antigens on target cells (e.g., T_H cells and macrophages) initiates infection. Replication of the viral genome in infected cells causes dysfunction of cells that play a central role in immune responses. The loss of CD4+ cells that follows is accompanied by progressive reduction in immunological capacity.

4. Treatments of AIDS endeavor to control clinical symptoms (e.g., antiviral agents), restore immune function, or both. In addition, vaccines are being developed in an effort to manage AIDS among infected individuals and provide protection against future infections.

Acquired immune deficiency syndrome, or AIDS, was first recognized as a disease in 1981 by the Centers for Disease Control (CDC) in Atlanta, Georgia. AIDS leaves an individual vulnerable to illnesses that a healthy immune system would readily overcome. As the name implies, this fatal disease is acquired, not inherited; the immune system is deficient and not able to combat disease; and, as a syndrome, this disease has a definite spectrum of signs and symptoms that characterize it. Once contracted, there is a *progressive loss of immune responsiveness* in the individual, and death results from opportunistic infections or cancer. The current epidemic of AIDS is predominantly among the homosexual male and intravenous (IV) drug using populations in the United States and the heterosexual central African population. However, the incidence of AIDS is increasing among other groups (e.g., heterosexual males and females) as well.

EPIDEMIOLOGY OF AIDS
Causative Agent of AIDS

An intensive research effort, led by Robert Gallo at the National Cancer Institute and Luc Montagnier at the Pasteur Institute, has implicated an RNA retrovirus as the causative agent of this debilitating disease. This virus, fomerly identified as human T lymphotropic virus type III (HTLV-III [by American investigators]) and lymphadenopathy virus (LAV [by European investigators]), is now called **human immunodeficiency virus (HIV)**.

HIV is a member of the subfamily of retroviruses known as lentiviruses. Retroviruses are enveloped viruses that possess an RNA genome and use reverse transcriptase to copy this genome in an infected host. There are two antigenic types of lentiviruses in humans, HIV-1 and HIV-2. These are the causative agent in AIDS; however, the pathological consequences of infection by HIV-2 remain undefined.

The fine structure of HIV-1 is shown in figure 15.1. The virion consists of two major regions: (1) a central core composed of RNA and reverse transcriptase and (2) an envelope comprised of two membranes. Certain proteins have been identified which appear to be diagnostic of HIV. These include two envelope glycoproteins (gp) designated gp-120 (MW of 120 kD) and gp-41 (MW of 41 kD), and the core proteins designated p-24 (MW of 24 kD) and p-18 (MW of 18 kD).

Origin and Transmission

HIV is believed to have *originated in central Africa* (probably being transmitted initially from monkeys to humans). From here, it spread to the rest of the world. Of the two strains of HIV identified thus far, HIV-1 has spread throughout the world, while HIV-2 is endemic mostly in West Africa.

AIDS is a pandemic (a worldwide epidemic) and epidemiologists have classified countries into one of three groups, based on the prevalent means of transmission found in each area (fig. 15.2). Countries displaying pattern 1 transmission include North and South America, western Europe, Scandinavia, Australia, and New Zealand. In these countries, AIDS is mainly a disease of homosexual males and IV drug abusers. Countries displaying pattern 2 transmission include central and eastern Africa, the Caribbean, and some areas of South America. Here AIDS is primarily transmitted through heterosexual contact. Pattern 3 transmission occurs in eastern Europe, North Africa, the Middle East, Asia, and the Pacific. In these regions, the number of AIDS cases is low, and persons afflicted seem to have contracted the disease in countries displaying pattern 1 or pattern 2 transmission.

HIV is *transmitted primarily by sexual contact* (where there is an exchange of body fluids) *and by exchange of blood products* (from an infected to an noninfected individual). AIDS is not a disease that can be casually transmitted. Transmission of the virus seems to be limited to blood, semen, and breast milk, in which relatively high concentrations of virus can be found. Nevertheless, HIV can be found in other body fluids, such as saliva. However, AIDS is not transmitted by these other fluids, suggesting that large volumes of free virus (or infected lymphocytes) might be required to transmit an infection.

Although AIDS in the United States was originally confined to homosexual males, IV drug users, Haitian immigrants, and hemophiliacs, it now appears to be spreading to the population at large. Nevertheless, sexually active homosexual and bisexual men, IV

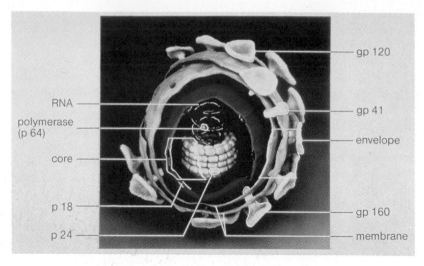

FIGURE 15.1   Model of human immunodeficiency virus. (Reprinted with permission, Organon Technica Corp., Durham, NC.)

drug users, persons transfused with infected blood, and sexual partners of a person with AIDS remain at highest risk. Moreover, it has recently been shown that AIDS can be transmitted by heterosexual females to male sexual partners. Since the disease can have a 10-year incubation period, it is a sobering thought that an AIDS epidemic throughout the entire population might be a reality by the turn of the century.

One theory for the increased susceptibility of homosexual men and IV drug users to AIDS is that exposure to other viruses indigenous to these populations compromises their immune system, leaving the individuals too weak to ward off infection by HIV. For example, a study among homosexual men in San Francisco showed that 95% of those tested had Abs to cytomegalovirus (CMV), a sign that they had once been infected with this herpes-type virus. Only 25% of the heterosexuals tested had these Abs. Perhaps heterosexuals have been exposed to the AIDS virus too, but have been able to resist AIDS because they had not been weakened immunologically by CMV infection. If this hypothesis is correct, then a CMV vaccine might help protect the immune system against being weakened and thus enable it to better handle exposure to HIV.

The hypothesis that CMV infection sets the stage for AIDS is not the only possible explanation for the present epidemics in central Africa and among homosexual males and IV drug users in America. Other predisposing factors to AIDS include nutritional deficiencies (particularly protein-caloric malnutrition), parasitic and gastrointestinal infections, and hepatitis. These factors also might be more prevalent within the susceptible populations mentioned above.

Infants and children who have AIDS either were exposed before or during birth or have had a history of blood transfusions. Not everyone who has been exposed to HIV-1 develops AIDS, however. Nevertheless, those who develop AIDS display numerous symptoms, and usually die two to four years after initial diagnosis.

Symptoms of AIDS

What are the symptoms of AIDS? Many of the symptoms are commonly present in minor illnesses, such as colds, bronchitis, and stomach flu. But unlike these minor illnesses, the AIDS symptoms are usually persistent or recurrent, and may be more severe. Early symptoms include unexplained increasing and persistent fatigue, periodic chills and fever, unexpected weight loss, swollen lymph glands, persistent diarrhea, and unusual skin rashes. As the disease continues to overwhelm the immune system, AIDS permits a variety of more severe infections to develop throughout the body. These opportunistic infections, only rarely seen in non AIDS persons, are listed in order of frequency in table 15.1.

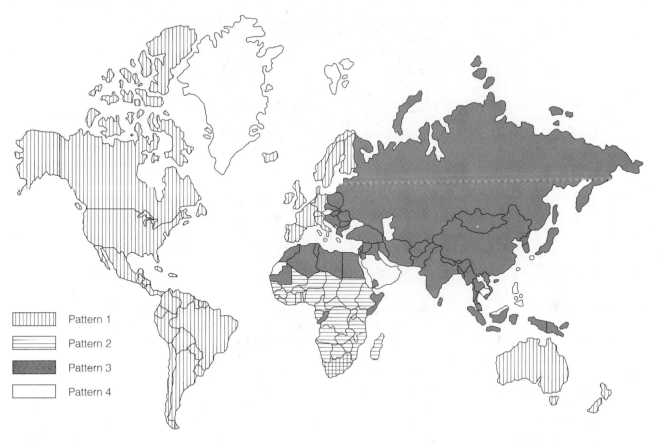

FIGURE 15.2 Patterns of transmission of HIV-1. Principal modes of transmission of HIV-1 in different regions of the world are indicated. Pattern 1 (*vertical lines*) represents transfer of HIV-1 predominantly by homosexual males and intravenous drug abusers; pattern 2 (*horizontal lines*) identifies countries in which heterosexual contact is the primary means of HIV-1 transfer; pattern 3 (*shaded*) denotes transfer of HIV-1 by varying degrees of expression of patterns 1 or 2; other countries (*without shading or pattern*) have no reported incidence of HIV-1 transmission. (Adapted from Lord, J. *Infection, Your Immune System, and AIDS.* © 1989 Enterprise for Education Inc., Santa Monica.)

TABLE 15.1 Opportunistic Infections Associated with AIDS

Infection	Opportunistic Agent
Manifested Early	
Pneumonia	*Pneumocystis carinii*
Oral fungal infections	*Candida albicans*
Body sores	Herpes simplex virus
Chronic diarrhea	*Cryptosporidium*
Appear Late; Potentially Fatal	
Cancer	Kaposi's sarcoma (cytomegalovirus [?])
Encephalitis	*Toxoplasma gondii*
Meningitis	*Cryptococcus neoformans*

Common among AIDS victims are pneumonia, oral fungal infections (e.g., candidoses of the mouth and esophagus), body sores (e.g., anal and oral sores caused by herpes simplex virus), and cryptosporidiosis, leading to chronic diarrhea. These opportunistic infections are very debilitating. As the disease progresses, more severe and life-threatening symptoms emerge. Among these are Kaposi's sarcoma (a virulent skin cancer), toxoplasmosis (caused by a protozoan that can fatally infect the brain [encephalitis] and lungs), and cryptococcosis (which can cause meningitis). Thus, as HIV destroys the immune system, it leaves the victim defenseless against cancer, fungal, bacterial, viral, and protozoan infections. This can lead to the destruction of lungs, brain, gastrointestinal tract, liver, and, ultimately, the individual.

There is also an **AIDS-related complex,** or simply **ARC.** This syndrome has appeared in persons who test positive for Abs to HIV-1 and have some of the early symptomology of AIDS, but not the "full-blown" disease. Persons with ARC are capable of transmitting AIDS and are followed clinically since they usually develop AIDS.

Thus, the wide range of symptoms in AIDS underscores the role of host resistance in host-parasite relationships. Since these relationships are in dynamic equilibrium, even a slight imbalance (as seen in the early stages of AIDS, where the immune system is weakened but not yet destroyed) can allow a sudden explosion in the population of organisms normally present at controlled levels. These parasites, now present in numbers that are out of normal control, can cause disease in the host.

Stages of AIDS

There are several ways in which the stages of HIV infection can be defined; however, there appear to be three broad phases: (1) the early or acute, (2) the middle or chronic, and (3) the final or crisis stages.

The **early,** or **acute, stage** begins with *initial exposure to HIV* and can last several weeks or months. Flulike symptoms are commonly encountered during this stage. While in this stage, the immune system responds with Ab production against the virus. In the **middle,** or **chronic, stage,** the infected individual can be asymptomatic but is nevertheless still infective. During this phase, which can last for years, the *immune system undergoes minimal but discernible pathological change.* The **final,** or **crisis, stage** is characterized by displays of the symptoms of ARC and AIDS. This stage can last for several months or years. During this time, there is a *steady depletion of CD4+ T cells,* and the infected individual usually experiences numerous opportunistic infections (fig. 15.3).

Each stage is also characterized by definite changes in lymphocyte numbers and reactivity. As noted in figure 15.3, T cell numbers display a rebound to near normal levels after initial exposure to HIV; however, neither T memory cells not T cell reactivity are fully restored during the chronic stage. In addition, titers of HIV and its Ags (e.g., p-24), as well as Abs to HIV Ags (e.g., anti-gp-41 and anti-p-24 Abs), vary with time after exposure to HIV. Implications of these changes to immunological function and the progression of AIDS are discussed in later sections of this chapter.

IMMUNOBIOLOGY OF AIDS

How does HIV take over the immune system and make it unresponsive to invasion by pathogenic cells or agents? To answer this question, we must first understand the characteristics of the HIV-1 virus.

Lymphocyte Infection

AIDS is caused by an RNA retrovirus, HIV-1. Attachment of the virus to the host cell occurs through **ligand-specific interaction** between *gp-120 envelope proteins* of HIV-1 and *CD4 molecules* on the cell surface. Subsequently, the virus can be internalized, apparently through receptor-mediated endocytosis, and uncoated. Once internalized, the HIV's reverse transcriptase transcribes viral RNA into proviral DNA. An integration protein then incorporates the proviral DNA into the host chromosome, where it can profoundly affect the infected cell. This alteration to the host cell's genome produced by viral infection enables the infected cell to transcribe and translate the viral genes. These genes now can be used to assemble new viruses that can be released to infect more cells.

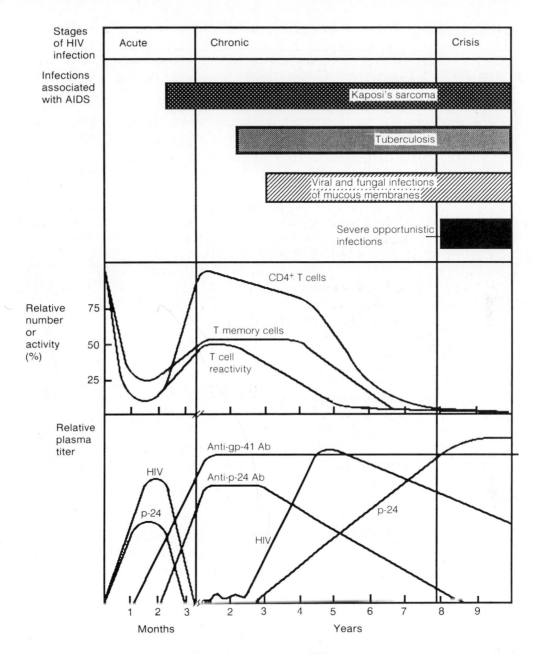

Time after exposure to HIV

FIGURE 15.3 Events associated with the progression of AIDS. The four successive panels of this figure depict (*top*) major stages in the progression of AIDS; (*second*) principal infections associated with each stage; (*third*) the relative number of CD4+ T cells and T memory cells and the relative degree of T cell reactivity plotted as a function of progression of the HIV-1 infection; (*bottom*) the relative plasma titers of HIV, p-24 Ag, and Abs against p-24 and gp-41. (Source: Lord, J. *Infection, Your Immune System, and AIDS.*, 1989 Enterprise for Education, Inc., Santa Monica; and Rosenberg, Z. F. and Fauci, A. S. Immunopathogenic mechanisms of HIV infection: cytokine induction of HIV expression. *Immunology Today* 11:70, 1990.)

How the HIV-1 Genome Operates

HIV-1, which can cause AIDS in humans, has an unusual genome for a retrovirus. Understanding how the genes work could be important in developing therapeutic agents targeted toward neutralizing or altering the actions of these unique genes or their products.

The genome of HIV consists of the usual structural genes of retroviruses and genes peculiar to HIV. The genes common to all retroviruses are (1) *gag* (group Ag gene), which encodes the viral core proteins; (2) *env* (envelope glycoprotein gene), which encodes gp-120 and gp-41; and (3) *pol* (polymerase gene), which encodes several enzymes required for replication of the viral genome (e.g., reverse transcriptase, a protease, and an endonuclease). These structural genes are flanked by regions called long terminal repeat (LTR) sequences, which contain regions responsible for initiating replication of the viral genes. In addition, HIV possesses several other genes called **accessory genes.** The accessory genes include three regulatory genes: (1) *tat* (transactivating), (2) *rev* (regulator of expression of virion proteins), and (3) *nef* (negative regulator factor). Of these three regulators, only *nef* appears to have a negative effect on HIV-1 replication. When this gene is deleted, viral replication increases up to 10-fold. Thus, a possible function of *nef* is to hold HIV replication in check or permit the virus to remain latent. Moreover, there are at least three other genes present: (1) *vpr*, which encodes viral protein R; (2) *vpu*, which encodes viral protein U (both with undefined functions); and (3) *vif*, which encodes a viral infectivity factor. The accessory genes are presumably responsible for the unique ecologic niche that HIV-1 has acquired, namely, the ability to uncouple integration from replication, which permits infection of nondividing cells.

The product of *tat* is a trans-activator protein that increases expression of viral genes, especially those for structural proteins. It seems to regulate both transcription and translation. Another transacting HIV gene is *rev* (also known formerly as *art* [antirepressor transactivator] or *trs* [transrepressor of splicing]), whose product seems to negate the effects of repressors of viral transcription. Haseltine's group at Harvard University has proposed that this gene acts to remove negative genetic regulation, whereas Wong-Staal of Gallo's group at the National Cancer Institute suggests that it represses genetic activity. However, regardless of which interpretation is correct, the end result is the same—the gene product allows the accumulation of certain proteins, but not of others, in the infected CD4+ T lymphocyte.

The regulatory genes appear to interact with one another. *Nef* encodes a protein that is phosphorylated and can bind GTP. It acts as a negative regulator of HIV expression. *Tat,* in contrast, is a positive regulator that can increase transcription of HIV mRNAs and stimulate the preferential translation of viral proteins. *Rev* can act as a two-way switch. On the one hand, its expression favors viral expression by activating virion genes; on the other hand, its repression reduces viral replication. It has been suggested that interaction of *nef* and *rev* might lead to viral latency, while the pairing of *tat* and *rev* can lead to active lytic expression of HIV. The consequences of the different patterns of interaction among these genes are depicted in figure 15.A.

Understanding how these regulatory genes act is critical for designing therapeutic agents to deal with HIV-1 infection. It might be possible in the future to design drugs that could block the action of *tat* or *rev*, or enhance the expression of *nef,* thereby blocking further expression of HIV.

Chakrabarti, S., Robert-Guroff, M., Wong-Staal, F., et al. Expression of the HTLV-III envelope gene by a recombinant vaccinia virus. *Nature* (London) **320**:535, 1986.

Goh, W. C., Rosen, C., Sodroski, J., et al. Identification of a protein encoded by the *trans* activator gene *tat* III of human T-cell lymphotropic retrovirus type III. *Journal of Virology* **59**:181, 1986.

Greene, W. C. Regulation of HIV-1 gene expression. *Annual Review of Immunology* **8**:453, 1990.

Haseltine, W. A. and Wong-Staal, F. The molecular biology of the AIDS virus. *Scientific American* **259**:52, 1988.

Marx, J. L. The AIDS virus—well known but a mystery. *Science* **238**:390, 1987.

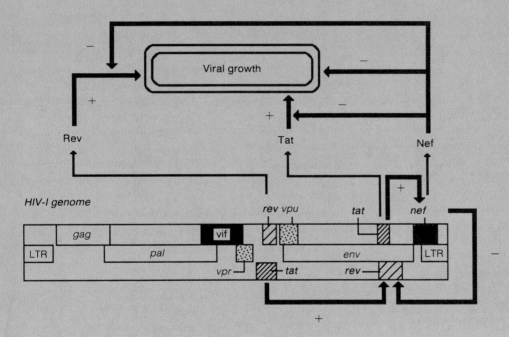

FIGURE 15.A Role of HIV genes in regulation of viral growth. Several viral genes exert positive (i.e., stimulate) and negative (i.e., suppress) influence on viral growth. These genes (*italic*), their products (*roman, capitalized*), and their sources of action are indicated. (From Haseltine, W. A., and Wong-Staal F. The molecular biology of the AIDS virus. *Scientific American* **259**:52, 1988 and Mitsuya, H., Yarchoan, R., and Broder, S. Molecular targets for AIDS therapy. *Science* **249**:1533, 1990.)

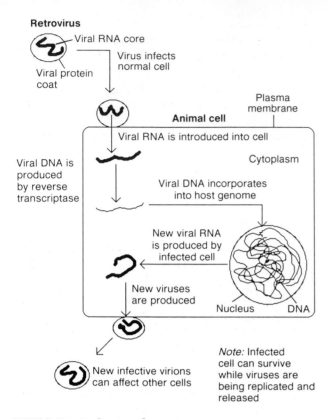

Retrovirus

Viral RNA core

Virus infects normal cell

Viral protein coat

Plasma membrane

Animal cell

Viral RNA is introduced into cell

Cytoplasm

Viral DNA is produced by reverse transcriptase

Viral DNA incorporates into host genome

New viral RNA is produced by infected cell

New viruses are produced

Nucleus   DNA

New infective virions can affect other cells

Note: Infected cell can survive while viruses are being replicated and released

FIGURE 15.4 Replication of retroviruses.

Unlike cells infected by many DNA viruses, those infected by RNA viruses need not die immediately, but might continue to survive, albeit crippled, to produce infective viruses (fig. 15.4). One trigger for virus activation is a T cell protein, nuclear factor κB, which is produced when $CD4^+$ cells are activated by Ag. Once activated, the HIV DNA directs the $CD4^+$ cell to make copies of virus RNA and proteins, assemble the viral parts, and release (by "budding") the completed infective HIV virus. Eventually, the host cell will die. However, before this occurs, it remains alive for a long period of time, serving as an HIV factory.

Although HIV-1 infects and kills primarily T_H cells, it can also infect other cells. In fact, *HIV-1 can infect any $CD4^+$ cell,* including monocytes, macrophages, and gut chromaffin cells. It seems that these cells can act as reservoirs for the virus in its latent form. However, infection by HIV can also disturb the normal function of these cells.

The fact that HIV can invade a variety of cells has broad clinical implications. For example, AIDS-infected macrophages can destroy tissue in the gastrointestinal tract. In addition, several neurological symptoms can be brought on by HIV infection. These can range from mild confusion and poor coordination to profound dementia. The target cells in these instances appear to be the endothelial cells of the brain's blood vessels and the macrophagelike glial cells (astrocytes and oligodendrocytes). Neurons themselves do not seem to be infected. Nevertheless, direct damage might be caused by infected macrophages, producing toxic factors bringing about neuronal death. Damage might be caused indirectly through inhibition of normal support functions. For example, suppression of neuroleukin secretion (needed for neuronal survival) or impairment of myelin (white matter of the brain) production by oligodendrocytes could account for the coordination problems of some AIDS patients.

Interestingly, the $CD8^+$ (T_S and T_C) cells are *not attacked by the AIDS virus.* In fact, $CD8^+$ lymphocytes have been shown to control HIV-1 infection *in vitro* by suppressing viral replication. Thus, it may be possible to treat AIDS patients by autologous therapy, in which their own T_S cells could be removed and amplified *in vitro* and then reintroduced into the host to control the spread of the disease.

Evading Immune Destruction

HIV appears to avoid destruction by the immune system by detrimentally affecting the cells that could mount an effective response against the virus, the $CD4^+$ lymphocytes. This is accomplished in three ways as follows:

1. Infected $CD4^+$ cells secrete a soluble suppressor factor, lymphotoxin, that acts as a generalized immunosuppressant.
2. In addition, the virus might also synthesize a membrane protein, which could interfere with the receptor functions of the $CD4^+$ cells. This renders the infected $CD4^+$ cells incapable of recognizing foreign Ags presented to them.
3. Moreover, the virus eventually kills the $CD4^+$ cells, thereby reducing their numbers in the immune network (fig. 15.5).

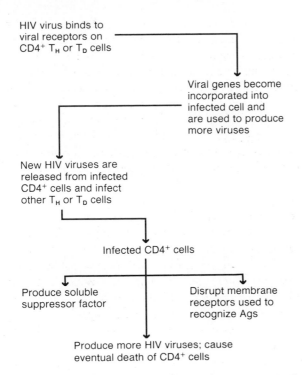

HIV virus binds to viral receptors on CD4+ T_H or T_D cells

Viral genes become incorporated into infected cell and are used to produce more viruses

New HIV viruses are released from infected CD4+ cells and infect other T_H or T_D cells

Infected CD4+ cells

Produce soluble suppressor factor

Disrupt membrane receptors used to recognize Ags

Produce more HIV viruses; cause eventual death of CD4+ cells

FIGURE 15.5 Possible mechanism of action of HIV on CD4+ cells.

There is an interesting phenomenon in this disease. In the terminal phase of the disease, there is *total T cell ablation* when in fact only few CD4+ T cells are infected with HIV-1. How can many die but few be actually infected? Two major possibilities seem to account for this phenomenon: (1) infected cells release lymphotoxin that can kill other CD4+ cells and (2) infected CD4+ cells can fuse with up to 100 non-infected CD4+ cells, forming a unit called a syncytium, which can be caused by gp-120 binding to CD4 molecules. This will lead to the death of the entire unit. The ability to direct cell-to-cell contact can also provide a mode of transmission and explain why there is a paucity of free virus in sera of persons with AIDS.

HIV-1 also has an amazing capacity for demonstrating antigenic variability. This means that the virus has the capability of changing the Ags on its surface coat. This makes it difficult for the immune system to mount an effective defense. A virus that can create many coats can shield itself from recognition at appropriate times in order to shield itself from whatever de-

fense the immune system is currently using against it. Furthermore, a therapeutic nightmare is created by this ability of the AIDS virus to undergo "antigenic drift." This ability to change its coat presents considerable difficulty for the production of an effective vaccine. A vaccine is only effective if we can identify invariant antigenic regions, which can be used to immunize large populations against viral invasion; otherwise it is futile, and mass immunization is impossible. The development of an AIDS vaccine will have to elicit immune cells capable of recognizing and killing specifically infected cells, in addition to eliciting neutralizing Abs.

Although it can be many years between initial infection with HIV and the symptoms of AIDS, it seems unlikely that a true state of latency exists. In persons tested, virus production was demonstrable throughout pre-AIDS stages. In particular, HIV replication is high during the early, acute stage. In addition, persistent, low-level virus production was detectable during the middle, chronic stage. These findings imply that there is continual dialogue between HIV and the immune system. For example, after infection, virulent clones of HIV (i.e., forms that can cause massive T cell depletion via syncytium formation) might be suppressed by normal humoral and cellular immune mechanisms. However, less virulent strains of HIV might continue to replicate and, over time, compromise immune responsiveness of the host. Although the infected individual might remain asymptomatic, selective loss of memory T cells and reduction of T cell and Ag-presenting cell (APC) function could contribute to the eventual breakdown of immune responsiveness. Subsequently, restraints preventing replication of more virulent forms of HIV might be lifted. This could promote rapid T_H cell elimination with the concomitant development of the symptoms of full-blown AIDS. Several of these factors are diagrammatically portrayed in figure 15.3.

Alternatively, HIV genes integrated into the host genome might be activated by superinfection with other viruses (e.g., herpesvirus or CMV). For example, herpesvirus can transactivate the long terminal repeat (LTR) of HIV in human T cells. In addition, a strain of herpesvirus has been found capable of coinfecting with HIV, leading to accelerated HIV expression and cell death. Of special interest is the observation that

Acquired Immune Deficiency Syndrome **387**

Acceleration of HIV Expression

HIV integrates its proviral genome into the host chromosome and appears to persist at a low level of expression for extended periods. This behavior prompts the question, What signals activate the integrated viral genome from a latent state to one of high expression?

Recent cell culture studies of HIV-infected T cells noted enhanced viral expression following mitogen stimulation. Mitogens, like phytohemagglutinin (PHA), can stimulate mRNA synthesis in eukaryotic cells. They might also be able to stimulate viral RNA transcription in HIV-infected cells. In T cells stimulated by mitogens or Ag, there is an induction of certain transcription factors, which bind to particular enhancer elements. One of these enhancer elements, designated κB, is present in both the IL-2 and IL-2 receptor genes. In addition, this enhancer appears in the LTRs of HIV. Consequently, induced κB-binding proteins could interact with the integrated HIV genome, thereby up-regulating the transcription of HIV mRNA. This could lead to amplified levels of HIV replication and ultimate T cell destruction.

Since cytokines also can activate T cell expression, some investigators have suggested that cytokines might be involved in the activation of HIV expression in infected CD4$^+$ cells. One candidate for such a role is tumor necrosis factor alpha (TNF-α). The observation that TNF-α, which is normally produced by macrophages during infection, is present at elevated levels in the serum of AIDS patients is consistent with such a role. Further support for this hypothesis can be found in the behavior of CD4$^+$ T cells, which are the primary targets for HIV. For example, the number of TNF-α receptors on the surface of CD4$^+$ cells is increased in cells infected with HIV. In addition, TNF-α can induce factors that bind to the κB enhancer. Thus, all the elements are present for TNF-α activation of HIV replication in infected cells (fig. 15.B).

Thus, the activation of HIV replication could be an inevitable consequence of normal immunological responses to Ag challenge, which unwittingly leads to increased pathogenesis of HIV infections. However, the observations cited above do not prove that cytokines accelerate HIV replication in the course of AIDS. Nevertheless, these data provide insights into regulation of HIV pathogenesis at the cellular and subcellular levels.

Greene, W. C., Bohnlein, E., and Ballard, D. W. HIV-1, HTLV-1 and normal T-cell growth: transcriptional strategies and surprises. *Immunology Today* 10:272, 1989.

Rosenberg, Z. F., and Fauci, A. S. Immunopathogenic mechanisms of HIV infection: cytokine induction of HIV expression. *Immunology Today* II:176, 1990.

Virelizier, J. L. Cellular activation and human immunodeficiency virus infection. *Current Opinion in Immunology* 2:409, 1990.

certain cells infected this way were CD4$^-$. This may be a way in which cells lacking CD4 molecules become infected with HIV-1.

Destruction of Immune Competence

Impairment of T Cell Function

A major reason that AIDS is such a devastating disease is the particular target cell of HIV-1, namely CD4$^+$ T cells. CD4$^+$ T cells are helper/inducer lymphocytes that play a central role within the intact immune network. Their malfunction or depletion can have far-reaching consequences for proper immunological response. For most immune responses, the CD4$^+$ T cells are the first cells to recognize the Ag presented by macrophages (or other APCs). Once the Ag is recognized, CD4$^+$ T cells are essential for the activation of both humoral and cell-mediated immune responses. In humoral immunity, CD4$^+$ T cells specifically stimulate the proper B lymphocytes to clone into Ab-producing plasma cells and memory B cells. The Ab (with or without serum complement) can specifically attack and

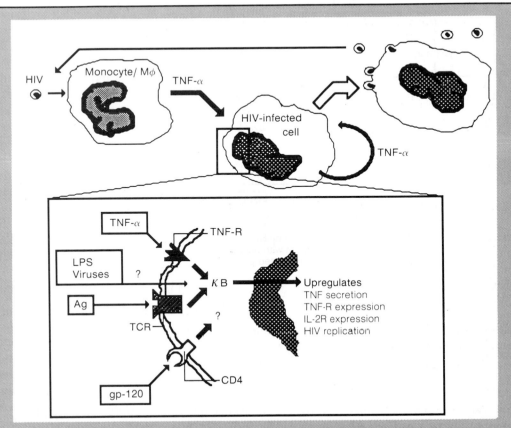

FIGURE 15.B Signals that can accelerate HIV replication. TNF-Rs are upregulated in HIV-infected cells, setting the stage for autocrine stimulation which can enhance HIV replication. This pathway can interact with other signals or with other viruses with the same consequences. (Abbreviations: κB, transcriptional activator protein; LPS, lipopolysaccharide; MΦ, macrophage; TCR, T cell receptor; TNF-R, TNF receptor.)

kill (or inactivate) the foreign (or transformed) cell or virus that is attacking the host. In cell-mediated immunity, CD4$^+$ T cells are responsible, in part, for the clonal formation and expression of T_D cells, T_C cells, and T memory cells. These activated T cells can directly battle the foreign cell either by direct killing (T_C cells) or recruitment of phagocytes (T_D cells) (fig. 15.6).

The host cells can become efficient producers of new HIV, which can be shed from the infected cell, until the cell is spent and dies. However, normal functioning of CD4$^+$ cells infected by HIV might be af-

fected long before T cell depletion occurs. At the cellular level, there can be several direct pathological consequences of HIV infection. These include interference with synthesis of normal cellular products during the manufacturing and assembly of viral particles, destruction of the cell membrane due to prolific viral budding, and interruption of cell signaling.

For example, T cell regulation can be disrupted at the level of Ag recognition. CD4 molecules on T_H cells can bind both HIV gp-120 and MHC class II molecules on APCs. Consequently, gp-120 might

functioning, (2) hyperactivity of B cells, and (3) normal CD8$^+$ T cell function. Another model makes use of immune deficient mice (the **scid mutant**) into which human immune cells are transplanted. The transplanted cells reconstitute a functional immune system in the host mice. Moreover, these transplanted human cells can be infected by HIV, which can replicate. Other murine models make use of HIV-murine hybrids. In one case, HIV-1 was injected into mouse embryos. These infected embryos subsequently developed into mice displaying skin and immune system abnormalities similar to human AIDS. In another model, transgenic mice were constructed that contained HIV genes. In this latter model, genes from HIV-1 were inserted into the mouse genome using recombinant DNA technology. This model should prove useful in more fully understanding how regulatory and structural HIV genes interact and express themselves during the pathogenesis of AIDS.

These and other animal models are being developed to augment *in vitro* studies being conducted with HIV-1. Although studies conducted in tissue culture can elucidate the molecular events associated with HIV infection, animal studies are critical to characterizing the biological and clinical events associated with AIDS. Moreover, animal models provide the most effective means for exploring therapies and vaccines for use in the management and prevention of AIDS.

TREATMENTS OF AIDS

What therapies are available to victims of AIDS? The most common initial strategy is to treat the symptoms, for example, give antibiotics for bacterial infections, antifungal drugs for fungal infections, aspirin for fever, morphine for pain. Table 15.2 lists some means for treating AIDS. Certain of these are currently in use while others are only potential candidates.

Conventional Therapies

The list of different drugs to treat opportunistic infections of AIDS has expanded in recent years. Individuals with AIDS suffer from a number of opportunistic infections, and drug therapies are now being used not only to treat any active infections, but also prophylactically as treatments to prevent projected infections (primary prophylaxis) and to prevent recurrences (secondary prophylaxis). However, there is *no effective cure* for AIDS.

Opportunistic viral infections can devastate a person with AIDS, as seen in CMV infections. This herpes virus can cause blindness as well as life-threatening ulcers in the gastrointestinal tract. A generalized problem with drugs used to treat opportunistic infections in AIDS arises because the pathogens are intracellular parasites. Those drugs that are effective in eradicating the parasite leave the person's own healthy cells at risk of being destroyed as well. Nevertheless, numerous agents have been found that provide some assistance in managing AIDS and its associated symptoms.

Antiviral drugs have also been used with some success in treating individuals afflicted with AIDS. For example, AZT (azidodeoxythymidine), suramin, dideoxyinosine (ddI), and dideoxycytosine (ddC) are nucleoside analogues that show some promise as antiviral therapeutic agents. These drugs act early in the viral life cycle and block viral reproduction (production of proviral DNA). However, they can have harmful side effects in humans. New antiviral drugs, such as ganciclovir and foscarnet (both interfere with viral DNA synthesis) show promise. Their use also is limited by toxic reactions in some individuals. Another antiviral agent, acyclovir (an antiherpes agent), is less toxic, but unfortunately is less effective when used alone. However, when combined with AZT, acyclovir seems effective in halting the progression of, but not in curing, AIDS. Other drugs, such as interferon (IFN-α and IFN-β), and ribavirin interfere with later viral translational events. It was hoped that combining early and late antiviral agents would produce more effective therapy. However tests performed *in vitro* showed that the two drugs were antagonistic, but alone were effective in stemming the continued onslaught of the disease. Nevertheless, antiviral IFN-α can combat both HIV infection and the AIDS-related cancer, Kaposi's sarcoma. Related drugs are being developed, such as CS-85, CS-87 and CS-91, which have fewer side effects.

Another approach employs a protease inhibitor called A-74704 as an antiviral agent. Therapy with this agent is based on the observation that HIV-1 pro-

TABLE 15.2 Possible Means of Treating AIDS

Treatment	Mode of Action
Conventional Drug Therapies	
Antibiotics (e.g., rifamycin, pentamidine isethionate)	
Antiviral agents e.g., AZT, ddI, ddC, suramin	Inhibit multiplication of opportunistic bacteria and fungi Inhibit early replication of HIV
e.g., ribavirin, IFN (α and β)	Inhibit late stages of viral replication
Immunomodulation	
Anti-HIV antibody	Neutralizes free HIV
Bone marrow transplant	Replaces infected CD4$^+$ cells by uninfected precursors
Cyclosporin	Suppresses infected CD4$^+$ cells
IFN-γ/ILs	Restore/stimulate immune function (?)
Biotechnology Products	
Immunoadhesins	Block HIV binding, promote clearance by ADCC and related reactions
Ribozymes	Block viral replication by degrading HIV mRNA
Soluble CD4 antigen	Blocks HIV attachment to CD4$^+$ cells
AIDS Vaccines	
Attenuated/killed HIV	Stimulates generalized immunity
Antiidiotype	Produces anti-CD4 Abs, blocks HIV binding
HIV subunits or products plus adjuvant	Induce Abs to interfere with selected steps in HIV infection or replication
HIV/vaccinia recombinant	Induces Abs to interfere with selected steps in HIV infection or replication

tease is essential for the proper assembly and maturation of the HIV-1 virus. It has been effective in cell culture in inhibiting viral replication, and it is hoped that the same efficacy will be seen *in vivo*.

A problematic bacterial infection, caused by *Mycobacterium avium,* can account for the fever, night sweats, weight loss, and fatigue in AIDS. This pathogen can be treated with the rifamycin group of antibiotics used against tuberculosis. This treatment is effective both against active infections and as a prophylactic measure. Other measures also show promise for primary and secondary prophylaxis. For example, pentamidine isethionate is used in the management of pneumonia caused by the fungus, *Pneumocystis carinii.* This drug inhibits the synthesis of microbial DNA and can be dispensed as an inhalant for use as a primary and secondary prophylactic agent. Treatment of acute infections is accomplished by cotrimoxazole (a combination of sulfamethoxazole and trimethoprim), which inhibits folic acid synthesis in microbes.

Other opportunistic infections present additional challenges. For example, in toxoplasmosis, a parasitic infection of the brain, the blood-brain barrier presents an obstacle to treatment. Few drugs can cross the blood-brain barrier. Nevertheless, a combination of coenzyme inhibitors, pyrimethamine and sulfadiazine, seems to suppress the infection. On the other hand, cryptococcal meningitis is caused by a fungus. The usual treatment is an antifungal agent, amphotericin B, which can be highly toxic. Recent clinical trials with less toxic antifungal compounds, such as the imidazoles, show promise in suppressing this fungal disease.

Immune Restoration

Other strategies are to try to restore immune function. Bone marrow transplantation is one course open to AIDS patients in an attempt to replenish functioning $CD4^+$ cells by donor bone marrow stem cells. Other attempts at immune restoration employ immune modulators in an effort to recover or restore function in the remaining uninfected immunocytes. One such drug is inosine pranobex, an immune modulator that can enhance the function of various cells of the immune system, perhaps through increased production of IL-1 and IL-2. Early in HIV infections, treatment with this drug has enhanced T cell and NK cell expression and appears to delay the progression to full-blown AIDS. Other immune system boosters that have shown promise are thymostimulin, granulocyte-monocyte–colony-stimulating factor, amplugen (which boosts IFN production), and peptide T (which prevents HIV-1 from entering cells *in vitro*). In contrast, natural immune response modifiers such as the ILs and IFN-α or IFN-β have not proved that successful in halting the course of the disease.

Some AIDS therapies include aggressively attacking the disease at an early stage by combining antiviral drugs and immune stimulators. Currently, however, there is no effective cure for AIDS.

Therapies from Biotechnology

One approach to managing AIDS entails efforts at destroying HIV. This is accomplished by engineered substances called ribozymes, which are enzymatic RNA molecules that can cleave other RNA molecules. Using cultured human cells infected by HIV, ribozymes were shown to be capable of blocking the expression of certain viral gene products. This suggests that ribozymes might be capable of blocking viral replication. If so, they might provide an effective antiviral therapy in the treatment of AIDS.

Another approach under study focuses on preventing virus entry into the target cell. HIV specifically interacts with T_H cells through an interaction between gp-120 envelope protein and CD4 on the lymphocyte surface. A soluble form of CD4 has been produced that can bind to gp-120, thereby blocking viral entry. This prevents the spread of HIV from infected to noninfected cells. In addition, soluble CD4 has been found to be effective in binding to envelope gp-120. This interaction neutralizes this binding protein and blocks interaction with CD4 on T cell surfaces. Furthermore, altering HIV envelope proteins (e.g., gp-120) could also render the virus incapable of infecting its host cell. Extracts from seeds of an Australian chestnut tree can interfere with the glycosylation of gp-120. Studies *in vitro* have shown that virions with nonglycosylated (or underglycosylated) gp-120 can bind to CD4 but cannot enter T_H cells.

Combination Therapies

Combination therapies might prove useful in the management of AIDS. This approach seems reasonable in view of the virus' capability of adapting to the chemotherapeutic roadblocks presented to it. For example, combination of antiviral AZT with soluble CD4 should diminish the extent of effective binding between HIV and target T cells, on the one hand, and of effective replication, on the other. Alternatively, CD4 can be combined with IgG and IgM to produce a hybrid molecule known as an immunoadhesin. The Ig serves two important functions: (1) it extends the half-life of soluble CD4 in plasma and (2) it provides a second reactive focus for clearing bound HIV, since it is capable of attaching to Fc receptors. A third approach links soluble CD4 with a toxin. This reagent should selectively eliminate infected T cells displaying the gp-120 Ag on their surfaces (where budding HIV virus will concentrate this viral envelope Ag).

VACCINES

Another area of intensive research is the development of AIDS vaccines. In spite of the fact that HIV can mutate rapidly, many investigators are endeavoring to produce vaccines against it in an effort to prevent the spread of AIDS. Several strategies for developing an AIDS vaccine have emerged.

Along traditional lines, Jonas Salk (who developed the Salk polio vaccine) has produced a whole killed virus vaccine, while Essex and Kanki at Harvard University are experimenting with a less deadly form of the AIDS virus, HTLV-IV. Interestingly, there are indications that the immune system of persons already infected with HIV-1 can be boosted by vaccination with the Salk vaccine of inactivated virus. Animal models are also being used in vaccine development. Rhesus monkeys, when infected by SIV, develop an AIDS-like disease. Treatment of rhesus monkeys with a killed viral preparation conferred immunity to infection for a significant period of time.

Passive immunotherapy is also being tested. Hyperimmune plasma with high levels of anti-HIV Abs have been administered to persons with AIDS in hopes that the administered Abs might boost ADCC reactions against the virus. The treatments did result in increased Ab synthesis and the clearance of certain HIV Ags from the blood. However, further studies must be performed in order to more critically evaluate the efficacy of human HIV immune globulin in the treatment of HIV infections.

Certain other groups attempting to produce an AIDS vaccine have focused their attention on virus coat proteins. One approach makes use of extracted pieces of the protein coat (gp-120 and gp-160) from live virus to make the vaccine. Since gp-120 can bind to CD4 Ag on T_H cells, it is hoped that Abs raised to the vaccine will interfere with the adsorption of HIV-1 to CD4$^+$ lymphocytes. In fact, using recombinant DNA technology, many biotechnology companies have synthesized the gp-120 protein coat and have used the product as the basis of the vaccine. Others have inserted the gene for the outer coat of HIV-1 into live vaccinia virus. Vaccinia virus is an avirulent poxvirus that can replicate in the host and secrete the surface proteins encoded in the HIV gene fragment spliced into its genome. The Abs raised against this vaccine should also neutralize the HIV and prevent the expression of AIDS. However a drawback to this approach is the possibility that the body could produce an autoimmune attack on APCs that share some epitopes with gp-120. A third approach under study entails raising antiidiotypic Abs to components of the virus outer coat or CD4. It is hoped that these antiidiotype Abs will block viral penetration into host cells.

Early clinical trials of a subunit vaccine made from the HIV-1 protein, gp-160 (the precursor molecule for the envelope glycoproteins), appear promising. Immunization with this vaccine has induced immune responses that result in the killing of HIV-infected CD4$^+$ T cells grown in culture. The use of vaccines with neutralizing epitopes is important because of the concern that killed viral preparations might still contain infectious particles. Besides gp-120, another neutralization target is the envelope protein gp-41, which can regulate the interaction between gp-120 and CD4. It is hoped that the Abs produced against these epitopes will promote ADCC reactions against the virus.

DIAGNOSTIC EVALUATION OF HIV

Several methods are available for detecting Abs to HIV and HIV Ags, genes, and gene products. The prevalent method for screening for HIV Abs is the *enzyme-linked immunosorbent assay* (ELISA). Positive results are confirmed by the *Western blot* technique. In the ELISA, test wells are coated with HIV Ags. Serum to be tested is then added, incubated, and washed. Ab specific for human Ig, which is linked to an enzyme, is added and then a color assay initiated. If anti-HIV Ab is present in the serum, it will bind to the Ag-coated wells. The enzyme-linked second Ab will then bind to it, and a color change occurs when the substrate is added. A positive result would be confirmed by the more costly and time-consuming Western blot technique. With this latter method, HIV-1 viral Ags are separated by electrophoresis and then transferred onto nitrocellulose paper, which is then incubated with the serum to be tested. If the person is seropositive, then Ab binding would be detected by addition of a secondary enzyme-linked antihuman Ab followed by a colored product reaction.

The presence of HIV-1 Ag can be detected by a variety of methods. This is an important assay for individuals who are HIV positive but Ab negative. This can be accomplished with an ELISA developed for Ag detection in serum. Wells are coated with monoclonal Abs (MAbs) to the p-24 core protein. Serum is added, followed by the sequential addition of the probe Ab and enzyme substrate. The resulting color reaction in a positive test can provide a quantitative estimate of the HIV Ag in the serum tested. In addition, infectious viral particles can be detected in cell culture using techniques that assay HIV reverse transcriptase. Moreover, immunofluorescence assays can be used to detect HIV Ag in noninfected cells. This is accomplished with the use of MAbs to core proteins, followed by exposure to fluorescent secondary Abs.

Advances in genetic technologies have made it possible to detect the presence of the viral genes as well as their products. Methods such as *in situ* hybridization, filter hybridization, Southern blot analysis, and DNA amplification enable virus to be detected even when it is latent and its production is minimal. A new technique, the *polymerase chain reaction* (PCR), can be used to detect HIV proviral DNA. The PCR amplifies specific nucleic acid sequences to detectable levels through repetitive cycles of DNA synthesis. Amplification of HIV provirus DNA requires primer sequences complementary to the target DNA sequence, DNA polymerase, nucleoside triphosphate substrates, and a DNA sample extracted from mononuclear leukocytes of the person to be tested. Although not widely used, this test could provide a highly sensitive and specific means for detecting the presence of HIV-1. In addition, it could be used to evaluate both false-positive and false-negative ELISA results.

S U M M A R Y

1. Acquired immune deficiency syndrome is caused by the retrovirus, HIV, which infects and impairs the functioning of T_H (CD4$^+$) lymphocytes, and leads to the complete breakdown of the immune network. [p. 379]
2. AIDS is believed to have originated in central Africa and initially been transmitted to humans by monkeys. The virus is usually transmitted among humans through body fluids (sexual contact), contaminated blood products, and placental transfer. [p. 379]
3. The symptoms of AIDS include recurrent, chronic viral, bacterial, fungal, and protozoan infections, as well as cancers like Kaposi's

sarcoma. Progression to AIDS following initial infection with HIV proceeds through several stages over a period of several years. [p. 380–382]
4. HIV gains entry to target cells through ligand-specific binding to the CD4 molecule on the cell surface. Once within the cell, it produces proviral DNA, then either inserts into the host genome (silent) or initiates a lytic cycle (active). Host cells appear to become nonfunctional when the virus is involved in an active lytic cycle. Although T lymphocytes are primarily affected, any CD4$^+$ cells can serve as targets. As more cells become infected, immunological function progressively decreases. [p. 382–390]
5. Evidence has emerged that there might be a genetic component to the development of AIDS following exposure to HIV. In addition, several animal model systems are being explored as tools for acquiring greater understanding of the cellular events and clinical progression of HIV infections. [p. 391–392]
6. Current therapies have not been able to stop the fatal course of AIDS, but future success might lie in aggressively attacking the disease with antiviral drugs and immune stimulators early after initial infection. Efforts at development of vaccines against HIV-1 are also in progress in hopes of preventing AIDS. [p. 392–395]
7. Several diagnostic tests are available for detecting HIV, its products and components, and antibodies against them. The most widely used tests are the ELISA and Western blot assay. [p. 395–396]

R E A D I N G S

Allan, J. S. A new HTLV-III/LAV encoded antigen detected by antibodies from AIDS patients. *Science* **230:**810, 1985.

Baltimore, D., and Feinberg, M. B. HIV revealed: toward a natural history of the infection. *New England Journal of Medicine* **321:**1673, 1989.

Brookmeyer, R. Reconstruction and future trends of the AIDS epidemic in the United States. *Science* **253:**37, 1991.

Capon, D. J., and Ward, R. H. R. The CD4-gp120 interaction and AIDS pathogenesis. *Annual Review of Immunology* **9:**649, 1991.

Chang, D. D., and Sharp, P. A. Messenger RNA transport and HIV *rev* regulation. *Science* **249:**614, 1990.

DiMarzo-Veronese, F., Copeland, T. D., DeVico, A.L., et al. Characterization of highly immunogenic p66/p51 as the reverse transcriptase of HTLV-III/LAV. *Science* **231:**1289, 1986.

Fauci, A. S. The human immunodeficiency virus: infectivity and mechanisms of pathogenesis. *Science* **239:**617, 1988.

Gallin, J. T., and Fauci, A. S. (eds.). *Advances in Host Defense Mechanisms* (Vol. 5) *AIDS.* Raven Press, New York, 1985.

Gardner, M. B., and Luciw, P. A. Animal models of AIDS. *FASEB Journal* **3:**2503, 1989.

Gottlieb, M. S., and Groupman, S. E. (eds.). *UCLA Symposia on Molecular and Cellular Biology* (Vol. 16) *AIDS.* Alan R.Liss, Inc., New York, 1984.

Greene, W. C. The molecular biology of human immunodeficiency virus type 1 infection. *New England Journal of Medicine* **324:**308, 1991.

Groopman, J. E. et al. Collection of articles on "Current advances in the management of AIDS." *Reviews in Infectious Disease* **12:**908, 1990.

Huang, M., Simard, C., and Jolicoeur, P. Immunodeficiency and growth of target cells by helper-free defective retrovirus. *Science* **246:**1614, 1989.

Kestler, H., Kodama, T., Ringler, D., et al. Induction of AIDS in rhesus monkeys by molecularly cloned simian immunodeficiency virus. *Science* **248:**1109, 1990.

Khan, N. C., and Chatterjee, S. Transmission of human HIV. *American Clinical Laboratory* **9:**10, 1990.

Lawrence, J., Saunders, A., and Kulkosky, J. Characterization and clinical association of antibody inhibitory to HIV reverse transcriptase activity. *Science* **235:**1501, 1987.

Letvin, N. L., and King, N. W. Immunologic and pathologic manifestations of the infection of Rhesus monkeys with simian immunodeficiency virus of macaques. *Journal of Acquired Immune Deficiency Disease* **3:**1023, 1990.

Lo, S.-C., Tsai, S., Benish, J. R., et al. Enhancement of HIV-1 cytocidal effects in CD4+ lymphocytes by AIDS-associated mycoplasmas. *Science* **251:**1074, 1991.

Mak, T. W., and Wigzell, H. (compilers of several reviews). AIDS: ten years later. *FASEB Journal* **5:**2338, 1991.

McCune, J., Kaneshima, H., Krowka, J., et al. The SCID-hu mouse: a small animal model for HIV infection and pathogenesis. *Annual Review of Immunology* **9:**399, 1991.

Mitsuya, H., Yarchoan, R., and Broder, S. Molecular targets for AIDS therapy. *Science* **249:**1533, 1990.

Murray, H. W., Rubin, B. Y., Masur, H., et al. Impaired production of lymphokines and immune (gamma) interferon in AIDS. *New England Journal of Medicine* **310:**883, 1984.

Murray, H. W., Gellene, R. A., Libby, D. M., et al. Activation of tissue macrophages from AIDS patients: in vitro response of AIDS alveolar macrophages to lymphokines and interferon. *Journal of Immunology* **135:**2374, 1985.

Norman, C. AIDS therapy. *Science* **230:**1355, 1985.

Orentas, R. J., Hildreth, J. E. K., Obah, E., et al. Induction of CD4+ human cytolytic T cells specific for HIV-infected cells by a gp-160 subunit vaccine. *Science* **248:**1234, 1990.

Piel, J. (ed.). *The Science of AIDS: Reading from Scientific American Magazine.* W. H. Freeman, New York, 1989.

Rosenberg, Z. F., and Fauci, A. S. Immunopathogenic mechanisms of HIV infection: cytokine induction of HIV expression. *Immunology Today* **11:**170, 1990.

Vaishnav, Y. N., and Wong-Staal, F. The biochemistry of AIDS. *Annual Review of Biochemistry* **60:**577, 1991.

CHAPTER *16*

Autoimmunity

OVERVIEW

In this chapter, the mechanisms of breakdown in self-tolerance and the promulgation of autoimmune diseases are explored. Genetic influences and clinical associations between autoimmune diseases are elaborated, as are the associated mechanisms of tissue damage. Selected autoimmune diseases are also examined.

CONCEPTS

1. A breakdown in the immune network that monitors the expression of "self" can lead to pathological expression of an autoimmune disease state.

2. The mechanism of tissue damage brought about by autoimmune reactions can include Type II (e.g., thyroiditis), Type III (e.g., rheumatoid arthritis), and Type IV (e.g., juvenile diabetes mellitus) hypersensitivity reactions.

3. Some autoimmune disorders produce autoantibodies, which bind to cell-membrane receptors (e.g., myasthenia gravis) and cause dysfunction by blocking normal receptor binding and impairing subsequent physiological responses of the cell.

Normally, individuals do not form potentially destructive Abs to their own cells, but only to foreign Ags. This is because the body has developed a tolerance to the Ags (other than Igs) normally present within itself. This state of immune tolerance to self-Ags is maintained by a complex network of T and B lymphocytes and their regulatory products. However, in certain diseases, we can produce Abs to our own cell or tissue components. This type of Ab is called an auto-Ab, and the diseases associated with auto-Abs are called autoimmune diseases.

This chapter examines possible reasons for pathological auto-Ab formation and mechanisms of cellular, tissue, and organ damage in autoimmune diseases. Diagnostic tests for the presence of auto-Abs are outlined. In addition, genetic factors associated with several autoimmune disorders and the pathogenesis of selected autoimmune diseases are explored.

It is essential that the body be able to recognize self from nonself for survival. For example, the immune system can distinguish self-MHC Ags on its own cells from those on foreign cells. Yet some physiological autoimmune reactivity against self-Ags (Abs) can occur and is normal. The auto-Abs produced by this action serve as physiological regulators of the immune system. Thus, auto-Abs can exist at normal physiological levels as components of the body's homeostatic mechanisms. It has been postulated that auto-Abs might also act as "biological taxis," transporting cellular breakdown products for their ultimate disposal. For example, after myocardial infarction (e.g., heart attack), we find apparently harmless auto-Abs to heart tissue, whose function is to clear away damaged heart tissue. Yet the appearance of normal auto-Abs is a carefully controlled event; if it goes awry and lymphocytes proliferate and large quantities of auto-Abs are produced, autoimmune disease can occur. It is this latter state, this pathological breakdown in self-tolerance, that is examined in this chapter.

THEORIES OF BREAKDOWN IN SELF-TOLERANCE

There are several ways that auto-Ab formation can be triggered. Scientists have been able to identify either the precipitating event that takes place just prior to the expression of disease, or the underlying events that seem to eventually lead to a disease state, but not both. What was originally thought to be a simple matter of one common biological trigger for many autoimmune disorders is now known to be a puzzling assortment of triggers, which have to occur in the right space and time for disease to occur.

For example, in juvenile diabetes, complement-fixing auto-Abs to the insulin-producing islet cells (β cells) of the pancreas cause their immune destruction, with subsequent expression of the clinical symptoms of diabetes. When siblings of diabetics were tested, many possessed the same IgG auto-Abs directed against pancreatic β cells, but they showed no signs of disease. However, within three to seven years, the siblings who tested positive for auto-Abs became frankly diabetic. This would indicate that there were other triggers that had to occur before the disease manifested itself; it was not just the presence of cytotoxic Abs that brought on the disease. But the final sequence of events is still unknown.

Another example suggesting that the presence of auto-Ab alone is not sufficient to cause disease is autoimmune hemolytic anemia. In this disease, monoclonal auto-Abs are formed against normal red blood cell constituents. The Abs coat the erythrocytes, causing clumping, lysis, and premature clearance by the spleen. The immunological test used to diagnose this condition is called the **Coombs' test,** which can assesses whether an individual's red blood cells are coated with IgG Ab. However, a positive Coombs' test occurs without any evidence of hemolytic disease in a small percentage of healthy blood donors. Thus, although it is necessary for red blood cells to be coated with auto-Ab in hemolytic anemia, other factors also must be involved in order for the disease to manifest itself.

From these and other autoimmune diseases, it is clear that multiple factors are at work in bringing about the pathology seen in these conditions. The triggers for autoimmune diseases are diverse and include immunological, genetic, viral, drug-induced, and hormonal factors, acting singly or in combination, in time and space. At present many individual mechanisms have been identified (tables 16.1 and 16.2), but how they interact with the immune network has not yet been elucidated. Mechanisms that have been shown to

TABLE 16.1 Inducers of Autoimmune Diseases

Inducer	Mechanism
Viral infection	Virus integrates into host genome; causes expression of altered cell-surface markers, polyclonal activation of B lymphocytes, etc.
Drugs	Binding of drug alters Ags and elicits immune response
Antigen crossreaction	Abs directed against infective agent (e.g., *Treponema pallidum* [in syphilis]), also react with normally expressed Ags on healthy cells (e.g., erythrocytes, causing their unintended autoimmune destruction)
Expression of novel antigenic determinants	Newly exposed determinants in Fc region of Abs (IgG) can evoke immunological attack (e.g., attack by rheumatoid factor [IgM and IgG] against portions of certain IgGs)

eventually cause a **breakdown of self-tolerance** include (1) infection of somatic tissue by viruses, (2) development of altered self-Ags due to binding of certain drugs to cell surfaces, (3) crossreactivity of some Abs to bacterial Ags and self-determinants, (4) development of newly exposed Ags in the body, (5) the influence of hormones, and (6) breakdown in the immune network that recognizes self.

A major focus of the immune system is to maintain self in the body. An event that could lead to a breakdown in self is **viral infection.** Since viruses can cause the *display of viral Ags* on the surface of body cells, viral antigenic expression could act to induce autoimmune diseases. Many animal viruses can enter a latent state, where they remain hidden and noninfective for long periods of time. However, in this state they might still influence the cell-surface markers, which could lead to an autoimmune response. Viruses can also induce autoimmune disease by *polyclonal activation* of lymphocytes, the *release of subcellular organelles* after viral lysis of the cell, by *antigenic mimicry,* or by *functional impairment of regulatory immunocytes* such as T_S or T_H cells. Viral infections prior to disease have

been associated with systemic lupus erythematosus (SLE), multiple sclerosis, and diabetes.

Another way to alter cell-surface antigenic determinants is by **binding of certain drugs.** Hemolytic anemia can be produced in susceptible people taking the antibiotic penicillin. Penicillin can bind to the erythrocytes, and the Abs that develop to the drug can then bind to the foreign antigenic penicillin molecules. It has been suggested that the membrane-bound penicillin can initiate events that lead to the activation of lymphocytes, previously silenced by immune suppressor activity. Subsequent Ab formation against erythrocyte Ags and complement activation can lead to hemolysis and the onset of anemia.

Autoimmune diseases can also be caused by the **formation of Abs that crossreact** with the host's Ags. Many microbial products have Ags that crossreact with self-Ags in human somatic tissue. For example, in syphilis, caused by the spirochete *Treponema pallidum,* many people develop hemolytic anemia. It has been suggested that Abs raised against *Treponema* Ags can also crossreact with certain erythrocyte blood group Ags, thus bringing about the anemia. Antigenic mimicry is also seen in the pathology of Chagas' disease. There is evidence that the Ags common to its causative agent, *Trypanosoma cruzi,* and human cardiac muscle produce the immunopathological lesions seen in this disease. In addition, crossreactions of Abs against *Streptococcus* Group A bacteria with human cardiac muscle are responsible for the myocardial effects of rheumatic fever.

Yet another way of triggering autoimmune diseases is the **development of new antigenic determinants.** This happens in rheumatoid arthritis (RA), where rheumatoid factors (RFs) (IgM or IgG) are directed against newly exposed antigenic determinants on Igs. In affected individuals, when Ags bind to certain IgG Abs, new antigenic determinants are exposed in the Fc region of the molecule, and these new determinants stimulate the formation of RF.

Hormones seem to *influence the expression of certain autoimmune disorders* as well. It is known that hormones of the hypothalamus, thyroid, and adrenal glands affect the homeostasis of the lymphoid system and responses to Ags, by as yet uncharacterized mechanisms. SLE and RA preferentially afflict women,

TABLE 16.2 Means Through Which the Immune Network Might Break Down in Autoimmune Diseases

Production defects	Somatic mutation or alteration of lymphoid progenitor cells
	Thymus and bone marrow defects
Modified expression	Contrasuppression of T cell function
	Enhanced T_H activity
	Polyclonal B cell activation
	Breakdown in idiotypic network
	Defects in macrophage function
	Breakdown in lymphokine release
	Abnormal gene expression

whereas more men develop myasthenia gravis. The predisposing factors in these instances appear to be the sex hormones. It is known that testosterone is immunosuppressive and estrogen is immunoenhancing; but how these hormones contribute to the disease state has not been elucidated.

Last, and perhaps most important, autoimmune diseases can be triggered by some **breakdown in the immune network** that strictly monitors the expression of self (table 16.2). A breakdown in the immune network can occur at many different levels. It could be at the level of production of immunocytes or at the level of expression of a defect in the functioning of the immunocyte.

At the level of **production defects,** there is also the possibility that *germline or somatic mutations of B or T lymphocytes could alter their roles.* The result might be abnormal expression, improper recognition, or harmful interaction with self-Ags. Defects in thymus and bone marrow could also influence the competency and development of the T or B lymphocytes, by adversely affecting the microenvironment of either the stem cells, some other precursor cell, or the differentiating lymphoid cell. It is known that thymic hormones, such as thymosin and thymopoietin, are essential for the differentiation of T cells and their helper, inducer, suppressor, and cytotoxic subsets. Thymic atrophy is often encountered with SLE, but whether it is a cause or an effect has yet to be established.

Defects in Ag recognition might also contribute to the expression of autoimmune diseases. For example, it has been suggested that the number of immunoreactive cells recognizing self-peptides and MHC molecules within the developing thymus might not be properly regulated. Consequently, cells (which should have been clonally deleted) might remain. These cells later could be stimulated inappropriately by combination with self-components altered by disease or other factors. Furthermore, malfunction in the regulation of T cell expression could lead to contrasuppression of T cell function. It is believed that T_S lymphocytes play an essential role in maintaining immune silence to certain self-components found in somatic tissue cells. Interference with (or contrasuppression of) T_S cell activity could lead to autoimmune diseases by allowing the immune system to interact positively with self-Ags. Alternatively, enhanced T_H cell activity could also disrupt the immune network. Unresponsiveness to self-Ags could be maintained by self-tolerance at the level of the T_H cell. If activated, these tolerant T_H cells could be induced to activate B cells to produce auto-Abs.

The induction of autoimmunity could also be accomplished by bypassing T cells. For example, *self-reactive cells could be directly stimulated by* **polyclonal activators,** such as lipopolysaccharides (LPS), which can directly activate B lymphocytes. In this way, we could circumvent the tolerant T cells and bypass the regulatory mechanisms. This could lead to the direct activation of specific B cells, with subsequent formation of Abs to self-components. This has led to the suggestion that autoimmune diseases arise through a combination of polyclonal and Ag-specific stimulation. For example, polyclonal stimulation could cause expansion of B cell clones expressing surface receptors for self-Ags. Subsequent encounter with Ag would lead to activation. Moreover, it is possible that specific activation and self-Ag-driven selection of autoreactive B cells could occur.

Breakdown in the idiotypic Ab network would be another means of activating the immune system against self-elements. Abs raised against the variable, idiotypic Fab region of an Ig molecule are called antiidiotypic Abs, as proposed by Jerne. Abs against the newly formed antiidiotypic Abs, so called anti-antiidiotypic Abs, can be raised experimentally.

What results from this is an idiotypic immune network of Abs that can bind to each other. Jerne has hypothesized that such idiotypic networks can act either as inhibitors or activators of the immune response, depending on the information received. It is, therefore, theoretically possible to envision a situation in which signals could be received by this network that lead to an aberrant autoimmune response to self-Ags.

Since proper Ag presentation is essential for Ab production by B cells and T cell expression of its subsets and effector molecules, it is possible that **macrophage defects** could produce an autoimmune response. *Defects in Ag presentation* could tip the scales to effect a choice of T_H over T_S cells in response to a self-Ag. There is little information of the functional state of macrophages in autoimmune disorders, yet it is accepted that mononuclear phagocytes play an essential role in determining how Ag is processed and presented to lymphocytes, which underlies immune competency.

Ag-processing macrophages also produce factors that influence the activities of lymphocytes. One of these is the monokine interleukin 1 (IL-1), a mitogenic regulatory molecule that stimulates T_H activity. If pathological signals *cause an inappropriate release of lymphokines,* the immune system could become primed to react to self-Ags in a way that would lead to tissue destruction and disease.

Genetic factors can also ultimately influence the operation of the immune system. It is known that certain MHC alleles are associated with certain autoimmune diseases (e.g., DR4 with RA). But the trigger for an autoimmune disorder has not been mapped to a single genetic locus. Yet genetic aberrations in the expression of class II MHC Ags could certainly be the trigger in the breakdown of the self-immune network. In a murine model system, Ia Ags altered by T cells can lead to an SLE-like illness.

Thus, a variety of defects of T and B cells could lead to the expression of autoimmune diseases. Most likely, a number of these mechanisms come into play in a certain temporal and spatial framework to override the cardinal rule of the immune system, that is, to preserve the integrity of self.

TABLE 16.3 Mechanisms of Tissue Damage in Autoimmune Diseases

Mechanism	How Damage is Induced
Complement-fixing Abs	Binding of complement to Ab attached to cell-surface Ag; causes cytolysis
Ab binding to cell receptor*	Binding of Ab to cell-surface receptor impairs normal function by blocking access of normal ligand to its receptor
Immune-complex formation	Formation of immune complexes between self-Ags and self-Abs trigger inflammatory reaction, which can damage local tissues
T_C cells	Activation of T_C cells against normal surface Ags leads to their destruction

*This is considered a form of hypersensitivity (Type V) by some; see chapter 14 for further discussion.

MECHANISM OF TISSUE DAMAGE IN AUTOIMMUNE DISEASES

There are a variety of ways in which an autoimmune response can cause tissue damage (table 16.3). Details of certain disease states are discussed in a later section of this chapter; however, their general mechanisms of action can be classified into the following groups: (1) damage by complement-fixing Abs raised against auto-Ags; (2) compromise of cellular function when auto-Abs bind to cell surface receptors which mediate, degrade, or block expression of differentiated function; (3) tissue damage when auto-Abs and soluble self-Ags form immune complexes and initiate a destructive inflammatory response; and (4) damage to cells through specific T_C cell responses activated to destroy self cellular Ags.

Auto-Abs directed against self-Ags located on the membrane of body cells might bind to these Ags, **activate serum complement,** and cause cytolysis. This occurs in autoimmune hemolytic anemia, when IgG auto-Abs bind to certain blood group Ags, fix complement, and destroy the erythrocytes, thereby causing anemia.

Auto-Abs can form against cell-surface receptors, for example, hormone receptors. (Recall that this mechanism also can be considered as a Type V hypersensitivity reaction [refer to chapter 14 for additional discussion.]) These auto-Abs can either *mimic the function of the normal hormone, block hormone binding, or even degrade the receptor site.* Thus, the formation of a receptor-auto-Ab complex alters the function and activity of the receptor. In myasthenia gravis, auto-Abs are produced to myocyte acetylcholine (ACh) receptors located at the neuromuscular junction. These Abs interfere with proper neurotransmission, diminish the contractility of the muscle cells, and cause fatigue and weakness. In contrast, in thyrotoxicosis, binding of auto-Abs stimulates the thyroid gland, mimicking the action of the normal hormone.

Auto-Abs can be produced against soluble self-Ags, which can **form immune complexes.** This might lead to activation of the complement cascade, with the formation of the anaphylactic and chemotactic fragments, C3a and C5a. Histamine is then released and phagocytic activity is increased, causing an inflammatory response that is destructive to tissues at the site of immune-complex formation. This is the usual series of events during acute episodes in SLE, when auto-Abs to DNA generate anti-DNA:DNA immune complexes, with subsequent inflammation (fig. 16.1).

The *recognition of self-Ags as immunostimulatory* can lead to the **initiation and expansion of T lymphocyte subsets.** Populations of phagocytic cells and T_C cells would be drawn to the antigenic site and proceed to destroy cells displaying the specific self-Ags. An example of this type of immune mechanism is autoimmune thyroiditis, where accumulation of phagocytic and cytolytic cells can be found in the thyroid lesions.

In summary, there are several ways in which the immune system, stimulated to eliminate certain self-Ags, can effect its own end. The four mechanisms mentioned above can act either independently or in concert in bringing about autoimmune disorders. The severity of the disease often lies in which tissue, organ, or system is adversely affected by the resulting tissue

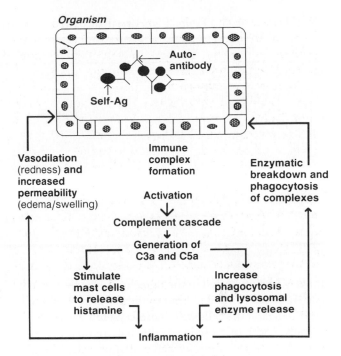

FIGURE 16.1 Complement-mediated inflammatory response to immune-complex formation. Immune complexes can activate the complement system. Consequences of this activation lead to inflammation and possible tissue damage.

damage. Specific autoimmune diseases and the course of immune pathology are covered in greater detail later in this chapter.

DIAGNOSTIC TESTING

Although selective methods can be employed to detect each autoimmune disease, testing generally falls into three categories: (1) immunofluorescence, (2) agglutination, and (3) radioimmunoassay.

The indirect **immunofluorescence** (IF) test is usually used in the detection of autoimmune disorders. This test may be employed to determine the presence of auto-Abs in serum. Frozen tissue samples, displaying the suspected self-Ag, are incubated with a sample of the person's serum. If the serum contains auto-Ab, the Ig binds to the surface self-Ags. Then anti-human IgG Ab, tagged with a fluorescent dye, is added.

TABLE 16.4 Tests Used to Diagnose Autoimmune Diseases

Test	Autoantibody Detected	Autoimmune Disease
Coombs test	Antierythrocyte Ab	Autoimmune hemolytic anemia
Immunoprecipitation	Abs to ACh receptors	Myasthenia gravis
IF	Abs to islet cells	Diabetes mellitus (juvenile)
	Abs to myelin	Multiple sclerosis
RIA	Abs to TSH receptors	Graves' disease
IF and RIA	Anti-basal lamina Abs	Goodpasture's syndrome
	Abs to thyroglobulin	Hashimoto's thyroiditis
	Anti-γ-globulin Ab	RA
	Antinuclear Ab	SLE

IF, immunofluorescence.

If auto-Abs are bound to the tissue cells, the fluorescent anti-IgG molecule will bind to the Fc portion of these auto-Abs, and the cells will fluoresce when viewed with a fluorescence microscope. Cells that are unaffected by auto-Ab will not fluoresce and will appear dark against the glowing cells that are affected by autoimmune disease. This type of testing is used to diagnose autoimmune diseases like Hashimoto's thyroiditis, juvenile diabetes, Goodpasture's syndrome, myasthenia gravis, RA, and SLE (table 16.4).

In the direct **agglutination test,** serum is added to a suspension of cells that have the surface self-Ag to be tested (fig. 16.2). If the individual's serum contains the specific auto-Ab, Ig will bind and, at the appropriate Ab concentration, the cells will become crosslinked. This will cause agglutination, and the cells will form a mat at the bottom of the test well. Auto-Abs attached to a patient's cells can be detected by the addition of a second Ab (anti-IgG to Fc portion of IgG) and observed for agglutination.

Selective soluble self-Ags can also be used to assay auto-Abs by attaching them to the surface of red blood cells. This latter type of agglutination test is called passive or indirect hemagglutination. Agglutination tests are commonly used to detect RFs (RA), thyroglobulin auto-Abs (thyroiditis), and red blood cell Abs (autoimmune hemolytic anemia).

The **radioimmunoassay** (RIA) is a very sensitive technique for detecting small quantities of auto-Abs in the serum of persons suspected of having au-

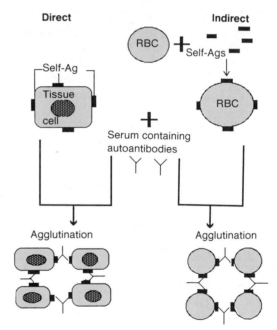

FIGURE 16.2 Detection of immune complexes by direct and indirect agglutination.

toimmune disease (fig. 16.3). Ag can be adsorbed onto the inner surface of a plastic tube and test serum can then be added. If the serum contains auto-Abs specific for the bound Ag, it will bind to the Ag. A radioactively labeled secondary Ab (anti-human IgG) can then be added which attaches only to the Fc portion of IgG. The tube is washed and then the radioactivity in the

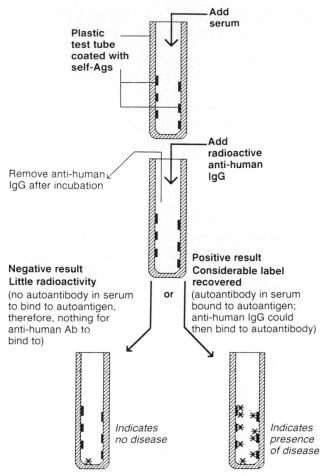

Plastic
test tube
coated with
self-Ags

Add
serum

Remove anti-human
IgG after incubation

Add
radioactive
anti-human
IgG

Negative result
Little radioactivity

(no autoantibody in serum
to bind to autoantigen,
therefore, nothing for
anti-human Ab to
bind to)

or

Positive result
Considerable label
recovered

(autoantibody in serum
bound to autoantigen;
anti-human IgG could
then bind to autoantibody)

Indicates
no disease

Indicates
presence
of disease

FIGURE 16.3   Quantifying autoantibody by RIA.

tube is measured in a gamma counter. If the serum does not contain auto-Abs, then none of the radioactive anti-IgG should bind, and there should be little radioactivity in the tube. However, even small amounts of auto-Ab in the serum should lead to the binding of labeled anti-IgG, which can be detected in the gamma counter. RIAs are used to determine the presence of intrinsic factor (pernicious anemia), anti-DNA Abs (SLE), and antithyroglobulin IgG (thyroiditis).

These tests can also be used to screen people who are considered at risk for a specific autoimmune disease. These include relatives of patients and the elderly (whose risk increases as immune function declines with age).

GENETIC FACTORS IN AUTOIMMUNE DISEASES

Certain autoimmune diseases run in family trees. For example, juvenile diabetes, pernicious anemia, and Hashimoto's thyroiditis are apparently caused by inherited traits that can be passed on in certain families. These familial relationships are also affected by environmental factors. The **genes** play an important role in *predisposing the person* to developing an autoimmune disease, while the **environmental factors** might present the *precipitating events* leading to the expression of the disease.

Autoimmune diseases afflict women almost twice as frequently as men. This might suggest that the differential expression in the sex chromosomes (Barr body; the inactive, second X chromosome) or differences in sex hormones (testosterone/estrogens) play important roles in the etiology of autoimmune diseases. The incidence of autoimmune diseases also increases with age, especially after the age of 60. Somatic mutations increase with age and might play an essential role in age-related increases in autoimmune disorders, but this is yet to be established.

There are also very close *links between certain histocompatibility Ags and autoimmune diseases* (table 16.5). The risk of contracting the disease increases for individuals bearing the histocompatibility Ags associated with the disorder. Nearly all autoimmune diseases have an association with some HLA specificity, *usually the D/DR locus* of HLA. For example, the greatest risk for developing juvenile diabetes is associated with the HLA genotype DR3/4 (heterozygous), which actually might be the disease's "susceptibility gene pair" region. Environmental, hormonal, age-related, and other physiological factors can also play a role in determining whether or not the person of that genotype will become a diabetic. Nevertheless, the genetic predisposition will be there for the person's lifetime. This places the individual at higher risk than the general population. In addition, the HLA genotype might be passed on to the next generation.

Most autoimmune diseases are associated with the HLA alleles DR2, DR3, DR4, and DR5. Interestingly, there can be multiple autoimmune disease expression associated with the same allele in the same

TABLE 16.5 Autoimmune Diseases Associated with Histocompatibility Antigens

Antigen	Disease	Disease Risk*
DR2	Goodpasture's syndrome	5
	Multiple sclerosis	5
DR3	Juvenile-onset diabetes	5
	Graves' disease	5
	Myasthenia gravis	10
	SLE	5
DR4	RA	10
DR5	Hashimoto's thyroiditis	5

*Disease risk defines likelihood of disease occurring when particular histocompatibility Ag is expressed, as compared with the general population at large, whose risk factor is assigned a value of 1.

individual. A case in point is the overlap between the organ-specific diseases, autoimmune thyroiditis and pernicious anemia. Individuals with pernicious anemia have a greater chance of developing autoimmune thyroiditis (and vice versa) than the general population. This phenomenon also occurs in systemic diseases. The alleles DR3 and DR4 seem associated with SLE and RA. The probability of a person with one of these diseases developing the second is higher than for individuals not possessing these HLA genotypes.

Genes involved in Ig synthesis can also play a role in autoimmune disease. In RA, RF has a specificity for the Fc region of Ig. Ag binding could reveal these altered Fc sequences, inducing the formation of RFs.

There are a number of interesting animal model systems for studying the genetic influence on autoimmune expression. One is a New Zealand black (NZB) mouse that spontaneously develops autoimmune hemolytic anemia. Understanding the mechanisms behind the expression of autoimmune disorders in animals that are genetically programmed for the disease will lead to a better understanding of the genetic input and how other factors influence genetic predisposition in the expression of autoimmune disorders.

CRITERIA FOR CLASSIFICATION AS AN AUTOIMMUNE DISEASE

Through the foregoing discussion we have provided general characteristics of autoimmune diseases. In addition, we have examined theories and mechanisms for breakdown of tolerance to self. However, not all instances in which some manifestation of breakdown in self-tolerance exists qualify as true autoimmune diseases. This realization led to the establishment of criteria that must be satisfied in order to classify a disorder as an autoimmune disease. These criteria, which parallel Koch's postulates, were formally enunciated by Witebsky in the 1950s. Accordingly, they have been designated as Witebsky's criteria.

A disorder can be properly considered as an autoimmune disease if **Witebsky's criteria** can be met as follows:

1. In association with the disorder, an *Ab must be demonstrable,* either by direct or indirect means.
2. A specific *Ag must be identified,* in the individual displaying the disorder, *against which this Ab is directed.*
3. It must be possible to *experimentally induce an Ab against the Ag.* For example, inoculation of an experimental animal with the Ag should provoke an immune response, with development of symptoms paralleling those of the disorder.
4. The symptoms must be *inducible in an experimental model.* The disorder should be reproducibly demonstrable in test subjects. In addition, the disorder should be transmittable through the transfer of serum or lymphoid cells from an immunized (autoimmune) animal to a nonimmunized animal.

SELECTED AUTOIMMUNE DISEASES: ORGAN SPECIFIC

In this section, we explore the development of certain autoimmune disorders that affect specific organs and organ systems in the body. The tissue destruction that occurs is restricted to the specific Ags localized in that organ. Hence, the specific auto-Ab will not attack other

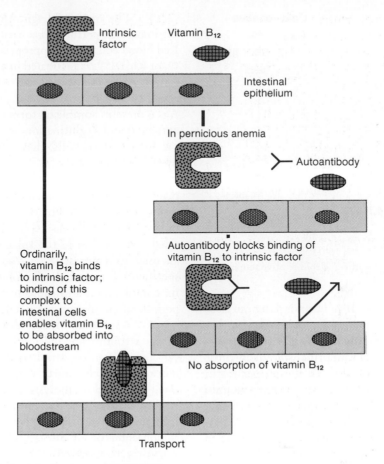

Intrinsic factor

Vitamin B₁₂

Intestinal epithelium

In pernicious anemia

Autoantibody

Autoantibody blocks binding of vitamin B₁₂ to intrinsic factor

Ordinarily, vitamin B₁₂ binds to intrinsic factor; binding of this complex to intestinal cells enables vitamin B₁₂ to be absorbed into bloodstream

No absorption of vitamin B₁₂

Transport

FIGURE 16.4 Immunological mechanism in pernicious anemia.

organs. There can be overlap with other organ-specific diseases, which predispose the individual to other autoimmune diseases. However, in such cases the auto-Abs are separate and the organ destruction is distinct. An example of this situation occurs with the increased predisposition of individuals with pernicious anemia to developing thyroiditis. The auto-Abs and organs affected are different, but the expression of one disease seems to lead to further breakdown in self-tolerance in other organ systems. In this section, we discuss the immune pathogenesis of organ-specific autoimmune diseases affecting the blood, brain, thyroid, pancreas, and muscle.

Autoimmune Anemias

The autoimmune anemias that are discussed in this section include pernicious anemia, autoimmune hemolytic anemias, and drug-induced hemolytic anemias. All present different clinical symptoms but share the common feature of auto-Ab production against specific self-Ags.

In **pernicious anemia,** an IgG auto-Ab can be made that binds to a specific receptor secreted by stomach cells that is responsible for transporting vitamin B₁₂ in the small intestine (fig. 16.4). The receptor is a membrane-bound protein called intrinsic

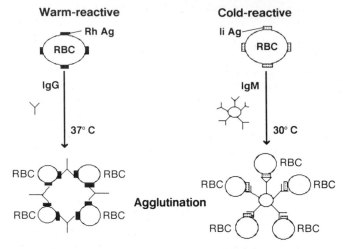

Warm-reactive

Rh Ag

RBC

IgG

37° C

RBC — RBC

RBC — RBC

Cold-reactive

Ii Ag

RBC

IgM

30° C

RBC

RBC — RBC

RBC — RBC

RBC

Agglutination

FIGURE 16.5   Comparison of warm- and cold-reactive autoimmune hemolytic anemias.

factor. The *binding of auto-Ab to intrinsic factor can block transport of vitamin B$_{12}$.* Vitamin B$_{12}$ cannot be synthesized by the body, but is supplied by diet and is transported across the intestinal wall principally by intrinsic factor. Vitamin B$_{12}$ is essential for the proper maturation of erythrocytes. Depriving the body of vitamin B$_{12}$ leads to the release of immature erythrocytes that do not function well as transporters of oxygen. If pernicious anemia is not treated with injections of vitamin B$_{12}$ (delivered to the bloodstream, thus bypassing intestinal absorption), the individual can die.

Factors leading to the formation of auto-Abs to instrinsic factor are not yet known. The use of some immunosuppressants, for example, corticosteroids, has improved vitamin B$_{12}$ absorption, enhanced intrinsic factor secretion, and decreased levels of auto-Abs in some patients, but complete reversal of the disease has not yet been accomplished.

Autoimmune hemolytic anemias encompass a wide spectrum of disease states that are typified by the production of *auto-Abs that can bind to erythrocyte blood group Ags.* Autoimmune anemias that are not drug induced fall into two major classes: warm and cold Ab types. Warm Abs are mainly IgG auto-Abs, but can also include IgM auto-Abs that will optimally agglutinate erythrocytes at body temperature (fig. 16.5). Cold Abs are IgM auto-Abs that agglutinate erythrocytes only when the blood is chilled.

The immunodiagnostic test for either is the Coombs' test, performed at the different temperatures. Red blood cells of the appropriate serotype (A, B, AB, O, or Rh[D]$^+$) are incubated in a sample of the person's serum. After removal of the serum, the cells are exposed to anti-human IgG. If auto-Ab to erythrocyte Ags is present, complexes form (erythrocyte–auto-Ab–anti-IgG) and agglutination occurs. If no Ab is present on the red blood cells, they will not be agglutinated by the anti-human Ig.

Although the etiology is unknown, warm-reactive auto-Abs are usually formed against the Rh system Ags. The binding of the Ab to the erythrocytes in the body usually results in rapid clearance of sensitized erythrocytes in the spleen, thereby causing the anemia. In contrast, cold-reactive auto-Abs, whose specificity is against the Ii blood Ag system, can bind, fix complement, and cause hemolysis in areas where peripheral circulation temperatures fall below 37° C.

Agglutination can also occur. Consequently, in the extremities (hands, feet, and ears), erythrocytes can agglutinate in peripheral capillary beds, causing blockage and leading to tissue destruction. Complement-mediated hemolysis can occur as well, provoking intravascular lesions in these regions. Thus, the IgM auto-Abs in cold-reactive hemolytic anemia cause a different type of disease from that caused by IgG warm-reactive auto-Abs.

Treatment of warm autoimmune hemolytic anemia makes use of immunosuppressive corticosteroid therapy. The disease can go into long periods of remission. The prognosis of the disease depends on its underlying cause, that is, whether it is a primary cause (good prognosis) or if it is secondarily associated with other disorders, such as SLE or lymphoma (poor prognosis). Treatment of cold autoimmune hemolytic anemia is much simpler. Usually the cure for cold hemolytic anemia consists of keeping the person's extremities warm and waiting for spontaneous remission, unless the underlying cause is cancerous lymphoma.

Drug-induced immune hemolytic anemia occurs when certain drugs associate themselves with erythrocytes. If Abs are formed to the drug's antigenic determinants, the association with red blood cells results in Ab binding to erythrocytes, causing hemagglutination or hemolysis. This leads to anemia. The

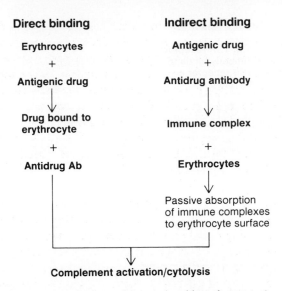

Direct binding	Indirect binding
Erythrocytes	Antigenic drug
+	+
Antigenic drug	Antidrug antibody
↓	↓
Drug bound to erythrocyte	Immune complex
+	+
Antidrug Ab	Erythrocytes
	↓
	Passive absorption of immune complexes to erythrocyte surface

Complement activation/cytolysis

FIGURE 16.6 Mechanisms of drug-induced hemolytic anemia.

association with the red blood cell membrane can be either direct binding or indirect adsorption (fig. 16.6). *Direct binding of the antigenic drug to the erythrocytes can lead to Ab binding and complement-mediated cytolysis.* Hemolysis can be either due to Ab, specific for the drug, or auto-Ab, specific for certain blood group Ags on the erythrocyte surface. In the latter case, it is believed that direct binding of the drug somehow induces a breakdown in tolerance, leading to the formation of auto-Abs to erythrocyte surface determinants, with subsequent immune lysis of the affected erythrocytes.

In indirect binding, previously formed immune complexes (drug:IgG Ab) can be passively adsorbed onto the erythrocyte, which is an innocent bystander damaged in the subsequent complement-mediated lysis. Many antibiotics, antihistamines, and even aspirin can lead to these immune events. Fortunately, the symptoms usually resolve themselves spontaneously once the person discontinues use of the drug.

Autoimmune Encephalomyelitis

Encephalomyelitis is a rare disorder of the nervous system that is becoming more common because of the practice of vaccination. Encephalomyelitis refers to an inflammatory condition of the brain and spinal cord. One example is a reaction to a certain type of rabies vaccine. Formerly, if a person was bitten by a rabid animal, vaccine would be given through the so-called Pasteur treatment (not widely used today). The rabies virus was injected into a rabbit, where it multiplied in the brain and spinal cord. The virus was subsequently harvested from the rabbit's brain tissue, inactivated, and injected abdominally through a series of injections over a three-week period. In some instances, an immune reaction against myelin in neural tissues resulted, thereby inducing autoimmune encephalomyelitis in the treated individual (explained below). Rabies vaccines currently in use are safer and do not induce this autoimmune reaction.

Although this treatment immunizes some against rabies, it can produce fatal encephalomyelitis in others. The vaccine is often contaminated with rabbit brain Ags, which can be seen as antigenic by some individuals. Unfortunately, the *Abs raised can also cross-react with human brain self-Ags.* These crossreacting Abs bind to human brain and spinal cord tissues, fixing complement, destroying the antigenic cells, and causing a massive inflammatory reaction with macrophage and lymphocyte infiltration. Brain lesions develop, along with demyelination and axon damage. Death can rapidly ensue from a vaccine-induced autoimmune response.

This immune reaction can also be experimentally induced in animals by injecting them with brain tissue emulsified in Freund's complete adjuvant. Similar responses have been noted in some individuals after receiving attenuated vaccine therapy to prevent other viral diseases such as measles, rubella, mumps, and influenza. In these cases, it has been suggested that the live, attenuated virus infects the cells of the brain, causing the display of new antigenic determinants. The resulting neo-Ags could lead to the formation of Abs and activated lymphocytes, causing the life-threatening inflammatory response. People so afflicted often respond favorably to corticosteroid treatment, which can suppress further inflammatory encephalomyelitic attacks.

Autoimmune Thyroid Diseases

The thyroid is an endocrine organ that synthesizes hormones, such as thyroxine, that are essential for proper body growth and metabolism. Thyroid diseases fall into three clinical categories: (1) Graves' disease,

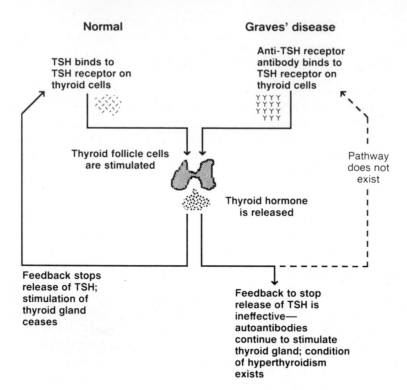

Normal

TSH binds to
TSH receptor on
thyroid cells

Thyroid follicle cells
are stimulated

Thyroid hormone
is released

Feedback stops
release of TSH;
stimulation of
thyroid gland
ceases

Graves' disease

Anti-TSH receptor
antibody binds to
TSH receptor on
thyroid cells

Pathway
does not
exist

Feedback to stop
release of TSH is
ineffective—
autoantibodies
continue to stimulate
thyroid gland; condition
of hyperthyroidism
exists

FIGURE 16.7 Immunological mechanism in Graves' disease. The thyroid gland is stimulated to release thyroid hormones by TSH. However, binding of antibodies against the TSH receptor can also trigger the release of thyroid hormones. In this latter situation, the normal feedback that halts continued stimulation of the thyroid gland is not effective in blocking the signal (Ab) responsible for stimulating thyroid hormone release.

or hyperthyroidism (hyperactive); (2) Hashimoto's disease, or hypothyroidism (underactive); and (3) myxedema, where there is a near loss of thyroid function. The primary cause for any autoimmune thyroiditis is unknown. Interestingly, there can be a steady progression from Graves' disease to Hashimoto's disease to myxedema in the same individual.

With **Graves' disease,** we can find the presence of an *auto-Ab to thyroid-stimulating hormone (TSH) receptors,* which can be detected by IF. The thyroid cells are normally stimulated when TSH from the pituitary gland binds to cell receptors. When combined with the thyroid TSH receptor, auto-Ab can also stimulate the thyroid cells to secrete hormones (fig. 16.7). This would produce the hyperactive thyroid condition of Graves' disease. Treatment may include surgical removal of the thyroid, with subsequent hormone therapy or use of antithyroid drugs.

The progression to **Hashimoto's disease** involves further complications. Here the *thyroid gland becomes infiltrated with lymphocytes and phagocytes,* causing inflammation and appearance of a goiter (enlargement of the thyroid). Different *auto-Abs appear that can either bind to the protein thyroglobulin (antithyroglobulin Ab) or to a cytoplasmic constituent located in thyroid epithelial cells (antithyroid cell microsomal Ab).* It is believed that complement-mediated Ab lysis plays a vital role in the destruction of thyroid cells coated with thyroglobulin or thyroid microsomes. In addition, cell-mediated immune responses also influence the course of this disease, as evidenced by the infiltration of phagocytic neutrophils, macrophages, and cytotoxic lymphocytes. Both humoral and cell-mediated reactions lead to the diminished function of the thyroid gland. Antithyroglobulin and antithyroid cell microsomal Abs can be

Immune Regulation in Autoimmune Thyroid Disease

From the study of autoimmune thyroid diseases, it has been proposed that self-reactive lymphocytes exist in the body. For example, a small percentage of normal B cells bind self-thyroglobulin to surface membranes, and lymphocytes cultured with thyroid tissue can become autosensitized. How are normal controls on autoreactivity bypassed? Organ-specific autoimmune diseases, such as Graves' disease and Hashimoto's thyroiditis, appear to be excellent model systems to explore this question. Researchers in this field have discovered a number of interesting points on immune regulation that may be applied to the etiology of other autoimmune disorders.

First, there seems to be intense signaling between the thyroid cells and the immune system. Treatment of Graves' disease with the drug methimazole (which inhibits the synthesis of thyroid hormones) increases the number of CD8 (suppressor/cytotoxic) cells and decreases CD4 (helper/inducer) cell numbers. The reduction in auto-Ab levels seems to be a consequence of thyrocyte-immunocyte interactions, especially T_S cells. Studies showing that thyroid cells themselves are capable of presenting Ag directly to the pool of T lymphocytes in the thyroid, causing their activation, provide further evidence of this interaction.

Second, normal thyroid cells can be induced to express the HLA-DR (class II) Ag. However, in persons with autoimmune thyroid disease, the HLA-DR expression is aberrant. In normal thyrocytes, the expression of class II Ag is transient, but expression persists in autoimmune diseases. This persistence might be an indicator of a larger disturbance in immune regulation. The chief destabilizing factor appears to be a defect in the T_S lymphocyte pool. Thus, autoimmunity can be induced through a bypass of regulatory mechanisms resulting from a defect in Ag-specific T_S cells. The inappropriate expression of MHC class II Ags on a cell (T_S) carrying an auto-Ag (thyroglobulin) can convert that cell into an Ag-presenting cell to the autoreactive T_H cell.

This bypass mechanism could explain why the administration of thyroxine reduces thyroid auto-Ab synthesis in Hashimoto's thyroiditis (hypothyroidism). The auto-Ag expression of thyroid cells can decrease without the inductive effects of TSH, whose levels diminish with the administration of thyroxine. The decline in the levels of the auto-Ag, thyroglobulin, halts Ag presentation to T_H cells producing the auto-Ab.

Thus, a more comprehensive understanding of the mechanism of thyrocyte-immunocyte signaling can lead to developing ways of correcting the immune disturbances in thyroid and other organ-specific autoimmune diseases.

Bottazzo, G. F., Pujoll-Borrell, R., Hanafusa, T., et al. Role of aberrant HLA-DR expression and antigen presentation in induction of endocrine autoimmunity. *Lancet* **2**:1115, 1983.

Iwatani, Y., Gerstein, H. C., Itaka, M., et al. Thyrocyte HLA-DR expression and interferon-gamma production in autoimmune thyroid disease. *Journal of Clinical Endocrinology and Metabolism* **63**:695, 1986.

Tötterman, T. H., Karlsson, F. A., Bengtsson, M., et al. Induction of circulating activated suppressor-like T cells by methimazole therapy for Graves' disease. *New England Journal of Medicine* **316**:15, 1987.

detected by IF or agglutination techniques. Hormone replacement therapy is the primary means of treating Hashimoto's disease.

The symptoms of **myxedema** are manifested because of a near loss of thyroid function and thyroxine synthesis. Because thyroxine plays such an important role in the body's metabolism, lack of this hormone seriously upsets the balance of many bodily processes, including reproductive, immune, cardiovascular, and digestive functions. Myxedema can be diagnosed by IF techniques detecting the presence of thyroglobulin auto-Abs. It is treated by administration of thyroid extract or synthetic thyroid hormones. If treatment is started soon after the symptoms first appear, recovery can be complete.

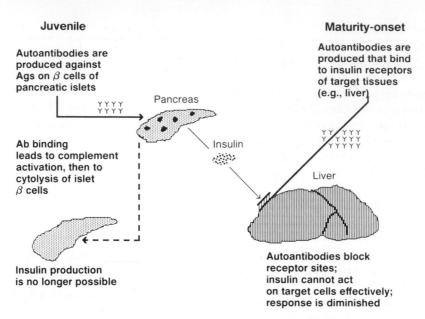

Juvenile

Autoantibodies are produced against Ags on β cells of pancreatic islets

Pancreas

Ab binding leads to complement activation, then to cytolysis of islet β cells

Insulin

Insulin production is no longer possible

Maturity-onset

Autoantibodies are produced that bind to insulin receptors of target tissues (e.g., liver)

Liver

Autoantibodies block receptor sites; insulin cannot act on target cells effectively; response is diminished

FIGURE 16.8 Autoantibody actions in juvenile and maturity-onset diabetes. Although autoantibodies appear in both of these forms of diabetes, the Ags against which they react differ and, accordingly, so do the consequences induced.

The more progressive destruction seen in myxedema seems to involve several immune mechanisms including auto-Ab production, B and T cells, and various Ags released from the damaged thyroid tissue. The cytotoxic responses are so dramatic that they lead to almost complete destruction of the glandular tissue. Histological examination reveals a chronic inflammatory response, with tissue destruction mediated by monocytes and macrophages. Eventual fibrosis occurs. Yet, unlike Hashimoto's disease, in myxedema the thyroid does not become a goiter, rather it shrinks.

Most people have only one form of autoimmune thyroiditis, but the fact that all three forms can develop in one individual indicates that the steady progression in the loss of immune tolerance to self-Ags can lead from altered thyroid function to complete destruction of the organ.

Diabetes Mellitus

There are different forms of diabetes mellitus, for example, juvenile and maturity-onset diabetes. In all cases, the hormone insulin is prevented from playing its metabolic role as a mediator of glucose transport across cell membranes. This can compromise basic metabolic functions of cells and, if left untreated, can lead to a number of organ pathologies and even to death. What typifies many forms of diabetes is the pathological role of the immune system, where the formation of auto-Abs can lead to the clinical symptoms.

In one form of **maturity-onset diabetes,** the number of free insulin receptors is reduced due to binding of auto-Ab directed against them (fig. 16.8). *Auto-Ab binding to insulin receptor* sites can diminish cellular responses to insulin since few sites remain free for the hormone to bind. This *insulin-resistant* form of diabetes can be treated with injections of insulin at concentrations many times higher than normal in order for the insulin to better compete for receptor sites.

In **juvenile diabetes,** also called **insulin-dependent diabetes mellitus** (IDDM), *auto-Abs to self-Ags located on the islet cells* of the pancreas can lead to cytolysis. These IgG auto-Abs can fix complement and mediate the lysis of the insulin-producing β cells in the islets of Langerhans of the pancreas. Detection of the auto-Abs can be made by RIA or IF techniques. Several auto-Abs have been isolated. These include a cytoplasmic islet cell auto-Ab (designated ICA), and Ab to a 64 kD islet cell protein (designated 64-K), and an auto-Ab to insulin. Of these, the 64-K Ab might serve as an important predictor of IDDM since it appears before symptoms of diabetes are expressed.

The cause for loss of self-tolerance is unknown, but it is associated with certain MHC loci and may also be induced by certain enterovirus infections. For example, certain alleles in the HLA-DQ, HLA-DR3, and HLA-DR4 loci on chromosome 6 (see chapter 7, Histocompatibility Systems) appear to be associated with increased susceptibility to IDDM. On the other hand, the HLA class II Ag, DQw1.2, appears to confer protection against development of IDDM. This locus apparently is altered in individuals with IDDM.

Auto-Abs seem not to be the only mode of cellular destruction since the *islets become infiltrated with lymphocytes, activated monocytes, and T_C cells.* According to one prevailing hypothesis, β cell destruction begins when a genetically predisposed individual is exposed to an Ag that mimics a cell-surface protein found on β cells. For example, structural similarities have recently been found between Ags in Epstein-Barr virus (EBV) and rubella viruses (mimics) and a subunit from the DQ locus (self-Ag). Processing of the Ag mimic by APCs leads to activation of T_C cells directed against β cells (auto-Ag), as well as cells carrying the mimicking (foreign) Ag. Subsequently, T_H cells are also stimulated. This amplifies the autoimmune response against the β cells in the islets of Langerhans. As this process continues, diabetes eventually ensues.

Treatment of IDDM usually entails insulin replacement therapy at physiological concentrations. More recently, attempts have been made to correct the physiological consequences of IDDM. Transplants of islet cells have been somewhat successful in recent clinical trials. In addition, immunosuppressive agents such as cyclosporine, prednisone, and azathioprine have improved the survival of remaining functional β cells. However, a relapse can result when immunosuppressant therapy is halted. There may also be promise in developing alternative modes of treatment. For example, antiidiotypic monoclonal Abs (MAbs) might be developed, which could prevent the onset of the disease in susceptible individuals. Alternatively, T cell vaccines (anti–T cell receptor Abs or blocking peptides) might be used to prevent activation of T_C cells directed against β cells. In addition, gene therapy might be invoked. Recent studies have observed suppression

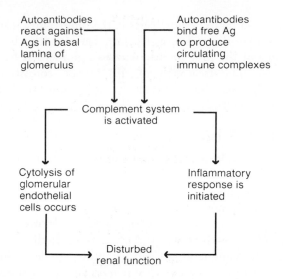

FIGURE 16.9 Steps to glomerular destruction in Goodpasture's syndrome.

of diabetic symptoms in transgenic offspring of non-obese diabetic (NOD) and normal mice. As the genetic component(s) of diabetes become more fully characterized, effective gene therapy might become possible and practical.

Goodpasture's Syndrome

The kidney is an organ whose proper function is essential for survival. Chronic renal failure can lead to lethal complications if left untreated. One form of chronic renal failure is rapidly progressive glomerulonephritis resulting from inflammation of the functional unit of the kidney, the nephron. **Goodpasture's syndrome** is a good example of this type of disease. It is a rare autoimmune disease that usually affects young men. Its etiology is unknown, but IF techniques demonstrate the presence of *autoimmune Abs against the glomerular basement membrane* (basal lamina). The glomerulus is a part of the nephron unit that is a capillary network where filtration of the plasma takes place. The IgG auto-Ab can fix complement and so cause necrosis of the glomerulus with loss of renal function (fig. 16.9). Immune complexes (self-Ag:auto-Ag) form an even layer on the basal lamina and lead to Type III hypersensitivity reactions. Ig deposits can also be found along the basal lamina in the alveoli of the lung, leading to hemorrhages in the lung. Thus, it appears that there is crossreaction between the basal lamina of the lung and the kidney's glomerular basal lamina. The treatment of this disease consists of hemodialysis, but individuals often die of lung hemorrhage.

Multiple Sclerosis

Multiple sclerosis (MS) is a demyelinating disease of the central nervous system (CNS). It is characterized by patchy inflammatory lesions scattered throughout the myelin-containing areas (white matter) of the CNS. Myelin is a fatty, insulating substance that forms an interrupted sheath around certain neurons. It allows for the faster conduction of nerve impulses. In demyelinating disease, the removal of myelin (and possible formation of scar tissue in its place) can lead to a slowing down of the nerve impulse in the affected neurons. Since temporal and spatial interactions among neurons are common, upsetting the timing in even partially demyelinated neurons can lead to gross neurological dysfunction.

In MS, the demyelination appears to have an immunological, autoimmune component. This is interesting since neural cells do not normally express either class I or class II MHC Ags. The triggering mechanism is not clear, but prior exposure to a virus seems one way autoimmune demyelination might be induced. It has been shown, in some animal systems, that infection with certain viruses induces class I MHC Ags on brain glial cells. Glial cells are accessory cells of the brain that normally do not express these Ags on their surfaces. This induction might occur through soluble factors (e.g., H-2 inducing factor) released by infected glial cells and could set the stage for a breakdown in self-tolerance, leading to virus-induced, immune-mediated demyelination in the CNS.

Demyelination seems to be mediated by immune responses to the self-Ag, myelin. The resulting *antimyelin Ab can bind and initiate complement-mediated destruction of the myelin sheath* (forming sclerotic plaques) as seen in early active disease (fig. 16.10). Activation of the complement cascade releases fragments C3a and C5a that can mediate an inflammatory response, causing further local tissue damage. Cell-mediated cytotoxic responses also seem to be involved

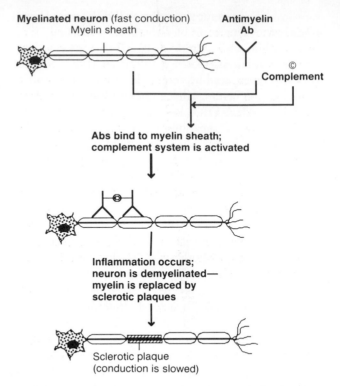

FIGURE 16.10 Autoimmune demyelination in multiple sclerosis.

in the immune pathogenesis of this disease in later, older lesions. It has been noted that in animal models, such as experimental autoimmune encephalitis (EAE), relapses during remission are accompanied by elimination of T_S cells. Ag-processing macrophages have been shown to release IL-I, γ-interferon, and prostaglandins in this system, with accompanying release of mitogenic IL-2 by T_H cells. This could lead to clonal expansion of other effector T cell clones and their products, which could further the cytotoxic mechanisms in demyelinating diseases.

There also seems to be an MHC component to this disease. Increased risk is associated with a specific haplotype in the HLA-DR2 (MHC class II) region located on chromosome 6. If environmental factors, such as viral infection, are added to the picture, the risk is statistically greater. It has been suggested that a childhood viral infection may become latent and reappear in adult life to activate MHC-restricted Ags and initiate subsequent responses.

Elevated levels of IgG in the cerebrospinal fluid, accompanied by neurological symptoms, indicate a positive diagnosis for MS. The progression of the disease is unpredictable. There are often long periods of remission, interrupted by acute periods of relapse. Antiinflammatory, immunosuppressive corticosteroids are commonly used during acute attacks in this disease. However, long-term corticosteroid therapy has not proven valuable either in treating the symptoms or preventing relapse. One future hope is the use of anti-Ia Ab therapy. Treatment of mice having EAE with MAbs for the Ia antigen on T lymphocytes specific for myelin Ag has led to arrest of the disease. Pathogenic autoreactive T cells that respond to myelin basic protein express very few markers. If clonal expansion of these cells could be suppressed, neurological impairment might be limited.

Myasthenia Gravis

The name **myasthenia gravis** means grave muscle weakness. Skeletal muscles thus affected become rapidly fatigued and have a prolonged recovery time. The cause of this disease is unknown. Initial symptoms involve the eye muscles, causing droopy eyelids, with gradual involvement of other skeletal muscles. Death can result if the respiratory muscles become affected.

Skeletal muscle cells are innervated by somatic motor neurons that release the neurotransmitter, ACh, into the neuromuscular junction where it diffuses over to the muscle membrane. Located on the skeletal muscle membrane are ACh receptors. When enough of these receptors are loaded with neurotransmitter, a signal can be initiated, leading to the contraction of the skeletal muscle cell (myofiber). Rapid destruction of ACh is brought about by a membrane-bound enzyme, cholinesterase, located next to ACh receptor sites. Thus, enough ACh must be released at one time to counteract cholinesterase and load enough receptors to effect a contraction response. In myasthenia gravis, the proper sequence of events at the neuromuscular junction does not occur, leading to the physiological symptoms of aberrant muscle contraction (fig. 16.11). The basic abnormality is a reduction in the number of ACh receptors on muscle membranes at the neuromuscular junction, brought about by an Ab-mediated autoimmune attack. The *auto-Ab formed is against the ACh receptor*. These anti-ACh receptor Abs can activate complement, form immune complexes, promote Ab-dependent cellular cytotoxicity (ADCC) responses, and cause endocytosis of these receptors. All of these events lead to the reduction in the number of ACh receptors. If enough receptors are destroyed, muscle contraction cannot be triggered unless cholinesterase activity is inhibited so that the receptor sites remaining can be continually stimulated by ACh.

Interestingly, the thymus can show changes during the manifestation of the disease. It is known that thymic tissue can undergo rapid proliferation and the levels of the thymic hormone, thymopoietin, can rise during the course of the disease. Thymopoietin has been shown to have biological activity that can block certain neuromuscular events. Thymectomy in these individuals has brought about partial or total remission of myasthenia gravis.

IF techniques can be used to diagnose the disease and detect the anti-ACh receptor Abs. Individuals often respond favorably initially to anticholinesterase drug therapy. Patients who become resistant to this therapy can receive immunosuppressive agents such as corticosteroids, followed by plasmapheresis, which can remove large amounts of the auto-Abs from the circulation. The ultimate cure of myasthenia gravis might require the elimination of immunocytes involved in the responses against the auto-Ag. One approach would be the induction of T_S cells specific for ACh receptors. This has been accomplished in rats with experimental autoimmune myasthenia gravis by culturing lymphocytes with the immunosuppressive drug, cyclosporin A, and the ACh receptor. When mixed with lymphocytes from afflicted rats, the auto-Ab response is suppressed, without impairing Ab responses to unrelated Ags. Assay results showed the presence of functional T_S cells. This appears to be the mechanism by which the abnormal immune response is brought under control.

This strategy could be applicable to humans suffering from myasthenia gravis or other autoimmune diseases for which Ag is available. The response appears to be both highly specific and physiologically normal. Another approach would be the development of a specific immunotoxin that would eliminate only

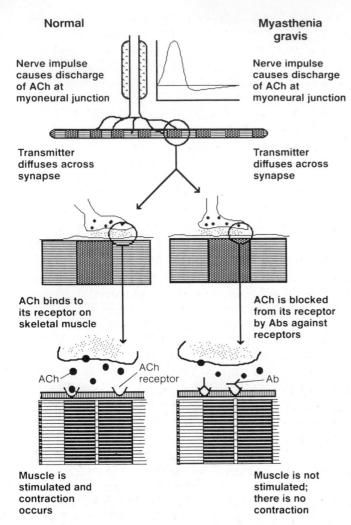

Normal

Nerve impulse causes discharge of ACh at myoneural junction

Transmitter diffuses across synapse

ACh binds to its receptor on skeletal muscle

ACh

ACh receptor

Muscle is stimulated and contraction occurs

Myasthenia gravis

Nerve impulse causes discharge of ACh at myoneural junction

Transmitter diffuses across synapse

ACh is blocked from its receptor by Abs against receptors

Ab

Muscle is not stimulated; there is no contraction

FIGURE 16.11 Alteration of muscle stimulation in myasthenia gravis. In myasthenia gravis, the functional characteristics of neurons (signal conduction and neurotransmitter release) remain intact. However, the presence of autoantibodies against the ACh receptor, which are formed in this disease, prevent normal stimulation of the muscle that is innervated by cholinergic (use ACh) neurons.

the lymphocytes involved in this autoimmune response. In experimental animals, the disease can be inhibited by treatments with an Ag-specific MAb tagged with a toxin. In this way, the toxin would be targeted only for cells producing auto-Ab. This strategy might also prove successful in human myasthenia gravis in the future.

SELECTED AUTOIMMUNE DISEASES: SYSTEMIC DISEASES

Systemic autoimmune diseases can invade many regions of the body. Often circulating immune complexes are deposited in several different organ regions. This occurs when immune complexes become lodged in small capillary beds as the blood flows through the vascular system. Auto-Abs to soluble self-Ags complex with each other and migrate to preferred sites that differ depending on the disease state. Two autoimmune disorders are explored in this section, namely RA and SLE. Immune complexes are preferentially found in the joints of the skeletal system in RA and mainly in the kidney, joints, and skin in SLE. As organ-specific diseases overlap with each other, systemic diseases can too. In fact, RA is frequently associated with SLE. Thus, this type of autoimmune disease is typified by immune complexes being deposited systemically to give rise to the more disseminated feature of these nonorgan-specific diseases.

Rheumatoid Arthritis

RA is a progressive debilitating inflammatory disease of connective tissues. The most common sites affected by this disease are joints. This disease can be characterized by acute phases, followed by periods of remission. Other organs that can be involved in this systemic disorder include the lung, eye, skin, and nervous system. The course of the disease is variable, but can lead to death in active progressive forms, usually due to infection or complications of therapy.

One diagnostic test for RA is an RIA to detect the presence of RFs (IgM and IgG) in the serum. RF is an *anti-γ-globulin auto-Ab*. The cause of the disease is uncertain, but it has been suggested that infection with EBV may lead to the activation of a synovial B lymphocyte to produce an abnormal IgG Ab. The immune response to the novel Fc region of this IgG may be the production of RF, which can subsequently lead to immune-complex formation in the synovial fluid (fig. 16.12).

RA usually affects the freely movable joints of the hand and feet first and then moves to other joints in the body. In freely movable joints, the ends of the

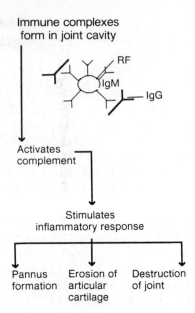

Immune complexes
form in joint cavity

RF

IgM

IgG

↓

Activates
complement

↓

Stimulates
inflammatory response

Pannus
formation

Erosion of
articular
cartilage

Destruction
of joint

FIGURE 16.12　Immune response in RA.

bone are covered with articular cartilage and are held together by a capsule of fibrous tissue called a joint capsule. This joint capsule is composed of an outer layer of ligaments and an inner lining of synovial membrane that secretes synovial fluid, which acts as a joint lubricant. In RA, the formation of immune complexes (RF:IgG) can activate the complement cascade, which initiates and amplifies an inflammatory response, causing synovial membrane damage and cell lysis.

Complement fragments, C3a and C5a, have anaphylatoxic and chemotactic properties. The anaphylactic activity leads to the localized release of histamine by mast cells and monocytes, producing symptoms like swelling of the joints (edema), redness, and pain. Chemotactic factors can cause an influx of phagocytes to the site. These cells can also be provoked to release lysosomal enzymes into the synovial space, which furthers the inflammatory and proliferative response of the synovium.

As inflammation worsens, T and B cells can also be detected (along with their products) and their interaction may ensure the continued production of Igs, continuing the vicious cycle of this immune-complex syndrome. Circulating lymphocytes can enter the joint tissue from venules called the high endothelial venules

(HEVs). There appears to be a specific recognition system of lymphocyte-endothelial interactions that controls lymphocyte traffic into the inflamed synovium. Interestingly, the interaction is different from other lymphocyte-endothelial associations in the body (e.g., lymphocyte entry into lymph nodes). The differences are reflected in the types of lymphocytes bound and in the receptors on HEV to which they attach. This might have future clinical implications. It should be possible to raise specific MAbs against the specific receptor, thereby selectively blocking lymphocyte infiltration into the synovium and thus eliminating a key player in the disease process.

During an acute episode, the proliferating cells of the synovium can grow into the joint cavity and form pannus. Pannus is composed of vascularized fibrous scar tissue that can invade the joint cavity and spread the inflammation to the articular cartilage. The hydrolytic enzymes released can erode the cartilage leading to joint destruction and other complications. There are a number of substances that can activate synoviocytes, including IL-1 and monocyte-derived tumor necrosis factor-α (TNF-α). Alternatively, the nervous system can also be involved with the release of the neuropeptide substance P, which can stimulate synoviocyte proliferation. This suggests a link between the nervous and immune systems in the expression of this disease state. Substance P is normally involved in the transmission of pain signals, but, when released into joint tissue by sensory nerves, can stimulate the release of prostaglandins and collagenase from the rheumatoid synoviocytes. These results can also be obtained from IL-1 and TNF-α. Perhaps pannus formation is enhanced with the stimulation of synoviocyte proliferation by long-term exposure to these immune and neuronal factors.

This disease might also have a genetic component, associated with the HLA DR4 region. The MHC appears to have an important role in controlling immunological defense mechanisms. In autoimmune disorders, there is a loss of this control. Thus, altered HLA Ag expression might impart a genetic predisposition that interacts with environmental factors (e.g., viruses), leading to initiation of the disease process. Of interest is the finding that many individuals with RA also have auto-Abs to IgD. The function of IgD has yet to be clearly defined, but it has been proposed that

Autoantibodies Secreted by Human Leu-1$^+$ B Cells

The mechanisms behind the breakdown of self in autoimmune diseases seem to be as diverse as expression of the disease states themselves. Autoreactive B cells are believed to be present but not active under normal circumstances. In systemic diseases, such as RA and SLE, auto-Abs are made by a B cell subpopulation that expresses the cell-surface Ag Leu-1$^+$. What is unusual about this subpopulation is that it exists in normal adults and can be induced to produce auto-Abs in amounts comparable to those seen in persons with autoimmune diseases. Moreover, large numbers of Leu-1$^+$ B cells are found early in development (as well as in patients with systemic autoimmune diseases) but not in normal adults.

In one study of RF (IgM) release from human Leu-1$^+$ cells, these B cells were shown to represent an independent B cell population, not just an activated form of another population (e.g., Leu-1$^-$B cells). *In vitro* stimulation of Leu-1$^+$ B cells with a polyclonal activator resulted in increased secretion of RF, regardless of the cell source (e.g., normal individuals, cord blood, or persons with autoimmune disease).

Leu-1$^+$ cells can also be transformed into Ig-secreting cells by infection with EBV. The Igs produced by this subpopulation include RF and anti-DNA auto-Abs. The source can again be from the serum of either normal or diseased individuals.

These preliminary studies suggest that the trigger to the development of certain autoimmune disease states is not merely the expression of self-Ags. Auto-Ab production might result from the continued effects of a polyclonal activator and auto-Ag stimulation. The fact that Leu-1$^+$ cells are present in normal B cell populations and can be induced to produce auto-Abs should enable researchers to explore the effects that a variety of factors (oncogenes to growth factors) have on the expression of auto-Abs.

Casali, P., Burastero, S. E., Nakamura, M., et al. Human lymphocytes making rheumatoid factor and antibody to ssDNA belong to Leu-1$^+$ B-cell subset. *Science* **236**:77, 1987.

Dziarski, R. Autoimmunity—polyclonal activation or antigen activation? *Immunology Today* **9**:340, 1988.

Hardy, R. R., Hayakawa, K., Shimizu, M., et al. Rheumatoid factor secretion from human Leu-1$^+$ B cells. *Science* **236**:81, 1987.

IgD is necessary for B cells to respond to T-dependent Ags. That raises the possibility that interfering with IgD function might alter T cell modulation of Ab response, and lead to production of an abnormal Ig, against which RF is made.

At present, the symptoms, but not the underlying cause, of RA can be treated. Drug treatments include antiinflammatory agents such as aspirin, slow-acting gold salt injections (which reduce the release of lysosomal enzymes), and immunosuppressive agents (only in severe cases due to their generalized depression of the immune system). A better understanding of the molecular underpinnings of RA could lead to successful immunotherapy techniques, such as the use of antiidiotypes or immunotoxins, to cure this disease in the future.

Systemic Lupus Erythematosus

SLE is a multisystem, chronic, autoimmune disease. It involves immunological reactions to a number of self-Ags, resulting in an inflammatory process. The disease mainly affects middle-aged women and is characterized by acute flare-ups and remissions. The prognosis is very individualistic, but death can result if the inflammatory response compromises the function of certain organs, as occurs in lupus nephritis. The name *lupus* (Latin for wolf) was given to describe the characteristic butterfly facial rash, resembling the coloring of a wolf, that can occur. Systemic refers to the multiorgan involvement and erythematosus to the redness of the skin rash.

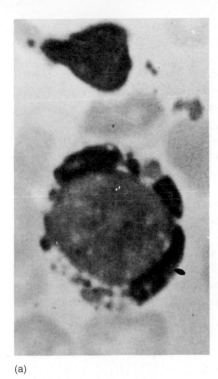
(a)

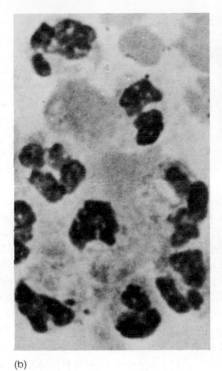
(b)

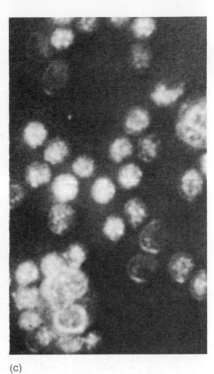
(c)

FIGURE 16.13 Diagnostic features of SLE. Laboratory diagnosis of LE traditionally has been based on the observation of the characteristic "LE cell" (*a*). The presence of rosettes (*b*), although not definitive, is strongly suggestive of LE. More recently, IF testing for antinuclear Abs has been employed. Demonstration of positive IF around the nuclei of affected cells *(c)* also provides confirmatory diagnosis of LE. See plate 3 for color photographs of LE cell and IF reaction with antinuclear Abs. (From Hyun, B. H., Ashton, J. K., and Dolan, K. *Practical Hematology.* 1975. W. B. Saunders Co., Philadelphia.)

Diagnosis of SLE has traditionally been based on the observation of a characteristic "LE cell" (fig. 16.13*a*). Immune diagnosis of the disease also can be made by RIA techniques detecting the main auto-Ab in lupus, namely, antinuclear Ab (fig.16.13*b*). If kidney involvement is suspected, then IF studies on kidney tissue can reveal "lumpy" deposits of complexes along glomerular basal lamina. Other common symptoms, beside the skin rashes, are pleurisy, arthritic joint pain, and kidney damage.

SLE is a puzzling autoimmune disease because of the great *variety of Abs against tissue and cellular components,* such as DNA, RNA, and cytoplasmic elements, found in the serum. It is not a monoclonal disease and perhaps reflects a more generalized loss of tolerance to a number of self-Ags, as seen by the wide range of auto-Abs formed. In many individuals, there is a deficiency of T_s cells, which suggests that the loss of tolerance might be due to a release of inhibition imposed by suppressor cells and their products. HLA and viral involvement in triggering the apparent contrasuppression of the B plasma cell system has been proposed. The MHC gene region, HLA-DR3, is suspect in SLE, as are latent viral infections (e.g., measles and parainfluenza).

The main auto-Ab found in SLE is anti-DNA (IgM and IgG), which can complex with free DNA (released in cell lysis) to form immune complexes. The resulting circulating immune complexes can become deposited at any number of tissue sites in the body. Once deposited, the ensuing activation of complement can bring about generalized inflammation, ADCC, and activation of the phagocyte systems (fig. 16.14). Neutrophils and mononuclear cells can be provoked to release degradative hydrolytic enzymes, which only further the tissue damage, until the immune complexes are removed (usually by the mononuclear phagocyte system). The disease goes into remission

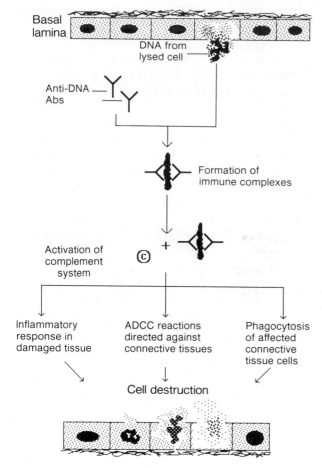

Basal lamina

DNA from lysed cell

Anti-DNA Abs

Formation of immune complexes

Activation of complement system

+

ⓒ

Inflammatory response in damaged tissue

ADCC reactions directed against connective tissues

Phagocytosis of affected connective tissue cells

Cell destruction

FIGURE 16.14 Immunological activities in SLE.

only when synthesis of the auto-Ab downshifts, and the majority of immune complexes are cleared away.

If the complexes form in the kidney's glomeruli, they can cause glomerulonephritis, while in arterioles they can produce hemorrhage and fibrosis. If these complexes appear in the synovia of the joints, they provoke the symptoms of RA. When they are found in the myocardium, they can cause fatal myocarditis. Thus, the pathology of this disease can injure many different organs and compromise a variety of organ systems.

In both RA and SLE, there are circulating idiotype-antiidiotype complexes. The importance of this lies in the suspicion that antiidiotypes can perpetuate the autoimmune state once it is initiated, perhaps

by acting as a surrogate auto-Ag or by acting as a positive inducer of auto-Ab expression. This also makes immunotherapy possible. If the premise is correct, then a deeper understanding of how these reactions control immune expression could make it possible to correct defects in the immune network maintaining tolerance to self-Ags.

Most treatments of SLE are geared only to relieve the unpleasant symptomology, depending on the course of the disease during a crisis. Aspirin is used to reduce arthritic inflammation, topical corticosteroids can heal the skin rashes, and systemic corticosteroids are used if organs, such as the kidney, become involved. Alternative future strategies for addressing SLE might include (1) development of cytotoxic MAbs directed against autoreactive lymphocytes or (2) administration of blocking Ags designed to compete with activating Ag. Yet the ultimate solution will be treatment that would reestablish immune tolerance to the self-Ags, and this has not yet been accomplished.

EXPERIMENTAL MODELS FOR AUTOIMMUNE DISORDERS

Several animal models for autoimmune disorders have been described. In some instances, the disorder arises spontaneously. In fact, certain inbred strains of mice display high frequencies of autoimmune disorders. Spontaneously arising autoimmune disorders seem to have a genetic basis, which often is associated with the MHC. Other models have been developed by induction of disorders resembling human autoimmune disorders in otherwise healthy animals.

Among spontaneously arising autoimmune disorders are the murine models for autoimmune hemolytic anemia, SLE, and IDDM. For example, NZB mice can spontaneously develop an *autoimmune hemolytic anemia*. In addition, an *SLE-like syndrome* can arise in offspring produced by crossing NZB and New Zealand white (NZW) mice, designated NZB/NZW mice. Secretion of anti-DNA auto-Ab can occur in NZB/W mice. *Diabetes* is expressed in the NOD mouse and the BioBreeding (BB) rat. These animals develop an IDDM-like disease in which pancreatic cells are destroyed by T_C cells. The NOD mouse is of particular interest because it also secretes insulin auto-Ab.

Other experimental models are artificially produced by inducing the disease in healthy animals. This can be accomplished in several ways. For example, cells from diseased animals can be transferred into healthy ones. In this manner, IDDM-like symptoms can be induced in healthy animals that receive spleen cells from NOD mice. Similarly, transfused lymphocytes from diabetic humans can induce insulitis in nude mice. An alternative means of creating autoimmunelike disorders is to immunize with anti-idiotypic Abs. In this fashion, an SLE-like disease can develop in mice after immunization with a pathogenic idiotype of anti-DNA auto-Abs. In addition, RA-like symptoms can be induced in monkeys exposed to collagen Ags. Moreover, rats receiving suspensions of CNS tissue develop allergic encephalomyelitis. These animals display demyelination similar to that encountered in MS. A third method is effective in inducing certain forms of autoimmunelike disorders, on occasion. This method employs a virus as a provocative agent. For example, neonatal mice can be infected with temperate viruses, such as lymphocytic choriomeningitis virus. Subsequently, infected mice develop a chronic infection, which leads to the expression of self-Ags. In turn, this can lead to autoimmune disorders, such as autoimmune hemolytic anemia.

The development and exploitation of experimental models should provide researchers with powerful tools for understanding the various dimensions of autoimmune disorders. On the one hand, they will augment our understanding of the etiology of these disorders. For example, what factor(s) lead to a genetic predisposition to particular disorders? What roles do lymphocyte activities play in the progression of these disorders and the expression of symptoms? On the other hand, these models can lead to the development of new therapies addressing the underlying causes of these disorders, not merely their symptoms.

S U M M A R Y

1. The immune system usually maintains a state of tolerance to self-antigens, but in autoimmune disease, there is a breakdown in self-tolerance. This can lead to the production of autoantibodies and expression of disease. [p. 399]

2. Theories of breakdown in self-tolerance include (a) virus induction, (b) drug induction, (c) microbial products crossreacting with human antigens, (d) development of new antigenic determinants, (e) hormonal induction, and (f) breakdown in the immune network. [p. 399–400]

3. Factors that could lead to an imbalance in the immune network include (a) contrasuppression of T cell function, (b) enhanced T_H activity, (c) polyclonal B cell activation, (d) breakdown in the idiotypic antibody network, (e) macrophage defects, (f) abnormalities in the expression of lymphokines, (g) abnormal gene expression, (h) thymus or bone defects, and (i) expression of germline or somatic mutations of B or T lymphocytes. [p. 400–402]

4. The mechanism of tissue damage in autoimmune disease can be classified under four headings: (a) damage by complement-fixing antibodies (antibody-dependent cellular cytotoxicity reactions), (b) impaired cell function by autoantibodies binding to cell-surface receptors, (c) damage by Type III hypersensitivity (immune complex), and (d) damage through T_C cell responses. [p. 402–403]

5. The three main types of diagnostic tests for the presence of autoantibodies are (a) immunofluorescence, (b) agglutination, and (c) radioimmunoassay. [p. 403–405]

6. Genetic factors in autoimmune disease include links to the major histocompatibility complex, which are the HLA alleles in humans. The genes in the DR locus of HLA can express altered antigens in some individuals, which could lead to predisposing a person to autoimmune disease when confronted with additional environmental factors (e.g., viral infections). [p. 405–406]

7. Witebsky established criteria, paralleling Koch's postulates, for determining that diseases are of an autoimmune nature. [p. 406]

8. Autoimmune diseases tend to fall into two broad categories: organ specific and systemic. Organ-specific diseases include autoimmune anemias, autoimmune encephalomyelitis, autoimmune thyroid diseases, diabetes mellitus, Goodpasture's

syndrome, multiple sclerosis, and myasthenia gravis. Organ-specific diseases are typified by the production of an autoantibody whose immune destruction is restricted to one organ. [pp. 406–407]

9. Autoimmune anemias include pernicious and autoimmune hemolytic anemias. In pernicious anemia, autoantibody to intrinsic factor inhibits the absorption of essential vitamin B_{12}, needed for erythropoiesis, thus giving rise to anemia. Autoimmune hemolytic anemias are characterized by the production of autoantibodies that can bind to erythrocyte blood group antigens (usually Rh). These include warm antibodies, cold antibodies, and antibodies induced by certain drugs binding to erythrocyte surfaces. Complement-fixing autoantibodies can cause agglutination and hemolysis in autoimmune hemolytic anemias. [p. 407–409]

10. Autoimmune encephalomyelitis is an acute disorder of the nervous system that can be induced by vaccination or following certain viral infections. The loss of tolerance to brain antigens can lead to the formation of autoantibodies and activated lymphocytes that can lead to life-threatening inflammatory responses. [p. 409]

11. Autoimmune thyroid diseases fall into three categories: Graves' disease (hyperthyroidism), Hashimoto's disease (hypothyroidism), and myxedema (loss of thyroid function). With Graves' disease, autoantibodies are formed against thyroid-stimulating hormone receptors. Binding of autoantibody to this receptor causes hyperactivity. Hashimoto's disease involves the production of antithyroglobulin antibody, and the resulting ADCC reactions cause inflammation, thyroid cell destruction, and the formation of a goiter. The near loss of thyroid function and mass manifested in myxedema appears to be mediated by ADCC reactions primed by antithyroglobulin autoantibodies. [p. 409–412]

12. There are different forms of the autoimmune disease, diabetes mellitus. In maturity-onset, insulin-resistant diabetes, there are a reduced number of available insulin receptors due to competitive binding with the hormone by the autoantibody. In juvenile, insulin-dependent diabetes, complement-fixing autoantibodies to surface antigens on insulin-producing β cells can lead to the destruction of these cells in the pancreas. [p. 412–413]

13. Goodpasture's syndrome is usually a fatal disorder characterized by the production of anti–basal lamina antibodies specific for the kidney's glomeruli and lungs. The IgG autoantibody can fix complement and initiate antibody-dependent cellular cytotoxicity reactions that can result in irreversible damage to kidneys and lungs. [p. 413–414]

14. Mutiple sclerosis is a demyelinating disease of the central nervous system. Antimyelin antibodies can mediate reactions that result in the removal of myelin sheaths from neurons, which causes the subsequent disruption of nerve impulses and neurological function. [p. 414–415]

15. The autoantibody formed in the skeletal muscle disease, myasthenia gravis, is an antiacetylcholine receptor antibody. The antibody successfully competes with the neurotransmitter for the receptor site at the neuromuscular junction, causing muscular fatigue and weakness. This disease is also influenced by pathological changes in the thymus, and thymectomy has been very successful in treating this disease. [p. 415–416]

16. The systemic autoimmune diseases include rheumatoid arthritis and systemic lupus erythematosus. The autoantibodies formed in systemic disease can invade many regions of the body. The circulating immune complexes formed cause damage only when deposited into tissue regions where complement fixation initiates a variety of antibody-dependent cellular cytotoxicity reactions and can cause tissue damage. [p. 416]

17. Rheumatoid arthritis is a progressive inflammatory disease of connective tissue, mainly affecting the joints of the skeletal system. Rheumatoid factors (IgG and IgM) are formed against an altered immunoglobulin, forming immune complexes in the synovium of the joints. During an acute episode, inflammatory reactions, caused by the activation of the complement cascade by immune complexes, can lead to cell lysis, edema, pannus formation, and joint destruction. [p. 416–418]

18. Systemic lupus erythematosus is another systemic inflammatory disease in which autoantibodies to nuclear antigens, DNA, RNA, and cytoplasmic elements can form circulating immune complexes that can deposit in a number of organs including the skin, kidney, and joints. The ensuing inflammatory reactions can lead to the destruction of the cells in the affected organs. Damage to the glomerular nephron structure can cause irreversible loss of function and life-threatening kidney failure. Treatment of this, as in many other autoimmune diseases, is mainly symptomatic, but future hope may lay in immunotherapy, as we further our understanding of how tolerance is maintained and lost. [p. 418–420]

19. Several animal models for autoimmune diseases have been developed. Certain of these diseases arise spontaneously. However, others are induced by immunizing animals with pathogenic antigens or cells. Subsequently, autoantibodies are produced leading to expression of clinical, serological, immunological, and pathological features paralleling those found in the human disease. [p. 420–421]

READINGS

Ada, G. L., and Rose, N. R. The initiation and early development of autoimmune diseases. *Clinical Immunology and Immunopathology* **47**:3, 1988.

Barisch, J. M., Weeks, T., Giles, R., et al. Analysis of HLA-DQ genotypes and susceptibility to insulin-dependent diabetes mellitus. *New England Journal of Medicine* **322**:1836, 1990.

Bohme, J., Schuhbaur, B., Kanagawa, O., et al. MHC-linked protection from diabetes dissociated from clonal deletion of T cells. *Science* **249**:293, 1990.

Bottezzo, G. F., and Doniech, D. Autoimmune thyroid disease. *Annual Review of Medicine* **37**:353, 1986.

Brinkman, K., Termaat, R., Berden, J. H. M., et al. Anti-DNA antibodies and lupus nephritis: the complexity of crossreactivity. *Immunology Today* **11**:232, 1990.

Cohen, P. L., and Eisenberg, R. A. *Lpr* and *gld*: single gene models of systemic autoimmunity and lymphoproliferative disease. *Annual Review of Immunology* **9**:243, 1991.

Cruse, J. M., and Lewis, R. E. (eds.). *Autoimmunity: Basic Concepts; Systemic and Selected Organ-Specific Diseases.* S. Karger Publishers, New York, 1985.

Diener, E. Tolerance and autoimmunity. *Immunology Today* **7**:5, 1986.

Harley, J. B., Reichlin, M., Arnett, F. C., et al. Genes interaction at HLA-DQ enhances autoantibody production in primary Sjögren's syndrome. *Science* **232**:1145, 1986.

Harris, E. J., Jr. Rheumatoid arthritis: pathophysiology and implications for therapy. *New England Journal of Medicine* **322**:1277, 1990.

Haskins, K., and McDuffie, M. Acceleration of diabetes in young NOD mice with a CD4+ islet-specific T cell clone. *Science* **249**:1433, 1990.

Jalkanen, S., Steere, A. C., Fox, R. I., et al. A distinct endothelial cell recognition system that controls lymphocyte traffic into inflamed synovium. *Science* **233**:556, 1986.

Kennedy, R. C., Melnick, J. L., and Dreesman, G. R. Antiidiotypes and immunity. *Scientific American* **255**:48, 1986.

Lambert, P. H., Perrin, L., and Izui, S. (eds.). *Recent Advances in Systemic Lupus Erythematosus.* Academic Press, Inc., New York, 1984.

Lander, L. L., and Phillips, J. H. Evidence for three types of human cytotoxic lymphocyte. *Immunology Today* **7**:132, 1986.

Marx, J. Testing of autoimmune therapy begins. *Science* **252**: 27, 1991.

McIntosh, K. R., and Drachman, D. B. Induction of suppressor cells specific for AChR in experimental autoimmune myasthenia gravis. *Science* **232**:401, 1986.

Nepom, G. T., and Erlich, H. MHC class-II molecules and autoimmunity. *Annual Review of Immunology* **9**:493, 1991.

Palliard, X., West, S. G., Lafferty, J. A., et al. Evidence for the effects of a superantigen in rheumatoid arthritis. *Science* **253**:325, 1991.

Rennie, J. The body against itself. *Scientific American* **263**(6):106, 1990.

Rose, N., and Mackay, I. (eds.). *The Autoimmune Diseases.* Academic Press, Inc., New York, 1985.

Scarlato, G. (ed.). *Multiple Sclerosis.* Plenum Publishing Co., New York, 1984.

Schoenfeld, Y., and Mozes, E. Pathogenic idiotypes of autoantibodies in autoimmunity: lessons from new experimental models of SLE. *FASEB Journal* **4**:246, 1990.

Sinha, A. A., Lopez, M. T., and McDevitt, H. O. Autoimmune diseases: the failure of self-tolerance. *Science* **249**:1380, 1990.

Souroujon, M., White-Scharf, M. E., Andre-Schwartz, J., et al. Preferential autoantibody reactivity of the pre-immune B cell repertoire in normal mice. *Journal of Immunology* **140**:4173, 1988.

Walfish, P., Wall, J., and Volpe, R. (eds.). *Autoimmunity and the Thyroid.* Academic Press, Inc., New York, 1985.

Wilkin, T. J. Receptor autoimmunity in endocrine disorders. *New England Journal of Medicine* **323**:1318, 1990.

Winter, W. E., Muir, A., Maclaren, N. K., et al. Heritable origins of type I (insulin-dependent) diabetes mellitus: immunogenetic update. *Growth, Genetics, and Hormones* **7**:1, 1991.

Young, M., and Geha, R. S. Human regulatory T-cell subsets. *Annual Review of Medicine* **37**:165, 1986.

6

Cancer and Transplantation

This unit examines the body's response to two curious forms of challenge: (1) challenges presented by cells that are part of the individual but that deviate from their normal roles (i.e., cancer cells) and (2) challenges presented by foreign cells and tissues that are needed in order to ensure the survival and well-being of the individual (i.e., tissue grafts). Chapter 17, Cancer, presents a general discussion of tumors, the processes through which they arise, and how they differ from the "normal" cells of the body from which they arose. Chapter 18, Tumor Immunology, explores the ways in which the immune system interacts with tumors. The problems associated with transplantation, and some attempts at resolving them, are the focus of chapter 19, Transplantation Immunology.

17

Cancer

OVERVIEW

The general nature, distribution, and major causes of cancer are outlined. Comparisons are made between normal and neoplastic cells. In addition, mechanisms of oncogenesis and metastasis are explored. Furthermore, methods for treating and preventing cancer are described.

CONCEPTS

1. Cancer represents an altered condition typified by a failure of cells to respond to normal regulatory control.

2. Transformation of a normal cell to a cancerous, or tumorous, state can be accomplished by several factors that lead to a heritably modified pattern of cellular behavior, which include chemical and physical agents, viruses, oncogenes, and antioncogenes.

3. Any tissue can potentially give rise to tumors; however, those that have an active proliferating (dividing) population are most commonly affected.

F ew diseases have the impact on us that cancer has. This is a form of disease that seems to be everywhere and is capable of evading all our efforts at controlling it. Although there are certain patterns of distribution, this disease, or rather family of diseases, can affect any race, social class, or age group. No one seems to be free of its scourge, regardless of the precautions taken. Nevertheless, we are constantly counseled about ways to lessen our chances of becoming a "cancer victim." Yet, if we stop to consider for a moment why we react the way we do whenever the topic of cancer arises, we readily discover that we are reacting emotionally and often out of ignorance.

What, then, is cancer? Is there justification for the fear that it strikes? This chapter explores some of what has been learned about this disease. Exploring how cancer cells differ from their normal counterparts, and how they might have been modified, enables us to place this disease in perspective. In addition, an increased understanding of cancer can help us see where we might look to find yet greater insight into this area.

■ ■ ■ ■ ■ ■ ■ ■ ■ ■ ■ ■

DISTRIBUTION AND CAUSES OF CANCER
Incidence of Cancer

Less than 100 years ago, infectious diseases were the primary cause of death in the United States. On average, one of every two deaths recorded was due to infections such as pneumonia, tuberculosis, diphtheria, and influenza. Presently, infectious disease is the cause of only one in 20 deaths in the United States. As control over infectious diseases increased, the average life span was expanded from less than 50 to greater than 70 years of age. Cancer predominantly affects the elderly, with half of the current cancer deaths occurring in individuals over 60 years old. This, in part, undoubtedly accounted for the strikingly lower incidence of cancer a century ago, as compared with today, when one out of every five deaths is caused by malignancies. Another important factor is the remarkable increase and variety of cancer-causing agents that have been introduced into our environment since that time.

Analytical observers predict that one out of every four Americans now alive will develop some form of cancer. Each year more than 450,000 people in the United States and up to 4 million people throughout the world die from cancer. A bit of optimism and hope following these grim figures is offered by health experts, who estimate that perhaps half of all cancers can be prevented and more than half of those that cannot be prevented are at least curable. This can be illustrated by trends in survival for various forms of cancer as seen between 1960–1963 and 1977–1982 (table 17.1).

Although cancer appears to be a more prominent threat to us now, it has apparently existed since ancient times. Contemporary examination of Egyptian mummies has revealed evidence of bone cancers in those who lived thousands of years ago. Inca Indians, during the pre-Columbian period, had skin cancers as well as bone cancers. Since then, cancers have been found to affect peoples throughout the world, with the incidence of cancer being higher in some areas than in others. For example, rates are generally higher in densely populated and industrialized countries, and lower in developing nations. This is in contrast to the situation involving parasitic diseases (see chapter 11, Agents of Infectious Disease).

It soon became evident that the incidence of cancer was directly related to the prevalence of carcinogens, or cancer-causing agents, in the environment. Certain forms of cancer that were seen to strike peoples of some countries more severely than others appeared linked to the customs and environmental factors peculiar to that country. For example, in certain parts of India there are abnormally large numbers of people suffering from mouth cancer, which is related to the custom of eating betel leaves spread with lime, betel nut, and tobacco flakes. Although considered a delicacy, the juices may irritate the oral cavity and, over long periods of time, initiate or promote transformation of cells in the mouth. In addition, the very high incidence of lung cancer in the United States and Great Britain is attributed to the degree of cigarette smoking and industrial pollution in these countries.

Variation in the frequency of certain cancers in different parts of the world definitely implicates environmental agents as primary causes of malignancy. Furthermore, the genetic constitution of peoples in any

TABLE 17.1 Trends in Five-Year Survival Rates for Selected Forms of Cancer

Cancer	Relative 5-Year Survival (%)								Increased Survival (%)	
	1960–63*		1970–73*		1973–76†		1977–82†			
	W	B	W	B	W	B	W	B	W	B
Bladder	53	24	61	36	74	47	76	56	23	32
Breast (female)	63	46	68	51	74	63	75	63	12	17
Colon	43	34	49	37	50	46	53	47	10	13
Leukemia	14	—‡	22	—‡	33	29	34	29	20	≥0
Lung/bronchus	8	5	10	7	12	10	13	10	5	5
Lymphomas (non-Hodgkin's)	31	—‡	41	—‡	46	48	49	49	18	≥1
Ovary	32	32	36	32	36	40	37	37	5	5
Prostate	50	35	63	55	67	57	72	62	22	27
Rectum	38	27	45	30	48	39	51	37	13	10
Uterine										
Cervix	58	47	64	61	68	64	68	59	10	12
Corpus	73	31	81	44	89	59	85	56	12	25

W = white; B = black.

Source: Biometry Branch, National Cancer Institute.

*Rates are based on data from a series of hospital registries and one population-based registry.

†Rates are from SEER Program and include patients diagnosed through 1982 and follow-up on all patients through 1983. They are based on data from population-based registries in Connecticut, New Mexico, Utah, Iowa, Hawaii, Atlanta, Detroit, Seattle-Puget Sound, and San Francisco-Oakland.

‡No rates calculated because of insufficient number of cases.

Modified from *Cancer Facts and Figures–1986.* American Cancer Society.

of these areas causes some inhabitants to be more, or less, susceptible to a carcinogen. Susceptibility to cancer appears to run in families, and the inheritance of a predisposition of susceptibility to cancer has been unequivocally demonstrated in inbred laboratory animals.

Cancers are not restricted to humans and other mammals. Recently, a cancer "epidemic" in fish from a number of lakes and rivers in the United States has been reported. Cancer rates of up to 80% have been recorded from just about every chemically polluted body of water examined. Eating fish fillets from contaminated waters is not recommended, since fish concentrate pollutants such as polychlorinated biphenyls (PCBs) in their tissues.

Carcinogens

Carcinogenic, or cancer-causing, agents in our external and internal environment include chemicals, hormones, radiation, and viruses. About 75 years ago, Yamagiwa and Ichikawa showed that cancer could be induced by chemicals. These Japanese researchers painted the skin of rabbits with coal tar repeatedly over a period of months. They observed that skin cancers developed in treated animals, but not in untreated control animals living in the same environment. Recently, fish were painted with chemicals extracted from river sediments, and many developed cancers after a year.

Since that time, many chemicals have been tested for cancer-causing properties. In fact, many of us probably tend to exhibit a cancerphobia on learning of the many carcinogens that may be present in the air we breathe, fluids we drink, food we eat, clothes we wear, and the drugs or medications we take. We are also alarmed by either the potential dangers of radiation (from prolonged exposure to the sun or diagnostic x-rays) or the possibility that the viruses we encounter or inherit may initiate or promote cancer. Furthermore, we are warned of occupational hazards, such as the danger to carpenters from prolonged exposure to wood dusts; to automobile mechanics from petroleum products; to chimney sweeps from soot and coal products; to farmers from ultraviolet light; to miners from arsenic, asbestos, coal, iron oxide, and uranium; to painters and shoemakers from benzene; and to welders from cadmium.

One means of determining that a substance is carcinogenic is to actually demonstrate that its administration causes cancer in an experimental animal. This is usually achieved by administering the maximum tolerated dose (MTD [the highest dose that causes no more than 1% mortality]) of that substance to animals (usually mice or rats) daily throughout the animals' lives, and examining them for evidence of cancer. Initially, all carcinogens were believed to be mutagens, which was assumed to be the common basis for their cancer-causing properties. This gave rise to a second test for carcinogenicity, the **Ames test,** which is a sensitive, short-term screening procedure that measures the ability of a chemical to induce mutations in a special strain of *Salmonella typhimurium* (a bacterium). Accordingly, this test provides a meaningful indication of a chemical's potential as a human carcinogen. (See highlight 17.1.) In recent years, many substances have been identified as carcinogenic by animal experiments (when given at MTD), but have been found not to be mutagenic. These include substances that naturally occur in certain vegetables. The need to reconcile these discrepancies has called for a reevaluation of the criteria used to label substances as potential carcinogens.

Although we can be overwhelmed with the growing list of potential cancer risks, we should not develop a "what's the use, everything causes cancer" attitude, for the situation is certainly not hopeless. Most cancers are caused by only a handful of major carcinogens. Health experts further point out that about half of all cancers are preventable. Prominent carcinogens

such as cigarettes, high-fat diets, heavy alcohol consumption, and excessive sun exposure should be avoided, and greater precautions should be used in the workplace. The number of lives that might be saved by exercising these measures could be dramatically increased, since any one of these cancer-causing agents can potentially initiate or promote transformation of a normal cell into a cancer cell.

TUMORS

Cells within a tissue display functional variation over time. These variations generally represent modifications in the level of activity characteristic of the cell type. This modification of cellular activity reflects change in extrinsic characteristics; that is, the cell's environment has been modified. For example, the cyclical modifications that the uterus of a mature female undergoes reflect changes in the hormonal composition of the internal environment throughout the menstrual cycle. This leads alternatively to a buildup and sloughing of the endometrium as the final stages of oogenesis and ovulation occur.

On occasion, however, functional variations are encountered that are not in response to modifications in the cells' immediate external environment. Rather, these variations occur because of intrinsic modifications of the cells themselves. The consequence of these modifications is the formation of a *pathological overgrowth within the tissue*—a mass known as a **tumor.** There is considerable variation among tumors (discussed below); some show little deviation from normal tissue, while others bear no obvious similarity to normal tissues either structurally or functionally. The former are referred to as benign tumors and the latter as malignant tumors or cancers. Nevertheless, all tumors share the characteristic that they *originated through inappropriate growth.*

Hyperplasia and Neoplasia

When the modification in cellular behavior leads to *increased total activity* by the tissue or organ because of increased cellular mass (without increased cell numbers), we describe this change as **hypertrophy.** If the modification leads to an *increase in cell number* of an adult

The Ames Test

Rapid and efficient evaluation of the carcinogenic potential of suspected cancer-causing agents encountered in the workplace has become increasingly important. The Ames test provides the most widely used screening tool for this purpose. This test relies on the fact that carcinogenic substances are also mutagenic; that is, they can cause mutations.

Specifically, the Ames test makes use of several mutant strains of *S. typhimurium,* which are incapable of synthesizing the amino acid histidine. Such mutants do not grow and multiply in histidine-depleted culture media. However, histidine-minus mutants, as a consequence of rare "back mutation," can regain the ability to synthesize histidine and hence regain the ability to thrive in histidine-depleted media. This forms the basis of the Ames test.

In performing the test, small quantities of the chemical to be tested are added to culture dishes containing histidine-minus bacteria in histidine-depleted media. If mutagenic, the chemical induces many types of mutations, some of which might restore the ability of histidine-minus bacteria to synthesize histidine. If so, these cells grow and divide and produce visible colonies in culture in one to two days.

With appropriate standardization, the degree of colony formation can be equated with the mutagenic and, hence, carcinogenic capability of the agent in question.

The Ames test, as outlined above, is extremely sensitive, rapid, and cost-effective. However, some potential carcinogens might not be discerned by this simplified procedure. These are substances that become carcinogenic only following appropriate *biochemical or metabolic modifications* (or activation) within an animal cell. Certain of these substances can be demonstrated to have carcinogenic properties by performing the Ames test using a rat liver extract, S-9, containing metabolizing enzyme activity. Incubation of the suspected carcinogen with this extract can often accomplish this "activation."

In addition to the Ames test, other bacterial tests have been developed to measure carcinogenicity. Among these are the **inductest** and the **lambda mutatest.** Both make use of prophages—yet, as with the Ames test, require a mutagenic effect of the test substance to determine carcinogenic potential. These latter tests are potentially more sensitive than the Ames test but have not been as extensively tested and validated.

Ames, B. N., McCann, J., and Yamasaki, E. Methods for detecting carcinogens and mutagens with the Salmonella/mammalian-microsome mutagenicity test. *Mutation Research* **31:**347, 1975.

Devoret, R. Bacterial tests for potential carcinogens. *Scientific American.* August 1979.

Moreau, P., Bailone, A., and Devoret, R. Prophage (lambda) induction in *Escherichia coli* K 12 *envA uvrB:* a highly sensitive test for potential carcinogens. *Proceedings of the National Academy of Sciences* (USA) **73:**3700, 1976.

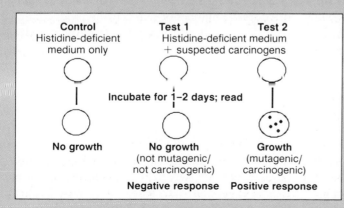

FIGURE 17.A Ames test.

tissue or organ, we identify this as **hyperplasia.** Both represent responses on the part of cells of the tissue to external signals.

A tumor, or **neoplasia,** arises through increased cellular proliferation. In a sense, it reflects hyperplasia in the affected tissue. However, this increased proliferation represents an intrinsic change in the tumor cells rather than a response to extrinsic (external) signals. This change is heritable; that is, it can be passed on to future cell generations. This kind of heritable transformation is called *metaplasia*. In addition, pathologists recognize an intermediate type of change. This alteration is characterized by atypical hyperplasia and, although not itself neoplastic, is believed to represent a step toward neoplasia. This apparent shift to a "preneoplastic" state is referred to as *dysplasia*.

Hyperplasia can occur as the result of either of two different processes. The first involves an *increase in the number of dividing cells* that remain replicative. The second mechanism represents an *increase in cell longevity, divisional rate, or both*. In the formation of a tumorous mass, these mechanisms need not be mutually exclusive.

When cellular proliferation yields two daughter cells, one of which differentiates and no longer divides while the other retains its proliferative potential, little if any growth occurs. Under these conditions, the first cell becomes a functional part of the tissue and adds no new cells to its mass. The second cell essentially replaces the parent cell as part of the "growth fraction" and can be called upon to provide replacement cells at some later time. As long as the growth fraction remains constant, increases in cell numbers occur very slowly, if at all. Should the number of cells that retain proliferative potential increase, then an increase in the number of cells in a tissue can occur rapidly (fig. 17.1). For example, when both daughter cells retain their proliferative potential (i.e., neither differentiates), then the growth fraction increases leading to eventual hyperplasia.

This illustration shows that only five cells will be produced over the span of five generations under normal circumstances (fig. 17.1*a*). Yet there will be no net gain if these cells are produced to replace others that have died out. In contrast, 11 offspring will result over this same span if the pattern depicted is followed

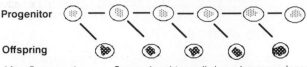

(a) Stable growth fraction: Normal replacement

After 5 generations have elapsed — *5 new daughter cells* have been produced; single progenitor cell still remains

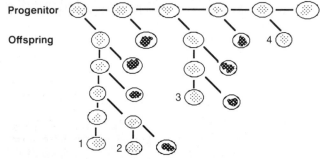

(b) Expanding growth fraction: Hyperplasia

After 5 generations — *11 new cells* have been produced; 7 of these are nondividing; 4 are *new progenitor cells*; original progenitor cell still remains

Growth fraction has *expanded 5-fold*

FIGURE 17.1 Hyperplasia due to enlargement of growth fraction. (*a*) In normal replacement, one daughter cell replaces the parent in the growth fraction, while the other replaces a lost tissue cell. No net growth results. (*b*) When both daughter cells retain the ability to divide, the growth fraction expands. Each additional progenitor cell increases the number of progeny that can be produced.

(fig. 17.1*b*). In this situation, some, but not all, of the offspring retain their ability to proliferate. This not only increases the number of cells actually produced but also increases the size of the growth fraction, thereby further increasing the rate of expansion of the tissue.

Even more progeny will be produced, however, if all of the descendants of the first offspring cell remain as permanent members of the growth fraction. This cell alone will contribute 16 daughter cells over the four generations that follow. This might occur if the first offspring cell were transformed to a malignant tumor cell. But the maximum number of cells that can be produced (2^n, which represents the rate of exponential expansion) will appear if all of the progeny of the original progenitor cell become part of the growth fraction. Now a total of 32 cells will be produced. This

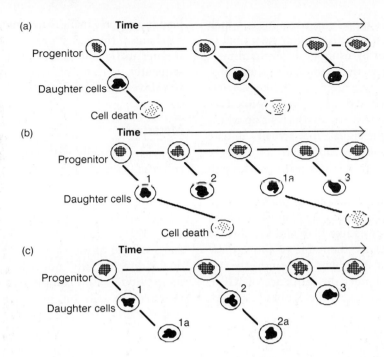

FIGURE 17.2 Hyperplasia due to altered rate of replacement or loss. (*a*) Ordinarily, new cells are produced to replace cells that die or are damaged. (*b*) When cells are produced before they are needed as replacements, tissue growth (hyperplasia) results. Cells 2 and 3 are extra, cell 1a replaces cell 1. This occurs if the cell division cycle is initiated prematurely. (*c*) When cells are produced in anticipation of a need for replacement that does not occur because of increased longevity, tissue growth occurs. Cell 2 should replace cell 1, and cell 3 should replace cell 2; however, all three cells remain. This presupposes that the cell division cycle is preprogrammed at a set rate.

reflects an expansion of tissue at a rate that is more than six times that of the normal tissue over the five generations represented. This is a probable result of transformation of the progenitor cell into a tumor cell.

The second mechanism through which hyperplasia comes about represents an alteration in the rate of replacement within the tissue (fig. 17.2). Ordinarily, cells will die after a certain period of time and be replaced by new progeny from the growth fraction (fig. 17.2*a*). If the frequency at which new cells are produced should be accelerated (increased mitotic rate), then the number of new products becomes accelerated, leading to increased cell numbers (fig. 17.2*b*). Alternatively, if cell death does not occur as scheduled (increased longevity), but production of new cells continues on schedule, then an increase in the number of cells must result (fig. 17.2*c*).

A dividing cell's life history can be presented as a cycle comprised of four basic stages: G_1, S, G_2, and M. While the duration of the cell cycle is quite variable for the many different types of normal cells in the body, it generally lasts for approximately 16 to 24 hours, with G_1 ranging from 5 to 12 hours, and S, G_2, and M lasting about 8, 2, and 0.7 hours, respectively. Although cancer cells usually do not divide or replicate more rapidly than normal cells, the elevated cell numbers associated with a tumor are a consequence of the *lack of constraints that regulate the proliferation of normal cells.*

Normal cells and tissues appear to precisely regulate their own population size. This can be achieved through a positive control by the action of growth factors (e.g., nerve growth factor [NGF], epidermal growth factor [EGF]) and hormones (e.g., erythropoietin). In addition, there are negative control factors. Negative control might be achieved through cell-to-cell contact (contact, or density-dependent, inhibition), by producing specific biochemical factors (e.g., chalones, mitosis-suppressing hormones), which impede the proliferation of cells of their own kind in the immediate locale, or by using both mechanisms.

Those substances that stimulate cellular proliferation act in either of two ways. Some, like platelet-derived growth factor (PDGF), are **competence factors.** These substances act by making the cells on which they act responsive to the signals that actually initiate the proliferation cycle. Other substances act on these "competent" cells, causing them to progress through the cell cycle. They can be considered as **progression factors** by comparison. For example, PDGF acts on nonproliferating fibroblasts, moving them from a G_0 to a G_1 status. Other factors like EGF and insulin-like growth factor I (IGF-I) are then able to move these proliferation-competent fibroblasts through the G_1 stage of the cell cycle. Under the influence of IGF-I, the fibroblasts finally enter into the S phase and replicate their DNA.

Substances that act as *growth inhibitors* will block the action of the competence or progression growth factors. For example, interferon (IFN) blocks the transition of fibroblasts from G_0 to G_1 following stimulation by PDGF. In blocking the action of this "competence-inducing factor," IFN prevents the fibroblasts from initiating DNA replication, and cell proliferation does not occur. Some substances can act as either positive or negative growth regulators. Transforming growth factor-β (TGF-β) is one example. Although originally named for its ability to mediate oncogenic transformation of rat fibroblasts, this peptide can antagonize and suppress proliferation induced by several other growth factors. In addition, it is capable of enhancing the differentiation of connective tissue. The specific manner in which it acts appears to be determined by the particular conditions that prevail.

Cancer cells do not respond to these normal proliferative controls. Consequently, they continue to proliferate, but not necessarily at greater than normal rates. The ultimate result is the generation of a mass we recognize as a tumor.

Both mechanisms for promoting hyperplasia might be at work in the development of a tumor. Characteristically, the second mechanism (increased longevity/mitotic frequency) seems to predominate in benign and early malignant tumors. In contrast, the first mechanism (increased growth fraction) predominates in later malignant tumors. A malignant tumor, consequently, is characterized by the presence of more primitive undifferentiated cells.

Metastasis

In general, rapidly dividing, undifferentiated cancer cells can "crowd out" the less rapidly dividing or nondividing differentiated normal cells of the body. Consequently, cancer cells compete for vital nutrients and hence "starve" normal cells. As a result, normal tissues, organs, and organ systems might eventually fail and succumb to the cancer. Accordingly, cancer cells do not directly "kill" normal cells *per se,* but indirectly do so through their competition for vital nutrients and resources. In addition, malignant tumors can also obstruct blood vessels, the alimentary tract, or the urinary tract. These, in turn, can prevent food absorption (causing wasting), destroy tissues, and perhaps subject the affected individual to infectious diseases.

In addition to their competition with normal tissues for essential nutrients, some tumors have a tendency to spread to diverse sites. This property of tumor cells to *disseminate to other sites* is called **metastasis.** This is perhaps the most widely feared property of tumors. However, it is not a property associated with all tumors. In fact, this feature is one means of discriminating between benign and malignant tumors.

Benign tumors exhibit a *slower growth rate* than malignant tumors and, since they become encapsulated, their cells do not invade blood vessels or metastasize (fig. 17.3). Although they normally cause little tissue damage when compared with malignant tumors, they can be fatally damaging if they occur in vital areas such as the heart or brain. Thus, most benign tumors are not life threatening as many of us know from experiencing common warts, which is a virus-induced epithelial benign tumor. The cells of benign tumors still retain some similarity to normal cells, morphologically and physiologically. Thus, they present a somewhat more *differentiated appearance* than do cells of a malignant tumor.

Malignant tumors tend to be more aggressive. They display *significant growth rates* and a greater

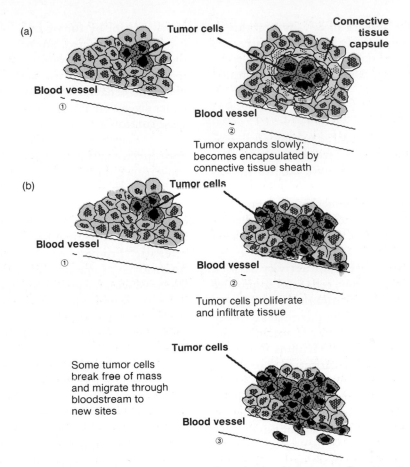

(a)

Tumor cells

Connective tissue capsule

Blood vessel

①

Blood vessel

②

Tumor expands slowly; becomes encapsulated by connective tissue sheath

(b)

Tumor cells

Blood vessel

①

Blood vessel

②

Tumor cells proliferate and infiltrate tissue

Some tumor cells break free of mass and migrate through bloodstream to new sites

Tumor cells

Blood vessel

③

FIGURE 17.3 Tumor progression: benign versus malignant tumors. (*a*) Benign tumors grow slowly and become encapsulated by connective tissues. They consequently do not display invasive tendencies. (*b*) Malignant tumors grow rapidly, do not become encapsulated, but rather invade the surrounding tissue. In addition, malignant cells display a tendency to break free of the parent tumor and metastasize to other sites, thereby causing the cancer to "spread."

tendency toward *metastasis*. In addition, they are typically characterized by a population of cells that appear generally *undifferentiated* and display few characteristics of their normal counterparts. The aggregate of these features is sometimes termed anaplasia.

Although cancer can develop in almost any cell of the body, some cells are more susceptible than others. When normal cells divide, they do not necessarily produce two exact copies of themselves; instead, some cells differentiate into specific types (e.g., brains cells or skin cells or blood cells, and so forth). Some cells never mature fully, such as the renewable stem cells of the bone marrow, although they possess the potential to differentiate into blood cells. Other cells differentiate

and retain the ability to proliferate, producing exact copies of themselves, if healthy and normal. Some other cells, however, stop duplicating at maturity. Skeletal muscle cells, for example, can increase in size, but their maximum numbers are acquired before birth. Nerve cells, including brain cells, multiply rapidly until birth and then no longer replicate. Cells that are actively multiplying are the ones that are most susceptible to cancer. Specific brain or nerve cells, for example, almost never become cancerous, although supportive tissue in the brain may become malignant. For similar reasons, blood, skin, and lung cancers are common because the cells of these tissues must be continuously replaced. Although the genetic composition of a nondividing cell can be altered, in the absence of cell division this alteration is limited to the affected cell. Obviously, a cell that is not dividing, although it might become transformed into a cancer cell, cannot lead to the formation of a tumor mass.

Biochemical Features

The heritable changes that give rise to tumor cells produce several alterations. As discussed above, there is loss of normal responsiveness to growth control mechanisms. In addition, there are other biochemical changes that occur. There have been numerous efforts to characterize these changes in an attempt to gain further insight into the properties of tumors. Four general features about these changes stand out.

First, **increased glycolytic activity** has been associated with tumors. Tumor cells tend to produce greater amounts of lactic acid from the breakdown of glucose than do normal cells. This increased glycolytic activity has been attributed to greater anaerobic metabolism in tumors because of limitations in oxygen delivery, especially where vascularization is poor. Although this might be true, it is not the full explanation since tumors still display elevated glycolytic activity in the presence of an ample oxygen supply. There appear to be alterations in energy metabolism in tumor cells. Despite the considerable attention focused on this issue since its discovery by Otto Warburg in the 1920s, the significance of this metabolic change in tumors remains controversial and unclear.

Second, there is a tendency for the biochemical activities of tumor cells, particularly malignant tumors, to be very similar. In other words, there is **convergence in the display of biochemical characteristics.** In comparing the activities of cells from different tissues, we expect to encounter variation in biochemical activities—for example, the biochemical activities of kidney cells will differ from those of liver cells. However, with malignant neoplasias, these differences are reduced, if not abolished. Consequently, renal (kidney) and hepatic (liver) neoplasias might display very similar biochemical features.

Third, there is **metabolic rigidity.** This means that tumor cells are less variable and flexible in their metabolic expression. This reduced flexibility provides additional evidence of loss of normal regulatory control by tumor cells. When environmental conditions are altered, normal cells adapt the rates of their metabolic pathways accordingly, chiefly in response to controls exerted on these pathways. Since the metabolic behavior of tumor cells is more invariant under diverse environmental conditions, it means that these controls are not functioning properly.

Fourth, tumor cells are characterized by **inappropriate cell products.** In conjunction with the convergence in biochemical expression mentioned above, tumor cells stand out from the surrounding normal tissue because of the products that they make or fail to make. For example, highly malignant carcinomas of the skin might fail to produce keratin, a characteristic product of normal epidermal cells. Alternatively, some tumors of the digestive tract are associated with the production of carcinoembryonic Ag (CEA), a product that is normally expressed by embryonic endodermal tissues but that is inappropriate in adult tissues. Certain of these are manifested as antigenic markers in the cell membrane and might be identified by the immune system as foreign. In addition, modifications in the expression of histocompatibility genes can occur. For example, mice have been found to have altered expression of class I MHC genes, which encode for the transplantation Ags (see chapter 19, Transplantation Immunology). These alterations include (1) loss or reduced expression of certain genes, (2) expression of genes in the H-2 and Qa/Tla regions, and (3) generation of novel Ags through mutation. These surface modifications can profoundly influence interactions between tumor cells and the immune surveillance system (see chapter 18, Tumor Immunology) and appear to play a role in metastasis.

These features reflect a condition in which behavior is inappropriate and independent of normal regulatory influence. They are associated with cells that have been intrinsically modified. The extent to which these altered characteristics are displayed by benign and malignant tumors is compared in table 17.2.

Classification

Benign tumors are named for the type of tissue from which a tumor arises. This is accomplished by adding **-oma** to the tissue name. Thus, an adenoma is a tumor ("oma") affecting glandular tissue. Malignant tumors

TABLE 17.2 Characteristics of Tumors

Normal Tissues	Benign Tumors	Malignant Tumors
Appearance		
Cells/tissues display stable, differentiated appearance	Cells and tissues tend to retain differentiated features	Cells display primitive, undifferentiated appearance
Function		
Metabolic activities respond to regulatory signals (e.g., fluxes in extrinsic metabolites)	Metabolic activities appear somewhat normal	Metabolic activities are variably altered; changes are intrinsic, reflecting loss of control by normal regulatory factors
Cell products typify tissue and its role	Cell products are essentially normal	Cell products are often inappropriate (absent, overexpressed, or out of character for tissue)
Growth		
Mitosis is absent to regular (depending upon tissue type)	Mitotic activity shows limited deviation from that of tissue of origin	Mitotic activity is uncontrolled; mitosis is frequent
No net growth occurs (proliferation is limited to cell replacement)	Growth is very slow	Growth is sustained/rapid
No expansion occurs beyond limits of organ	Metastasis is rare (tumor is often encapsulated)	Metastasis is common

are named according to the embryonic origin of the tissue that is affected. For example, the suffix **-carcinoma** describes those tumors that are endodermal or ectodermal in origin, and **-sarcoma** describes mesodermally derived tumors. Accordingly, an adenocarcinoma represents a malignant tumor of a gland. In general, during metastasis, carcinomas have a tendency to spread first through the lymphatics, while sarcomas tend to spread first through the vasculature.

This scheme for naming tumors has a few exceptions, however. These are (1) blastoma (malignant tumor that resembles embryonic tissues), (2) melanoma (malignancy of pigment-forming cells), (3) hepatoma (malignant tumor of the liver), and (4) myeloma (plasma cell malignancy).

ONCOGENESIS

Transformation of a normal cell into a cancerous cell, referred to as oncogenesis, can involve several steps. The word **initiator** is used at times in reference to a mutagen that *genetically changes or transforms a normal*

cell to a cancer cell, whereas the word **promoter** designates agents or possibly conditions that *promote malignancy by triggering changes in gene expression.* The distinctions are often difficult to see. Nevertheless, a rather coherent view of how a cell can become cancerous has been developed.

Several hypotheses have been proposed to account for the transformation of a normal cell into a cancer cell (table 17.3). Certain of these proposals are more favored than others; however, it is not unlikely that each of these can account for at least one form of cancer or another. A simplified way of considering these hypotheses groups them into (1) chemical and physical induction, (2) the threshold hypothesis, (3) error accumulation, (4) viral induction, and (5) oncogenes and antioncogenes.

Chemical and Physical Induction

Transformation of a normal cell to a tumor cell can be accomplished by chemical or physical agents capable of producing heritable alterations in cellular behavior.

Cellular Immortality

T here has been considerable interest expressed over the years in understanding cellular function. Among some of the most intensely studied questions are those that relate to gene expression and cellular behaviors associated with proliferation, differentiation, and aging. Investigators have sought to learn: What caused certain cells to express one set of genes and not another, thereby becoming different from another population of cells? What factors control the initiation and execution of cell division? What signals direct a cell to choose a pathway leading to differentiation as opposed to proliferation? What changes in cellular function and gene expression are associated with, and responsible for, the apparent breakdown that occurs during aging?

Studies with isolated vertebrate cells in tissue culture have proved instrumental in advancing our understanding of these important issues. Within the context of the tissue culture vessel, the investigator has considerable control over the variables affecting the cells being studied. Through the manipulation of the tissue culture environment, investigators have uncovered a number of factors that are responsible for the regulation of proliferation and differentiation. In addition, considerable insight has been gained about the ways in which these factors exert their influence.

One especially interesting point relating to cancer and to aging has emerged from certain of these studies. In his investigation of numerous established cell lines during the 1960s, Leonard Hayflick observed a curious phenomenon. Normal cells, it seemed, had a definable lifespan. Although some variability existed among the cell lines tested, normal human diploid cells persisted for approximately 50 generations. Mouse cells had shorter lifespans, 20 to 30 generations. Then, regardless of the steps taken to preserve them further, the cultures died. No explanation has yet been found to account for this particular phenomenon. Nevertheless, some clues are beginning to emerge.

In contrast to this limited lifespan displayed by normal cells, transformed cells appeared to be immortal. Cells taken from the same cultures, but infected by oncogenic viruses, became transformed and proliferated— the cell culture equivalent to becoming a tumor. But, more importantly, they outlived their normal counterpart cultures.

A similar ability to live indefinitely is associated with cancer cells. This display of apparent immortality by cancer cells suggests that normal cells need not have a discretely limited lifespan. What changes occurring during transformation of a normal cell into a cancer cell are responsible for this immortality?

Studies of a tumor suppressor gene whose dysfunction gives rise to retinoblastoma (RB) might shed light on this question. Recent studies have disclosed that the RB gene product might play a central role in the regulation of cell proliferation and senescence. Increased phosphorylation of the RB gene product coincides with progression through the G_1/S interface. Underphosphorylation of the RB gene product is associated with aborted progression through this interface. Moreover, senescent human fibroblasts display a failure to both phosphorylate the RB gene product and proliferate. From these studies, the suggestion has emerged that aging might be genetically controlled and be expressed as a dominant trait.

Burnet, F. M. Immunology, Aging and Cancer. W. H. Freeman & Co., Publishers, San Francisco, 1976.

Goldstein, S. Replicative senescence: the human fibroblast comes of age. Science 249:1129, 1990.

Hayflick, L. The limited in vitro lifetime of human diploid cell strains. Experimental Cell Research 37:614, 1965.

Mihara, K., Cao, X.-R., Yen, A., et al. Cell-cycle-dependent regulation of phosphorylation of the human retinoblastoma gene product. Science 246:1300, 1989.

Stein, G. H., Berson, M., and Gordon, L. Failure to phosphorylate the retinoblastoma gene product in senescent human fibroblasts. Science 249:666, 1990.

TABLE 17.3 Some Proposed Cancer-Producing Mechanisms

Hypothesis	Mechanism of Carcinogenesis
Chemical/Physical Induction	
Carcinogen induction	Certain classes of chemical substances bring about transformation of cells by altering DNA or its expression
Hormone induction	Repeated stimulation of target tissue by its hormone can lead to eventual transformation over extended period
Physical induction	Physical insult, such as ionizing radiation, causes genetic alteration and transformation
Threshold Theory	Repeated insult or injury to cells progressively leads to inherited functional change and transformation
Error Accumulation	With advancing age, cells produce increasing numbers of errors, finally leading to transformation of normal cells into cancer cells
Viral Induction	Tumor viruses infect cells and cause their transformation
Oncogenes/Antioncogenes	Tumor genes, believed by some to be viruses that are now integrated into the gene pool, and tumor suppressor genes, which, when inappropriately expressed lead to cellular transformation

The inducing agents include an extensive list of carcinogenic substances, hormones (under certain circumstances), and ionizing radiation.

Chemical Carcinogens

The chemical carcinogens fall into two categories: (1) those that cause tumors where they are applied and (2) those that do not induce tumors locally but rather lead to tumor formation at some remote site. The first group includes substances that are very reactive, such as alkylating agents (e.g., dialkylnitrosamines, ethionine, and urethane) and polycyclic aromatic hydrocarbons (e.g., 3-methylcholanthrene). The latter group contains substances that are not themselves carcinogenic, but which can be modified within the body to potent carcinogenic substances. Substances such as 2-naphthylamine, which must be converted to an N-hydroxy derivative in order to become active, illustrate the second group. In either case, it appears that the ability to induce tumor formation is dependent upon the existence of an active electrophilic molecule. The electrophilic derivative of the original substance, in turn, interacts with nucleophilic groups in DNA, RNA,

protein, or all three to bring about oncogenic transformation. The ultimate result is a heritable alteration in the affected cell.

Hormones

Hormones do not ordinarily lead to tumor formation; however, under unusual circumstances they can do so. The conditions that lead to oncogenesis generally involve chronic and extensive overstimulation of the target tissue by its regulating hormone. This stimulation leads first to hyperplasia, but eventually progresses to neoplasia. In 1949 G. R. and M. S. Biskind were the first to demonstrate this by transplanting ovaries of young adult mice and rats to their spleens and subsequently observing the formation of neoplasias. In this rather unusual site, the ovaries were still functional, but were unable to provide feedback to the pituitary gland—the liver metabolized all estrogens secreted. As a result the pituitary continued to secrete gonadotropins, eventually provoking hyperplasia, then neoplasia, in the transplanted ovaries. Similar demonstrations of hormonally induced neoplastic transformation have since been achieved for essentially all target organs.

Physical Agents

The means through which physical agents (e.g., ultraviolet radiation, x-rays) cause the induction of tumors is not entirely clear. One way in which radiation produces oncogenic transformation is by inducing mutational change. For example, radiation can produce thymidine-dimers (two adjacent thymidine residues in DNA become linked chemically). Repair mechanisms are then initiated that excise (remove) the dimer and replace the bases that are discarded. If substitution, rather than replacement, of the bases occurs, then a modified DNA sequence is produced. This change is heritable and might lead to a deviation away from normal function, if it is not lethal.

Alternatively, some believe that radiation might only indirectly lead to tumor formation. Since radiation can be immunosuppressive, tumor formation might result from a defect in immune surveillance (see chapter 18, Tumor Immunology) rather than a direct effect of radiation damage on somatic cells.

Threshold Hypothesis

The threshold theory of oncogenesis considers that cancer is a complex, multifactorial disease. In order for tumor transformation to occur, a certain minimal level (or threshold) of induction by several factors acting in conjunction must be reached. No single agent acting alone is responsible for the transformation of a normal cell into a cancerous cell according to this notion.

The apparent need for repeated exposure to chemical carcinogens, ionizing radiations (low level, at least), and hormones before tumor expression occurs can be taken as evidence that a certain threshold of "insult" is required before a normal cell transforms into a tumor cell. Breast cancer in mice provides an excellent illustration of the participation of several factors in the genesis of a tumor. Although breast cancer was originally considered a genetic disease in mice, in the 1930s it was shown by C. C. Little at the Jackson Memorial Laboratories (Bar Harbor, Maine) to require the participation of an "extrachromosomal factor." Through extensive experimentation, it was determined that three "factors" played a role in the expression of breast cancer in mice. These were (1) the genetic constitution of the individual (there are high- and low-tumor strains of mice), (2) the presence of an RNA-containing virus (transmitted in the milk; more virus is transmitted by high-tumor-strain mothers), and (3) the hormonal environment (chronic administration of estrogens and prolactin could induce breast cancer in male mice).

Error Accumulation

This hypothesis is slanted toward the apparently greater incidence of tumors with advancing age. It proposes that the expression of cancer is enhanced, if not caused, by the progressive accumulation of uncorrected errors in cellular behavior. Each time DNA is replicated, RNA is transcribed, or protein is translated there is a definable chance of a mistake being made. The more frequently these events occur, the greater is the chance for error. Eventually, a situation will arise when such an error occurs that is passed on. The result might be a transformed cell. In addition, the possibility for a defect in surveillance, leading to the escape of a deviant (cancer) cell, also increases with age. Thus, oncogenesis occurs when there is a catastrophe, or major error, that allows deviant cells with heritable defects to remain and reproduce. Although raising some interesting notions, this hypothesis does not enjoy much popularity.

Viral Induction
Tumor Viruses

In 1910 Peyton Rous reported the discovery of an RNA virus that could cause tumors (sarcomas) in chickens. If the tumor was harvested from a diseased chicken, Rous found that he could prepare a cell-free filtrate, which when inoculated into a normal chicken would give rise to another sarcoma. This was an epoch-making discovery. Since that time, viruses have been shown to cause numerous malignant tumors in animals, including primates. Such viruses are referred to as oncogenic, or tumor-causing, viruses.

The search for a human cancer-inducing virus has been intense. Viruses cause certain benign tumors in humans, such as warts, and there is increasing evidence suggesting a close association between certain herpes and hepatitis B viruses and human cancers. A recently developed hepatitis B virus vaccine, in the view of some, will not only protect us against viral hepatitis, but probably against certain liver cancers as well. Only recently (1978) have viruses been demonstrated conclusively to cause human cancers. The first demonstration was a virus that causes a rare form of leukemia. Since that time two other related retroviruses have been identified. The first retrovirus has been called HTLV-I for human T cell lymphotropic virus, type I. Accordingly, the second and third have been designated as HTLV-II and HTLV-III. HTLV-III (also called LAV [lymphadenopathy virus] and more recently HIV [human immunodeficiency virus]) has been implicated as the cause for AIDS (see chapter 15).

Tumor viruses contain genetic information in the form of either RNA or DNA. In either case, they possess very few genes compared with normal animal cells whose genes number in the thousands. Of momentous interest, for understanding oncogenesis, is the recent discovery that some tumor viruses possess one or perhaps several genes that are capable of changing a normal cell into a cancerous cell following viral infection. Since these genes are thought to be responsible for cell transformations, they are called oncogenes. Viruses possessing oncogenes can transform cells both outside the host (e.g., *in vitro*), as well as inside the host (*in vivo*). The viruses that have oncogenes are mostly RNA viruses.

Oncornaviruses

Oncornaviruses are RNA-containing viruses that have served as an experimental model for human cancer. In order to produce a protein, cells first produce an mRNA transcript from the appropriate segment of DNA, then translate this message into a protein on the ribosomes. How are virally specified, or coded, proteins synthesized by RNA viruses, since there is no viral DNA? This puzzle was resolved when researchers discovered that, in these viruses, the process is initially reversed. That is, the viral RNA has the blueprint for transcribing viral DNA and with the help of a biocatalyst, an enzyme, known as reverse transcriptase, this extraordinary feat can occur (described in greater detail under Acquired Immune Deficiencies in chapter 14, Immune Deficiencies). This property of oncornaviruses has given rise to the alternative name of retrovirus for this group. The newly formed viral DNA

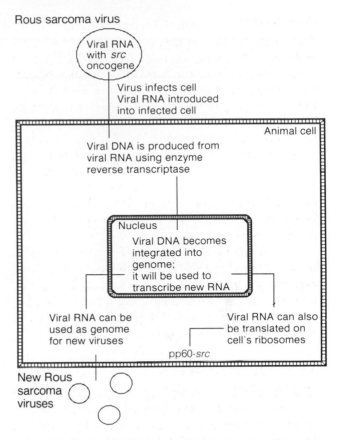

FIGURE 17.4 Events leading to oncogene expression. Retrovirus genes must first be converted into DNA before being incorporated into the host genome. Once incorporated, these genes can be transcribed. As viral genes, the RNA produced can be used to produce new viruses. Alternatively, as *oncogene* transcripts, they can function as mRNA and be translated to yield oncogene proteins, for example, pp60-*src*, the protein kinase encoded in the *src* gene of the Rous sarcoma virus. (Adapted from Bishop, J. M. Oncogenes. *Scientific American* **246**:80, 1982.)

becomes integrated or inserted into the DNA of the host cell, and the two genomes coexist in relative synchrony. The viral oncogene becomes rapidly active, once integration takes place, and readily dominates the activity of the other genes.

In the Rous avian sarcoma system, a single viral oncogene (called *src*) transcribes the code for a specific protein to be formed, which is referred to as pp60v-*src* (fig. 17.4). This protein apparently causes a normal cell to be transformed into a cancerous cell. The transformation protein was called pp60v-*src* because it is a

TABLE 17.4 Some Oncogenes and Their Sites of Action

Class of Oncogene Product	Site of Action	Oncogene	Virus Source
Tyrosine-specific protein kinase	Plasma membrane	src	Chicken sarcoma
		yes	Chicken sarcoma
		fps	Chicken sarcoma
		abl	Mouse leukemia
	Cytoskeleton (?)	fes	Cat sarcoma
	Undefined	ros	Chicken sarcoma
		fgr	Cat sarcoma
Potential protein kinase	Membranes	erb-B	Chicken leukemia
		fms	Cat sarcoma
	Cytoplasm	raf	Mouse sarcoma
		mos	Mouse sarcoma
		mil	Chicken carcinoma
Growth factor	Secreted	sis	Monkey sarcoma
GTP-binding protein	Plasma membrane	Ha-ras	Rat sarcoma
		Ki-ras	Rat sarcoma
		N-ras*	—
Nuclear-binding protein	Nucleus (DNA ?)	myb	Chicken leukemia
		myc	Chicken leukemia
		ski	Chicken sarcoma
		fos	Mouse sarcoma
		B-lym†	—
Unclassified	Undefined	erb-A	Chicken leukemia
		ets	Chicken leukemia
		rel	Turkey leukemia

*Not isolated from a retrovirus, but oncogene or proto-oncogene has been identified with human leukemia and carcinoma, although not caused by a virus.
†Not isolated from a retrovirus, but oncogene or proto-oncogene has been identified with human and chicken lymphomas, although not caused by a virus.
Source: Adapted and modified from Hunter, T. The proteins of oncogenes. *Scientific American,* August, 1984.

phosphoprotein (pp) with a molecular mass of 60,000 daltons (60) and is derived from a sarcoma virus gene (v-src). The avian sarcoma oncogene, src, is one of many oncogenes that have been identified (table 17.4).

This RNA virus can reproduce in the cell and be released in the process of transformation. Thus, not only can the released virus transform more fresh cells, but the transformed cell can also replicate and give rise to identical cancerous copies of itself. As noted above, DNA viruses do not replicate in the cells that they transform. Accordingly, cell-free extracts of DNA virus-induced tumors do not contain viruses, whereas similar extracts from RNA virus-induced tumors do contain viruses. These points are important to keep in mind for our later consideration of immunological control (chapter 18, Tumor Immunology).

Oncogenes and Antioncogenes

Transformation of a normal cell into a cancer cell can be considered the result of either a somatic mutation or a disturbance in the regulation of proliferation and differentiation. Chemical and physical carcinogens transform the cell through somatic mutation; they alter the DNA. The threshold and error accumulation theories presume distortion of the normal expression of the differentiated character of the affected cells. Tumor viruses induce cancer through mutation as well; however, they accomplish this by adding new DNA rather than altering existing DNA.

Two additional hypotheses for oncogenesis have emerged that are similar in that neither requires any alteration of the genetic composition of the cells that undergo transformation. These are the plasmagene theory and the oncogene theory. They contrast in that the plasmagene theory proposes that the initial transformation occurs through somatic alteration, whereas the oncogene theory requires only a special modification in the pattern of gene expression by the transformed cell.

In his *plasmagene theory,* Darlington (1948) suggested that the transformed cell might have experienced some extragenic mutation or modification that was heritable. According to this scheme, cytoplasmic or membrane factors that could be passed on intact through mitosis were responsible for the traits of the transformed cells. Support for this hypothesis came from a variety of organisms, mostly invertebrates, in which patterns of cytoplasmic inheritance could be demonstrated during embryonic development. Sonneborn provided even stronger support for this hypothesis by demonstrating, in 1964, that certain surgically induced cell surface alterations could be inherited in paramecia.

More recently, another hypothesis for cellular transformation has been proposed that does not require any alteration in the genetic constitution of the affected cell. The **oncogene theory,** formulated by Huebner and Todaro in 1969, proposes that the information for oncogenic proteins (the same as are induced by retroviruses) is included within the DNA of normal cells. In a sense, normal cells already contain latent viruses. Although these oncogenes are carried from cell generation to cell generation, there is no manifestation of the traits of cancer because these genes are not ordinarily expressed. It is only when they are activated, and expressed, that transformation of a normal cell into a tumor cell occurs. These oncogene-like sequences that are used by normal cells, but which can be shifted to cancerous expression, are now called proto-oncogenes. The oncogene hypothesis currently enjoys great popularity and broad support.

Numerous oncogenes have been characterized from retroviruses (table 17.4). Retroviruses have also been recovered from tumor cells and have been shown to be capable of reinfection. In addition, oncogenes have been found associated with some tumors that have not been shown to be caused by viruses. Examples of these include *abl* and *myb* with human leukemias; *mos* with mouse leukemia; Ha-*ras* with human and rat carcinoma; Ki-*ras* with human carcinoma, leukemia, and sarcoma; N-*ras* with human leukemia and carcinoma; *myc* with human lymphoma, and B-*lym* with chicken and human lymphomas. However, the association of retrovirus oncogenes with transformed (cancerous) cells is not sufficient proof that inherent oncogenes exist or that they can cause cancer.

Evidence that oncogenes can cause cancer was provided by DeLorbe and Luciw. They isolated the *src* oncogene from Rous sarcoma virus, cloned it, then introduced it into normal cells (fig. 17.5). Cells infected with this cloned gene were transformed, thus demonstrating that a single oncogene was capable of inducing oncogenic transformation.

In the early 1970s, **James Bishop, Harold Varmus,** and their co-workers sought oncogene sequences in normal cells using radioactively labeled v-*src* RNA probes. If an oncogene existed in normal cells, then there should be a sequence in the DNA that was complementary to the probe. Their experiments found that such a sequence existed. This "gene" was designated c-*src* to differentiate it from the viral oncogene. Note the prefix used in each case: v-*src* denotes the viral oncogene and c-*src* denotes the cellular oncogene. Further exploration of the "oncogene" sequence in the normal cells disclosed some startling revelations: (1) the cellular gene was divided into several domains, (2) there was considerable conservation of the gene sequence among varied vertebrate groups (fish, birds, and mammals), and (3) the gene was actually active in normal cells. For their efforts in defining oncogenes and their roles in regulating cell function, Bishop and Varmus were awarded the 1989 Nobel Prize for Physiology or Medicine.

Within the last few years, some genes have been described whose absence, rather than expression, is associated with oncogenic transformation. These genes have been called **antioncogenes** or **tumor suppressor genes.** These genes appear to play a role as *negative regulators of cell proliferation.* When these genes fail to act, suppression of proliferation is lifted. Consequently, inappropriate proliferation occurs. Thus, the normal expression of these genes is incompatible with tumor growth; hence their designation as tumor suppressor genes.

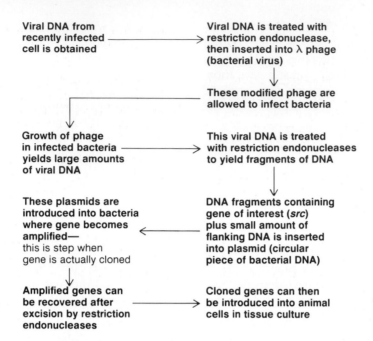

Viral DNA from recently infected cell is obtained → **Viral DNA is treated with restriction endonuclease, then inserted into λ phage (bacterial virus)**

↓

These modified phage are allowed to infect bacteria

Growth of phage in infected bacteria yields large amounts of viral DNA → **This viral DNA is treated with restriction endonucleases to yield fragments of DNA**

↓

These plasmids are introduced into bacteria where gene becomes amplified— this is step when gene is actually cloned ← **DNA fragments containing gene of interest (src) plus small amount of flanking DNA is inserted into plasmid (circular piece of bacterial DNA)**

↓

Amplified genes can be recovered after excision by restriction endonucleases → **Cloned genes can then be introduced into animal cells in tissue culture**

FIGURE 17.5 Procedure for isolating, cloning, and testing suspected oncogenes. Oncogenes can be recovered from infected cells using a procedure such as the one outlined. When this particular procedure was followed using the *src* gene, the cloned gene was found to be capable of transforming normal cells into tumor cells and the oncogene product, pp60-*src,* was recoverable.

Transformation Proteins

In order for these oncogenes to exert their influence, they must be translated into functional proteins. The protein products of these genes then bring about changes in cellular function. To date, the means through which these **transformation proteins** alter cellular behavior seem limited to only a few mechanisms (see table 17.4). These few mechanisms include (1) protein phosphorylation, (2) metabolic regulation of GTP-binding proteins, (3) control of gene expression, and (4) acting as growth factors.

A large number (up to half of those listed in table 17.4) of transformation proteins exert their influence through phosphorylations, adding phosphate groups to particular amino acids in target proteins. Phosphorylation of a protein leads to an alteration in the functional status of that molecule. Proteins that mediate phosphate transfer to other proteins, using ATP as a substrate, are known as protein kinases. These protein kinases can be further classified on the basis of the amino acids that receive the phosphate. Many transformation proteins characterized thus far appear to be *tyrosine- or serine/threonine-specific protein kinases.*

Although several oncogenes are known to code for protein kinases, the identities and functions of the proteins that are phosphorylated are not as well characterized. Nevertheless, some candidates do exist. For example, three potential target sites for the Rous sarcoma virus transformation protein (p60*src*) have been proposed by different investigators. Erickson, Cantley, and their associates at Harvard University have suggested that p60*src* phosphorylates the lipid phosphatidylinositol (a major component of cell membranes). This, in turn, leads to accelerated production of diacylglycerol, which is implicated in the activation of cellular proliferation (mitosis) in several systems. J. M. Bishop, at the University of California at San Francisco, suggested that p60*src* might dismantle adhesion plaques by phosphorylating one or several of their component proteins. This leads to decreased cell adhesion, which some believe can contribute to metastasis. Both of these proposals have the cell membrane as the immediate site of action for the protein kinases. In contrast, Tony Hunter, of the University of California at San Diego, has suggested that protein kinases, like p60*src* and *fes,* might alter the cytoskeleton of the cell. Through phosphorylation of cytoskeletal proteins like vinculin, cell shape and function can be affected.

In addition to suggesting potential sites of action for the protein kinases, other studies have excluded certain proteins as likely targets for these transformation proteins. For example, since cancer cells are known to produce large amounts of lactic acid, the enzymes involved in regulating glucose breakdown through glycolysis would be likely candidates. However, examination of the major enzymes of this pathway revealed little phosphorylation of tyrosine residues by p60*src*. Since this transformation protein is a tyrosine-specific kinase, it seems unlikely that p60*src* acts by altering the rate of glycolysis.

Other transformation proteins alter cellular function through mechanisms that involve tight binding of GTP. The result of this binding is the intracellular transmission of a signal. Ordinarily, this would be encountered as a step in relaying information following hormonal stimulation through a cell-surface receptor. For example, glucagon stimulation of liver cells to promote gluconeogenesis (formation of glucose from lactic acid or amino acids) or glycogenolysis (breakdown of glycogen) leads to the production of cyclic adenosine monophosphate (cAMP) as an intracellular second messenger. This glucagon-stimulated production of cAMP can be enhanced by reactions involving binding of GTP to a "G protein" in this system. In the case of transformation proteins that bind GTP, this might lead to the generation of a continuous, rather than a regulated, signal. The family of proteins encoded by the *ras* oncogenes seems to be of this type.

A third way in which transformation proteins alter cellular function is through modifications in gene expression. These transformation proteins can be isolated from the nucleus of affected cells, rather than from the cytoplasm or in association with cellular membranes, as would be the case with the two groups discussed above. For example, products of the *fos, jun, myc,* and *myb* oncogenes fall into this category. Since these substances play a role in regulating transcriptonal activity, they are designated *transcription factors.*

In a very few instances, the oncogene products are proteins that appear to *function like growth factors.* The product of the *sis,* and related, oncogenes exemplify this group. Their action appears to be mediated by phosphorylation of molecules at specific sites in the infected cells that leads to a stimulation of proliferation—which mimics that induced by other growth factors such as EGF and PDGF. Both EGF and PDGF appear to increase the amount of phosphorylation of tyrosine residues in their target cells.

The *sis* oncogene encodes a protein that is almost identical to PDGF. Therefore, it can act like a growth factor, inducing proliferation in responsive target cells. Other oncogenes mimic growth factor action through other mechanisms. For example, the *erb*-B oncogene produces a protein that resembles the EGF receptor, at least in part. It is thus able to interact with the intracellular machinery activated by this receptor in evoking cellular proliferation. The proteins of the *src* and *ros* genes act even farther downstream. As mentioned above, these proteins are kinases and are directly involved in phosphorylating other proteins. Thus, these oncogene products might cause effects similar to those of growth factors by phosphorylating the same, or related, target proteins, thereby giving rise to an inappropriate activation of cellular proliferation.

Oncogenes and Normal Cells

In the early 1970s, Huebner and Todaro, of the National Cancer Institute, proposed the oncogene hypothesis of cancer formation. They suggested that all vertebrate cells, including human cells, contain oncogenes as part of their DNA. These oncogenes had been acquired through virus infection(s) of ancestors, thousands and perhaps millions of years ago. Somehow they survived evolutionary pressures, suggesting that the oncogenes had some selective value to the host organism. It was further proposed that these oncogenes were normally quiescent or innocuous, but could be stimulated into activity by a carcinogenic agent, whereupon they could transform normal cells to cancer cells.

Studies of the Rous sarcoma gene, *src,* led to the realization that oncogenes did appear in the genomes of eukaryotic cells. However, of greater interest was the demonstration by Bishop's group that the c-*src* gene consisted of several interrupted sequences when compared with the v-*src* gene. That is, the gene as it appeared in eukaryotic cells (chickens) consisted of seven exons (DNA sequences coding for parts of the gene product) separated by six introns (DNA sequences that do not appear translated in the final product) (fig. 17.6).

Subsequent studies indicated that the c-*src* gene was active, not silent, in normal cells, although the protein product (pp60c-*src*) was formed in very small quantities. Studies of other cellular oncogenes have revealed a similar pattern of relatively low-level activity in normal cells. Moreover, the products of several of these oncogenes (e.g., c-*sis,* c-*erb* B, c-*fms,* and c-*fos*) have been implicated in mediating cellular responses to growth factors or mitogens. Consequently, these genes are activated only periodically.

These observations have given rise to the interesting proposal that the oncogenes originated in eukaryotic cells. Their presence in oncogenic retroviruses, therefore, is believed to have occurred through later incorporation into the viral genome after excision of the introns and splicing of the exons.

Tumor Suppressor Genes

In retinoblastoma (RB) it was learned the absence of a gene was responsible for tumor expression (see highlight 17.3). This led to the realization that genes exist that exert negative influence on tumor expression. These genes have been alternatively designated as tumor suppressor genes, since they suppress tumor growth, or antioncogenes, because they seemingly oppose the actions of oncogenes which promote tumor growth.

There is evidence that tumor suppressor genes can function in one of three ways: (1) maintenance of chromosomal integrity, (2) regulation of differentiation and senescence, and (3) regulation of proliferation. For example, in Bloom's syndrome, a defective DNA ligase apparently exists that is incapable of properly repairing DNA. This is associated with an increased incidence of chromosomal abnormality.

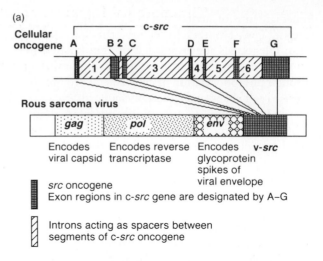

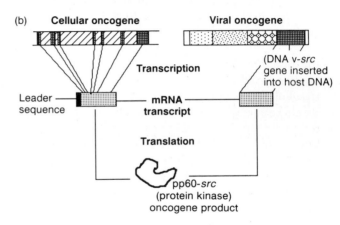

FIGURE 17.6 Relationship between cellular and viral *src* oncogenes and their products. (*a*) The c-*src* gene occurs as an interrupted DNA sequence (exons) with intervening (introns) regions of DNA. In contrast, the v-*src* gene contains only the exon portions of the c-*src* gene. (*b*) In producing the oncogene product, pp60-*src,* the exon portion of the c-*src* gene is used to transcribe the functional mRNA molecule. The v-*src* gene, after incorporation into the host genome, is used to transcribe an equivalent mRNA; however, there are no introns to be deleted. Both mRNAs can be translated to yield the same functional protein product.

Deletion (or mutation) of the RB gene is associated with expression of RB, while underphosphorylation of the RB gene product has been implicated in senescence of fibroblasts *in vitro.* From other studies it appear that the RB gene product might be involved in the regulation of proliferation in several cell systems.

Putative tumor suppressor genes have been localized to several chromosomes (table 17.5). Several of

TABLE 17.5 Chromosomal Locations of Selected Putative Tumor Suppressor Genes

Putative Gene	Chromosomal Location	Confirmed by Genetic Studies	Gene Cloned
Cutaneous melanoma	1p	**Yes**	No
Neuroblastoma	1p	No	No
Breast carcinoma	1q	No	No
Uveal melanoma	2	No	No
Cervical carcinoma	3p	No	No
Renal cell carcinoma	3p	**Yes**	No
Small-cell lung carcinoma	3p	No	No
Hepatic carcinoma	4q	No	No
Colorectal carcinoma	5q	**Yes**	No
Familial adenomatous polyposis	5q	No	No
Ovarian carcinoma	6q	No	No
Glioblastoma multiforme	10	No	No
Adrenal adenoma	11p	**Yes**	No
Breast carcinoma	11p	No	No
Cervical carcinoma	11p	No	No
Embryonal rhabdomyosarcoma	11p	**Yes**	No
Hepatoblastoma	11p	**Yes**	No
Transitional-cell bladder carcinoma	11p	No	No
Wilms' tumor	11p	**Yes**	**Yes**
Insulinoma	11q	**Yes**	No
Ductal breast carcinoma	13q	No	No
Osteosarcoma	13q	**Yes**	No
Retinoblastoma	13q	**Yes**	**Yes**
Small-cell lung carcinoma	13q	No	No
Stomach carcinoma	13q	No	No
Astrocytoma	17p	No	No
Breast carcinoma	17p	No	No
Colorectal carcinoma	17p	No	No
Osteosarcoma	17p	No	No
Colorectal carcinoma	18q	**Yes**	**Yes**
Meningioma	22q	**Yes**	No
Neurofibroma	22q	**Yes**	No
Pheochromocytoma	22q	No	No

Source: Miller, J. A. Genes that protect against cancer. *BioScience* **40**:563, 1990.

these have been confirmed by genetic studies; however, only three have been cloned thus far. These are the genes for RB, colorectal cancer, and Wilms' tumor.

Oncogenes, Antioncogenes, and Cancer

Cellular oncogenes and antioncogenes (tumor suppressor genes) are normal components of typical cells that are ordinarily expressed at low levels. These genes, and their products, appear to be involved in the regulation and expression of growth by normal cells. Their inappropriate expression and failure to be controlled is the characteristic feature of their expression in transformed, or cancerous, cells. How does such perversion of normal function and expression occur?

In the case of **virus-induced carcinogenesis,** there appear to be two contrasting explanations for this transformation in behavior as follows:

1. The mutational hypothesis, which suggests that there are subtle, but extremely important, differences between cellular and viral oncogenes. This hypothesis argues that although the gene products encoded within these genes are very similar, they nevertheless have different targets within the cell. The result of these differences is an altered pattern of cellular behavior.
2. The dosage hypothesis, which proposes that there is a difference in the amount of oncogene products associated with transformation. For example, following infection by an oncogenic retrovirus the affected cell is overwhelmed by transformation proteins and is "forced" into a cancerous state.

Tumorigenic activation of cellular oncogenes can be accomplished through **mutations.** One form of mutational change, called insertional mutagenesis, occurs as the result of introduction of viral genes. This brings the cellular oncogenes under the influence of viral promoters or regulators. This form of mutagenesis can occur whether or not the tumorigenic virus possesses an oncogene. In a similar vein, other carcinogens might induce mutations in a target cell, leading to activation of cellular oncogenes or alteration of a second gene that regulates oncogene expression.

Modification of the chromosomes through translocations, inversions, deletions, and amplifications can also lead to transformation of a normal cell into a cancer cell. For example, the Philadelphia chromosome, a diagnostic indicator of chronic myelogenous leukemia, involves a reciprocal translocation of portions of chromosomes 9 and 22. This repositioning of chromosomal material fuses a segment of the oncogene c-*abl* with a new locus designated *bcr* (breakpoint cluster region). The result of this fusion is a protein that retains the functional specificity of the c-*abl* gene product, but which is enzymatically more active. Thus, enzymatic activity, rather than gene expression, is affected; but the ultimate consequences are the same nevertheless. Breast cancer provides an example in which gene amplification can occur. In this system, the oncogene HER-2/*neu* codes for a cell-surface receptor for an unidentified growth factor. Through amplification of this gene, the number of receptors is greatly increased. This leads to an enhanced response to the growth factor and exaggerated growth of the breast tissues. It is of some interest to note that there is an apparent correlation between the degree of amplification and the prognosis for the patient—specifically, the greater the amplification of HER-2/*neu* the poorer is the prognosis.

On the other hand, cell transformation associated with dysfunctioning antioncogenes arises as the result of decreased gene expression. For example, in the case of RB, expression of the tumor state occurs because of a failure in gene expression. The RB gene is a recessive gene located in band q14 on chromosome 13. When both alleles of the cell are recessive, some product that affects growth control does not appear and transformation into a tumor cell occurs. Alternatively, if the recessive state of this same gene occurs in bone cells, then osteosarcoma will result. In the case of hereditary RB, the child is born with one recessive allele and one normal allele. If a mutation affects the normal allele, growth control is lost in the affected cell. For a normal child, mutations would have to alter both alleles within the same cell before transformation could occur. (See highlight 17.3 for additional information about the RB system.)

Endogenous Oncornavirus Genes

Thus far we have briefly considered exogenous tumor viruses that spread horizontally, that is, from one animal to another. Surprisingly, some oncornaviruses are inherited and transmitted vertically, namely through germ or sex cells (i.e., spermatozoa and ova). Viral genetic information that is an integral part of the DNA of normal cells is said to be endogenous. It is believed that cellular genes determine whether or not endogenous viral genes are expressed.

Many vertebrates including chickens, mice, cats, and baboons possess endogenous viral gene sequences. Some can have multiple endogenous virus genes. These genes are often present in the sex or germ cells and are therefore inherited. Physically or chemically induced tumors in these animals can be shown, by hybridization techniques, to contain virus-specified DNA sequences. However, most endogenous viruses that are extracted from transformed cells or tumor-bearing animals have a very low disease-producing potential. Moreover, the majority of the endogenous viruses have not been shown to transform cells in culture or to be oncogenic in the host. The significance, if any, of inherited oncornavirus genes for normal cell function or natural oncogenesis, therefore, remains unclear.

METASTASIS

One of the most dreaded features of cancer is the property of **metastasis,** *the ability of tumor cells to dislodge from the primary tumor and seed secondary tumors at other tissue sites.* This is a characteristic of malignant, but not benign, tumors. Metastases are more common for larger tumor masses than for small ones. In addition, there appear to be preferred sites of metastasis for different primary tumors. For example, lung tumors frequently tend to metastasize to the brain, while adenocarcinoma of the breast metastasizes to regional lymph nodes, lungs, liver, bones, adrenals, and ovaries (in descending order of frequency). Other tumors, like melanoma, are more unpredictable. Since the dislodged tumor cells must be conveyed to the new "seed site," it is not unreasonable to find that sites of secondary tumors are located downstream (along lymphatic or vascular channels) from the site of the primary tumor. Alternatively, metastasis can occur if the tumor cells successfully seed sites within body cavities, giving rise to ascites tumors.

In order for metastasis to occur, a number of steps must be completed successfully. These represent hurdles over which many tumor cells cannot rise and, thus, help to limit the frequency of metastatic tumors encountered. The *steps that must be accomplished in metastasis* are (1) invasion of the surrounding tissue, (2) penetration into vessels (lymphatic or vascular) or body cavities, (3) dislodgement from the original tumor mass, (4) transport to and invasion of a new site, and (5) appropriate manipulation of the new environment.

The means whereby tumor cells invade the surrounding tissues is not fully understood. Simple physical crowding as a result of a higher rate of proliferation of the tumor cells, however, is not sufficient by itself to account for the penetration that occurs. Efforts to find other explanations have led to the discovery that many tumors have greater concentrations of certain enzymes, cathepsins and hyaluronidase. These enzymes degrade extracellular matrix and can loosen tissue associations. The activities of these enzymes are also not sufficient to fully account for the invasiveness of the tumor. Other, as yet unidentified, factors must also be employed.

Penetration of the vessel wall is perhaps facilitated by these enzymes or by other factors that reduce the intimacy of association among the endothelial cells of the blood vessels. Dislodgement of individual tumor cells from the parent mass can be explained by the reduced binding affinity that tumor cells possess. Normal tissue cells will associate with each other in aggregates if placed in suspension cultures. When cells from different tissues are mixed in these cultures, cells from the same tissue will sort out from those of other tissues. The tightness of the association displayed by the cells is a measure of their affinity. Through this type of manipulation, we can rank cells from different tissues on the basis of higher to lower affinities. Compared with normal cells, cancer cells do not show any marked tendency to associate with one another (fig. 17.7).

On The Trail of a Cancer Gene

R **B** is a tumor of the eye. It appears in one out of 20,000 births, afflicting children under four years of age. Although first described in 1597, it was not until 1886 that it was perceived that RB was an inheritable form of cancer. Since that time, *two forms* of RB have come to be recognized: one that is inherited and the other that occurs spontaneously. These two forms differ in two important features. First, inherited RB is usually manifested before the end of the first year of life, whereas the spontaneous form does not usually emerge until approximately 18 months. Second, the inherited form characteristically presents with several tumors in both eyes, while children with spontaneous RB typically have but a single tumor in one eye.

Genetic analysis had revealed that the RB gene was probably in the q14 band of chromosome 13 since this region always seemed to be defective in RB. All the cells of children with hereditary RB had defects in chromosome 13, which also rendered them prone to the manifestation of osteosarcoma. In contrast, only the affected cells from children with spontaneous RB displayed defects in chromosome 13.

The q14 region of chromosome 13 contains 5 million DNA base pairs and might be expected to hold some 250 genes. Nevertheless, with the use of recombinant DNA technology, the RB gene was pursued through the 1970s in the same way that other oncogenes were being pursued. Ultimately, it was determined that the RB gene was a recessive gene and that its *absence* (or failure to perform), rather than its activation, gave rise to the tumorous state.

Thus, the *two-hit hypothesis,* first proposed by Alfred Knudson in 1971, now meant that both alleles for this trait had to be silenced in order for RB to occur. Children with hereditary RB start life with one allele already compromised.

Intense competition arose among several laboratories to isolate, clone, and sequence the RB gene. In October 1986, after years of effort making DNA probes to different portions of the q14 region, the Weinberg (Whitehead Institute at MIT) and Dryja (Massachusetts Eye and Ear Infirmary) laboratories reported that they had isolated and cloned the RB gene. Their principal evidence was the demonstration that two patients, one with RB and the other with osteosarcoma, lacked a portion of chromosome 13 which occurred within the cloned gene. Using the more painstaking approach of "walking along" the chromosome, in March 1987, workers in Lee's laboratory (University of California at San Diego) confirmed the location of the gene in chromosome region 13q14. Confirmation of the identity of their gene consisted of the demonstration that the mRNA encoded by the gene was either not detectable, or that a reduced mRNA was variably expressed in six RB cases examined. In contrast,

---

Transport to a new site is accomplished in many cases passively; that is, the tumor cells are merely borne to the new sites by the flow of blood or lymph. This, nevertheless, exacts a severe toll since only a small fraction of the cells that dislodge ever survive to establish a secondary tumor.

Actually seeding the new site requires that the tumor cells pass, once more, through the vessel wall to gain entry to a new tissue environment. For this to occur, the tumor cells must stop their migration through the circulation. This can be accomplished in a few ways. If a small tumor mass is circulating, the mass might actually become trapped in a capillary through which it cannot pass. Alternatively, smaller masses and individual tumor cells might induce the formation of small fibrin clots in which they can become enmeshed and then attached to the vessel wall. There is also evidence that tumor cells can interact with extracellular matrix components, like fibronectin, and become anchored to a position on a vessel wall. Determination of sites where tumor cells will attach is not necessarily a random process. Tumor cells possess a variety of receptors in their membranes. Certain of these

five other neural tumors, normal retina, and placenta expressed the full-length mRNA. Moreover, Lee's group reported sequencing of the gene. Their results disclosed that the RB gene contains over 12 exons and encodes a 4.6 kilobase mRNA. A hypothetical protein containing 816 amino acids, but as yet undefined function, is the proposed gene product.

More recent attention has been directed at determining the role of the RB gene in normal cell function. Certain of these studies suggest that phosphorylation of the RB gene product is important for regulation of cellular proliferation. In addition, age-related changes in phosphorylation of the RB gene product might contribute to senescence.

Angier, N. Light case on a darkling gene. *Discover* **84,** March 1987.

Friend, S. H., Bernards, R., Rogelj, S., et al. A human DNA segment with properties of the gene that predisposes to retinoblastoma and osteosarcoma. *Nature* **323:**643, 1986.

Goldstein, S. Replicative senescence: the human fibroblast comes of age. *Science* **249:**1129, 1990.

Lee, W.-H., Bookstein, R., Hong, F., et al. Human retinoblastoma susceptibility gene: cloning, identification and sequence. *Science* **235:**1394, 1987.

Mihara, K., Cao, X.-H., Yen, A., et al. Cell-cycle-dependent regulation of phosphorylation of the human retinoblastoma gene product. *Science* **246:**1300, 1989.

Stein, G. H., Berson, M., and Gordon, L. Failure to phosphorylate the retinoblastoma gene product in senescent human fibroblasts. *Science* **249:**666, 1990.

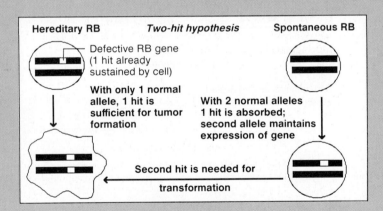

Hereditary RB   *Two-hit hypothesis*   **Spontaneous RB**

— Defective RB gene (1 hit already sustained by cell)

With only 1 normal allele, 1 hit is sufficient for tumor formation

With 2 normal alleles 1 hit is absorbed; second allele maintains expression of gene

Second hit is needed for transformation

FIGURE 17.B   Expression of retinoblastoma.

might actually be employed by tumor cells during metastasis to identify suitable environments. Such interaction between membrane receptors of tumor cells and other tissues could account for the preferential metastasis of tumors to particular sites.

Once attached, passage through the vessel wall can then be achieved. Some tumor cells have been shown to be capable of inducing changes in the adhesion between vascular endothelial cells, causing them to create a gap in the vessel wall. The tumor cells can then migrate through this portal.

Survival of the tumor cells, and the successful formation of a secondary tumor, require manipulation of the environment to the tumor's ends. This new tumor must now confront the same problems originally encountered by the parent tumor, in fact by the cell that was originally transformed. If the environment is hospitable, survival of the tumor cell will not present any serious obstacle. However, in order for the tumor to grow, the needs of all of the cells of the tumor mass must be satisfied. This will require modification of the environment.

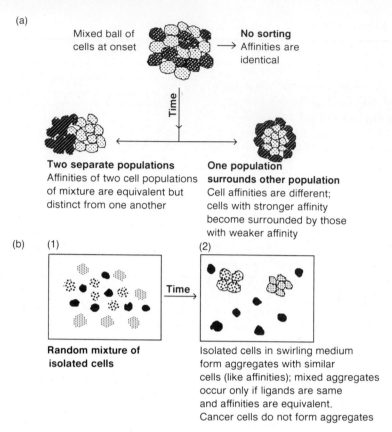

(a)

Mixed ball of
cells at onset

No sorting
Affinities are
identical

Time

Two separate populations
Affinities of two cell populations
of mixture are equivalent but
distinct from one another

**One population
surrounds other population**
Cell affinities are different;
cells with stronger affinity
become surrounded by those
with weaker affinity

(b) (1)   (2)

Time

**Random mixture of
isolated cells**

Isolated cells in swirling medium
form aggregates with similar
cells (like affinities); mixed aggregates
occur only if ligands are same
and affinities are equivalent.
Cancer cells do not form aggregates

FIGURE 17.7 Cellular adhesion affinities in cell sorting and aggregation. (*a*) When cells from different tissues are mixed into an aggregate and allowed to sort, one of three results can be obtained: (1) they remain randomized, (2) they sort into two populations that might eventually separate from each other, (3) one population surrounds the other. (*b*) If isolated cells are placed in a rotating vessel, their occasional collisions lead to the formation of aggregates. Cells from the same tissue preferentially associate because they possess the same adhesion ligands and affinities. Cells from different tissues aggregate if their affinities are closely matched and they possess similar ligands. However, malignant cells display diminished adhesion and do not aggregate.

All cells must remain close to a capillary bed in order to obtain nutrients and oxygen. This imposes a serious constraint on solid tumor growth. Once a tumor has grown to be approximately 1 to 2 mm³, further growth is not possible. This obstacle is overcome by tumors through the elaboration of substances called tumor angiogenesis factors (TAFs). TAF causes the production of new blood vessels. These new vessels in the tumor restore the necessary proximity between the tumor cells and the blood supply. As a result, further growth of the tumor becomes possible.

Several substances have been identified that have angiogenic properties (table 17.6). These factors affect the proliferation or motility of vascular endothelial cells, which are required for the formation of new blood vessels. Certain of these factors, the fibroblast growth factors (FGFs) and TGF-α, appear to act directly on the endothelial cells. Others exert their influence indirectly, possibly by inducing the mobilization of growth factors from other sources such as macrophages and vascular endothelial cells. Angiogenic factors have been found in normal tissues where they seem to be closely regulated. In addition, excessive expression of angiogenic potential has been found in several nonneoplastic diseases.

TABLE 17.6 Substances with Angiogenic Properties

Substance	Actions
Direct-Acting Factors	
Fibroblast growth factors (both acidic and basic)	Stimulate proliferation and motility of endothelial cells
Transforming growth factor-α	Stimulates proliferation of endothelial cells; effect on motility has not been determined
Transforming growth factor-β	Stimulates increases in macrophages, fibroblasts, collagen production, and new capillary formation *in vivo; inhibits* proliferation of endothelial cells in culture; effect on motility has not been determined
Indirect-Acting Factors	
Angiogenin	Has no effect on proliferation of endothelial cells; effect on motility has not been determined; target remains unknown
Polar lipids (from 3T3-derived adipocytes)	Stimulate motility of endothelial cells; have no effect on proliferation
Prostaglandins (E series)	Have no effect on endothelial cell proliferation; effect on motility has not been determined; have indirect action exerted through macrophages (?)
Wound fluid	Stimulates motility of endothelial cells; has no effect on proliferation

Source: Adapted from Folkman, J., and Klagsbrun, M. Angiogenic factors. *Science* **235:**442, 1987.

CANCER THERAPY

According to the American Cancer Society, cancer management is becoming increasingly individualized with respect to detection and the type or combination of therapies being employed. Many cancers are being cured because of recent therapeutic advances. These cancers include acute lymphocytic leukemia, adult myelogenous leukemia, Hodgkin's disease, histiocytic lymphoma, Burkitt's lymphoma, nodular mixed lymphoma, Ewing's sarcoma, Wilms' tumor, rhabdomyosarcoma, choriocarcinoma, testicular cancer, ovarian cancer, breast cancer, and osteogenic sarcoma. Unfortunately, little progress has been made in treating the most deadly form of the disease, lung cancer, which of course is largely preventable.

Surgery

Effective removal of malignant tumors by surgery depends upon early detection, before metastasis has occurred. Skin cancer, for example, is usually detected earlier than most other cancers and can be effectively treated by surgery. Obviously, the goal of any surgical procedure is the removal of every single cancer cell.

Some tumors, however, occur in multiple foci or locations, which complicates total removal of tumor cells. Nevertheless, with the aid of improved diagnostic procedures and laser instrumentation, surgery has become more precise. This increased precision can lessen the consequences for a patient. Many patients with bone cancer are apparently being treated successfully by removing and replacing a section of bone, rather than by amputating a complete limb.

In addition, surgery is often combined with other regimens, for example, drug treatment or radiation. Intense drug therapy is sometimes given before surgery, for example, in the treatment of children with bone tumors. Drugs and radiation are also being used following surgery to destroy residual tumor cells that may not have been removed. These approaches are intended to improve the overall effectiveness of surgical intervention. Nevertheless, reduction of tumor load is also a rationale for tumor extirpation.

Radiotherapy

Both x-rays and radioactive substances, such as cobalt-60, are used in radiotherapy. Postoperative irradiation, as noted above, might be used in attempts to eliminate cells not removed by surgery. Irradiation can also be used to destroy tumors that are inoperable for one reason or another. Most common tumors, such as those of the lungs, breasts, and colon, however, are not well controlled by irradiation. Accordingly, hyperthermia, or the superheating of the body tissues, can be used to increase the effectiveness of radiotherapy and chemotherapy. Nevertheless, for certain, well-defined forms of cancer, perhaps pinpointed by ultrasound, radiotherapy may be chosen by the therapist. If the cancer has metastasized, however, the problem becomes much more difficult.

Ionizing radiation is usually more destructive to rapidly dividing cancer cells than to most normal cells. Moreover, some tumor cells are more radiosensitive than others. However, normal cells have a differential radiosensitivity as well. As examples, a nondividing nerve cell is quite radioresistant when compared with either blood-forming cells in the bone marrow or the rapidly dividing cells that line the intestine, either of which may be more radiosensitive than a slower growing cancer cell.

Unfortunately, radiotherapy can produce radiation sickness: anemia, nausea, vomiting, diarrhea, hair loss (follicle damage), and damage to the bone marrow and intestinal mucosa. This occurs since ionizing radiation preferentially destroys actively dividing cells, normal as well as cancerous. Hence, radiotherapy of cancer suffers from a general lack of specificity. In view of the extreme radiosensitivity of lymphocytes, the immune response is generally depressed following radiotherapy, and patients are rendered more susceptible to infection. Irradiations can, unfortunately, also incite the formation of new tumors while being used to destroy tumor target tissue. The decision to use radiation must be carefully weighed by the cancer therapist.

Chemotherapy

Chemotherapy refers to the use of chemicals in the treatment of diseases such as cancer. Chemotherapy is perhaps the primary choice of treatment of cancer and can be employed as an ancillary measure in combination with other therapies. Ideally, drugs should selectively inhibit or destroy cancer cells and be harmless to normal cells. As yet, this ideal has not been realized,

although anticancer drugs, appropriately employed, cause more damage to cancer cells than to normal cells.

Selectivity is based on the premise that cancer cells are more metabolically active than most normal cells and, therefore, will be more sensitive to drug action. In principle, drugs are used that block DNA formation, bind and inactivate DNA, inhibit RNA formation, block protein synthesis, and/or inhibit cell division. These activities that are targeted for interruption are not peculiar to cancer cells and, therefore, normal actively dividing cells can likewise be injured. An antibiotic, such as penicillin, can inhibit bacterial cell wall synthesis, leaving host cells unharmed because they do not possess or require cell walls. Obviously, this antibiotic drug, used to treat certain infectious diseases, is more selective than one that blocks DNA synthesis—a process common to both cancer cells and normal cells.

Biochemical differences between cancerous and normal cells that might be exploited have been sought for decades. These differences might permit investigators to design and synthesize drugs that would affect only cancer cells. This search has met with little success.

Although side effects from the current lack of drug specificity tend to complicate the use of most chemotherapeutic agents, as many as 50 drugs have been proven effective against certain cancers. Others are continually being developed and tested, and attempts have also been made to develop specific drug delivery systems. A particular drug, for example, might be enclosed in a membrane package, which then could be coated with monoclonal Abs (MAbs) raised against cancer Ags. Theoretically the package, once introduced into the body, would "stick" specifically to cancer cells and "unload" the cytotoxic drug. In practice, however, phagocytes often engulfed the packages before they reached their tumor targets. Nevertheless, other avenues are constantly being explored.

Hormones

Some cancers are sensitive to hormones. Charles Brenton Huggins, a Nobel laureate (1966), was the first to demonstrate the importance of hormones in the development and treatment of cancers of the prostate and the breast. For example, some breast cancers require estrogens to grow and are actively inhibited by testosterone. Prostatic cancer can frequently be controlled by the administration of estrogens, often in combination with removal of the testes, the major source of testosterone.

Immunotherapy

To date, immunotherapy has only been selectively employed in the treatment of cancer. Results of clinical trials suggest that there is considerable promise in enlisting either the patient's own immune system or the immune components of an exogenous system to destroy cancer cells. Accordingly, immunological response modifiers, which manipulate the immune system and application of MAb technology for potential detection and treatment, are being intensely investigated. (See chapter 18, Tumor Immunology, for a further discussion of this topic.)

Cancer Cells to Normal Cells?

Tumor cells arise as a result of an alteration in cellular expression and behavior. These changes are stable and heritable. However, these are features of a process that normally occurs throughout development, namely differentiation. What is anomalous about the transformation that occurs during oncogenesis is that the change(s) produced a cell that did not fit into the "normal" pattern. Nevertheless, the question might be raised, Is this change irreversible?

In the case of cellular differentiation during development, it is not likely that a cell will retrace its steps. Thus, differentiation appears to be a one-way street toward ever-increasing specialization. Yet occasionally, conditions can be contrived that allow an expression of a somewhat earlier stage of development to be manifest. Such manifestations are extremely rare among mammals, but seem somewhat more commonplace among amphibians (during the process of epimorphic regeneration). Perhaps such a reversal of the events of transformation is not impossible.

For some tumors, transformation does not entail loss of differentiated features as much as loss of normal growth control. This applies to highly proliferative cells that remain immature. These cells, when transformed, fail to respond to signals that should direct them to differentiate. Current investigations suggest that these cancer cells might be "transformed" into essentially normal cells with appropriate treatment. As an example, human myeloid leukemia cells have been induced to differentiate into essentially normal cells upon exposure to phorbol esters. These present exciting possibilities yet to be realized at the clinical level.

CANCER PREVENTION

Since only a few prominent environmental agents cause most human cancers, it would appear more sensible to prevent cancer than to cure it. This is also the case with parasitic diseases. However, individuals faced with potential exposure to cancer-causing agents can use more help from the regulatory agencies having designated responsibility for the identification, regulation, and/or elimination of environmental carcinogens. For example, tobacco smoke, containing perhaps 2,000 chemicals, is probably the most important single source of environmental carcinogens—yet the production and use of tobacco products remain uncontrolled in most countries. In fact sale of tobacco, including export, may be government subsidized. Furthermore, government efforts to control carcinogens may be strongly opposed politically by agricultural and industrial lobbyists, for economic reasons.

Prescott and Flexer, authors of *Cancer, the Misguided Cell,* suggest that personal actions are the first line of defense against cancer. They recommend the following: "Don't smoke, drink alcohol only in moderation (and never when you smoke, if you must); avoid nonessential x-rays and other forms of radiation including excessive sunlight; eat a low fat, high fiber diet; avoid carcinogenic foods such as charred foods and charred meat in particular; and avoid occupations that entail exposure to known carcinogens." Sounds easy. But how many of us heed this advice?

SUMMARY

1. The incidence of cancer has progressively increased in recent years. The rate of cancer-related deaths has risen dramatically during this century, while the death rate for infectious diseases has dropped markedly. This seems to

correlate with (a) increased longevity, (b) greater prevalence of carcinogens in the environment, and (c) improved management of infectious diseases. [p. 428–429]

2. Carcinogens, or cancer-causing agents, are major factors in oncogenesis; nevertheless genetic predisposition or susceptibility also play important roles. [p. 429–430]

3. Tumors are masses of cells that have been diverted from their normal pattern of behavior. They arise through hyperplasia. [p. 430]

4. Hyperplasia represents growth resulting from increased cellular proliferation. This can occur as a normal response to external signals. In the formation of tumors, hyperplasia reflects an intrinsic disturbance. This leads to either (a) an increase in the growth fraction or (b) increased longevity or mitotic frequency. [p. 430–434]

5. Tumors can be benign or malignant. These can be discriminated by the extent to which they (a) lose the characteristic appearance of normal tissues, (b) behave atypically, and (c) metastasize (i.e., give rise to secondary tumors). Benign tumors are closer to normal and rarely metastasize. Malignant tumors differ radically from normal and frequently metastasize. [p. 434–436]

6. Cancer cells display four major biochemical departures from normal cells: (a) increased glycolytic activity, (b) biochemical convergence, (c) metabolic rigidity, and (d) inappropriate cell products. [p. 436]

7. Oncogenesis is the conversion of a normal cell into a cancerous cell. Numerous mechanisms for oncogenesis have been proposed. These suggest transformation by (a) chemical or physical induction, (b) attaining a transformation threshold, (c) accumulation of functional errors, (d) viral induction, or (e) oncogene/ antioncogene activity. [p. 437]

8. Chemical and physical induction often occurs through somatic mutations in a proliferating population. However, in certain instances, overstimulation by otherwise normal effectors can lead to permanently altered cellular behavior and hyperplasia. [p. 437–440]

9. The threshold and error accumulation hypotheses consider that cancerous transformation occurs only after a critical level of alteration has been achieved. They differ in that the threshold hypothesis requires the cooperative interaction of several predisposing factors to obtain oncogenic transformation, while the error accumulation hypothesis proposes a more generalized breakdown in normal regulatory functioning. [p. 440]

10. Oncogenic (oncorna- or retro-) viruses have been shown to cause tumors in virtually all animal hosts. These are principally RNA-containing viruses which possess oncogenes, short segments of genes that can effect the transformation of a normal cell into a cancerous cell. [p. 440–442]

11. The oncogene theory proposes that sequences of DNA normally occur in animal cells that correspond to the viral oncogenes. These "latent viruses" if activated give rise to tumor transformation. [p. 442–443]

12. Efforts to test the oncogene theory disclosed that oncogene sequences did exist in animal cells. However, it was further demonstrated that these genes played a normal role in animal cells. These proto-oncogenes might have appeared in animal cells first and been later acquired by viruses. Transformation into a cancerous cell involves the inappropriate expression of these oncogenes. [p. 443]

13. "Transformation proteins" is the name used to describe the protein products of the oncogenes. All transformation proteins appear to act in one of four ways: (a) through protein phosphorylation, (b) by metabolic regulation of GTP-binding proteins, (c) through the control of gene expression, or (d) as growth factors. [p. 444–445]

14. Transformation of normal cells into tumor cells involves the inappropriate expression of oncogenes and antioncogenes (tumor suppressor genes), most of which appear to affect the expression of a cell's proliferation potential. This is accomplished either by mutations directly

affecting the oncogene, rearrangement of chromosomes, or gene amplification. However, in some instances, the emergence of cancer is associated with reduced gene expression. [p. 445–449]

15. Metastasis, the expansion of a tumor to secondary sites, requires the successful completion of several steps. These include (a) invasion of local tissue, (b) separation from the parent mass, (c) relocation to a distant site, (d) effective manipulation of the new local environment. [p. 449–452]

16. Some forms of therapy include surgery, radiotherapy, chemotherapy, hormones, and immunotherapy. Early detection, prior to metastasis, is critical for successful treatment. [p. 453–455]

17. Cancer cannot be prevented completely; however, avoiding factors that are known to promote or exacerbate cancer expression provides the best assurance for preventing cancer. [p. 455]

READINGS

Azarnia, R., Reddy, S., Kmiecek, T. E., et al. The cellular *src* gene product regulates junctional cell-to-cell communication. *Science* **239:**398, 1988.

Bishop, J. M. The molecular genetics of cancer. *Science* **235:**305, 1987.

Bishop, J. M. Molecular themes in oncogenesis. *Cell* **64:**235, 1991.

Cohen, S. M., and Ellwein, L. B. Cell proliferation in carcinogenesis. *Science* **249:**1007, 1990.

Fearon, E. R., Cho, K. R., Nigro, J. M., et al. Identification of a chromosomal 18q gene that is altered in colorectal cancer. *Science* **247:**49, 1990.

Folkman, J., and Klagsbrun, M. Angiogenic factors. *Science* **235:**442, 1987.

Friedberg, E. C. (ed.). *Cancer Biology* (Readings from *Scientific American*). W. H. Freeman & Co., New York, 1986.

Graves, D. T., Jiang, Y. L., Williamson, M. J., et al. Identification of monocyte chemotactic activity produced by malignant cells. *Science* **245:**1490, 1989.

Hollstein, M., Sidransky, D., Vogelstein, B., et al. p53 mutations in human cancer. *Science* **253:**49, 1991.

Kimchi, A., Wang, X.-F., Weinberg, R. A., et al. Absence of TGF-β receptors and growth inhibitory responses in retinoblastoma cells. *Science* **241:**196, 1988.

Klein, G. Multistep emancipation of tumors from growth control: can it be curbed in a single step? *BioEssays* **12:**347, 1990.

Koth, R., and Herlyn, M. Molecular biology of tumor antigens. *Current Opinion in Immunology* **1:**863, 1989.

Lee, W.-H., Bookstein, R., Hong, F., et al. Human retinoblastoma susceptibility gene: cloning, identification, and sequence. *Science* **235:**1394, 1987.

Lyons, J., Landis, C. A., Harsh, G., et al. Two G protein oncogenes in human endocrine tumors. *Science* **249:**655, 1990.

Marshall, C. J. Tumor suppressor genes. *Cell* **64:**313, 1991.

Pitot, H. C., and Dragan, Y. P. Facts and theories concerning the mechanisms of carcinogenesis. *FASEB Journal* **5:**2280, 1991.

Prehn, R. T. Neoplasia. In *Principles of Pathobiology.* 4th ed. LaVia, M. F., and Hill, R. B. (eds.). Oxford University Press, Inc., New York, 1985.

Rez, A., and Fidler, I. J. Some biochemical properties associated with the metabolic potential of tumor cells. In *Receptors in Cellular Recognition and Developmental Processes.* Gorczynski, R. M. (ed.). Academic Press, Inc., Orlando, Fla., 1986.

Rice, G. E., and Bevilacqua, M. P. An inducible endothelial cell surface glycoprotein mediates melanoma adhesion. *Science* **246:**1303, 1989.

Sager, R. Tumor suppressor genes: the puzzle and the promise. *Science* **246:**1406, 1989.

Stanbridge, E. J. Identifying tumor suppressor genes in human colorectal cancer. *Science* **247:**12, 1990.

Sutherland, R. M. Cell and environment interactions in tumor microregions: the multicell spheroid model. *Science* **241:**177, 1988.

Taylor, G. M. Immunogenetics and cancer. *Current Opinion in Immunology* **1:**872, 1989.

Travali, S., Koniecki, J., Petralia, S., et al. Oncogenes in growth and development. *FASEB Journal* **4:**3209, 1990.

Tzen, C.-Y., Esterviz, D. N., Minoo, P., et al. Differentiation, cancer, and anticancer activity. *Biochemical Cell Biology* **66:**478, 1988.

Weiss, L., Orr, F. W., and Honn, K. V. Interactions of cancer cells with the microvasculature during metastasis. *FASEB Journal* **2:**12, 1988.

18 Tumor Immunology

OVERVIEW

Immune surveillance and host immune responses to tumors are examined in this chapter. The consequences of adaptive responses by the tumor to immunological defense are discussed. In addition, cancers of the immune system are described. Major nonspecific and antigen-specific tumor immunotherapies are also outlined.

CONCEPTS

1. The immune system employs several mechanisms that can enable tumor cells to be identified as "nonself" and cause their elimination.

2. Tumor cells can also interact with the immune system using defenses that allow them to evade detection and attack by the immune system.

3. Tumor immunotherapies exploit immune system–tumor interactions in attempting to eliminate cancers either by immune restoration or by circumventing tumor escape mechanisms.

4. Cancers of the immune system present a unique situation since B and T cell tumors act both as cancer cells and as disrupters of the immune network.

Despite the fact that cancer is the second leading cause of death in the United States, cancers are rare in terms of the numbers of cells in the human body that are actually involved. Nevertheless, tissue culture studies have shown that the frequency of neoplasms is far greater than would be expected from clinically detectable cancer. Thus, it seems likely that many transformed cells do not progress to become life-threatening cancers and, therefore, must have been destroyed by the body early after their transformation. So what happens in the stages between transformation into a tumor cell and the billion cell cancer mass? This chapter explores this question with respect to the theory of immune surveillance of tumors, probing how some cancers can escape surveillance, and how immunotherapy might be an approach to cancer management and elimination. In addition, this chapter describes specific cancers that arise within the immune system itself, thereby affecting both B and T cells. These cancers are a two-edged sword. On the one hand, they have the characteristics of neoplastic cells and should activate immunological defenses, but on the other hand, as immune cells gone awry, they disturb the immune network essential in combating the progression of the disease.

■ ■ ■ ■ ■ ■ ■ ■ ■ ■ ■

THEORY OF IMMUNE SURVEILLANCE

Immune surveillance is based on the concept that tumor cells display nonself, in this case tumor, Ags that can be recognized and reacted against by the host's immune system. Execution of an appropriate immune response would lead to the elimination of neoplastic cells. Thus, one reason that an individual frequently does not develop cancer derives from the cytotoxic immune reactions to early tumor growth. Cancer becomes a manifest disease and potentially life threatening only when these immune mechanisms break down and metastasis of the tumor occurs throughout the body.

The **immune surveillance hypothesis** states that (1) *transformed and normal cells possess different antigenic determinants* and that (2) the *immune system responds to cancer cells as it would to a pathogen or foreign graft.* Normal cells undergo cancerous transformation through a series of genomic alterations that are associated with the production of altered or unusual cell proteins (see chapter 17). But are transformed cells immunogenic?

It has been difficult to demonstrate that most tumors are immunogenic. In fact, one type of cancer immunotherapy involves the xenogenization (from the Greek, *xeno* = stranger and *gene* = birth; thus, to give birth to a stranger) of tumors. In this treatment, the immunogenic potential of a tumor is increased by the introduction of a novel, antigenic determinant, since many tumors are only weakly (or not) immunogenic. The indication that most tumors are not strongly immunogenic raises a challenge to the immune surveillance theory. This is due to the potential difficulty the immune system would have in surveying the body for neoplastic transformations if the resulting cancer cells did not carry a "foreign" antigenic marker.

Because of this objection, some scientists dispute an immune surveillance theory based on immunogenic cancer cells and propose immune surveillance of tumors without immunogenicity. This theory exploits the notion that the immune system can assist in regulating the differentiation of normal cells, by eliminating "self" cells that are expressing themselves in the wrong space or time. A prime example of this inappropriate expression could be cancer cells. The immune mechanisms for clearing these phenotypically irregular cells might actually be the same as suggested by the former immune surveillance theory (see next section). The persistence of cancers in some individuals could be explained by both theories if we look at the impairment of regulatory immune function as part of the tumorigenic process (which is, as yet, not completely understood).

The primary difference between the two theories of immune surveillance lies in the perception of cancer cells as self versus nonself. The **Ehrlich-Thomas-Burnet theory** of immune surveillance considers that the immune system is an *active guardian against* transformed cells carrying foreign, **nonself,** signals. In contrast, the **Grossman-Herberman theory** proposes an antitumor surveillance system that *regulates* **self** populations of cells and assures elimination of any quantitative or qualitative deviations from the norm.

If either theory of immune surveillance of tumors is correct, new vistas into cancer therapy will be open. The approaches may be different, but treatments that could modulate or restore immune function could direct the immune system to eliminate tumor cells, regardless of their nature or location in the body. In fact, as we learn to control the heterogeneity of tumor cells, it should be possible to immunize against tumor growth. But first we must better understand the biology of cancer cells, the biology of the immune system, and the interactions between tumors and the immune system. Only then can we hope to successfully alter the course of tumor growth by immunotherapy.

HOST IMMUNE RESPONSES TO TUMORS

According to the Ehrlich-Thomas-Burnet theory of immune surveillance of cancer, a person with an alert immune system responds to cells that carry nonself antigenic tags on their surfaces. The cells are seen as foreign, and appropriate reactions by the immune system result in their eradication. In virus-infected cells, the presence of a single foreign viral Ag can elicit a strong cytotoxic immune response despite the fact that all other surface Ags are self-Ags. The same reaction should hold true with a newly transformed neoplastic cell. Once a normal, differentiated body cell, the transformed cell now carries a new tumor Ag on its surface as a result of the events of transformation (see chapter 17). If this new tumor Ag is seen as nonself, foreign, the immune response should be swift and decisive. This intruder should be eradicated before being allowed to grow into a mass (through proliferation) or invade into other areas of the body (metastasis).

However, Richmond Prehn has proposed that *immunostimulation* might actually be needed to promote early tumor growth. He observed that certain tumors displayed poor rates of growth when implanted into immunosuppressed mice. In addition, some tumors actually can use stimulation of an immune response as a means of evading detection by the immune system. (This topic is addressed in greater detail later in the chapter.) Nevertheless, the body can address cancer cells under certain circumstances and, in the following sections, we explore the natural defenses that are invoked in response to cancer cells.

Specific Immune Responses

As with virus-infected cells and foreign grafts, the T lymphocyte plays a major role in the destruction of tumor cells in mammals. T cell activation includes the generation of **helper** (T_H), **sensitized** (T_D), and **cytotoxic** (T_C) subset clones. Of special interest is the role played by T_D cells. These cells can affect four important areas of tumor killing by means of the lymphokines that they release (fig. 18.1).

Lymphokines can be involved in *mobilizing and activating B cells* through B cell growth factors and B cell differentiation factors. The expression of foreign tumor Ags on the surface of a cancer cell can provoke activation of immunocytes. This activation leads to the formation of clones of plasma cells that produce Abs that are specific for determinants expressed on the surfaces of cancer cells. In turn, these give rise to a range of *Ab-dependent cellular cytotoxicity* (ADCC) reactions. On one level, complement-fixing Abs can directly bind to the tumor Ags and lyse the cells by complement activation. On another level, effector cells, such as cytotoxic killer cells and **macrophages** (Mϕs), carrying Fc receptors can be recruited for tumor killing by Fc binding to the cancer cell membrane coated with Ab receptors. The binding of Ab to the tumor cell would trigger opsonization, which would facilitate phagocytosis of the cancer cell. In addition, some lymphocytes, for example, **natural killer** (NK) cells and **lymphokine-activated killer** (LAK) cells, can be similarly *recruited*. Moreover, complement activation would lead to generation of complement fragments, C3a and C3b. C3a is chemotactic for neutrophils, while C3b induces Mϕ enzyme release. Thus, inflammatory activities of complement-activated neutrophils and Mϕs can lead to cytolysis of the tumor cells.

A second set of lymphokines can activate the phagocytes of the reticuloendothelial system. These lymphokines include migration-inhibiting factor

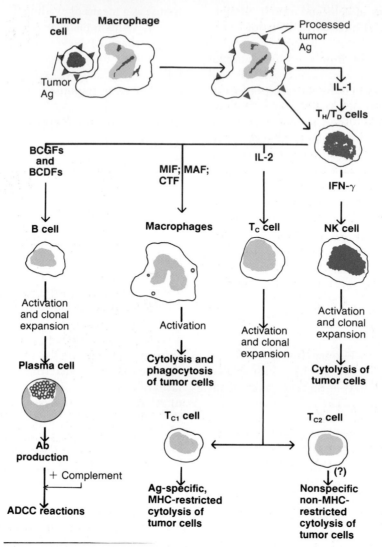

FIGURE 18.1 Host immune responses to tumors. Following tumor Ag processing by a macrophage, T_H or T_D cells set into motion mechanisms that lead to tumor cell destruction. Tumoricidal action of macrophages is primarily cytolytic; however, phagocytic destruc-

tion of tumors can also occur. The action of T_{C2} cells as nonspecific, non-MHC-restricted cytotoxic cells is designated by (?) because this function has not been unequivocally proved.

(MIF), chemotactic factor (CTF) and Mφ-activating factor (MAF). Monocytes and Mφs recruited and regulated by these lymphokines phagocytize the tumor cells, thereby engulfing, killing and digesting them.

Another lymphokine, interleukin 2 (IL-2), appears to be a growth factor and is essential in stimulating T and B cell populations to divide and expand their clones. IL-2 is produced by Ag-stimulated T lym-

phocytes and must be present in sufficient quantities in order to mount an effective counterattack against the cancer cell population. This is an important means of expanding the population of T_C lymphocytes. These killer cells can accomplish lysis of tumor cells through cell-to-cell contact. Two categories of this cell type are believed to exist, namely, (1) Ag-specific, MHC-restricted (well-established) and (2) broad specificity, non-MHC-restricted T_C lymphocytes (not unequivocally demonstrated). Thus, Ag-specific killer cells would recognize cells with specific tumor markers, whereas those with broad specificity could lyse a variety of tumor cell targets.

In addition, the lymphokine interferon (IFN) (type γ), may also be produced by the T cell immune response and this immunomodulator molecule can regulate T cell functions, B cell Ab production, and enhance NK cell and Mϕ tumoricidal activity. A very important regulatory role for IFN in tumor killing may be in amplifying the NK cell population. NK cells are a heterogeneous group of granular lymphocytes that appear very effective in lysing target cancer cells through cell-to-cell contact without prior sensitization. Tumor cells of various types might possess a unique set of tumor markers that can be recognized by NK cells; nevertheless, they appear to be activated by the *absence* of class I MHC self-Ags. In addition, the lytic process involves the release of cytotoxic factors for which there seem to be more receptors on the surfaces of target cancer cells than on nonmalignant body cells. Thus the efficiency of tumor killing by NK cells is both high and specific for tumor cells.

Nonspecific Immune Responses

Tumor cells can also be eliminated by Ag-nonspecific cell types, such as activated Mϕs and NK cells (fig. 18.2). These exert their tumoricidal effects through different mechanisms.

From *in vitro* studies, it appears that **Mϕs** can *eliminate tumor cells through both cytolysis and phagocytosis.* It has been shown that the efficiency of cytolysis of tumor cells by Mϕs is increased by the presence of activated lymphocytes or their product lymphokines. The events leading to cytotoxic Mϕ killing are still unclear but once elucidated have potential as a form of cancer immunotherapy.

Lysis of tumor cells by **NK cells** seems to be another important immune defense against cancer. NK cells are null cells, neither B nor T lymphocytes, comprising 5% to 15% of the total lymphocyte population of the blood that have been found in the spleen, lymph nodes, bone marrow, and blood. They *have a broad specificity, are non-MHC restricted,* and seem to recognize the cancer cell by an unidentified NK target receptor.

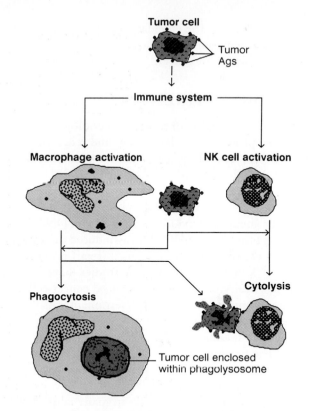

FIGURE 18.2 Nonspecific immune responses. Tumor cells can be attacked in Ag-nonspecific fashion by macrophages and NK cells. These can lead to destruction of the tumor cell either by phagocytosis or cytolysis. The tumoricidal action of macrophages is often cytolytic; nevertheless, there is evidence to support phagocytic elimination of tumors as well.

However, recent studies indicate that the degree of response by NK cells to tumor cells is inversely related to the expression of MHC class I Ags. In particular, tumor cells that express little or no MHC class I Ags are more readily attacked by NK cells than are those that express greater amounts of MHC class I Ags. Nevertheless, although NK cell killing is not MHC restricted, it appears to be influenced by MHC expression.

The killing mechanism is mediated by cell-to-cell contact leading to *cytolysis* where the target cell is destroyed but not the NK cell. *In vitro* studies have demonstrated that the NK cell is responsible for cytolytic activity against a variety of tumor cell lines. The role of immune modulators in regulating NK activity is still unclear but the elucidation of protocols for sustained augmentation of NK activity might lead to more effective therapy of cancer.

TUMOR ANTIGENS

Currently, in the area of tumor immunology, the most difficult problem is identifying and characterizing tumor Ags. The existence of **tumor-associated Ags (TAAs)** has been clearly established in animal systems, but the heterogeneity of the Ag population makes their classification difficult. TAAs include Ags (1) on physically or chemically induced tumors, (2) on DNA virus-induced tumors, (3) on RNA virus-induced tumors, and (4) associated with developmental (fetal) products.

Tumor transplantation studies have shown that physically or chemically induced cancer cells express a unique set of antigenic determinants, also called tumor-specific transplantation Ags (TSTAs). In contrast, virus-induced tumors often express common or viral-specific Ags on their surface. Oncofetal Ags present an interesting phenomenon. These are Ags that are expressed normally only during fetal development but are reexpressed abnormally in many adult tumors (table 18.1). There are some investigators who do not consider oncofetal Ags as tumor Ags, but rather as Ags that are expressed in addition to TAAs. Nevertheless, levels of expression of certain of these oncofetal Ags are increased in association with particular tumors.

Theoretically, tumor Ags should be new antigenic determinants on the surface of the transformed cell. In fact, the picture is much more complex. In the case of tumor-specific Ags *induced by physical or chemical carcinogens,* each tumor expresses unique cell-surface Ags. If a chemically induced tumor is removed from an animal and subsequently reinjected into the same animal, there is no recurrence of the cancer and there are signs of intense immune activity. Perhaps the response to the initial tumor was mounted too slowly and a tumor mass was established—while upon a second challenge, the heightened anamnestic response was able to destroy the cancer cells rapidly enough to eradicate the disease. These Ags are so unique that tumors chemically induced on different areas of the body will produce antigenically distinct cell populations. Thus, carcinogen-induced tumors carry cell-surface Ags

TABLE 18.1 Classification of Tumor Antigens

Tumor Type	Characteristics of Their Antigens
Chemically or physically induced	Unique tumor-specific Ags
Virus induced DNA viruses RNA viruses	Common TAAs Virus-specific Ags
Developmental	Oncofetal Ags (e.g., AFP and CEA)

unique to the specific tumor but not unique to the inducing chemical. This fact makes it impossible to use Ag-specific immunotherapy since resistance raised to one set of carcinogen-induced tumor Ags might not prevent the growth of a second tumor induced by the same chemical. This is unfortunate since many human cancers have been attributed to physical and chemical carcinogens in the environment, such as radiation, asbestos, smoke, and food additives.

Tumors *induced by oncogenic viruses* display cell-surface Ags that are coded from the viral genome. In the case of DNA viruses, these Ags are encoded by virion DNA sequences, but are not considered viral protein products, rather they are distinct to and expressed only on transformed cells. Yet no matter where the transformation takes place in the body, be it in a lung or liver, the DNA viral TAAs are always the same. In fact there is extensive crossreactivity between different oncogenic DNA viral Ags of the same viral class. Thus, Ags can be diagnostic of the specific DNA virus or group and can be dealt with by Ag-specific immunotherapy.

In contrast, cells transformed by RNA viruses, called oncornaviruses, display tumor Ags that are also viral protein products. Therefore, transformed and RNA virus-infected cells produce the same Ags. To complicate matters further, tumor cells induced by RNA viruses express both viral tumor Ags and normal host differentiation Ags. Within the oncornavirus tumor Ags themselves, we can find (1) group-specific determinants or common Ags that are shared by all viruses in that group, (2) type-specific products that are

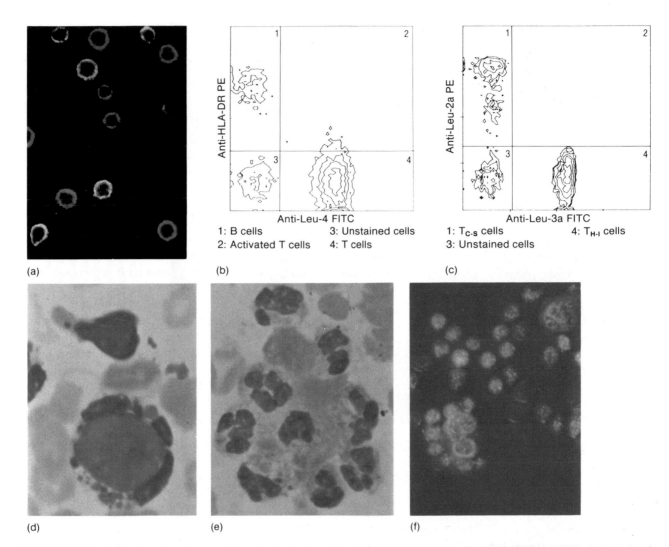

(a)

(b)

1: B cells
2: Activated T cells
3: Unstained cells
4: T cells

(c)

1: T_{C-S} cells
3: Unstained cells
4: T_{H-I} cells

(d)

(e)

(f)

PLATE 3 (a) Discrimination of lymphocyte subsets. Leukocytes can be distinguished one from another by unique differentiation antigens (Ags) displayed on their surfaces (discussed in Chapters 2 and 9). With the aid of monoclonal antibodies (MAbs) against these Ags and a fluorescence-activated cell sorter (FACS), we can quantify and separate these cells into their respective subclasses (see Chapter 5). This illustration depicts lymphocytes stained to discriminate T_{H-I} (CD4+) from T_{C-S} (CD8+) cells. T_{H-I} cells are stained with anti-Leu-3a FITC (labeled anti-CD4 Ab), which induces a greenish fluorescence, while T_{C-S} cells are stained with anti-Leu-2a PE (labeled anti-CD8 Ab), causing them to appear reddish orange under the conditions used. (b–c) FACS profiles of lymphocyte subsets. Using different combinations of fluorescently labeled MAbs, the FACS can discern various lymphocyte subpopulations. For example, B and T cells can be separated from each other (b). Alternatively, T_{H-I} cells can be resolved from T_{C-S} cells (c). (Refer to Chapter 5 for discussions of methods for identifying leukocytes on the basis of surface markers and the FACS.) *Key:* **PE** is phyocoerythrin label; **FITC** is fluoroscein isothyocyanate label; **anti-HLA-DR PE** is Ab against HLA-DR labeled with PE (monomorphic Ag appearing on up to 11% ± 4% peripheral lymphocytes); **anti-Leu-4 FITC** is FITC-labeled Ab against CD3 (T cell Ag); **anti-Leu-2a PE** is PE-labeled Ab against CD8 (differentiation Ag on T_{C-S} cells); **anti-Leu-3a FITC** is FITC-labeled Ab against CD4 (differentiation Ag for T_{H-I} cells). (d–f) Lupus erythematosus (LE) cell and immunofluorescence localization of antinuclear Ab. The characteristic LE cell (d), is a neutrophil that is engorged by a phagocytized nucleus (Wright's stain). Rosettes (e), formed by aggregates of neutrophils around nuclei of damaged cells, are not indicative of LE but suggest that further evaluation is warranted (Wright's stain). Alternatively, LE can be diagnosed by the presence of antinuclear Ab (f). This can be seen in the intense fluorescence around the nuclei of affected cells when a fluorescently tagged antinuclear Ab is used. Note the intense outline of the nucleus of the neutrophil in the field and the nuclei of the lymphocytes present. (a–c: Supplied courtesy of Becton Dickinson Immunocytometry Systems. d–f: From Hyun, B. H., Ashton, K., and Dolan, K. *Practical Hematology.* W. B. Saunders Co., Philadelphia, 1975.)

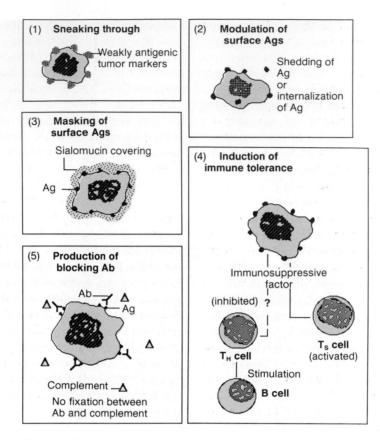

FIGURE 18.3 Tumor escape mechanisms. Shown here are five ways that a tumor cell evades detection and destruction by the immune system.

decreasing the expression of these substances, tumor cells can reduce the formation of stable contacts with cytolytic cells. Ag modulation can also be affected by redistributing the Ags within the cell membrane in such a way as to prevent immune reaction. Moreover, tumor Ags can be removed from the surface of the cancer cell by "shedding." This loss of tumor Ags desensitizes the cancer cell populations and protects them against subsequent cytolysis in the immune host.

Another strategy is to devise a cloaking mechanism that renders one invisible. This tool is realized in certain cancers by *production of a mucoprotein that coats and masks surface tumor Ags.* Tumor cells often produce copious amounts of a mucoprotein called sialomucin. This molecule binds to the surface of tumor cells, providing a protective shield against immune attack. Since sialomucin is a normal (self) component, the immune system cannot "see" through the surface slime layer to the tumor Ags below. Thus, the cancer goes undetected by natural defenses.

The observation that certain types of tumors can synthesize various immunosuppressants has led to speculation that some tumors might be able to actively suppress the immune response. By taking the offensive, cancer cells could activate specific T_S cell populations, thereby crippling effector T and B cell clones. This would induce a state of immune tolerance to the cancer, which could then be free to take over the body.

Cancer cells can also use weapons of their own against the immune system. They do this by somehow *invoking the immune system to produce blocking Abs against the tumor Ags.* If specific Abs that cannot fix complement are made in response to antigenic challenge by cancer cells, then their subsequent binding to tumor cells could be disastrous for the host. Blocking Abs cannot activate complement, so lysis of the cell is not possible. This also means that no C3a or C3b is formed, thus neutrophil- and Mϕ-mediated inflammatory reactions are never elicited. Blocking Abs also cover the surface of cancer cells, preventing T_C cells from binding to the hidden receptors. In this way, killing of tumor cells by complement, phagocytosis, and T_C cells is blocked. Production of these blocking Abs has actually been demonstrated to enhance tumorigenesis by hampering immune attacks on all levels.

Last, tumors can suppress immune responses, thereby impairing the inflammatory response, chemotaxis of phagocytes, and the complement cascade. Certain of these factors seem to be nonspecific and lead to a generalized decline of immunity. It is well known that cancer patients show a progressive decline in immune responsiveness to all foreign Ags as the disease progresses. Other factors provide specific protection for the tumor cells expressing them. For example, expression of H-2D (a murine class I MHC Ag) is associated with immune suppression. Thus, MHC-restricted tumor cell elimination by T_C cells can be influenced by the ratio of expression of H-2K (stimulatory) and H-2D (inhibitory or suppressive).

DIALOGUE BETWEEN TUMOR CELLS AND THE IMMUNE SYSTEM

Thus, the picture of the simple, primitive cancer cell is radically changing. On the one hand, it appears that tumor growth occurs because the cancer cells can react with an array of defense mechanisms that are put into play at appropriate times during immunological attack. On the other hand, there is also increasing evidence that cancer cells can interact with and benefit by response of the host's immune system. Those cancers that grow do so because they are "clever" enough to respond to each immunological probe and reaction. This creates a far more complex set of rules and regulations than previously thought. It seems that neoplastic cell populations are continually changing and are capable of both sending and receiving regulatory signals between themselves and immunocompetent cells. This ability to communicate with the host immune defense network is what might prevent their being identified as nonself and lead to an effective escape from immune destruction.

Defensive strategies for avoiding detection and attack by effectors of the immune system have been outlined in the preceding section. In addition, tumor cells can take positive steps to coax the immune system to assist in tumor growth.

Evidence has been accumulating that shows that tumors can actually *attract Mϕs* which then contribute to tumor growth. In particular, paracrine interaction between **tumor-associated Mϕs** (**TAMs**) and tumor cells is established that maintains both populations. For example, certain tumors have been shown to produce chemotactic factors that lead to the immigration of Mϕs to the vicinity. Moreover, these Mϕs retain their ability to proliferate (which contrasts them markedly from those which are actively phagocytic). In turn, TAMs apparently *produce growth and angiogenesis factors* that contribute to the expansion of the tumor cell population. Consequently, the tumor can enlarge.

IMMUNE DIAGNOSIS OF TUMORS

Immune diagnosis of cancer falls into two categories: (1) the detection of tumor "markers" and (2) the evaluation of the antitumor response of the host (fig. 18.4).

Tumor products that are secreted by cancer cells and find their way into the bloodstream are the best tumor markers. These include the oncofetal Ags, AFP (as found in pancreatic cancer) and CEAs (as occur in colon cancer). If Abs can be raised to specific tumor Ags, these can be subsequently radiolabeled and used to locate or image tumors by binding to the Ag markers on the tumor wherever it is in the body. This technique is called radioimmunoscintigraphy. It can also be helpful in determining if the primary tumor has spread into other sites in the body.

Detection of a tumor-specific immune response can also be important as a means of demonstrating the presence of a tumor in the host. Humoral responses can be assessed by testing for the presence of

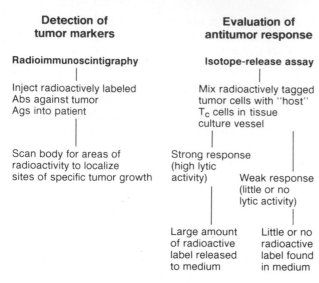

Detection of tumor markers	Evaluation of antitumor response
Radioimmunoscintigraphy	**Isotope-release assay**

Radioimmunoscintigraphy
|
Inject radioactively labeled Abs against tumor Ags into patient
|
Scan body for areas of radioactivity to localize sites of specific tumor growth

Isotope-release assay
|
Mix radioactively tagged tumor cells with "host" T_C cells in tissue culture vessel
|
Strong response (high lytic activity) — Weak response (little or no lytic activity)
|
Large amount of radioactive label released to medium — Little or no radioactive label found in medium

FIGURE 18.4 Immunodiagnosis of tumors.

certain Abs in serum which are diagnostic for certain tumors (e.g., melanomas and sarcomas). Cell-mediated responses can be measured after Ag stimulation of host T cells. In one such test, the isotope release assay, T_C cell activity can be measured. Lymphocytes from the cancer host are incubated with radiolabeled tumor cells. If the lytic activity of T_C cells is high, the levels of radioactivity in the tissue culture medium should also be high, since as tumor cells die, they lyse and release radioactivity into the medium.

Tumor markers and antitumor immune responses have proved useful in evaluating the progression or regression of the disease, a patient's responses to therapy, and in determining the recurrence of the disease. For example, it can be used to monitor AFP and CEA levels in patients with certain cancers following primary tumor removal. A rise in the levels of the oncofetal Ags postsurgery usually indicates a relapse, whereas low serum levels indicates continued remission.

TUMOR IMMUNOTHERAPY: NONSPECIFIC TREATMENTS

One approach to treating cancer is by directing the body's natural immune defense mechanism against the tumor. Immunotherapy may be used in conjunction with chemotherapy or radiation therapy, and seems to be most effective when the tumor mass is small (as in cancers, before metastasis). There are currently two broad categories of immunotherapy; Ag specific and Ag nonspecific. In Ag-specific treatments, the agents employed are directed against the tumor or tumor Ags, whereas Ag-nonspecific treatments use agents that activate the cells of the immune system in a generalized manner with the hope that tumor cells will consequently be destroyed. The biological complexity of the interaction between the cancer cell and immune system suggests that both approaches be used in a cancer patient, in an effort to activate or restore specific and nonspecific host resistance to foreign cells. In this section we deal with nonspecific treatments, such as immune restoration with microbial and synthetic products and immune modulation by thymic hormones, IFN, and bone marrow transplantation. Several of these are outlined in table 18.2.

Microbial and Synthetic Products

Treatment with certain bacterial products can produce regression of some neoplastic diseases. Especially successful is the use of an attenuated strain of *Mycobacterium bovis* called bacille Calmette-Guérin (BCG). When injected directly into certain solid tumors, BCG can produce striking tumor regression, especially when combined with chemotherapy. The effectiveness of BCG in treating certain cancers is probably related to the ability of the microbe to nonspecifically stimulate the immune system. As such, it is considered an immunoadjuvant. BCG has been shown to enhance Ab production and cellular immunity in certain parasitic infections as well. Although BCG modulates a wide variety of immune functions, the antitumor effect appears to result mainly from activation of Mϕs and NK cells. BCG is usually administered by the scarification technique, in which deep scratches are made in the thigh and the attenuated bacteria then applied to the site. This causes an intense local inflammatory response with some minor complications, such as fever and nausea. The cancers that have responded to this treatment include malignant melanomas, stage 1 lung cancer, certain leukemias, and bladder cancer.

Another gram-positive bacterium shown to have antitumor activity is *Corynebacterium parvum*. The

TABLE 18.2 Antitumor Actions of Selected Biological Molecules

Substance	Antitumor Action
Microbial and Synthetic Products	
Bacille Calmette-Guérin	Activation of Mφs and NK cells
Corynebacterium parvum	Activation of Mφs and B cells
Muramyl dipeptide Trehalose diester	Activation of Mφs
Levamisole	Generalized stimulation of lymphocytes and phagocytes
Azimezone	Immunorestoration; mitogenesis
Isoprinosine	Modulator of humoral and cell-mediated immune responses; enhancement of lymphocyte, Mφ, and NK activity
Thymic Hormones	Broad range of immunorestorative properties; alters T cell function
Cytokines	
Interferon (γ)	Enhancement of cytotoxicity of T and NK cells
Interleukin 2	Activation of LAK cells
Tuftsin	Activation of phagocytes
Tumor necrosis factor	Toxic to tumor cells (?)

immunological effects of *C. parvum* are diverse and involve Mφs, T cells, and B cells. Mφs appear to be activated while T cell function seems to be depressed. When used in conjunction with the chemotherapeutic agent, cyclophosphamide, a synergistic antitumor effect is achieved. This regimen has been beneficial, especially with various types of lung cancers and metastatic breast cancer. Unfortunately, it has many adverse side effects resulting from its high toxicity.

A way to circumvent many of the toxic side effects associated with using live bacteria is to use synthetic immunostimulants structurally derived from the bacterial cell walls of *M. bovis* and *C. parvum*. These adjuvant cell wall analogues include the muramyl dipeptides (*M. bovis*) and trehalose diesters (*C. parvum*). When used in combination, they act synergistically to give enhanced antitumor activity, an apparent consequence of activating Mφs against the cancer cell population.

Other substances that appear to be promising antitumor agents include levamisole, azimezone, iso-

prinosine, and tuftsin. Levamisole, an antihelminthic drug, has antitumor effects stemming from its generalized stimulation of both lymphocytes and phagocytes. This drug has been useful in treating certain leukemias and colon and breast cancers. An additional advantage is that this drug is relatively nontoxic. In contrast, azimezone is not used as an antitumor agent, but rather as an immunorestorative drug in conjunction with anticancer immunosuppressants like cyclophosphamide. Chemotherapy-induced immune suppression appears to be diminished following azimezone administration. This drug acts as a mitogenic agent, inducing the proliferation of leukocytes. Isoprinosine (Inosiplex) seems to have immunomodulating effects on both humoral and cellular immune responses. It enhances lymphocyte responses to Ags and acts as a mitogen to both lymphocytes and Mφs. It also increases NK cell activity, which is one mechanism in killing of cancer cells. With this drug, a heightened antitumor response has been seen in different types of leukemias.

Thymic Hormones

Other nonspecific immune modulators include the peptide **thymic hormones.** The best characterized are thymosin, thymopoietin, thymic humoral factor, and thymic serum factor. Since individuals with cancer frequently show abnormalities in both the numbers and function of T cells, thymic hormone therapy has been used to *restore immune competence.* Such agents have also been used to help reverse the significant immunosuppressive effects of chemotherapy and radiation therapy. Although there are differences in biological activity between different thymic fractions, they all can promote thymus-dependent immune responses and exhibit a wide range of immunorestorative properties. Clinical trials show that when coupled with chemotherapy, thymosin treatment can prolong survival time in lung cancer patients. However, the significance of thymic factors in cancer treatment will probably be more in providing a means of safely augmenting specific T cell functions in people with compromised cellular immunity. Many cancer patients die from bacterial and viral infections during treatment. This type of therapy should help these individuals survive such attacks while in chemotherapy.

Interferon, Tumor Necrosis Factor, and Tuftsin

IFN refers to a group of glycoproteins that interfere with viral replication and regulate immune reactivity. There are three major classes of human IFN: (1) IFN-α (derived from virus-infected leukocytes and activated NK cells); (2) IFN-β (derived from virus-infected fibroblasts, epithelial cells, and Mϕs); and (3) IFN-γ or immune IFN (derived from Ag-stimulated T lymphocytes and activated NK cells). The targets of **IFN-α** (class I) are cells exposed to viruses, where it *blocks viral replication.* **IFN-β** (class I) affects T$_S$ cells and *causes immune suppression*; while **IFN-γ** (class II) acts on T lymphocytes and NK cells, thus *enhancing the cytotoxicity* of these cells. In addition, IFN has anticellular activity, which also contributes to its anticancer properties.

Early clinical trials have shown that human leukocyte IFN may have potential use as an anticancer agent in breast cancer, multiple myeloma, and malignant lymphoma. Now that IFN can be produced by recombinant DNA technology, more of the various types of IFN will become available for testing. This should facilitate characterizing the nature and mechanism of the antitumor effects.

Another approach to the therapeutic use of IFN has involved the administration of synthetic drugs, such as synthetic poly I:C (inosinic and cytidilic acid polymer), which can induce the synthesis by host cells of its own IFN (i.e., it enhances endogenous production). However the IFN produced is different from virus-induced IFN both in size and chemical properties. Its use in cancer therapy is still in question.

Tumor necrosis factors (**TNFs**) are cytokines that have been shown to be *toxic for cancer cells in vitro.* Two forms have been identified: TNF-α (also called TNF or cachectin), which is produced by Mϕs, and TNF-β (lymphotoxin), which is produced by activated T cells. Both forms have very similar properties. Their production can be stimulated in mice infected with BCG, followed by injection with the bacterial endotoxin lipopolysaccharide (LPS). Then, if TNF-enriched serum is injected into mice with a tumor load, necrosis of the tumor can occur. Through recombinant DNA technology, human TNF can now be cloned and is being used experimentally in clinical trials with promising results. TNF appears to be most effective when it is used in combination with other agents, rather than as a single therapeutic agent.

Tuftsin is a naturally occurring tetrapeptide located in the H chain of γ-globulin that has been shown to *stimulate phagocytes.* Its tumoricidal activity, by means of Mϕ activation, has been documented in certain leukemias and melanomas. The following properties make tuftsin a unique immunoregulatory agent: (1) it is normally part of an Ab molecule that is released and activated by enzymes located in the spleen and phagocyte membranes, (2) there are specific receptors for it on target phagocytic cells, and (3) it stimulates all biological functions of these target cells from phagocytosis to Ab production.

Interleukin 2

The use of cytokines, such as the interleukins (ILs), as immunorestorative agents presents an exciting area of cancer research. IL-1 and IL-3 have been tested for anticancer activity but with only limited success. The IL that seems to offer the most promise as an antitumor treatment is **IL-2,** a glycoprotein that is derived from T_H cells. It has the ability to awaken the activity in many T lymphocyte subset populations. Dramatic *increases in the specific killing of cancer cells by T_C cells, NK cells, and Mϕs* are observed in animal systems after its administration. The specific antitumor effect of IL-2 seems to be its ability to stimulate the production of cytotoxic cells, such as NK and T_C cells, against tumor cells.

IL-2 receptors occur on many T cell subset populations, such as T_C and T_D lymphocytes. The binding of IL-2 to the surface receptors causes lymphokine production, cloning of T_C cells, and promotion of B cell functions. The appearance of lymphokines then stimulates Mϕ and NK cell activity against the tumor cells.

The levels of IL-2 are lower in cancer victims, and it is known that an appropriate level of IL-2 is essential for cytotoxic activities to be maintained by the immune system. By the administration of IL-2, the levels can be brought back to a normal physiological range, and the immune system can renew its attack on the invasive cancer cells. This is a practical strategy, since T lymphocytes that have been challenged with tumor Ags can be cultured for the production of IL-2 and other lymphokines. Moreover, the activity of IL-2 can be enhanced by inserting it into liposomes, which are biological membrane "sacs" that protect it from the body's degradative enzymes. Clinical trials of this antitumor, immunomodulating agent have just begun, and it seems to hold great promise from dramatic positive responses obtained in early trials (fig. 18.5).

Bone Marrow Transplantation and Other Treatments

Bone marrow transplantation is another approach to the treatment of some neoplastic diseases, such as leukemia. Between HLA-identical siblings there is the possibility of healthy donor bone marrow being transplanted to a recipient leukemic patient. Leukemic cells are destroyed by chemoradiotherapy, following which normal bone marrow is replaced with restoration of normal immune function. Marrow transplantation in-

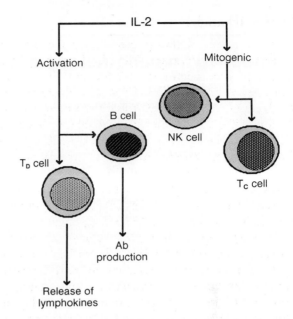

FIGURE 18.5 Immune modulation by IL-2. IL-2 can promote expression of Ag-specific immune responses by activating T_D cells (cell mediated) or B cells (humoral). Alternatively, IL-2 can stimulate Ag-nonspecific responses by acting as a mitogen for NK and T_C cells.

volves not only the transplantation of red blood cell precursors but also of the lymphoid and the monocyte-Mϕ systems.

The major complication of marrow transplantation is the possibility of the donor tissue causing a graft-versus-host disease (GVHD) (see chapter 19). If the match between donor and recipient is not close enough, the donor's immunocompetent marrow lymphocytes perceive the recipient body cells as foreign and mount an immune response against the immunoincompetent host. The principal target organs of GVHD in humans are the skin, gastrointestinal tract, and liver. Illness is due to an active immunological assault against the host tissues, and death from infection frequently occurs. However, if the immunologically competent foreign marrow graft does not mount a harmful reaction against the host, a stable graft-host tolerance can be maintained.

If matched donor marrow cannot be obtained, it is sometimes possible to use the person's own (i.e.,

Adoptive Immunotherapy in Treating Metastatic Cancer

A recent advance in cancer immunotherapy is the transfer of immune-activated lymphocytes to an individual with cancer. It is termed "adoptive immunotherapy" since the host adopts, or accepts, the stimulated lymphocytes into its own system. In 1985 Rosenberg reported use of a modification of this approach to treat 25 humans with metastatic cancer. The types of cancers differed, as did the previous chemotherapy and/or radiation treatments. The only common factor was that the cancers of these people had spread, and standard therapies had failed to contain the disease.

The treatment used had two parts. First, the host's own white blood cells were isolated by leukopheresis. The lymphocytes were then isolated and cultured in the presence of the immune-stimulating lymphokine, IL-2. The resulting autologous cells, called LAKs, were allowed to undergo clonal expansion. They were then harvested and reinfused into the host's body. Next, the host was injected with IL-2 for a prescribed time after the LAK infusion. Despite the toxicity of this therapy, regression of cancer was seen in about 50% of those participating in this clinical trial. Interestingly, it had been previously determined that neither LAK nor IL-2 therapy alone was sufficient to treat such cancers. However, as a combined therapy, it appears that combined LAK/IL-2 therapy might be useful in treating a variety of cancers at different stages of their progression. These studies are still considered preliminary, and further clinical trials are needed to evaluate the true efficacy of adoptive immunotherapy in humans.

Rosenberg has tried a different adoptive immunotherapy procedure initially using mice and more recently using human subjects. In the animal experiments, tumor-infiltrating lymphocytes (TILs) were isolated, activated by IL-2, and reintroduced into the host. Results showed that TILs were much more effective than LAK cells in mediating the regression of tumors. This subpopulation of lymphocytes has not been characterized, although it is likely that it contains a mixture of cells, including T_C and NK cells. In addition to TIL and IL-2 infusions, the hosts received injections of the immunosuppressant, cyclophosphamide. Cyclophosphamide has been shown to be effective in eliminating T_S cells, which could inhibit the effectiveness of the transferred lymphocytes. Treatment with any of these therapies alone produced negative results. However, together they provided a powerful tool in reducing, if not totally eliminating, the tumor load of the host. In the human experiments, a gene for neomycin resistance was introduced as a marker. The TILs had the desired effect in managing melanoma in the patients participating in this study. However, this study also demonstrated the feasibility of introducing a viable gene along with the lymphocytes. This represents the first step toward direct gene therapy in human subjects.

autologous) marrow. Autologous marrow transplantation consists of removing some of the person's own marrow, then administering chemoradiotherapy in an effort to eradicate the cancer. Subsequently, the marrow (treated by immunotherapy techniques to remove only the cancer cells) is returned to the individual. Usually, the marrow is removed while the person is in remission, and upon relapse, returned to the patient after immunotherapy and chemoradiotherapy.

Other nonspecific therapies include immune depletion therapy. This involves the removal of certain soluble tumor factors circulating in the blood.

Tumor cells are known to release immunosuppressive factors, which can inhibit the expression of tumor immunity by the host. Immunosuppressive factors released from tumor cells include prostaglandins, AFP, blocking Abs, and other ill-defined soluble factors that can block Mφ and lymphocyte activation or Ab production and induce T_S cells. One way these immunosuppressants can be removed is by a process called plasmapheresis (fig. 18.6). This technique makes use of a cell separator, which can remove certain circulating molecules such as blocking Abs and other immunosuppressing factors. In this way, the immune

The details of the protocols of adoptive immunotherapy will undoubtedly change, but the essential concept remains valid. Removing, activating, and reintroducing an individual's own lymphocytes eliminates the possibility of a transplantation reaction. This treatment's strength lies in trying to restore and rejuvenate the person's own immune system rather than replacing it. In this way, the body is allowed to cure itself, even when the cancer has spread. The above treatments might not yet be the magic combination, but pursuing this strategy should eventually lead us to it. Moreover, the ability to introduce normal genes with this method provides a means for correcting, even if only transiently, dysfunctions resulting from gene defects.

Rosenberg, S. A. Adoptive immunotherapy for cancer. *Scientific American* **262**(5):62, 1990.

Rosenberg, S. A., Aebersold, P., Cornetta, K., et al. Gene transfer into humans—immunotherapy of patients with advanced melanoma, using tumor-infiltrating lymphocytes modified by retroviral gene transduction. *New England Journal of Medicine* **323**:570, 1990.

Rosenberg, S. A., Lotze, M. T., Mul, L. M., et al. Observations on the systemic administration of autologous lymphokine-activated killer cells and recombinant interleukin-2 to patients with metastatic cancer. *New England Journal of Medicine* **313**:1492, 1985.

Rosenberg, S. A., Spiess, P., and Lafreniere, R. A new approach to the adoptive immunotherapy of cancer with tumor-infiltrating lymphocytes. *Science* **233**:1318, 1986.

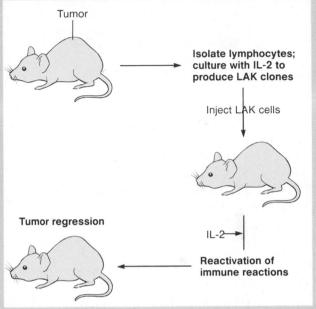

FIGURE 18.A Application of adoptive immunotherapy.

system might be able to return to peak efficiency and once more become active in eliminating the cancer cells. Another use of plasmapheresis is to remove circulating immune complexes. This can be important in cancer patients, since many develop immune-complex disease as a complication. This nonmalignant inflammatory condition, which usually affects the organ(s) afflicted with cancer, is possibly caused by antitumor Abs. These antitumor Abs could form complexes with tumor Ags or with specific antiidiotypes. Plasmapheresis can remove these immune complexes and thus reduce the source of inflammation.

TUMOR IMMUNOTHERAPY: ANTIGEN-SPECIFIC TREATMENTS

Another way of approaching immunotherapy is to direct the immune system against specific tumor Ags. In this way, the only immune mechanisms that would have to come into play would be those involved in removing the cancer cells. It would not be necessary to provoke a generalized activation of the immune system. Currently, these therapies include vaccination with tumor Ags, treatment with immune RNA, transfer

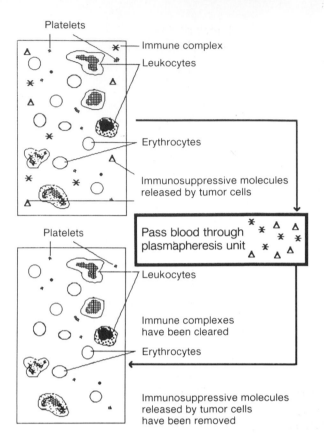

FIGURE 18.6 Immune depletion therapy by plasmapheresis. Passing a sample of blood through a plasmapheresis unit results in removal of immune complexes and immunosuppressive tumor products before it is returned to the patient.

factor, lymphokines or immunotoxins, and treatments involving the modification of tumor antigenicity (table 18.3).

Vaccination Against Tumors

In active immunization, cancer prevention is attempted by vaccinating with actual inactivated tumor cells or their Ags. Tumor cells are emulsified in Freund's adjuvant and injected prior to tumor challenge in animals. One oncogenic viral vaccine, feline leukemia vaccine, has been very effective in reducing the incidence of leukemia in the domestic cat population. However, immunization against the tumor itself depends on both the presence of tumor cell-surface Ags

TABLE 18.3 Some Means of Countering Tumors

Mode of Treatment	Effect
Vaccination against tumor	Provides immunity against specific tumor type
Immune RNA	Stimulates humoral and cell-mediated immune responses
Transfer factor	Stimulates cell-mediated immune response; stimulates release of lymphokines
Modification of tumor Ag	Increases immunogenicity of Ag, leading to heightened immune response
Immunotoxins (toxin attached to MAb)	Causes specific destruction of tumor cells

that can be "seen" by the immune system and on appropriate cytotoxic responses by the immune system. To date, most anticancer vaccines have failed—either because the tumor's antigenicity is somehow hidden or the immune system responds by producing blocking Abs that enhance tumor growth.

Immune RNA

Immunological information can be transferred from a sensitized animal to a nonsensitized one by an RNA extract, called immune RNA. RNA extracted from the lymphoid tissue of specifically immunized animals can amplify the immune responsiveness to that Ag in nonimmunized animals. This adoptive transfer of immunity by immune RNA is donor specific and cannot be transferred to a third party (fig. 18.7).

Immune RNA is actually a complex of Ag fragments complexed to small single-stranded molecules of RNA. Immune RNA acts as an informational molecule and evokes specific Ab and cell-mediated responses when injected into nonimmunized donors. It has potential use in cancer therapy. If immune RNA can be recovered from individuals cured of a specific cancer, then it could be used for immunization. Alternatively, immune RNA might be used to treat individuals with cancer as a means of reactivating the immune system against the tumor. Clinical trials have

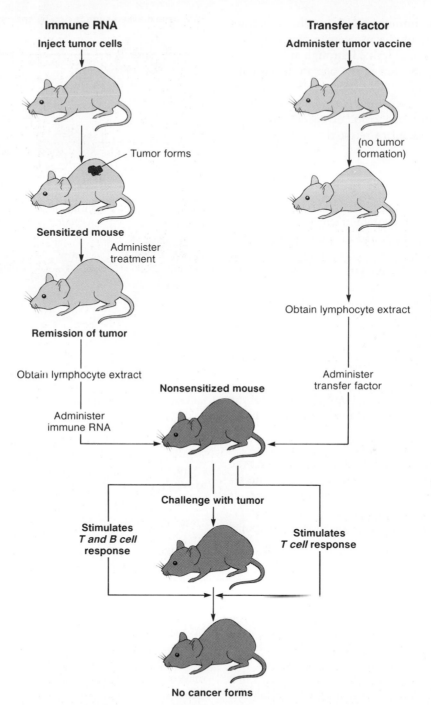

Immune RNA

Inject tumor cells

Transfer factor

Administer tumor vaccine

Tumor forms

(no tumor formation)

Sensitized mouse

Administer treatment

Obtain lymphocyte extract

Remission of tumor

Obtain lymphocyte extract

Administer transfer factor

Administer immune RNA

Nonsensitized mouse

Challenge with tumor

Stimulates
T and B cell response

Stimulates
T cell response

No cancer forms

FIGURE 18.7 Antitumor effect of immune RNA and transfer factor. The manner in which immune RNA and transfer factor are induced and their subsequent effects in preventing tumor formation are rep-resented. Note that in both instances, no lymphocytes are transferred to the nonsensitized recipient mouse.

already begun using immune RNA, but the results are not promising. Part of the problem is the source of immune RNA, which is derived through animal challenge or *in vitro* incubation of the person's own lymphocytes. Both methods yield only small amounts of immune RNA. Perhaps through recombinant DNA technology sufficient quantities of specific immune RNA might be obtained to retest the system and its potential promise.

Transfer Factor

If leukocytes from an immunized individual are disrupted, we can recover a soluble factor called transfer factor. If this extract is injected into nonsensitized individuals, it can evoke a cell-mediated response to that Ag. Transfer factor is a nucleopeptide whose mode of action is undetermined but appears to stimulate the release of lymphokines from sensitized T lymphocytes. It does not promote Ab synthesis and, therefore, does not have the range of immune RNA. Nevertheless, it can suppress tumor growth. A schematic representation of its production and use, as compared with immune RNA is presented in figure 18.7.

Clinical trials have been limited because of the problem of donor selection. It is known that household members of a cancer victim usually have cell-mediated reactivity to those tumor Ags. Transfer factor released from their leukocytes can be used to treat the cancer patient. Due to the paucity of donors, the effectiveness of transfer factor is not yet known. If transfer factor could be synthesized in the laboratory, it would offer a better chance of more widespread testing.

Modifying Tumor Antigenicity

Immunogenicity of the tumor cells can be increased in several ways (fig. 18.8). Among these are (1) treatment with the enzyme neuraminidase (to remove the sialic acid layer from the surface Ags), (2) introduction of antigenic foreign determinants by chemical or biochemical means, (3) infection with certain viruses that would promote a cytotoxic response, or (4) isolation and modification of the relevant tumor Ags to elicit an appropriate response from the immune system. Certain of these techniques show promise, especially

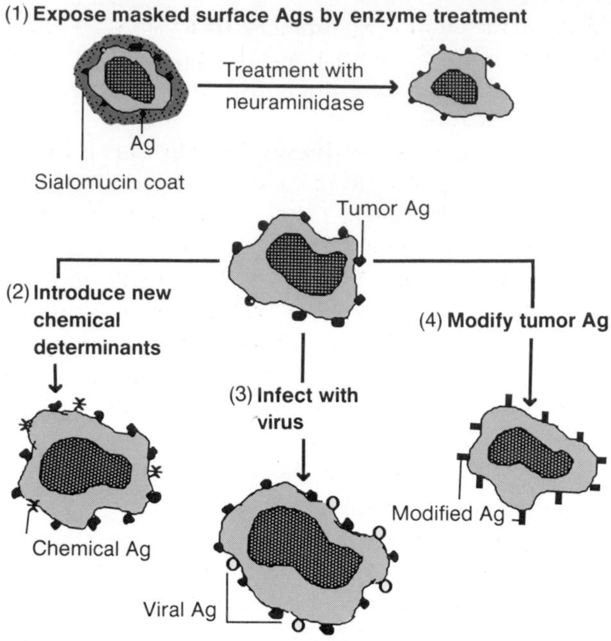

FIGURE 18.8 Ag-specific immunotherapy. (*1*) Neuraminidase removal of sialomucin coat exposes tumor Ags, thereby increasing immunogenicity. (*2*) Modulation of tumor immunogenicity can be achieved by the introduction of new chemical determinants, (*3*) virus infection, or (*4*) physicochemical modification of existing Ags.

against virus-induced tumors. However, vaccination will be limited to those cancers showing a nonmutable set of immunogenic tumor Ags. It might be possible to synthesize an effective vaccine against certain virus-induced cancers, but not against the highly variable carcinogen-induced tumor Ags.

Many tumors mask or modify their antigenicity in such a way as to make themselves inaccessible to immune attack. Because of this, many investigators have tried to find ways of *unmasking the tumor cells* so that the body's natural defense mechanisms can interact with and destroy the cancer cells. One approach is to use the enzyme neuraminidase, which can attack sialomucin. Sialomucin is made by many tumors and serves as a protective coating of the cell surface, masking the tumor Ags from the immune system. Clinical trials have focused on the effectiveness of neuraminidase-treated tumor cells in different types of leukemia. Leukemic cells are incubated with neuraminidase and injected into the person in an attempt to increase the immunogenicity of these cells. In combination with chemotherapy, the results have been positive, and significant increases in remission rates have been documented.

Other ways of **increasing the immunogenicity** of tumor cells include *x-irradiation, chemical modification, virus infection,* and introduction of foreign determinants by *somatic cell hybridization.*

Irradiation of tumor cells increases the immunogenicity of the tumor cells. This is achieved through the release of Ag from viable tumor cells and perhaps by modifying the chemical structure of the Ag as well, so that it is more easily seen by the immune system.

The preceding methods attempt to increase the immunogenicity of ordinarily weak tumor antigens. Another approach is to introduce some new foreign Ag into the tumor cell. Chemical modification of tumor cells is one way to incorporate more antigenic molecules onto the surface of these cells. Formaldehyde- and glutaraldehyde-treated cancer cells display modified immunogenicity; however, the immunogenicity remains weaker than that of irradiated tumor cells. Better results have been obtained with the use of hapten-carrier conjugates. The strategy is to attach tumor cells to antigenic foreign proteins as "carriers" and to elicit an immune response against weakly antigenic TAAs. Nevertheless, the stability of chemically modified tumor cell immunogenicity is poor, since the markers do not persist long after cell division.

Yet another way of modifying tumor cells is to infect them with viruses. Virus-infected tumor cells display viral surface markers which are very immunogenic. One advantage of using viral markers is that they are very stable. Tumor Ags modified by viruses can be maintained as genetically stable markers, even after several cell divisions, since the viral genome is replicated along with the host's DNA.

Hybrid tumor cells fused with either normal or tumor cells are also used to increase immunogenicity of tumor cells (fig. 18.9). The primary aim of this somatic cell hybridization technique is to increase expression of TAAs by fusing foreign Ag with tumor cells. Currently, the main use of hybrid tumor cells is as a viable cell vaccine for immunization, since most

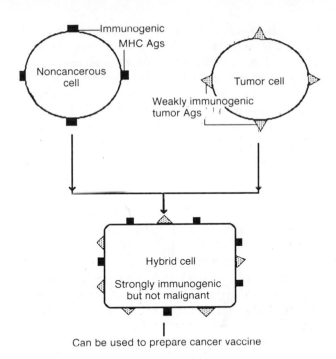

FIGURE 18.9 Somatic cell hybridization as a way of increasing immunogenicity of tumor cells. Fusing highly immunogenic noncancerous cells with weakly immunogenic cancer cells can create hybrids that enhance immunogenicity of tumor Ags.

hybrid tumor cells fused with normal or malignant cells lose their malignancy and cannot grow in the host. In other words, the hybrid cells are "attenuated" tumor cells, similar to a nonpathogenic form of a bacterium. However, the principal problem seems to be rejection of the somatic cell hybrids by the host. The presence of foreign histocompatibility Ags on the surface of the hybridoma cell can elicit a transplantation rejection reaction. Until this problem is resolved, this technique has only limited use.

Immunotoxins

There is now considerable interest in using Abs derived from antigenic challenge to deliver cytotoxic drugs to tumor cells. Hybridoma-produced monoclonal Abs (MAbs) can be raised against TAAs. Some of these are complement-fixing Abs that can be used to attach to and help destroy tumor cells directly, while others can be complexed to toxic drugs or radioisotopes. Since the delivery of these cytotoxic agents

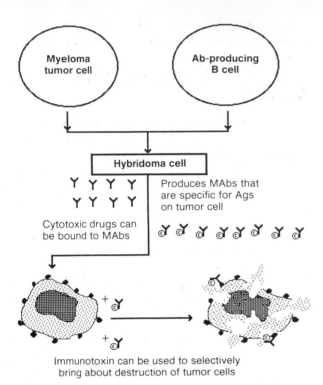

Myeloma
tumor cell

Ab-producing
B cell

Hybridoma cell

Produces MAbs that
are specific for Ags
on tumor cell

Cytotoxic drugs can
be bound to MAbs

+

+

Immunotoxin can be used to selectively
bring about destruction of tumor cells

FIGURE 18.10 Production of MAbs via hybridoma formation and their use as immunotoxins. Hybridomas can be formed to generate highly specific MAbs. These Abs then can be used to direct cytotoxins against selected targets, such as tumor cells.

bound to MAbs exhibits precise specificity, only tumor cells are destroyed, leaving healthy cells virtually untouched and unharmed.

With the recent development of somatic cell hybridization techniques, it is now possible to fuse a myeloma cell with an Ab-producing B cell to produce a hybridoma (fig. 18.10). The nonsecreting myeloma cell can grow indefinitely in tissue culture, but does not produce Abs. On the other hand, the Ab-producing B cell synthesizes small quantities of specific Ab in response to tumor Ags, but does not thrive under tissue culture conditions. However, the newly formed hybridoma cell can be successfully maintained and grown in tissue culture and can produce copious amounts of a single Ab that is specific to the tumor Ag. Alternatively, hybridoma cells can be inoculated into

the peritoneal cavities of mice where they produce hybridoma tumors (ascites) that secrete high levels of MAbs.

Hybridoma-produced MAbs have been developed against several different human tumors including malignant melanoma, colorectal carcinoma, leukemias, and lymphomas. Used alone, injection of MAbs should result in the specific binding to and complement-mediated lysis of the cancer cells. Clinical trials have demonstrated the need to select only tumor Ags that do not modulate or mutate on exposure to Ab and to select individuals without large tumor burdens and circulating Ags. Tumors that shed Ag upon attack by Ab present a two-fold problem in therapy. First, if the cancer cell sheds its antigenic marker, it is now impossible for the Ab to find its target. Second, when the shed Ag enters the circulation, it will combine with Ab to form harmful immune complexes, which can trigger an inflammatory reaction. Nonetheless, certain leukemias seem to respond positively to MAb therapy in that treatment significantly lengthens the periods of remission.

MAbs can also be used as carriers for cytotoxic agents. The resulting Ab-drug or Ab-radioisotope complex should be delivered only to cancer cells expressing the tumor Ag, while avoiding nonspecific effects on normal body cells otherwise susceptible to cytotoxic agents. The use of these immunotoxins have produced promising results in animal studies, where cytotoxic agents coupled to MAbs seem more effective than the cytotoxic drugs or Ab alone. Limited clinical trails are also being conducted. For example, one study reported that growth of human leukemic cells, *in vivo,* was suppressed by treatment with MAbs conjugated to the cytotoxic agent, ricin. The immunotoxin produced was highly specific and killed only leukemic cells. This technique is also being used in humans for the location of metastases (radioimmunoscintigraphy), but clinical trials are still in their early stages.

Another approach to the use of MAb-carrier conjugation has linked a MAb with a hormone. In this conjugate, MAbs specific for CD3 (an invariant component of the Ag-recognition complex) of T_C cells were coupled to an analogue of melanocyte-stimulating hormone (MSH). The MSH analogue (MSHa) is specific for MSH receptors found on melanoma cells. The resulting conjugate, therefore, displayed specificity for both tumor (melanoma) cells and effector T_C cells. In this way, the hormone was able to focus T_C cells on tumor cells for which they had no Ag specificity. Coupling of other hormones, or growth factors, with MAbs specific for various T cell populations has the potential for providing a new dimension to this approach to cancer management.

There are problems, however, in using MAbs as immunotoxic therapeutic agents. One that has already been mentioned is the antigenic modulation by cancer cells. If this occurs, the Ab's therapeutic effect is neutralized. Another problem is a phenomenon called MAb sensitization, which occurs in most individuals treated with the same MAb over several days. There can be an intense Ab response to the Fc fragment and to idiotypic determinants of the MAb that causes the formation of immune complexes in the blood. These complexes effectively stop the immunotoxic molecule from reaching the target and can cause serum sickness in the afflicted individual. Since MAb sensitization occurs in most people, long-term therapy, which would be necessary for most cancer victims, does not seem practical. One possible way to circumvent this problem is to administer, over consecutive days, different MAbs presenting the same specificity to tumor Ag binding but with distinct idiotypes. In this way, MAbs might be used on a long-term basis to eliminate tumors that did not undergo antigenic modulation.

In summary, there is, as yet, no "magic bullet" for eliminating only cancer cells from the body. Although the immune response might be recruited for the treatment of tumors, immunotherapy is not the treatment of choice, at present. The main problem seems to be the ever-changing cancer cell. It appears to have several mechanisms that it can invoke to outwit the defenses of the immune system: it can shed or mask its tumor Ags, induce the formation of T_S cells or the formation of blocking Abs, and produce immunosuppressants. None of the immunotherapies discussed in this section can overcome all of these tumor escape mechanisms. Until we can modify the tumor's re-

sponse, immunotherapy will be, at best, an adjunct to chemotherapy or radiotherapy in treating cancer.

CANCER OF THE IMMUNE SYSTEM

There are several types of malignancies of the immune system involving B and T lymphocytes. When lymphocytes become malignant, they give rise to leukemias, lymphomas, or myelomas. Most leukemias, lymphomas, and myelomas are of B cell origin, with T cells accounting for acute lymphocytic leukemia. Both B and T cells contribute to Hodgkin's disease. This section discusses both specific features of these disease states and their immunological impact on the host (table 18.4).

Cancers of the immune system are a two-edged sword, since the B and T cell tumors act as both cancer cells and specific disrupters of the immune network. Currently, immunotherapy has little effect in positively modulating the suppressed immune system. The immune response can become so profoundly depressed that many individuals with these cancers often die of secondary bacterial or viral infections that could be easily fought by a healthy, noncancerous immune system.

T Cell: Acute Lymphocytic Leukemia

Acute lymphocytic leukemia is a type of acute lymphoblastic leukemia that has two forms, one in children and the other in adults. Leukemia is a neoplastic disease, which affects white blood cells and is characterized by abnormal proliferation and maturation of hematopoietic cells (fig. 18.11a). The term acute refers to the sudden onset, aggressive progression, and limited time-course expected of this disease. The term lymphocytic specifies the cell type affected, while leukemia denotes that the disease state is characterized by the abnormal maturation and accumulation of these white blood cells.

In this type of leukemia, the *transformed lymphoid cells do not mature into functional lymphocytes.* Instead they accumulate in great numbers in the bone

Are Monoclonal Antibodies the Magic Bullets of Cancer Therapy?

The ultimate aim of immunotherapy is the generation of a treatment that will eliminate only the cancer cells of the body, no matter where they have spread, with minimal toxic side effects. Many investigators believe that MAbs, specific for tumor Ag, will eventually be these magic bullets in cancer chemotherapy.

Currently, there are three approaches in using these proposed magic bullets. The first approach uses MAbs raised against tumor Ags (or other foreign Ags inserted in the tumor cell membrane) that are tagged with a toxic molecule. Upon binding to the cancer cell, the tumor is selectively killed, while the neighboring cells are spared. The second approach is similar in general strategy; however, an enzyme is linked to the Ab. The Ab-enzyme conjugate is targeted to the tumor cell, where it can convert an inactive prodrug into an active cytotoxin capable of destroying the tumor cell. With the third approach, MAbs are made against tumor markers and used to target the tumor cells for ADCC, including participation of Mϕ and LAK cells.

MAbs have not yet been entirely successful as magic bullets because of several obstacles. The first is the difficulty in producing MAbs against unique TAAs. The second problem is antigenic modulation in which the foreign tag can be removed from the surface of the tumor cell, rendering it invisible to the attacking immune system. Third, MAb sensitization can occur by which the host makes anti-MAbs that reduce the efficacy of the treatment.

Despite these drawbacks, some success has been realized with animal models. For example, tumor cell destruction by alkaline phosphatase–MAb conjugates. In these experiments, the conjugate is targeted to the tumor cell where it becomes internalized. Subsequently, alkaline phosphatase converts etoposide-phosphate to etoposide, which proceeds to kill the tumor cells in which the reaction occurs. In other experiments, nude (athymic) mice injected with human melanoma cells showed regression of tumor growth when treated with LAK cells and MAbs raised against certain stable melanoma antigenic cell-surface markers. In these mice, there was a marked ADCC

marrow, blood, and lymphatic system, and functional normal blood cells are effectively crowded out. This leads to suppression of normal function of the bone marrow and peripheral blood with development of anemia (reduced oxygen-carrying capacity of the red blood cell mass), thrombocytopenia (reduced numbers of platelets, leading to reduced blood-clotting function), and granulocytopenia (diminished numbers of granulocytes, giving rise to overall impaired phagocytic function).

If left untreated, the course of the disease is very rapid, and death usually occurs only months after initial diagnosis. However, if detected early, radiotherapy and chemotherapy have yielded long-term re-mission and even cures. The causes of this leukemia seem to be multiple, including attack by oncogenic RNA viruses, radiation or carcinogens, and genetic predisposition. T cell leukemias are very prevalent in individuals with chromosomal abnormalities, specifically chromosomal rearrangements, such as translocations and inversions in chromosomes 8 and 14 in humans.

The immunological features of acute lymphocytic leukemia are (1) the appearance of leukemia-associated Ags, (2) the detection of Ags to leukemia-associated Ags, and (3) the presence of specific markers (the Ia T cell marker is found in the majority of childhood leukemias, while both T and B cell markers can

reaction, mediated primarily by the "armed" LAK cells. This latter treatment was effective in suppressing only the growth of human melanoma tumors (the target cells) in these mice. These approaches have yet to be tried in humans; nevertheless, preliminary results with animals have been promising.

Fanger, M. W., Segal, D. M., and Wunderlich, J. R. Going both ways: bispecific antibodies and targeted cellular cytotoxicity. *FASEB Journal* **4**:2846, 1990.

Ferrini, S., Melioli, G., and Moretta, L. Immunotherapy and immunity to cancer: cellular mechanisms. *Current Opinion in Immunology* **2**:683, 1990.

Honsik, C. J., Jung, G., and Reisfeld, R. A. LAK cells targeted by monoclonal antibodies to the disialogangliosides GD2 and GD3 specifically lyse human tumor cells of neuroectodermal origin. *Proceedings of the National Academy of Science* (USA) **83**:7893, 1986.

Schulz, G., Staffileno, L. K., Reisfeld, R. A., et al. Eradication of established human melanoma tumors in nude mice by antibody directed effector cells. *Journal of Experimental Medicine* **161**:1315, 1985.

Senter, P. D. Activation of prodrugs by antibody-enzyme conjugates: a new approach to cancer therapy. *FASEB Journal* **4**:188, 1990.

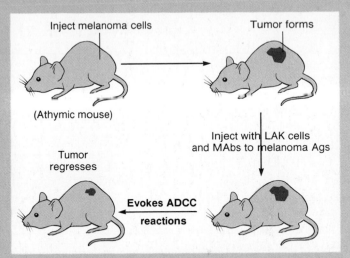

FIGURE 18.B Focusing cytotoxicity with MAbs.

be found in the more heterogenous adult form of the disease). The greater the amount of leukemia-associated Ags, antileukemic Abs, and reduction in immune function, the poorer the prognosis. Immunotherapy can be used in conjuction with radiotherapy and chemotherapy and is usually indicated when the individual is in remission. The immunotherapies that are the most successful in prolonging periods of remission include immunization with irradiated leukemic cells or bacterial products like BCG to stimulate the immune system and bone marrow transplantation following irradiation to replace the cancerous bone marrow. Complete remissions have been obtained using bone marrow transplantation.

B Cell: Chronic Lymphocytic Leukemia, Multiple Myeloma, and Burkitt's Lymphoma

The classification of the chronic leukemias is based on the identification of the predominant mature white blood cell found in the circulation (fig. 18.11*b*). In **chronic lymphocytic leukemia**, the major cell type is the B lymphocyte. This form of leukemia usually strikes only adults and, with or without radiotherapy or chemotherapy treatment, the average survival time after diagnosis is three years. This disease is manifested by a *proliferation and accumulation of small, abnormal B lymphocytes* in the bone marrow, blood, and lymph. It begins as a mild, almost asymptomatic disease that can

TABLE 18.4   Characteristics of Cancers of the Immune System

Cancer	Clinical Features	Immunological Features
T Cell Cancers		
Acute lymphocytic leukemia (ALL)	Presence of immature, nonfunctional lymphocytes; suppression of bone marrow function leading to anemia, thrombocytopenia, and granulocytopenia	Appearance of leukemia-associated Ags; presence of weak antileukemia Abs; presence of T cell markers on cancer cells
B Cell Cancers		
Chronic lymphocytic leukemia (CLL)	Accumulation of abnormal B cells in bone marrow, blood, and lymph; occurrence of numerous secondary infections	Demonstration of low Ig synthesis and depressed Ab response
Multiple myeloma	A lymphoproliferative B cell disorder; occurrence of bone marrow dysfunction with anemia, leukopenia, and thrombocytopenia	Display of excessive plasma cell proliferation and production of MAbs
Burkitt's lymphoma	A monoclonal B cell tumor affecting primarily the face and jaw with bone marrow and lymphatic involvement	Presence of Abs to tumor-specific Ags
B and T Cell Tumors		
Hodgkin's disease	Lymphoma of lymph nodes and spleen; occurrence of immunodepression; increased bacterial/viral infections	Accumulation of abnormal B and T cells

progress to the invariably fatal blast transformation stage in which lymphoblasts overwhelm the system. The abnormalities in the B cell lead to insufficient Ig synthesis and depressed Ab response, with resulting increases in the rate of secondary infections. Immunotherapy has not been successful in treating this form of leukemia.

Multiple myeloma is a lymphoproliferative disorder associated with *Ab-producing B lymphocytes*. It afflicts older adults (median age is 60) and arises in the bone marrow. Plasma cell proliferation is so rapid that it suppresses normal marrow elements causing bone destruction, leukopenia (low leukocyte count), anemia (low hemoglobin level due to a low red cell count), and thrombocytopenia (low platelet count). The *Ab that is produced by a single clone of malignant plasma cells* is of one type, monoclonal. The excessive production of this homogeneous Ab (which is usually IgG or IgA) suppresses the normal synthesis of the other Igs. Complications include recurrent infections (due to abnormal

Ab synthesis), renal failure (due to filtering problems of serum Ab overload), bleeding (due to low platelet count), and congestive heart failure (due to increased serum viscosity). Immunological diagnosis is based on serum electrophoresis and the subsequent detection of the monoclonal myeloma protein or, in some cases, the detection of Bence-Jones proteins (L chain myeloma). Bence-Jones proteins are actually the L chains of a MAb and are small enough to be filtered through the kidney and hence appear in the urine. As this disease progresses, the concentration of Bence-Jones proteins can become so great that the L chains crystallize out in the urine. Renal failure, due to filtering overload, is usually the cause of death. Radiation and chemotherapy are the preferred treatments in all types of multiple myeloma. As yet, there is no clear indication of the effectiveness of immunotherapy in multiple myeloma, but treatment with the immunorestorative drug, levamisole, has increased remission times slightly in some individuals.

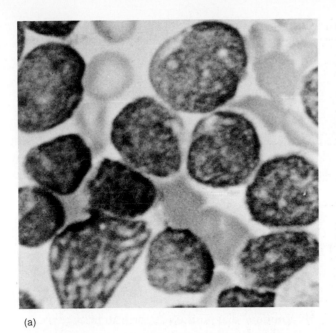

(a)

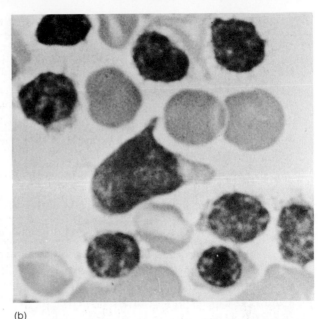

(b)

FIGURE 18.11 Abnormal blood cell composition in lymphocytic leukemias. (*a*) ALL. Note the presence of large numbers of immature lymphocytes (blast stage). (Contrast appearance with those of mature lymphocytes in *b*.) (*b*) CLL. Note the abundance of mature lymphocytes present. Ordinarily, granulocytes are the predominant leukocytes in adult peripheral blood. (From Hyun, B. H., Ashton, J. K., and Dolan, K. *Practical Hematology*. 1975. W. B. Saunders Co., Philadelphia.)

Burkitt's lymphoma is a *monoclonal B cell tumor* and mainly occurs in parts of Africa. The causative agent seems to be the Epstein-Barr virus, which can cause malignant transformations of B cells, resulting in tumors in the face and jaw. However, in terminal cases, there is lymphatic and bone marrow involvement. The disease responds to standard radiation and chemotherapy, and immunotherapy is still a promise of the future. However, individuals with Burkitt's lymphoma develop Abs to tumor-specific Ags which are expressed on all Burkitt tumors with surface Ig. Thus, it should be possible to develop a cytotoxic Ab that could bind to and destroy the tumor cells.

B and T Cell: Hodgkin's Disease

Hodgkin's disease is a type of cancer called a lymphoma, a lymphoproliferative disorder that initially affects the lymph nodes and spleen. It occurs mainly in young adults and seems to be of viral origin. The Epstein-Barr virus, seen in Burkitt's lymphoma, is often found. The malignant lymphocytes found in the secondary lymphatic tissue are usually of mixed cell type, including *B and T cells*. This cancer has three stages, and prognosis is best if diagnosed in stage I or II since the lymphocytes found in lymph node biopsies are still well differentiated. However, in stage III, the lymphocyte population is poorly differentiated, the cancer has spread into other organs, and the level of suppressor lymphocytes is extremely high. This causes an overall depression of the immune system, and death is often due to infection. Treatments used include radiation and chemotherapy, depending on the stage of the disease diagnosed. Various immunotherapies have been used in treating Hodgkin's disease. These include cytotoxic MAbs, the use of immunomodulating molecules (IFN and thymic factor), and bone marrow transplantation. Bone marrow transplantation seems to hold the greatest promise, if GVHD does not occur. Lethal irradiation of the primary and secondary lymphatic system, with subsequent bone marrow transplantation, should result in replacement of diseased lymphocytes with healthy, noncancerous ones and hence place the person in complete remission.

Tumor Immunology **483**

S U M M A R Y

1. Theories of immune surveillance suggest that cancer cells can be perceived as foreign and be subsequently destroyed by cytotoxic immune mechanisms. One function of the immune system is to continually "survey" the body for such malignant transformations. [p. 460–461]

2. The immune system responds to cancer cells displaying new or foreign tumor antigens with specific T and B cell responses. [p. 461]

3. T cell responses lead to the generation of T_C cells and NK cells and the release of lymphokines. The lymphokines include macrophage-activating lymphokines, interferon for NK cells, transfer factor capable of heightening T cell response to tumor killing, and IL-2 capable of activating T_C cells. [p. 461–463]

4. B cell responses include production of complement-fixing antibodies. Once the complement cascade is begun, by antibody binding to tumor surface antigens, complement fragments are generated that activate leukocytic phagocytes. The subsequent inflammatory antibody-dependent cellular cytotoxicity and opsonization responses can lead to cytolysis of tumor cells. [p. 463]

5. Ag-nonspecific defense against tumors is accomplished primarily by NK, LAK cells, and macrophages. NK and LAK cells display cytotoxicity for tumor cells that is not MHC restricted. [p. 463–464]

6. Tumor-associated antigens include physically or chemically induced tumors, DNA or RNA virus-induced tumors, and tumors associated with oncofetal protein products. [p. 464–465]

7. Tumor antigens produced by physical or chemical carcinogens display antigens unique for each specific tumor. Tumors induced by oncogenic DNA viruses synthesize a unique tumor antigen that is constant for all tumors raised by that class, whereas RNA oncornaviruses display antigens that are also viral protein products, which can range from common to unique tumor antigens. Oncofetal antigens are normal fetal, but abnormal adult, antigens associated with many cancers that are only weakly immunogenic but can be used diagnostically to detect tumor growth. [p. 465]

8. Tumor escape mechanisms play an important role in how certain tumors avoid immune detection. Such mechanisms include (a) escape by antigen modulation, where tumors can shed, rearrange, or internalize tumor antigens; (b) masking tumor antigens with a coating of sialomucin; (c) inducing tolerance by increasing T_S cell pools, (d) inducing the production of non-complement-binding, blocking antibodies; and (e) releasing suppressor factors that act as immunodepressants. [p. 465–467]

9. Paracrine interactions between tumor cells and tumor associated macrophages contribute to tumor growth. [p. 467]

10. Immune diagnosis of tumors can be used to either detect tumor markers or evaluate the antitumor response of the host. Tumor markers or antibodies to oncofetal proteins like AFP and CEA can be used to detect the presence of cancer in the host. The cytotoxic function of the immune system can be assessed by tests like the isotope release assay, which measures T_C cell activity. [p. 467–468]

11. Several nonspecific immunotherapies have been used in treating cancer, including (a) microbial and synthetic products to stimulate the immune response; (b) thymic hormones to restore T cell function; (c) interferon to awaken NK cells, and tuftsin to stimulate phagocytic cells; (d) treatments with IL-2 to stimulate the immune cytotoxic activities in the cancer host; (e) bone marrow transplantation to replace cancerous marrow and immune function; and (f) plasmapheresis as a way to remove tumor immunosuppressive factors from the blood. [p. 468–473]

12. Antigen-specific immunotherapies include (a) vaccination against tumors that would immunize an individual against certain cancers; (b) administration of immune RNA as a means of reactivating the immune system against the

tumor; (c) injections of soluble transfer factor to evoke a cell-mediated response to the tumor cells in a host; (d) modification of tumor antigenicity by treatment with neuraminidase, which removes sialomucin covering tumor antigens; and (e) immunotoxin therapy using antibodies raised against tumor antigens (either alone or tagged with a cytotoxic drug) that bind to and specifically destroy only cancer cells. [p. 473–479]

13. Cancer can also strike the immune system itself. These cancers present an unusual situation, since T and B cell tumors share the same destructive characteristics of all cancer cells while simultaneously specifically compromising the immune network that should challenge its growth. [p. 479]

14. Acute lymphocytic leukemia is one type of T cell cancer, of unknown etiology, that affects the bone marrow's production of competent T cells. [p. 479–481]

15. B cell cancers can take many forms including chronic lymphocytic leukemia, multiple myeloma, and Burkitt's lymphoma. In chronic lymphocytic leukemia, the bone marrow, blood, and lymph are flooded with mature, nonfunctional B lymphocytes. Multiple myeloma is associated with massive release of monoclonal antibodies into the serum by cancerous plasma cells. Burkitt's lymphoma is a monoclonal B cell tumor that results in tumors of the face and jaw. [p. 481–483]

16. Hodgkin's disease is a lymphoma affecting both B and T cells. This lymphoproliferative disorder mainly affects the lymph nodes and spleen. [p. 483]

READINGS

Baldwin, R., and Lyers, V. (eds.). *Monoclonal Antibodies for Cancer Detection and Therapy.* Academic Press, Inc., New York, 1985.

Blythman, H. E., Casellas, P., Gros, O., et al. Immunotoxins: hybrid molecules of monoclonal antibodies and a toxin subunit specifically kill tumor cells. *Nature* **290**:145, 1981.

Brandt, S. J., Peters, W. P., Atwater, S. K., et al. Effect of recombinant human macrophage-granulocyte colony-stimulating factor on hematopoietic reconstitution after high-dose chemotherapy and autologous bone marrow transplantation. *New England Journal of Medicine* **318**:869, 1988.

Burnet, F. M. The concept of immunological surveillance. *Progress in Experimental Tumor Research* **13**:1, 1970.

Erhlich, P. Uber den jetzigeb Stand der Karzinomforschung. In *The Collected Papers of Paul Erhlich,* (Vol. II). Himmelweit, F. (ed.). Pergamon Press, London, 1957.

Fathman, C., and Fitch, F. (eds.). *Isolation, Characterization and Utilization of T-Lymphocyte Clones.* Academic Press, Inc., New York, 1982.

Frankel, A. E., Houston, L. L., Issell, B. F., et al. Prospects for immunotoxin therapy in cancer. *Annual Review of Medicine* **37**:125, 1986.

Grossman, Z., and Herberman, R. B. "Immune surveillance" without immunogenicity. *Immunology Today* **7**:128, 1986.

Hara, H., and Seon, B. K. Complete suppression of *in vivo* growth of human leukemia cells by specific immunotoxins: nude mouse models. *Proceedings of the National Academy of Science* (USA) **84**:3390, 1987.

Herberman, R. (ed.). *NK Cells and Other Natural Effector Cells.* Academic Press, Inc., New York, 1982.

Kennedy, R. C., Melnick, J. L., and Dreesman, G. R. Anti-idiotypes and immunity. *Scientific American* **255**:48, 1986.

Killion, J. J., and Fildler, I. J. Evasion of host responses in metastasis: implications of cellular resistance to cytokines. *Current Opinion in Immunology* **2**:693, 1990.

Laurick, J. W., and Wright, S. C. Cytotoxic mechanism of tumor necrosis factor-α *FASEB Journal* **4**:3215, 1990.

Leith, J. T., and Dexter, D. L. *Mammalian Tumor Cell Heterogeneity.* CRC Press, Inc., Boca Raton, Fla., 1986.

Liu, M. A., Nussbaum, S. R., and Eisen, H. N. Hormone conjugated with antibody to CD3 mediates T cell lysis of human melanoma cells. *Science* **239:**395, 1988.

Mihich, E. (ed.). *Immunological Approaches to Cancer Therapeutics.* John Wiley & Sons, Inc., New York, 1982.

Montovani, A. Tumor-associated macrophages. *Current Opinion in Immunology* **2:**689, 1990.

Mosley, R. L., Styre, D., and Klein, J. R. Immune recognition by cytotoxic T lymphocytes of minor histocompatibility antigens expressed on a murine colon carcinoma line. *Cellular Immunology* **122:**200, 1989.

North, R. J. Down-regulation of the antitumor immune response. *Advances in Cancer Research* **45:**1, 1985.

Oppenheim, J., and Landy, M. (eds.). *Interleukins, Lymphokines and Cytokines.* Academic Press, Inc., New York, 1983.

Penn, I. Tumors of the immunocompromised patient. *Annual Review of Medicine* **39:**63, 1988.

Reif, A., and Mitchell, M. (eds.). *Immunity to Cancer.* Academic Press, Inc., New York, 1985.

Stevenson, F. K. Tumor vaccines. *FASEB Journal* **5:**2250, 1991.

Thurin, J. Characterization and molecular biology of tumor-associated antigens. *Current Opinion in Immunology* **2:**702, 1990.

Torrence, P. (ed.). *Biological Response Modifiers.* Academic Press, Inc., New York, 1985.

Wenz, B., and Barland, P. Therapeutic intensive plasmapheresis. *Seminars in Hematology* **18:**147, 1981.

West, W. H., Tauer, K. W., Yannelli, J. R., et al. Constant-infusion recombinant interleukin-2 in adoptive immunotherapy of advanced cancer. *New England Journal of Medicine* **316:**898, 1987.

CHAPTER 19

Transplantation Immunology

OVERVIEW

The immune mechanisms involved in self-nonself recognition are related to graft and organ rejection mechanisms in animals. In addition, different types of transplants are explored, and the mechanisms involved in the prevention of graft rejection are outlined.

CONCEPTS

1. Transplantation rejection mechanisms are activated mostly in response to foreign class I and II major histocompatibility antigens, which distinguish self from nonself.

2. The human major histocompatibility gene complex is located on chromosome 6 and codes for class I and II alloantigens (HLA). The better the HLA match between donor and recipient, the longer the graft will survive.

3. First-set rejection mechanisms involve mainly T_H and T_C cells; second-set reaction calls into play antibodies, NK cells, and T cells.

4. Graft rejection can be suppressed by immunosuppressant therapy, encompassing a number of treatments that try to induce a state of immune tolerance to the graft.

Experiments in transplantation during this century have given rise to a new medical era. Many situations have arisen in which clinicians have wanted to replace damaged tissues or organs of patients with similar healthy tissues or organs. It is now possible to surgically transfer a variety of tissues and organs from a healthy donor to an ailing recipient or from one site to another in the same individual. For example, the transplantation of skin or the cornea of an eye from one individual to another is usually accomplished successfully. In burn victims, the transplantation of skin from one region of the body to another is now a fairly common and successful procedure. However, transplantation of other organs such as heart, liver, or lung have proven to be more difficult.

Organ transplantation involves manipulating a complex collection of tissue and cell types. The cells of an individual express a unique set of membrane Ags called **allo-Ags,** which *immunologically define a person's cell type* as specifically as do fingerprints. The information about the synthesis of these unique proteins is stored in each person's chromosomal DNA. Thus, the expression of each individual's chromosomal DNA, which encodes for the allo-Ags, is unique.

This uniqueness of "self" is associated with a highly sensitive immune mechanism for sensing any foreign cell. Unfortunately, this also includes organs donated to a person whose life will depend upon accepting the new, healthy replacement for the diseased one. Since the cells of the transplanted organ will have a set of allo-Ags that are unique and different from the recipient, the transplanted organ will be seen as foreign and destroyed. The fact that the organ is needed for the host's continued survival is overruled by the body's immune defense system, which does not allow any foreign cell to prosper in the body.

The nonself cells of the transplanted organ will trigger a complex response that will activate both humoral and cell-mediated immune mechanisms. This rejection response can lead to the death of cells comprising the organ, unless the immune system is suppressed. Unfortunately, however, attempts to suppress this reaction with immunosuppressant drugs can also lead to the death of the transplant recipient due to complications related to drug treatment or infection.

The speed of rejection depends, in large part, on the degree of antigenic difference between donor and recipient. In general, the greater the difference, the faster and more acute the transplantation rejection reaction will be. Foreign tissues are usually killed and rejected approximately two weeks after transplantation. If a second transplant from the same donor is repeated, it is rejected much sooner (three to five days) than the first transplant. These are termed first-set and second-set reactions, respectively. A second transplant from a different, unrelated donor requires essentially the same time period for rejection as did the first transplant.

First-set reactions are chronic, being relatively slow and progressive. As a result, they have been referred to as delayed rejection reactions. They are typified by infiltration of the graft site by stimulated mononuclear cells that are cytotoxic to the transplanted cells bearing foreign surface Ags. In addition, Abs are believed to play a significant role in chronic rejection mechanisms. The blood vessels feeding the graft also are destroyed during rejection, leading to necrosis and sloughing of the graft (discussed later in this chapter). In **second-set** reactions, a hyperacute or immediate rejection response is elicited. This accelerated rejection of a graft is accomplished by cytolytic leukocytes and complement-mediated Ab lysis of transplanted cells. Destruction of the vascular supply to the graft is rapid and can be accompanied by thrombosis. In both immediate (hyperacute) and delayed (chronic) rejection, immune mechanisms are directed against determinants expressed on the surface membranes of the cells in the graft.

The success of transplantation depends on the amount of sharing of histocompatibility gene sets. As shown in figure 19.1, parents with HLA genotypes AA and BB will produce offspring with the hybrid genotype AB. The AB offspring can accept grafts from either parent, but the parents will reject grafts from their AB offspring. Thus, a graft is accepted only when *all* of the histocompatibility Ags are present in the recipient.

When tissue is transplanted from one site to another in the same individual, the transplant is termed an **autograft** (from the Greek, *auto* = self) When the transplant is from one individual to a genetically different individual, the graft is an **allograft** (from the

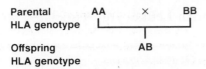

Parental
HLA genotype   AA   ×   BB

Offspring   AB
HLA genotype

**Ag (or pattern) must be present in order for
recognition as "self" to occur**

Transplants from AB cannot be integrated
into AA or BB because they lack horizontal
or vertical part of pattern

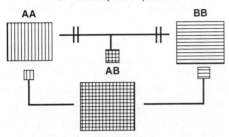

Transplants from AA or BB can be accepted
because horizontal or vertical lines can
be incorporated into pattern of AB

FIGURE 19.1 Mode of inheritance of HLA genes. Each parent contributes to the HLA identity (genotype) of the offspring. In terms of histocompatibility, the offspring of two homozygous parents recognize HLA Ags from each parent as self. However, each parent recognizes, as self, only part of the offspring's HLA genotype (namely, their own contribution); the other part of the genotype is identified as foreign.

Greek, *allo* = different). If the transplant is between identical twins, the graft is called an **isograft** (from the Greek, *iso* = equal). The graft between two different species, such as a human and baboon, is known as a **xenograft** (from the Greek, *xeno* = stranger). While autografts and isografts are often successful forms of transplantation, allografts and xenografts are usually not accepted. In fact, xenografts are rejected faster than allografts, since the level of genetic difference of cell-surface Ags is greater in transplants that cross species lines. These foreign grafted tissues will not remain viable since, immunologically, each of us is a rugged individual.

In the natural course of events, what would usually be lifesaving transplants of organs, are usually cast off because of subtle antigenic differences that exist among even closely related siblings. Unfortunately, this seems to be the price we have to pay in order to assure

that the immune system can recognize and destroy altered cells and tumors. As is discussed below, the humoral and cellular immune responses that are subsequently invoked in transplantation rejection reactions are directed against antigenic determinants on the cell membranes, which are products of distinct, but closely linked, genes of the cell's chromosomal DNA.

■　■　■　■　■　■　■　■　■　■　■

HUMAN TRANSPLANTATION ANTIGENS

The most important determinants responsible for graft rejection are the antigenic products of a closely linked cluster of genes located on chromosome 6, called the **major histocompatibility complex (MHC).** Histocompatibility systems have been discussed in detail in chapter 7; nevertheless, certain details are repeated here for emphasis.

Histocompatibility refers to the degree of antigenic likeness (or lack of it) between two given tissue types. In humans, the major histocompatability region has been designated **HLA.** The rejection process is largely directed against two types of major histocompatibility Ags designated class I and class II (table 19.1). Nevertheless, there are numerous minor histocompatibility loci, and differences in multiple loci may contribute significantly to the rejection process. For example, grafts between sexes (male to female) may also evoke a host response due to a histocompatibility Ag (H-Y) possessed by males and not females. (Review chapter 7, Histocompatibility Systems, for additional information.)

Class I Ags are found on cell membranes of *all nucleated cells* of the body. They are coded by three loci within the HLA complex, named A, B, and C. Specific T_C lymphocytes recognize and respond to foreign MHC class I Ags. Thus, class I HLA Ags control T_C lymphocyte responses. Since Abs can be raised against class I Ags, they have also been called serologically defined (SD) Ags. A class I Ag is a glycoprotein composed of a membrane-bound peptide, which is noncovalently linked to a microglobulin molecule.

TABLE 19.1 Characteristics of Class I and Class II Human Leukocyte–Associated Antigens

Characteristic	Class I Antigens	Class II Antigens
Alternate name	Serologically defined	Lymphocyte defined
Location	All nucleated somatic cells	Mϕs/monocytes; T and B lymphocytes
HLA loci	A, B, C	DO, DZ, DP, DQ, DR
Nature of Ag	Membrane-bound glycoprotein; β_2-microglobulin	Membrane-bound glycoprotein
Cells activated to foreign MHC Ags	T_C lymphocytes	$T_{H/I}$ lymphocytes

In contrast **class II Ags** are found mainly on the *surfaces of immunocompetent cells,* including macrophages (Mϕs), monocytes, and T and B lymphocytes. They are called lymphocyte-defined (LD) Ags. They are coded for by four loci in the HLA gene complex: the DO/DZ, DQ, DP, and DR regions. Class II Ags are cell-surface markers involved in immune regulation and are important in influencing graft rejection. The class II Ags are glycoproteins made up of two noncovalently-linked polypeptide chains that are both membrane bound.

Specific $T_{H/I}$ lymphocytes recognize and respond to foreign class II gene products. The closer the match of the SD and LD loci between donor and recipient cells, the longer the graft survives. Thus, both class I and class II Ags are important in mediating immune mechanisms involved in graft cell destruction (fig. 19.2).

Since the histocompatability Ags are encoded by DNA, their corresponding genes can be inherited. The MHC chromosomal unit, called a *haplotype,* is inherited in a codominant manner, like the blood groups. A family has only four haplotypes (fig. 19.3). Two are inherited from the father (e.g., units A + B) and two are inherited from the mother (e.g., units C + D). Therefore, the children can be either genotype AC, AD, BC or BD. If two children inherit the same pair of haplotypes (e.g., AD), they are called HLA-identical siblings. If two siblings share only one haplotype (e.g., AC and AD), they are HLA-haploidentical siblings. If they share neither (e.g., AC and BD), they are HLA-different siblings.

Siblings who have inherited the same pair of haplotypes and are HLA identical, reject grafts between themselves very slowly and require only small amounts of immunosuppressive drugs to prevent rejection. This occurs since there are only minor genetic differences that distinguish them as immunologically unique. On the other hand, grafts between haploidentical siblings show a wide variation in rejection time and in the amount of drug therapy needed to prevent rejection. Grafts between HLA-different siblings are rapidly rejected, and so transplants are rarely attempted under these circumstances.

It should be noted that there seems to be a strong correlation between certain HLA types and disease states. For example, many autoimmune disorders are known to be associated with particular HLA Ags. Diseases of endocrine glands, such as Graves' disease (thyroid gland) are most frequent in people carrying specific HLA-D or DR alleles. There is even evidence of differences between ethnic groups, which may explain differences in susceptibility of some races to infections while other populations are more resistant.

HISTOCOMPATIBILITY TESTING

When tissue transplantation is anticipated, typing and crossmatching of blood from donor and recipient are performed as a first step. If there exists any incompatibility in the ABO blood group, then the use of the prospective donor's tissue is absolutely contraindicated. Tissue typing for transplantation is also done

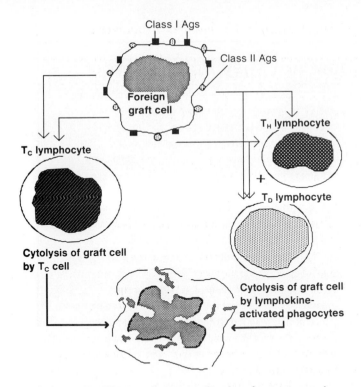

FIGURE 19.2 Class I and II Ag-mediated graft rejection mechanisms. Foreign tissue grafts interact with the immune system through class I and class II MHC Ags. Each class of MHC Ag stimulates specific effector cell populations that can cooperate, or act independently, to eliminate the source of foreign Ags.

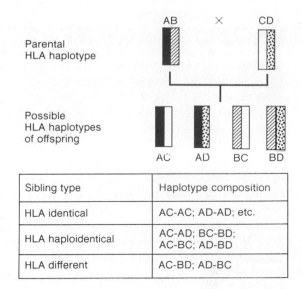

Sibling type	Haplotype composition
HLA identical	AC-AC; AD-AD; etc.
HLA haploidentical	AC-AD; BC-BD; AC-BC; AD-BD
HLA different	AC-BD; AD-BC

FIGURE 19.3 Codominant inheritance of MHC genes. The HLA genotype of an offspring reflects the HLA contributions from each parent. The offspring of heterozygous parents display different assortments of parental contributions, defined as haplotypes. The HLA haplotypes of the offspring can be compared with each other to determine the degree of their similarity. This simplified diagram depicts possible relationships among offspring HLA haplotypes. Those that are HLA identical are histo*compatible;* those that are HLA different are histo*incompatible.*

with leukocytes. Lymphoagglutination and lymphocytotoxicity tests are widely used. The principles of these assays are outlined in figure 19.4.

Abs can be made against HLA Ags that can lead to the agglutination of the foreign transplanted cells. The *lymphoagglutination test* can identify histocompatibility Ags present on donor and recipient lymphocytes when tested with a panel of specific antisera (Abs) to determine the degree of tissue match. In *lymphocytotoxicity or microcytotoxicity tests,* donor lymphocytes are similarly incubated with a panel of antisera directed against specific class I MHC Ags, followed by addition of complement. The percentage of cells lysed by each antiserum is measured, quantified, and the class I Ags that do not match are recorded. The greater the number of foreign class I Ags, the greater the risk of rejection.

The *mixed-lymphocyte culture (MLC) assay,* outlined in figure 19.4, can determine a possible match between donor and recipient class II MHC Ags. In this test, donor and recipient lymphocytes are mixed together in a tube containing a radioactive DNA precursor. Donor, or "stimulator," cells are irradiated to prevent DNA synthesis and proliferation. If the class II Ags are foreign, the responder cells will be stimulated to divide. As the stimulated cells replicate their DNA, they incorporate the radioactive precursor. The amount of radioactivity incorporated into cells can then be easily measured and quantified. The greater the amount of cell division (incorporation of labeled DNA precursor), the greater the degree of incompatibility between the cell sets and the greater the degree of rejection.

Non-MHC Transplantation Antigens: Are They Actually Minor?

The major criteria weighed in organ transplants are the ABO compatibility of the donor and recipient and the HLA (class I and II) compatibility. But even if there is a close match on those criteria, for example, between siblings with the same HLA haplotype, an allograft can still be rejected. The failure of HLA-compatible grafts to survive indefinitely seems to be due to the cumulative effects of a large number of minor histocompatibility antigenic differences. Thus, immunosuppressive drugs must be used, even between HLA-identical siblings.

The appearance of non-MHC (mH) transplantation Ags occurs during acute and chronic transplantation rejection reactions and elicits a T cell-mediated response that is MHC restricted. In contrast, mH Ags do not seem to elicit a B cell-Ab response. Each mH Ag has a characteristic immunogenicity, and when two Ags of equal strength are present, they can have an additive effect. The differences in the immunogenicity of certain organs (e.g., skin is more immunogenic than liver) may be attributed to differential expression of mH Ags.

Most of our knowledge of mH Ags comes from studies of congenic mouse strains. Genetically, the location of mH gene loci is disperse, and, in mice, is regulated by single genes. These cell membrane molecules seem to have a fluctuating association with MHC class I and II molecules, which is perhaps based on competition between individual mH molecules.

The current understanding of these minor Ags has led clinicians to examine donor and recipient mH Ag profiles. However, even in bone marrow donors who share about 50% of mH Ags with the recipient, the graft can still lead to fatal graft-versus-host disease. Thus, it is not enough to match the mH Ags, but rather we must understand how they interact with each other and how mH Ags associate with the MHC class I and II Ags on the surface of tissue cells. Until we can better identify and understand the regulation of mH Ags, there will remain a transplantation barrier.

Loveland, B., and Simpson, E. The non-MHC transplantation antigens: neither weak nor minor. *Immunology Today* **7**:223, 1986.

REJECTION MECHANISM

The major cell type involved in transplantation rejection of grafts is the T lymphocyte. One experiment that substantiates this view is portrayed in figure 19.5. This strategy demonstrates that certain rejection reactions can be transferred from an immunized donor to a nonsensitized recipient by T lymphocytes but not by serum (presumably, Abs). Further investigation has shown that the major immune components in early rejection reactions are T_H, T_C, and T_D (also called sensitized T) cells, and NK cells. Nevertheless, Abs are believed to play an important role in chronic rejection. Current evidence points to a primary dependence upon T_C cells in hyperacute rejection.

The mechanisms of graft rejection can be divided into two major types: first-set and second-set reactions. During first-set reactions, the recipient is immunologically sensitized to the donor's histocompatibility Ags. Sensitization involves the progressive activation of several T cell subclasses and their subsequent attack on the graft. In second-set reactions, there is immunological memory of the donor's Ags as evidenced by expanded clones of specific T and B cells. As a result, there is very rapid activation of lymphocytes which, in conjunction with Abs and complement, destroy the grafted tissues almost immediately.

First-Set Reaction

Presentation of foreign-cell MHC Ags is one of the initial events of a **first-set reaction.** Once blood vessels communicate with the graft, graft Ags can travel to the lymph nodes where they activate lymphatic T cells. The activated lymphocytes give rise to expanded clones of **specific T_C, T_H,** and **T_D** cells. T_C cells can

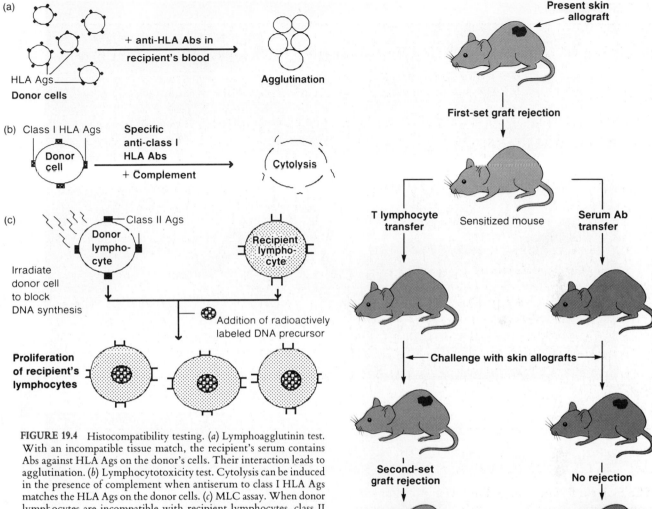

FIGURE 19.4 Histocompatibility testing. (*a*) Lymphoagglutinin test. With an incompatible tissue match, the recipient's serum contains Abs against HLA Ags on the donor's cells. Their interaction leads to agglutination. (*b*) Lymphocytotoxicity test. Cytolysis can be induced in the presence of complement when antiserum to class I HLA Ags matches the HLA Ags on the donor cells. (*c*) MLC assay. When donor lymphocytes are incompatible with recipient lymphocytes, class II foreign Ags stimulate proliferation of the recipient's lymphocytes.

FIGURE 19.5 T cell dependence for graft rejection. A mouse is sensitized to particular Ags contained in a skin allograft. Subsequently, T cells or serum (Abs) are transferred to naive mice that are isogeneic with the mice that provided the original graft. These naive mice, in turn, are challenged with skin grafts from the same source as the original graft. Mice that received the T cell transfer display a second-set graft rejection, although they have never been previously challenged. In contrast, mice receiving serum Abs fail to reject the graft. This demonstrates that sensitized T cells, not Abs, are required for graft rejection.

enter the circulation directly, while T_D cells remain in the lymph nodes and mobilize phagocytic leukocytes via the release of soluble lymphokines. Killer T_C cells eventually reach the transplantation site, enter the blood vessels of the graft, and proceed to destroy the grafted tissue by repeated cell-to-cell toxicity (fig. 19.6).

Histological studies reveal that the first cells to infiltrate the blood vessels of the graft are phagocytic *neutrophils,* followed by *lymphocytes* (T_C and NK) and *Mϕs.* (The histological picture of a first-set graft

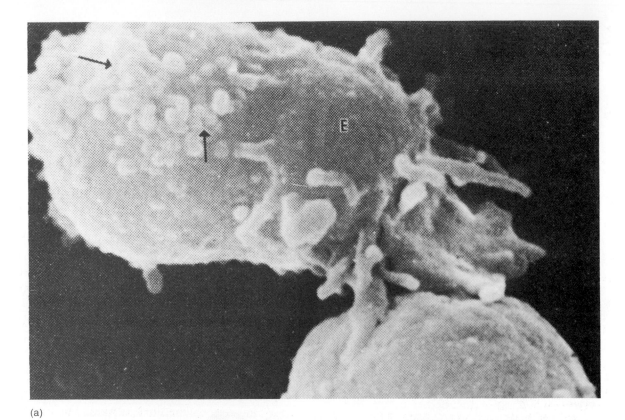

(a)

(b)

FIGURE 19.6 Interaction of effector T_C cell with target cells. (*a*) A stimulated effector cell (*labeled E*), with projections from its surface, is shown establishing contact with a target cell (*smooth surface*) (photograph made using a scanning electron microscope). (*b*) Higher resolution picture of interaction between a stimulated effector cell (*on left, labeled E*) and a target cell (*on right, labeled T*) showing penetration of the effector cell to the perinuclear region of the target cell (photograph made using a transmission electron microcope). (From Barber, T. A., and Alter, B. J. Ultrastructure of effector-target cell interaction in secondary cell-mediated lympholysis. *Scandinavian Journal of Immunology* **7:**57–66/fig. 1, 7. Blackwell Scientific Publications Limited. 1978.)

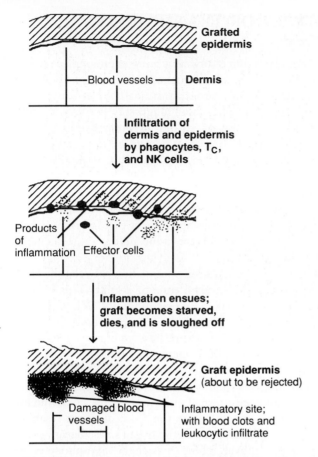

Grafted
epidermis

Blood vessels — Dermis

Infiltration of
dermis and epidermis
by phagocytes, T_C,
and NK cells

Products
of
inflammation   Effector cells

Inflammation ensues;
graft becomes starved,
dies, and is sloughed off

Graft epidermis
(about to be rejected)

Damaged blood
vessels

Inflammatory site;
with blood clots and
leukocytic infiltrate

FIGURE 19.7 *First-set rejection reaction. Events of a first-set graft rejection are diagrammatically portrayed. Compare with figure 19.8; note presence of effectors (phagocytes, T_C, and NK cells, middle panel) and intensity of inflammatory response (bottom panel).*

rejection reaction is diagrammatically represented in fig. 19.7.) Mφs play a supportive role by phagocytizing the foreign tissue cells. In addition, Abs produced against Ags in the graft can activate Ab-dependent and complement-mediated cytotoxic reactions. Yet, the rate of rejection does not seem to depend upon the presence of complement.

The first signs of damage at the tissue level are seen in the capillaries, vessels composed of a single layer of endothelial cells. Local hemorrhages and platelet aggregation may occur, with eventual blood clot formation and irreversible damage to the blood vessels feeding the graft. This cessation of capillary blood flow eliminates gas and nutrient exchange at the cellular level; death of the grafted cells occurs soon thereafter.

Second-Set Reaction

In **second-set reactions,** the *memory* of foreign antigenic cells is so vivid that the blood vessels of the second graft are destroyed almost as soon as they are established. This more rapid response is brought about primarily by T_C cells which are rapidly activated. The additional participation of circulating complement-fixing Abs and NK cells might contribute to graft rejection. Since these immune components are already present in the circulation, they can readily be mobilized to sites where foreign transplanted cells are located and immediately start the destruction of vascular endothelium. The infiltration of neutrophils, Mφs, and T_C cells, which soon follows, eventually serves to provide backup mechanisms to ensure the rapid and irreversible rejection of the foreign tissue transplanted to the host a second time. A second-set rejection reaction is diagrammed in figure 19.8.

Required Effector Cells

T_H and T_D cells are the *primary initiators* of allograft rejections. These cells are activated by class I HLA incompatible Ags on the donor tissues. The cytokines they produce recruit cytotoxic effector cells, which actually destroy the foreign tissues. They are indispensable for first-set rejection of foreign tissue grafts. These *effectors* include T_C cells, which recognize specific epitopes on the foreign graft, and **NK cells,** which are triggered by the absence of self class I HLA Ags in the foreign tissue.

In contrast, second-set rejection is more directly dependent upon T_C cells. Although T_H and T_D cells might still be involved in stimulating and recruiting T_C cells, they are not absolutely required. In the absence of these inducers, memory T_C cells are capable of rejecting foreign tissue grafts. These cells are directly activated by provoking class I Ags.

Activation of rejection appears to be dependent upon interleukin 1 (IL-1), since administration of soluble IL-1 receptor delayed allograft rejection. Presumably, circulating soluble IL-1 receptors in the test subjects bound physiologically released IL-1. The artificial reduction of IL-1 secretion that occurred, in turn, blunted activation of the rejection mechanism.

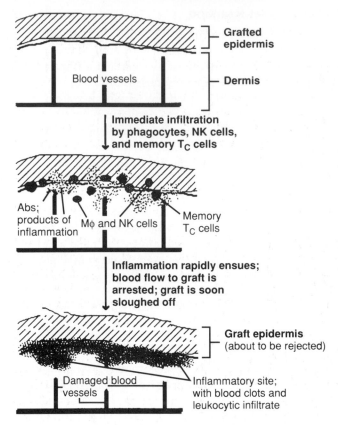

Grafted
epidermis

Dermis

Blood vessels

**Immediate infiltration
by phagocytes, NK cells,
and memory T$_C$ cells**

Abs;
products of
inflammation

Mϕ and NK cells

Memory
T$_C$ cells

**Inflammation rapidly ensues;
blood flow to graft is
arrested; graft is soon
sloughed off**

Graft epidermis
(about to be rejected)

Damaged blood
vessels

Inflammatory site;
with blood clots and
leukocytic infiltrate

FIGURE 19.8 Second-set rejection reaction. Events of a second-set graft rejection are diagrammatically portrayed. Compare with figure 19.7; note that effectors are generally similar, but include memory T$_C$ cells (*middle panel*) and intensity of inflammatory response (*bottom panel*).

This demonstration underscores the importance of Ag-presenting cells (APCs; the likely source of IL-1) in the initiation of rejection mechanisms.

In addition to physically presenting Ag and supplying monokines, the nature of the APCs might be important in activation of rejection mechanisms. Compatibility of HLA-D Ags (MHC class II) between donor and recipient often seems more important than compatibility of HLA-A, HLA-B, and HLA-C Ags (MHC class I) in predicting acceptance of a transplanted organ. This has prompted the suggestion that Ags provoking graft rejection must be presented to effector cells by APCs that are MHC compatible with the graft, not the host.

TYPES OF TRANSPLANTS
Organ

Transplantation of organs is fairly commonplace today. Although there are frequent public calls for organs for transplantation, the fact of a heart, heart-lung, liver, or kidney transplant is no longer newsworthy in itself. This reflects major strides in understanding tissue transplantation compatibility over the past several years. However, it should be recalled that transplantation of an organ from a living donor was not accomplished until 1954. In that year, **Joseph Murray** performed the first successful transplantation of a kidney from a living donor, an accomplishment that led to his being awarded the Nobel Prize in Physiology or Medicine in 1990.

There is a strong correlation between the HLA match and the survival time of a graft. This is especially true in human kidney allografts. When the siblings are HLA identical, the failure of the kidney graft is rare. If the kidneys from a parent or sibling are HLA different, it is actually better to use a kidney of a cadaver that is both HLA-A and HLA-B matched. In fact, if the cadaver's kidney is stored frozen, the chance of rejection is diminished even more. This phenomenon is thought to result from the death of donor lymphocytes that are trapped in the organ's vasculature at the time of removal. These "passenger" lymphocytes are far more immunogenic than other tissue cells, and their destruction by freezing would diminish the degree of foreignness of the transplanted tissue.

Another way to enhance the survival of an organ is to pretransfuse the recipient with blood that has an incompatible MHC Ag profile. It is thought that this "MHC-mismatched," pretransplant transfusion might provoke the formation of noncomplement-binding Abs that could bind to and "block" the MHC Ag site for T$_H$ recognition. Interestingly, this would enhance graft survival by preventing immune activation to the now masked foreign MHC Ags.

The need to crossmatch HLA Ags for a successful kidney transplant seems also to apply to other solid organ transplants such as the heart, liver, lung, and pancreas. But different tissues and organs vary in their ability to evoke an immune response. For example, liver and kidney organ transplants are less readily rejected, under similar circumstances, than heart, lung, or endocrine organs. However, with improved surgical techniques and drugs to more effectively prevent tissue rejection, the transplantation of these latter organs is becoming more successful.

If a first-set rejection reaction starts, the entire organ becomes gradually filled with lymphocytes, which first destroy the capillary beds of the organ. This vascular damage, including hemorrhages, blood clots, occluded blood vessel lumina, and necrotic tissue, becomes progressive and fatal. Once the blood supply has been cut off by destruction of these vessels, the tissue cells of the organ rapidly die as their oxygen and nutrient supply becomes irreversibly depleted.

Tissue

One of the most common tissue grafts is the skin graft. It is mainly used in the treatment of burns where a temporary cover is provided by an allograft, which is later permanently replaced by an autograft from another area of the burn victim's body. The transplanting of skin from one region to another in the same individual is a highly successful technique. This procedure is used for individuals, such as burn victims, who have experienced extensive skin destruction.

Since the tissue match in autografts is perfect, rejection reactions are rare. However, if a skin graft is not HLA matched, first- and second-set reactions can occur, as for any other transplant. However, rejection is slower than that for organs, because of the additional time needed to establish vascular and lymphatic communication between the graft and the host, or recipient. This may require several days as compared with an almost immediate establishment of vascular communication for grafted organs.

Once the vascular connections are made, the histocompatibility Ags can interact with the immune system, and the rejection process can begin. The grafted skin becomes infiltrated by neutrophils, lymphocytes, and Mϕs, causing damage to the blood vessels and tissue necrosis as the site is deprived of blood flow.

Cornea

Many individuals who are blind because of irreversible damage to the cornea can successfully receive a corneal transplant. Moreover, the cornea is located in an "immunologically privileged" site—a place in the body where the immune system cannot fully function. The cornea is housed in the anterior chamber of the eye and has little lymphatic or vascular supply. Instead, it receives its oxygen and nutrients from the atmosphere and the fluids bathing the interior of the eye (the aqueous and vitreous humors). It was formerly believed that the absence of lymphatic drainage prevented transplantation Ags from being exposed to the immune system, thereby causing sensitization. However, it is now known that Ags can escape from the anterior chamber and invoke an unusual form of immune response called anterior chamber–associated immune deviation (ACAID).

Studies of immune responses to intraocular Ags revealed this special form of immune response. In ACAID, delayed hypersensitivity (DTH) reactions, mediated by T_D cells, are suppressed in association with the induction of T_S cells. Nevertheless, humoral immunity and T_C cell function appear to remain intact. This selective suppression of DTH reactions seems to be related to an attempt to prevent inflammation of the eye, which could lead to other complications such as a detached retina and blindness. However, the protective effect of ACAID has potentially adverse consequences. Although ACAID provides protection against inflammation, it also deprives the eye of protection against intracellular pathogens, which DTH reactions effectively remove, for example herpes simplex virus, which can cause degenerative neural lesions. Thus, the suppression of DTH reactions by T_S cells in ACAID creates a "dangerous compromise" between maintaining the structural and functional integrity of the eye and the need to provide immunological protection against invading pathogens.

Since first-set transplantation reactions are cell-mediated (DTH) reactions, the high frequency of successful corneal transplants is understandable. Moreover, corneal grafts are usually permanently accepted without having to use immunosuppressant therapy. The only exception occurs with those individuals whose eyes were inflamed at the time of transplantation. Under these conditions, increased vascularization occurs, even in the anterior of the eye. The establishment of this vascular supply allows the host's immune system to become sensitized to the corneal HLA antigens and thus react against them. HLA matching is

Transplanting Brain Tissue

Parkinson's disease is a neurological disorder associated with such symptoms as muscle tremors and rigidity, difficulties in speech, and other severe problems that can lead to disability. The disease is caused by degeneration of the dopaminergic neurons in the area of the brain called the substantia nigra. Treatment consists of administration of L-dopa to increase the production of dopamine in the brain. However, there is one serious side effect, the appearance of schizophrenia symptoms.

In Sweden, an alternative treatment was tested. A group, directed by Lars Olson, transplanted dopamine-producing cells from the adrenal gland to the substantia nigra of the brain in persons afflicted with debilitating Parkinson's disease with the hope of reversing the symptoms of the disease. The symptoms were only partially alleviated. However, in Mexico City, Madrazo and Drucker-Colin discovered a more successful transplant procedure. The adrenal tissue was transplanted instead to a brain ventricle, a cavity filled with nutritive cerebrospinal fluid.

How is this possible? One reason is the presence of the blood-brain barrier, which prevents the entry or exit of many molecules from the brain. In addition, there is poor lymphatic drainage in the brain (especially in the meninges). This means that certain areas of brain are actually immunologically privileged sites, allowing the grafting of new brain tissue without the immune system fully reacting to the new foreign transplantation Ags and mounting a transplantation rejection reaction.

Although this is the first such transplant in humans, brain tissue transplant work has been done on rodents and primates. These studies showed that damaged neurons in adult animals could be successfully replaced by implanting neurons from fetal brains of the same strain. The implications of this work are far reaching. The ability to replace damaged brain tissue could be used to treat a wide variety of brain disorders from optic nerve blindness to Alzheimer's disease.

Kiester, E. Spare parts for damaged brains. *Science 86* **7**:32, 1986.

Madrazo, I. N., Drucker-Colin, R., Diaz, V., et al. Open microsurgical autograft of adrenal medulla to the right caudate nucleus in two patients with intractable Parkinson's disease. *New England Journal of Medicine* **316**:831, 1987.

Perlow, M. J., Freed, W. I., Hoffer, B. J., et al. Brain grafts reduce motor abnormalities produced by destruction of nigrostriatal dopamine system. *Science* **204**:643, 1979.

---

indicated, therefore, in cases of corneal transplantation when inflammation exists or when a previous cornea has been rejected.

Two additional immunologically privileged sites, defined by specialized vascularization, exist. These are the brain and the testes. Animal experimentation has shown that allogenic brain tissue can be transplanted successfully and that such tissue can function properly.

Bone Marrow

A child has acute leukemia in remission and has a very poor prognosis. What can now be performed is bone marrow transplantation from an HLA-identical sibling. Since the sick child's cancerous cells are derived from the bone marrow, the child is irradiated at a level that kills all cells in the bone marrow. Unfortunately, this procedure also destroys the hemopoietic stem cell procursors for other normal blood cells, which are required for continued survival. The only possibility for this child to survive is to receive a transplant of histocompatible bone marrow that will restore thrombocyte, erythrocyte, and leukocyte production.

Bone marrow transplants are also performed to treat nonmalignant disorders. Some infants with severe combined immunologic deficiency disease have been successfully treated with bone marrow from an HLA-identical sibling. Since these children possess neither functioning B nor T lymphocytes, they must either be treated with transplanted bone marrow (that will supply functioning lymphocytes) or be placed in a germ-free environment ("bubble chamber") to prevent the development of lethal viral, bacterial, or fungal infections. In addition, complication-free survival is high among children with β-thalessemia (congenital underproduction of hemoglobin β chain) who receive HLA-identical bone marrow transplants.

Bone marrow transplants are also used as a means of treating acquired aplastic anemia. In this disease, the bone marrow malfunctions and decreases its production of erythrocytes. In cases where the malfunction is irreversible and life threatening, bone marrow transplantation from a matched donor is usually successful but only if transplantation is carried out before blood transfusions are started (to prevent immune sensitization).

GRAFT-VERSUS-HOST REACTIONS

If transplantation of bone marrow to children with leukemia is successful, the cancerous bone marrow is replaced by normal bone marrow and the child is cured. On the other hand, if the graft is rejected, the child will die painfully from a **graft-versus-host** (**GVH**) reaction. This reaction occurs because the individual's lymphocytes (both B and T cells) have been destroyed by irradiation, thus rendering the person immunologically helpless. The transplanted bone marrow cells are "accepted" because there are no functioning B and T cells to recognize them as foreign. However, the grafted bone marrow (containing B and T cell stem cells) can perceive the host as foreign and begin to destroy the recipient's cells and tissues. In other words, the graft attacks the host, hence a GVH reaction.

GVH reactions are not limited to bone marrow transplants. Similar reactions can arise following transplantation of other tissues or organs. The requirement in each case, however, is the presence of immunological effector cells of donor origin.

Progress of Graft-Versus-Host Reactions

GVH reactions are dependent upon HLA incompatibility between the donor and the host (recipient). However, GVH reactions might not be limited to reactions induced by HLA Ags. Sensitization against non-HLA Ags can also play a role, according to some in-

TABLE 19.2 Stages of Graft-Versus-Host Reactions Induced by Non-HLA Antigens

Stage	Description	Characteristics
I	Priming	Production of Ag-reactive, sensitized T cells capable of reacting against Ags expressed by pathogens responsible for latent infections
II	Activation	Pathogens express Ags in immunosuppressed organ recipient Ag-reactive, sensitized lymphocytes of donor become activated
III	Recruitment, sensitization	Donor T cells become sensitized to non-HLA Ags of organ recipient
IV	GVH reaction	Recruited, sensitized T cells display widespread reaction against organ recipient's tissues

Source: deGast, G. C., Gratama, J. W., Ringden, O., et al. *Immunology Today* **8**:209, 1987.

vestigators. Nevertheless, expression of GVH reactions seems to be following a fairly orderly progression definable into distinct stages (table 19.2). The sequence leading to a GVH reaction is outlined in figure 19.9.

There is evidence suggesting that GVH reactions increase with age, that is, old organ recipients display more GVH reactions than do young organ recipients. This has prompted the suggestion that exposure to latent infections (e.g., viral or protozoal) prior to transplantation plays a role in GVH reactions. This constitutes **stage I** and *leads to the production of Ag-reactive, sensitized T cells.*

Stages II and III occur as a direct consequence of events associated with transplantation itself. **Stage II** occurs because of *immune suppression* of the organ recipient in preparation for transplantation. Organisms responsible for latent infections are able to express their Ags while the organ recipient is immunosuppressed. These Ags can activate Ag-reactive donor T cells. In addition to reacting against the activating pathogens,

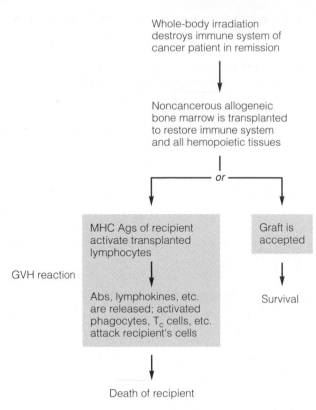

Whole-body irradiation
destroys immune system of
cancer patient in remission

↓

Noncancerous allogeneic
bone marrow is transplanted
to restore immune system
and all hemopoietic tissues

— *or* —

GVH reaction

MHC Ags of recipient
activate transplanted
lymphocytes

↓

Abs, lymphokines, etc.
are released; activated
phagocytes, T$_c$ cells, etc.
attack recipient's cells

↓

Death of recipient

Graft is
accepted

↓

Survival

FIGURE 19.9 GVH. This schematic outline shows the events leading to GVH reaction.

these cells can also recruit other T cells. Some recruited T cells can become sensitized to recipient non-HLA Ags. This *sensitization* constitutes **stage III.**

Stage IV occurs when *effector cells react against host* (recipient) tissues. For GVH reactions induced by HLA incompatibility, progression through stages I to III is not necessary. In these instances, the entire GVH reaction consists of expression of stage IV. However, for GVH reactions precipitated by non-HLA Ags, sensitization of an effector lymphocyte population of donor origin is accomplished through the events of stages I to III. Nevertheless, in all cases the cells that are most susceptible to GVH attack are cells of the skin, liver, and the gastrointestinal tract. This leads to diarrhea, anorexia, skin and mouth ulcers, jaundice, and liver destruction. The course of the reaction is relentlessly progressive, leading to organ and systemic failure and, ultimately, death.

Managing Graft-Versus-Host Reactions

GVH reactions have not remained as insurmountable obstacles to using bone marrow transplants clinically. The research efforts of **E. Donnall Thomas** led to the discovery that the drug, methotrexate, could reduce the occurrence of GVH reactions following bone marrow transplantation. This observation opened the way for more widespread clinical application of bone marrow transplantation and earned Thomas the 1990 Nobel Prize in Physiology or Medicine.

A theoretical way to circumvent fatal GVH disease in leukemic patients is the use of autologous marrow transplants that have been pretreated with cytotoxic monoclonal Abs (MAbs) specific for the leukemic tumor Ag. Autologous marrow transplantation consists of removing and saving a portion of an individual's bone marrow, administering radiotherapy, and returning the nonirradiated bone marrow explant to the individual. However, the explanted bone marrow may still possess leukemic cells, and so elimination of any tumor cells present in the marrow is essential.

One approach to this problem is the production of a MAb specific for the leukemic tumor Ag. Once obtained, the bone marrow removed from the person during remission could then be treated with this Ab and complement to specifically destroy *only* contaminating tumor cells (fig. 19.10). After treatment, the now noncancerous "self" bone marrow could be returned, with no chance of a fatal GVH disease developing, and the person would be cured! Animal studies are now underway, and the results look promising for clinical trials in the near future.

PREVENTION OF GRAFT REJECTION

Graft rejection may be prevented by (1) immune suppression with drugs or (2) development of immunological tolerance to the foreign transplanted tissue Ags.

Drug therapy can lead to nonspecific or specific immune suppression. **Nonspecific immune suppression** includes *x-irradiation* and the use of *corticosteroids* and *cytotoxic drugs*. All of these treatments lead to nonselective inhibition of rapidly dividing body cells, including active B and T lymphocyte populations.

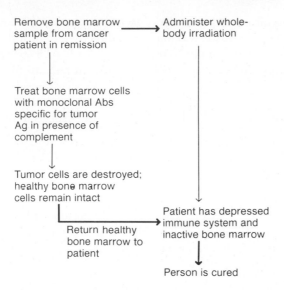

FIGURE 19.10 Use of monoclonal Abs to destroy leukemic bone marrow cells.

X-irradiation is more cytotoxic to actively replicating cells and is sometimes used with skin allografts. The main drawback is its nonspecific effect on all dividing cells, causing extensive damage to the tissues and organs comprising the gastrointestinal tract and bone marrow. This can lead to life-threatening complications.

Corticosteroids are antiinflammatory drugs that diminish the responsiveness of both B and T cell pools. This blanket immune suppression leaves the individual severely unprotected against even commonplace bacterial or viral infection. Cytotoxic drugs, such as azathioprine or cyclophosphamide, act on various stages of nucleic acid synthesis preventing replication of active lymphocytes. Their effects on the immune system are more specific than the corticosteroids. Azathioprine, used in renal transplants, inhibits T cell, but not B cell, responses; cyclophosphamide, used in bone marrow recipients, selectively prevents B cell replication. Although successful in suppressing immune sensitization, drug levels have to be carefully monitored to prevent damaging other organs with rapidly dividing cell populations such as the intestine and bone marrow.

Other nonspecific forms of immune suppression include depletion of certain T cell populations by antilymphocyte serum (ALS) and blocking T_H cell activation by the drug cyclosporin A. Antiserum can be produced by horses against human lymphocytes. This ALS or globulin, can destroy the body's T cell pools but leave Ab production intact. The effect of ALS is seen in transplants where subsequent reduced levels of T cells markedly diminish the rate of graft rejection. Unfortunately, the body's ability to fight viral infections is also impaired. One solution to the dilemma of using ALS in transplants is to produce cytotoxic MAbs to only those T cells that are specifically involved in reacting to the HLA Ags of the transplant. Then all other T and B cells would be able to remain viable and function normally. The technology for this alternative is currently unavailable but should be clinically possible in the near future.

One of the most promising immunosuppressive drugs presently in use is *cyclosporin A*. It is a chemical derived from a fungus and acts only on Ag-sensitive, dividing T cells where it blocks IL-2 production. This highly selective drug action means that B lymphocytes, resting T cells (e.g., T memory), or T_S cells are not affected. The individual is still susceptible to viral invasion and long-term treatment with cyclosporin A has produced kidney failure in some individuals. Yet despite the drawbacks, cyclosporin A therapy has given many organ transplant patients a better chance for long-term survival. Cyclosporin A has been shown to greatly reduce the risk of rejection of liver, spleen, heart, lung, and bone marrow grafts, especially when coadministered with corticosteroids. One promising area of cyclosporin research is the coupling of Ag with cyclosporin, causing a specific T_S response to just the transplantation Ag.

Ag-specific immune suppression can be obtained by *inducing tolerance* to MHC Ags in the individual receiving the transplant. Tolerance is a state of immune unresponsiveness to specific Ags such that an immune attack is never mounted or executed. In animal experimentation, antiidiotypic Abs can be induced against specific T cells, which view the graft tissue cells as foreign. These antiidiotype Abs will then bind to specific HLA T cell membrane receptors. Once the receptors are bound by Ab, the T cell is unable to interact with the MHC Ags on the graft cells (fig. 19.11). This type of Ag-specific immune suppression

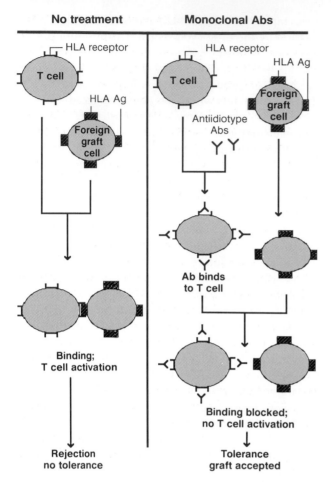

No treatment

HLA receptor

T cell

HLA Ag

Foreign
graft
cell

Binding;
T cell activation

Rejection
no tolerance

Monoclonal Abs

HLA receptor

T cell

HLA Ag

Foreign
graft
cell

Antiidiotype
Abs

Ab binds
to T cell

Binding blocked;
no T cell activation

Tolerance
graft accepted

FIGURE 19.11 Use of monoclonal Abs to induce tolerance to foreign graft. Interaction between the immune system and foreign graft cell Ags usually leads to sensitization against those Ags (*left panel*). However, presentation of antiidiotype Abs in conjunction with foreign graft cells can block interaction between T cells specific for the foreign Ag, thereby leading to a state of tolerance.

has been proven successful in certain animals but not yet in humans. The main problem has been that of maintaining a high level of antiidiotypic Abs for an extended period of time in order to maintain tolerance to the transplanted tissue.

Recent attempts to induce survival of grafted pancreatic islet tissue (which contains insulin-producing β cells) have employed direct transplantation to the host (recipient) thymus. These experiments demonstrated that islet tissue survived poorly (less than 10 days) when implanted into livers or under the renal

capsule of recipient mice. Survival was better (17 days) when islet tissue was implanted directly into host thymuses. Combining transplantation with ALS greatly improved survival of islet implants. In fact, 10 of 13 preparations implanted into thymuses were considered to have been accepted by recipients. This interpretation was supported by demonstrating survival of a second islet graft from the original donor, while islet tissue from another donor (third party) was rejected.

A treatment that is currently feasible and successful in some types of human transplants is that of *immune enhancement*. Prolonged graft survival is accomplished by preimmunizing the person with allogenic cells similar to those they will later receive in the graft. This induces a state of immune suppression that may operate in one of three ways:

1. The "enhancing" Ab, formed by preimmunization, might be non-complement fixing. By binding to the allo-Ags on the graft, it could block interaction with lymphocytes and, thus, prevent subsequent sensitization.
2. On the other hand, the Ab might bind to the highly antigenic "passenger" cells of the graft, and with complement, destroy these cells before they can sensitize the graft recipient.
3. Alternatively, immunization might provoke T_S cells, leaving the immune system unable to mount a response. The exact mechanism by which the enhancement occurs has not been elucidated, but this treatment has been used and shown to be effective in renal transplantation.

THE FETUS AS A GRAFT

When one looks at pregnancy, all the laws of transplantation seem to be broken. The fetus is always a genetic mosaic of maternal and paternal genes, and so the fetus' MHC Ags are certainly different from those of the mother. Yet the fetus is not seen as foreign transplanted tissue but, in fact, grows and prospers inside the mother's body for nine months. Therefore, despite great histocompatibility differences between the fetus, the placenta, and the mother, the fetal graft is not rejected. What interaction is occurring between the fetus and the mother's immune system (we presume the

(a) Placenta produces mucoprotein that coats fetal cells

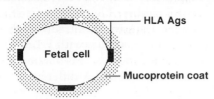

(b) Production of immunosuppressant hormones

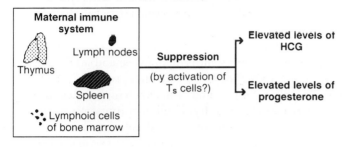

(c) Production of maternal non-complement-fixing Abs that block immune recognition

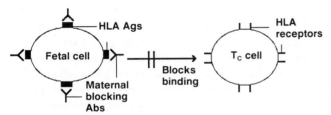

FIGURE 19.12 Immune mechanisms protecting fetus from rejection. The fetus can be protected from immunological rejection by several mechanisms that originate either in the fetus (and placenta) or the mother. These can limit exposure of fetal Ags (*a*), suppress maternal immune responses (*b*), or interfere with the expression of maternal immune responses (*c*).

fetus' developing immune system cannot respond) that allows for acceptance? It is known that the highly vascularized uterus is *not* an "immunologically privileged site," since other grafts are readily rejected in the uterus, yet the fetus appears to be an "immunologically privileged graft" (see chapter 20).

The protection of the fetus seems to come from three sources: the fetus itself, the trophoblast layer of the placenta, and the mother (fig. 19.12). All of these appear to employ both specific and nonspecific immune suppressive mechanisms as means to allow for the prosperity of the fetus as a graft.

One nonspecific defense mechanism is the secretion of mucoproteins by cells of the placenta, which come into direct contact with the maternal circulation. These secretions "mask" the histocompatibility Ags and prevent recognition. Placental giant cells can produce soluble inhibitory factor (SIF), which nonspecifically reduces T cell proliferation and Ab production, and induces a population of T_S cells. Immune suppression can actually come from the hormones produced during pregnancy. Human chorionic gonadotropin (HCG), produced by the placenta, and the high levels of maternal progesterone, act as generalized immune suppressants.

In addition, the mother produces specific "blocking" Abs to fetal Ags, which bind to the antigenic cells of the placenta. These cells are thereby protected against immune attack by interfering with T_C cell binding. The mother can also synthesize serum α-macroglobulins, which can inhibit certain cellular immunity responses. It is also believed that maternal T_S cells short-circuit the mother's immune system, preventing an attack on fetal transplantation Ags. The importance of these modes of immune suppression has led to the discovery that certain forms of infertility are actually due to defects in the mother's immune system, which lead to rejection of the conceptus (abortion). Administration of antiinflammatory steriods that depress immune reactivity is one way to sucessfully treat this problem.

The fetus is also actively involved in producing immunosuppressive factors that will ensure its continued success in the mother's womb. The major fetal serum protein, α-fetoprotein, can stimulate the formation of T_S cells, and the amniotic fluid contains immunosuppressive phospholipids. A glycoprotein of fetal origin, β_1-glycoprotein, can be found in maternal plasma and has been shown to inhibit certain maternal cellular immunity responses. The effect of all of these factors results in a depressed immune system in the mother, but it is usually not life threatening, since most of the response is localized in the uterus. An exception to this is the recent outbreaks of listeriosis. Improperly pasteurized milk and cheese products contain the infectious organism *Listeria monocytogenes*. This organism rarely causes disease in adults with competent immune systems; however, in infants, pregnant women, and the elderly, the disease is often fatal. Pregnant women who are not promptly treated with antibiotics usually die or abort their fetuses. Pregnant women should be aware of their impaired immune status and take more stringent precautions to protect their health.

SUMMARY

1. Transplanted tissue can introduce a different set of histocompatibility antigens into the host. The donor cell's antigens will be seen as foreign, and the host's immune system will begin a transplantation rejection reaction. [p. 488]

2. Tissues from a donor will be rejected faster the second time they are transplanted into the same host. The first reaction is called the first-set, and the next, the second-set reaction. The rate of rejection is determined, in part, by the degree of antigenic difference between the donor and recipient; the greater the difference, the faster the rejection. [p. 488]

3. An autograft involves grafting in the same individual from one site to another. An allograft is a graft from one individual to another. A xenograft is a graft of tissue from an individual of one species to an individual of a different species. [p. 488–489]

4. The human histocompatibility complex is located on chromosome 6 and gives rise to the human leukocyte antigens (HLA). Class I HLA antigens, or serologically defined antigens, are coded by HLA loci A, B, and C. Most CD8 ($T_{C/S}$) lymphocytes respond to these antigens. On the other hand, most CD4 ($T_{H/I}$) cells (which are also involved in graft rejection) respond to class II antigens (lymphocyte-defined antigens), which are coded by HLA loci DO/DZ, DP, DQ, and DR. [p. 489–490]

5. The MHC chromosomal unit is a haplotype, and the alleles are expressed codominantly. Two units are inherited from the parents, and the ability to accept a graft is dependent on the recipient sharing all the histocompatibility genes with the donor. HLA-identical siblings have the same pair of haplotypes; HLA-haploidentical

siblings share only one; and HLA-different siblings share neither. The most successful grafts occur between HLA-identical individuals, intermediate success occurs with HLA-haploidentical individuals, and the poorest rate of success is seen with HLA-different siblings. [p. 490]

6. The potential success of a graft can be assessed using (a) the lymphoagglutination test, which tests for agglutination reactions between donor and recipient cells; (b) the lymphocytotoxicity test, which measures the amount of cell injury to donor and recipient lymphocytes; and (c) the mixed-lymphocyte culture assay, which cocultures donor and recipient lymphocytes and measures labeled thymidine incorporation as an indicator of the rate of proliferation (where a lack of response suggests a close tissue match). [p. 490–491]

7. The mechanism of first-set rejection employs T lymphocytes, mainly T_C cells, which go to the transplant site and destroy the vasculature feeding the graft. This process cuts off the blood supply and starves the cells of the transplant, which soon dies. If the recipient receives a second graft from the same donor, a second-set reaction begins and calls into play antibodies and NK cells, as well as T lymphocytes. This leads to rapid destruction of the graft's blood supply, with subsequent death of the graft. [p. 492–496]

8. In organ transplantation, the better the HLA match, the longer the survival time of the graft. A graft is rejected through a classical first-set rejection reaction, in which reactions by T lymphocytes lead to the destruction of the capillary beds supplying the transplanted tissue, which results in the subsequent destruction of the foreign tissue. Survivability can be improved by (a) using frozen cadaver kidneys in which the antigenic "passenger lymphocytes" are killed prior to transplantation and (b) pretransfusing the recipient with the donor's blood, which seems to produce enhancing or blocking antibodies that suppress immune sensitization. [p. 496–497]

9. Skin grafts are used in burn patients. The first covering is an allograft, which is later replaced by an autograft from another region on the person's body. Rejections are rare, and this type of graft is highly successful. [p. 497]

10. If a transplant is made to a place in the body where the immune system in not wholly functional, called an "immunologically privileged site" (e.g., the cornea), rejection reactions are rare. The allogenic tissue is not rejected since the HLA antigens can avoid immune effector mechanisms. [p. 497–498]

11. Graft-versus-host (GVH) reactions occur when grafted bone marrow tissue reacts immunologically against the tissues of an immunoincompetent recipient, which are perceived to be "foreign" tissue cells. This occurs if there is not a close HLA match between the bone marrow transplant and the recipient's tissues. Complications of graft-versus-host disease often result in death. [p. 498–500]

12. Graft rejection can be suppressed by nonspecific and specific immunosuppressant therapies. Nonspecific treatments (e.g., x-irradiation and corticosteroids) are used to nonselectively inhibit active B and T lymphocytes, but they also affect other body systems (digestive, bone marrow, etc.) that possess rapidly dividing cells. Another therapy is the use of cyclosporin A, which selectively inhibits only dividing T lymphocytes, but leaves the person susceptible to viral infections. Specific therapies refer to antigen-specific immune suppression to the transplanted tissue, for example, the coupling of cyclosporin A to antigen results in the activation of antigen-specific T_s cells. [p. 500–501]

13. The use of antiidiotype antibodies to specific T cell receptors is a way to induce antigen-specific immune suppression in animals to transplanted grafts. Preimmunization with donor antigens may facilitate transplant survival by enhancing (or blocking) antibody formation, which stops sensitization to the foreign tissue. These antigen-specific procedures induce immune tolerance to the graft while leaving the rest of the immune system operational. [p. 501–502]

14. The fetus, composed of tissue expressing, at least in part, paternal foreign transplantation antigens, is a graft. However, it is not rejected because of immunosuppressant factors made by the fetus, placenta, and mother; blocking antibodies to placental antigens (that are non-complement fixing) produced by the mother; and the production of mucoproteins by the placenta that coat and mask the HLA antigens of the fetal placenta. These nonspecific and specific immune mechanisms ensure that the fetus can grow and mature in the mother, unimpaired by her immune system. [p. 502–504]

READINGS

Babbitt, B. P., Allen, P. M., Matsueda, G., et al. Binding of immunogenic peptide to Ia histocompatability molecules. *Nature* **317**:359, 1985.

Colver, R. B. Cellular and molecular mechanisms of allograft rejection. *Annual Review of Medicine* **41**:361, 1990.

Emmel, E. A., Verweij, C. L., Durand, D. B., et al. Cyclosporin A specifically inhibits function of nuclear proteins involved in T cell activation. *Science* **246**:1617, 1990.

Fanslow, W. C., Sims, J. E., Sassenfeld, H., et al. Regulation of alloreactivity in vivo by a soluble form of the interleukin-1 receptor. *Science* **248**:739, 1990.

Faustman, D., and Coe, C. Prevention of xenograft rejection by masking donor HLA class I antigens. *Science* **252**:1700, 1991.

Ferrara, J. L. M., and Deeg, H. J. Graft-versus-host disease. *New England Journal of Medicine* **324**:667, 1991.

Flye, M. W. (ed.). *Principles of Organ Transplantation.* W. B. Saunders Co., Philadelphia, 1989.

Guillet, J.-G., Lai, M.-Z., Briner, T. J., et al. Immunological self, nonself discrimination. *Science* **235**:865, 1987.

Kahan, B. D. Cyclosporine. *New England Journal of Medicine* **321**:1725, 1989.

Krensky, A. M., Weiss, A., Crabtree, G., et al. T-lymphocyte–antigen interactions in transplant rejection. *New England Journal of Medicine* **322**:510, 1990.

Krolick, K. A. Immunotoxins: current strategies for selective chemotherapy. *ASM News* **51**:569, 1985.

McVie, J. G., Dalesio, O., and Smith, I. E. (eds.). *Autologous Bone Marrow Transplantation and Solid Tumors.* Raven Press, New York, 1984.

Noga, S. J. Elutriation: new technology for separation of blood and bone marrow. *Laboratory Medicine* **19**:234, 1988.

Öhlén, C., Kling, G., Höglund, P., et al. Prevention of allogeneic bone marrow graft rejection by H-2 transgene in donor mice. *Science* **246**:666, 1989.

Posselt, A. M., Barker, C. F., Tomaszweski, J. E., et al. Induction of donor-specific unresponsiveness by intrathymic islet transplantation. *Science* **249**:1293, 1990.

Silvers, W. K., Kimura, H., Desquenne-Clark, L., et al. Some new perspectives on transplantation immunity and tolerance. *Immunology Today* **8**:185, 1987.

Stepkowski, S. M., and Duncan, W. C. The role of T_{DTH} and T_C populations in organ graft rejection. *Transplantation* **42**:406, 1986.

Strober, S. Approaches to human immune tolerance. *Immunology Today* **7**:153, 1986.

Tejani, A., Spitzer, A., and Nash, M. (guest eds.). Modulation of immune system in disease states and organ transplantation. *Journal of Pediatrics* **111**(6, part 2):995 (entire issue), 1987.

Whitley, D., Kupiec-Weglinski, W., and Tilney, N. C. Antibody-mediated rejection of organ grafts. *Current Opinion in Immunology* **2**:864, 1990.

Ontogeny and Phylogeny of Immunity

7 Developmental and Comparative Immunology

This unit provides a general survey of the origins of immune responses in adult mammals from two perspectives. Chapter 20, Development of Immunity, explores the development of the immune system and the maturation of cellular and humoral immune responses. In Chapter 21, Comparative Immunobiology, the immune systems and immunological capabilities of invertebrates and nonmammalian vertebrates are outlined. In addition, this chapter traces the evolutionary origins of mammalian cellular and humoral immune responses. As a result, this unit provides an account of the evolutionary and developmental origins of immunity in adult mammals.

Development of Immunity

20

OVERVIEW

Changes in the composition and competence of the immune system throughout life are explored. The formation and maturation of major lymphoid organs are described. In addition, immune status is traced through its several stages from fetal immune incompetence to adult immune competence. The changing capacities of the cellular effectors of immune responses are similarly outlined and described.

CONCEPTS

1. The mammalian fetus possesses an incompletely established, naive immune system that cannot properly discriminate self from nonself nor fully respond to the spectrum of insults to be encountered later in life.

2. As a result of extensive maturational change, the immune system becomes progressively more refined structurally and functionally and acquires the capacity for precise discrimination and decisive defense.

3. The several effectors of humoral and cellular immunity acquire sophisticated mechanisms for interacting with each other and with their environments to ensure effective protection for the individual.

he organization and function of the immune system has been discussed in detail in the preceding chapters. This discussion has presumed the immune system of the adult mammal, usually human, although some experimental examples have used mice. It is important to realize that the immune system of an individual is not always as represented in these chapters. Some indication of this has already been provided in the discussions of the effects of aging on immune expression (see chapter 16, Autoimmunity). Consequently, the reader should realize that the immune system undergoes change, not only in response to external challenge (as discussed throughout this book), but also as a function of age. This change is most dramatically apparent at the beginning of life.

This chapter explores the changes that occur in the organization of the immune system as the individual progresses through development, from fetus to adult, and differences in the ability to respond to immunological challenge throughout development. Significant advances in the acquisition of the full immune competence of adulthood is stressed in these discussions.

■ ■ ■ ■ ■ ■ ■ ■ ■ ■

IMMUNITY IN REPRODUCTION

Each individual had a similar beginning. Two allogeneic gametes had to unite to produce a diploid zygote. Subsequently, this cell had to implant in the mother's uterus in order to secure the necessary materials to support further development. Although the events of these processes are rather straightforward to describe and envision, each is fraught with pitfalls and dangers. The difficulties encountered by many couples in conceiving and carrying to term that have given rise to current explorations of *in vitro* fertilization and surrogate motherhood provide ample evidence of this. On the other hand, manipulation of immunity to reproductive cells or their factors has been the focus for efforts at inducing infertility or achieving contraception.

Fertilization

The first hurdle to scale in producing a child is that of uniting two genetically distinct gametes, a spermatozoan and an ovum, to produce a zygote. This process can be divided into two stages: first, producing the spermatozoa and ova through the process of gametogenesis and second, successfully bringing these gametes together through fertilization.

Gametogenesis, whether spermatogenesis or oogenesis, involves production of mature gametes from their precursors. These events are hormonally controlled: gonadotropin-releasing hormone (GnRH), secreted from the hypothalamus, regulates release of follicle-stimulating hormone (FSH) by the pituitary gland. In turn, FSH regulates oogenesis in the ovaries or spermatogenesis in the testes. This pathway has provided one focus for the production of *antifertility vaccines*. For example, contraceptive vaccines against GnRH and FSH are under investigation. These vaccines have the advantage of acting against substances directly involved in reproduction and have few side-effects on other physiological activities. However, long-term regulation of fertility is not yet possible. Naturally occurring Abs against these hormones have not been documented. Thus, immunological impairment of fertility does not seem to occur at this level.

Other antifertility vaccines under investigation focus on the developing gametes themselves. Vaccines targeting the zona pellucida or sperm Ags are under development. Within the zona pellucida, four glycoprotein regions (designated ZP1 through ZP4, by descending molecular weight) can be distinguished by two-dimensional gel electrophoresis. Abs against ZP3, which contains the sperm-binding protein, appear to be most effective in reducing fertility. However, as above, no naturally occurring Abs to zona pellucida glycoproteins are currently known.

In contrast, naturally occurring antispermatozoan immunity has been documented. For example, 30% to 60% of men undergoing vasovasostomy (reversal of vasectomy) display persistent infertility due to antisperm Abs. These Abs apparently were produced in response to exposure to sperm Ags made accessible to the immune system following vasectomy (since the testes are immunologically segregated sites not normally exposed to the immune system). In addition, T_S cells have been reported to occur within the male genital tract. These cells are believed to protect against autoimmunity. Furthermore, antisperm Abs have been detected in up to 33% of couples screened in one study. The presence of these Abs was associated with diminished sperm motility (which affects the ability of the sperm to reach the ovum) and poor *in vitro* fertilization.

Maternal-Fetal Interactions

After fertilization, the newly formed zygote goes through a series of cell divisions called cleavages to produce an embryo. Initially, the number of cells within the embryo increases; however, the mass of the embryo does not. As the early embryo develops, it migrates down the fallopian tubes into the uterus, where it must eventually implant if further development is to occur. This is known as the implantation stage.

The implantation stage embryo is a mass of tissue that is genetically distinct from the mother in whose uterus it implants and develops. Moreover, this mass (called a blastocyst) expresses Ags that are immunologically distinct from its maternal "host." Yet the implanted embryo is not rejected. Several features emerge as possible explanations for this. On the one hand, fetal and trophoblastic cells have a *sialoprotein coat* (similar to that found in tumors, see chapter 18, Tumor Immunology) and the trophoblast produces *chorionic gonadotropin (CG)*. Both are able to provide **protection against immunological detection or attack.** The sialoprotein coat provides a shield that masks fetal Ags, thereby reducing or preventing the maternal immune system from encountering them. CG is a hormone that inhibits immunological expression of maternal T cells that could react to paternally derived fetal Ags. Its protective effect appears to be mediated locally, that is, the hormone is associated with the trophoblast surface and impairs the action of T cells that might bind there.

On the other hand, factors are present in serum that **reduce immunoreactivity** of pregnant women (table 20.1). These factors include *α-fetoprotein (AFP)*, *α-macroglobulin, β₁-glycoprotein,* and *soluble inhibitory factor (SIF)*. Of the four, α-macroglobulin is produced by the mother. Its concentration in maternal plasma rises markedly during the first trimester and falls sharply after delivery. AFP and β₁-glycoprotein are produced by the fetus. Their levels rise progressively throughout pregnancy and decline after delivery. AFP levels may become as high as 550 ng/mL during the third trimester (normal = 2 to 10 ng/mL), while β₁-glycoprotein can rise to 300 μg/mL (normally not present). SIF is produced by the placenta, and might also be supplemented by maternal sources. All four of these substances can suppress immunological functions, at least *in vitro*. For example, α-macroglobulin inhibits several T cell functions, but does not interfere with B cell functions. AFP displays similar properties, but can also inhibit Ab production by murine spleen plaque-forming cells, while SIF suppresses lymphocyte proliferation and Ab synthesis nonspecifically. In contrast, β₁-glycoprotein appears to act more like CG in that it provides local protection. In addition to these factors, steroid hormones occasionally have been suggested as candidates for immunosuppressing maternal responses during pregnancy. However, although the levels of certain steroids (e.g., estrogen, progesterone, and 17-hydroxycorticosteroids) are elevated during pregnancy, their roles in suppressing immune reactions against the fetus are not widely supported.

Although most interactions between the implanted embryo and the maternal immune system end in peaceful coexistence, there are numerous instances in which the maternal immune system acts to the detriment of the embryo or fetus. In some instances, this leads to early termination of pregnancy. In other cases, fetal-maternal interactions lead to adverse, sometimes life-threatening, damage to the fetus and newborn. For example, the penetration of maternal lymphocytes into the fetus can provoke *graft-versus-host* disease. Alternatively, maternal Abs against fetal Ags might be transferred to the fetus with equally serious consequences—as occurs, for example, with the passage of anti-Rh Abs leading to erythroblastosis fetalis (hemolytic disease of the newborn).

A phenomenon has recently been designated as recurrent spontaneous abortion syndrome that might have an immunological basis. This syndrome is characterized by (1) recurrent spontaneous abortions in the first trimester (in 20% of the cases, this followed a successful first pregnancy); (2) subfertility and longer than normal interval between pregnancies; (3) double the normal frequency of ectopic pregnancy (implantation

TABLE 20.1 Factors in Maternal Serum Believed to Protect the Fetus Against Immunological Attack

Substance	Characteristics	Actions on Immune System
α-fetoprotein	Plasma protein of fetal origin	*Cellular immunity* Inhibits responses to PHA, Con A; suppresses responses to allogeneic cells in MLR; does *not* affect rosette formation *Humoral immunity* Inhibits primary IgM and secondary IgM, IgG, and IgA responses of mouse PFC to SRBC
α-macroglobulin	Group of high molecular weight plasma proteins of maternal origin (chiefly, α-glycoprotein)	*Cellular immunity* Inhibits response to T cell mitogens; inhibits migration and rosette formation *Humoral immunity* Has no demonstrated effect
β_1-glycoprotein	Glycoprotein of fetal origin found in maternal plasma; synthesized by trophoblast; localized on extracellular surfaces of trophoblast cells, suggesting local action	*Cellular immunity* Inhibits PHA- but *not* Con A–induced blastogenesis *Humoral immunity* Has no reported effect
Chorionic gonadotropin	Protein synthesized by trophoblast cells; associated with extracellular surface, restores protection after neuraminidase treatment	*Cellular immunity* Is believed to prevent T cell maturation after interacting with Ags at cell surface *Humoral immunity* Has no documented effect
Soluble inhibitory factor	Substance composed of 130–150 kD protein that is noncovalently linked to glycolipid (lipid suppressor substance); released by proliferating T and null cells and giant cells from normal human placenta	*Cellular immunity* Suppresses Ag- and mitogen-induced T cell proliferation; induces population of T_S cells *Humoral immunity* Nonspecific suppression of Ab production (indirect, through its induction of T_S cells)
Steroid hormones*	Corticosteroids, estrogen, and progesterone of maternal origin	*Cellular immunity* Has conflicting results and no conclusive effect *Humoral immunity* Has no reported effects

*Effects of steroids on immunological function reported in this table are limited to effects that appear to be associated specifically with pregnancy.
Con A = concanavalin A; MLR = mixed lymphocyte reaction; PFC = plaque-forming cell; PHA = phytohemagglutinin; SRBC = sheep red blood cells.
Sources: Loke, Y. W. *Immunology and Immunopathology of the Human Foetal-Maternal Interaction.* Elsevier Biomedical Press, Amsterdam, 1978; Wolf, R. L. *Pediatric Research* **23**:212, 1988.

outside the uterus); and (4) partner-specific association. Abortion in this syndrome can be prevented by immunization with paternal lymphocytes.

In addition to the potential for histoincompatibility reactions between the mother and the embryo, **positive interactions** appear to also occur between the maternal immune system and the developing conceptus. Numerous *cytokines have been found*

in the placenta. These include colony-stimulating factor 1 (CSF-1), granulocyte-monocyte–colony-stimulating factor (GM-CSF), interleukin 1 (IL-1), IL-2, IL-6, interferon-α (IFN-α), IFN-γ, and tumor necrosis factor-α (TNF-α). In addition, increased NK cell activity has been associated with increased fetal resorption. Based on these and other observations, Thomas Wegman, at the University of Alberta (Canada), has

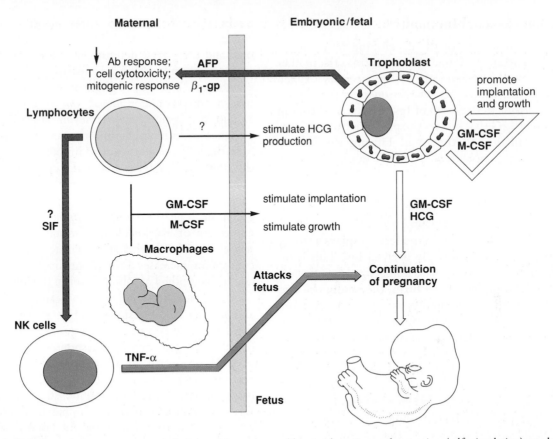

FIGURE 20.1 Dialogue between conceptus and maternal immune system during pregnancy. Trophoblast implantation and continuation of pregnancy depend upon interactions between the maternal immune system and the developing individual. Positive influences are denoted by *open arrows* while negative influences are indicated by *dark arrows*. Trophoblast-produced AFP and β_1-glycoprotein (β_1-gp) depress maternal immune responses. On the maternal side, lymphocytes and/or macrophages produce GM-CSF and macrophage-CSF, which favor the continuation of pregnancy by promoting tropho-blast implantation and autocrine (self-stimulating) production of similar factors. In addition, other undefined factor(s) (identified by ?) stimulate production of HCG. On the other hand, lymphocytes presumably produce some factor(s) (designated by ?) that suppress NK cells. SIF, found in maternal plasma, might be one such factor. If NK cells are not held in check, TNF-α can be released with adverse effects on pregnancy. (Adapted form Wegman, T. G. The cytokine basis for cross-talk between the maternal immune and reproductive systems. *Current Opinion in Immunology* **2:**765, 1990.)

proposed a *model for the dialogue between the maternal immune system and the embryo* that is required for subsequent development. Certain features of this model are outlined in figure 20.1.

According to this model, placental gland cells produce CSF-1, while lymphocytes and macrophages (Mϕs) associated with the placenta release GM-CSF. These cytokines promote placental growth, implantation, and initial growth of the embryo. The growing embryo, in turn, releases additional GM-CSF and CSF-1, which can act in an autocrine manner. However, CG and placental lactogen are also released, which

promote physiological responses in the mother that ensure continued placental maintenance and growth.

CHANGING STATUS OF IMMUNITY THROUGHOUT LIFE

During the nine months of gestation that we were guests of our mothers, we were acquiring independent identity. For much of this time we lacked an immune system or other independent means of defense. Nevertheless, as the weeks passed, we expressed our separate identity and acquired an effective immune system.

Fetal and Neonatal Immunity

In addition to effects of the developing fetus on the mother, there are profound influences from the mother on the fetus. Apart from providing necessary oxygen and nutrients, the *mother provides the fetus with immunological defense* in the form of Igs. This is primarily in the form of **IgG** that crosses the placenta from the maternal circulation to the fetus. During the last six months of gestation, IgG from the mother progressively accumulates in the fetal blood. This *passively acquired immunity* in the newborn infant serves as a first line of humoral defense while the infant's own Ab-producing cells begin to assume this role.

Thus, immunity in the fetus displays a strong dependence upon maternally derived Igs. This is reflected in the increasing levels of maternal IgG that are found in fetal plasma. After birth, the amount of maternal IgG diminishes rapidly, as the newborn infant begins to express its own immune capacity. Nevertheless, the maternal influence can continue for some time. In most newborn mammals and in infants that are nursed, passively acquired immunity continues to be maintained. This is accomplished by the Igs that are transferred in colostrum and mother's milk. This is mostly in the form of IgA in humans, whereas IgG can be transferred by this route in other species.

Curiously, passive immunity derived from the mother might actually contribute to suppressing, or delaying, the expression of active immunity in the fetus. Humoral immune capacity, in the form of IgM production, is not expressed until approximately 200 days' gestation in humans, and even later for other Igs. In addition, cellular immune responses, such as delayed hypersensitivity reactions ordinarily are not manifested until after birth. However, both humoral and cellular immune responses can be induced in human fetuses from 140 to 150 days' gestation.

Acquisition of Immune Competence

Three stages of immunological development can be described during the first months of development (table 20.2). The first is one of almost absolute *immune incompetence*. This exists during the embryonic stages of development, before the formation of hemopoietic tissues and the early circulatory system. This encompasses the first two to three months following conception (fertilization). During this period, embryonic and early fetal defenses are generally limited to native nonimmunological reactions by primitive phagocytes. The second phase of immunological maturation displays *transitional immunological capacity*. During this period, three to seven months' gestation, evidence of humoral immunity can be found. However, this is a passively acquired immunity, derived from the mother. The fetus does not display overt immunological expressivity of its own; however, this capacity can be induced beginning in the fifth month of gestation. The third stage is marked by progressive expression of *independent cellular and humoral immune competence.* This begins approximately 200 days after conception, increases through the first few years of life, and is maintained at a high level in the adult.

Fetal sheep and monkeys can reject allografts and produce Abs in response to foreign Ags during the first half of gestation. These responses show no delay or defect as compared with responses of adults. However, Ab production is not expressed uniformly to all Ags. That is, a certain level of maturity is required before responsiveness can be demonstrated to any given Ag. Prior to this stage of development, Ab production cannot be demonstrated to that Ag, but once that stage is attained, full competence is acquired. The stage of development required for full competence varies with the Ag used.

Despite the presence at birth of B and T cell populations, endogenous Igs, and complement activity, the human *neonate still does not possess a fully competent immune system.* Evidence for this derives from the increased susceptibility of newborn infants to a variety of infectious agents. Thus, although the components necessary for full and effective immunological expression are present at birth, the mechanisms for immune regulation or for efficient use of the effectors of humoral and cellular immunity might still be undeveloped. For example, Ab response to foreign Ags is often weak or absent. In addition, phagocytic and bactericidal activity of phagocytes appears to be less than that observed in older children and in adults. Moreover, skin tests and other assays to measure cellular immunity disclose slower or weaker responses. However, these apparent deficiencies of immunological function are

TABLE 20.2 Expression of Immune Competence During Intrauterine Life

Status	Gestational Age	Characteristics
Immune incompetence	Embryonic/early fetal period; 1–3 months	No hemopoietic tissues or circulatory system (0–1 month); no adultlike humoral or cellular immunity expressed
Transitional immune competence	3–7 months	Inherent phagocytic responsiveness exists, passively acquired humoral immunity is displayed; potential for independent cellular and humoral immunity is present but not expressed (begins approximately 140 days' gestation)
Progressive immune competence	Begins approximately 200 days' gestation, continues thereafter	Inherent phagocytic ability and passively acquired humoral immunity remain; independent expression of humoral and cellular immunity begin and progressively increase

rapidly corrected, and more characteristic expression of immune competence is acquired within the first year of life. Further maturation and refinement of immune competence occurs through childhood.

Maintenance of Immune Competence

Expression of immunological status depends upon three factors: (1) the *number of cells present,* (2) the *distribution of cellular subpopulations,* and (3) the *intrinsic properties of cells* themselves. It is fairly obvious that no effective immune response would be possible if there was an insufficient number of lymphocytes available. However, it is equally important that these cells be distributed adequately among the effector cell subpopulations required. For example, the distribution of T cells between T_H and T_S populations can profoundly affect the outcome of an immunological response. In addition, the cells must be competent to properly play their respective roles. APCs that cannot effectively interact with T cells or phagocytes with defective bactericidal capacities will not contribute constructively to an immune response.

Throughout adult life, these three criteria are satisfied. Through the interplay among the diverse cell populations and other regulatory factors an effective level of immune competence is maintained. However, as the individual ages, the efficiency of immunological defenses appears to diminish. What exactly happens to the immune system during aging is not understood. Nevertheless, humoral and cellular immune responses

decline, and the incidence of autoimmune phenomena increases. Aging appears to take its toll on both cellular and humoral immunity.

At puberty, with the onset of sexual maturity, the thymus begins to involute. Not only is there a reduction in thymic mass, but the production of thymic hormones declines as well. After the age of 30 in humans, a steady decline in the levels of thymopoietin can be demonstrated. However, *T cell numbers either remain stable or decrease with age.* Nevertheless, the nature of T cell subpopulations changes. For example, the number of thymocytes that bind sheep erythrocytes declines with age: 90% at age 20, 65% at age 50, and 50% at age 80. In addition, helper activity decreases, and there appears to be an *age-related increase in suppressor activity.* This increase in suppressor activity is believed, by some, to be a possible defense against the development of autoimmune reactions. Other manifestions of diminishing cellular immunity include reduced mitogenic responsiveness of T cells, possibly related to decreased production of lymphokines, and reduced manifestation of contact hypersensitivity responses. In contrast, auxiliary cells, like Mϕs, appear to retain their functional competence to respond to allo-Ags throughout adult life. However, in at least one series of experiments on mice, age-related decline in Mϕ activity was reported. In these experiments, Mϕ reactivity to infection by *Toxoplasma gondii* was diminished (delayed), while T cell function appeared to be unaffected in older mice (20 months old) when compared with young mice (4 months old).

Serum Ig levels and the number of available B cells do not appear to decline with age. However, primary, but not secondary, humoral responses appear to decline with age. This decline begins with thymus involution and progresses throughout the remainder of life. This raises the possibility that declining humoral response is related to alteration of T cell function rather than to intrinsic B cell defects. However, *B cells from older persons respond less effectively* to T cells from young individuals than do B cells from young individuals. Thus, there are age-related changes that affect B cell function intrinsically as well. Overall, it appears that the adverse effects of aging on the expression of immune competence affects cellular responses more than humoral immunity.

DEVELOPMENT OF HEMOPOIETIC AND LYMPHOID ORGANS

In adult mammals, hemopoiesis (blood cell formation) occurs principally in the bone marrow, and proliferation of activated lymphocytes occurs in various lymphoid tissues. However, during early development, these events occur elsewhere. Hemopoiesis occurs initially extraembryonically. Later, hemopoiesis shifts to the liver and lymphoid tissues before eventually becoming established in the red bone marrow compartments. For example, in humans, hemopoiesis begins in the yolk sac during the fourth week of gestation, then the liver and lymphoid organs become significant participants between the sixth week and seventh month of gestation, and finally the bone marrow assumes a progressively dominant role from the fourth month of gestation onward (fig. 20.2). In addition, lymphocytes migrate into the various lymphoid tissues at varying times during their development and maturation. The thymus gland (from 65 days) and the spleen (from 125 days) increase progressively in size throughout gestation. This correlates well with a parallel increase in the numbers of lymphocytes present, which begins at approximately 50 days' gestation. For a discussion of the structure and organization of these organs in adult mammals, review appropriate sections of chapter 2, Cells and Tissues of the Immune System.

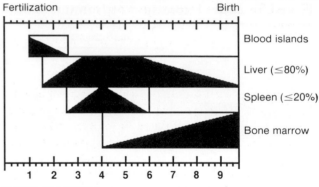

FIGURE 20.2 Hemopoiesis during embryonic and fetal development. Several organs play a central role in hemopoiesis during development. These include the blood islands in the yolk sac, the fetal liver and spleen, and the bone marrow. The period during gestation when each of these organs has a major role in hemopoiesis is noted. In addition, the *blackened area* reflects the magnitude of the contribution from each organ at any particular time in gestation. For example, we see a reduction in the contribution from the blood islands as that of the liver increases. Similarly, the contribution from the fetal liver can be seen to diminish as the bone marrow assumes its role as the primary hemopoietic organ.

Embryonic and Fetal Hemopoietic Organs

During development, *three phases of hemopoiesis* are identified. The first is known as the *mesoblastic* phase. This occurs in the extraembryonic blood islands. The second phase, known as the *hepatic* phase, occurs during the middle period of gestation, when the liver is the primary hemopoietic organ. The final phase begins near midgestation and continues through adulthood. This is the *myeloid* phase, when the bone marrow serves as the major site for hemopoiesis.

Blood Islands

Blood cells are produced initially outside the embryo, in specialized areas known as blood islands. These islands are small aggregates of hemoblasts (blood-forming cells) and mesenchyme (embryonic connective tissue) in the yolk sac. These islands appear during the fourth week of gestation and are the active hemopoietic tissue until approximately the tenth week of gestation. During this phase, erythropoiesis appears to be the sole hemopoietic activity. Nevertheless, cells derived from these blood islands appear to be capable of populating the thymus later in development and appear to possess other hemopoietic potencies as well.

Liver

The fetal liver then assumes a role as a significant blood-forming organ. In humans this role begins during the sixth week of gestation, while in mice it emerges at approximately 14 days' gestation (beginning of the third trimester). The liver's role increases progressively as that of the blood islands decreases. By the end of the first trimester, the liver is the major hemopoietic organ and accounts for 80% of hemopoiesis. The liver continues as the major hemopoietic organ throughout the middle trimester. During this period, leukopoiesis, as well as erythropoiesis, occurs. In fact, during the early portion of hepatic hemopoiesis, the liver is probably the major source of lymphocyte precursors for all lymphoid organs. The hemopoietic function of the liver diminishes during the last trimester of gestation, as this role is assumed by the developing bone marrow.

Adult Hemopoietic and Lymphoid Organs

Other organs develop at this time that will assume the functions of hemopoiesis in adulthood. These are supplemented by yet other organs that figure prominently in lymphocyte circulation and education throughout the remainder of life. The most significant of these are the bone marrow (and bursa of Fabricius, in birds), thymus, and spleen.

Bone Marrow

The bone marrow begins to form during the fourth month of gestation, in humans. It arises within highly vascularized areas of developing bones at about the time that ossification begins. The developing bone marrow cavity becomes populated by progenitor cells (stem cells?) for the various blood cell lines. Its role in hemopoiesis gradually increases during the second half of gestation, as the hemopoietic activities of all other organs decreases. Moreover, the bone marrow of mammals is believed to become the *site for B cell education/maturation*. In addition, lymphocyte precursors that will eventually become T cells also arise within the sinusoids of the bone marrow (fig. 20.3).

Bursa of Fabricius

Although this organ is unique to birds, its importance to understanding the initial differentiation and maturation of B cells and their role in humoral immunity justifies its inclusion. It originates as an evagination from the dorsal wall of the cloaca on the fifth day of incubation (hatching occurs at three weeks' incubation). However, it is not until approximately 12 to 13 days' incubation that cells resembling lymphoblasts are found in the bursa. These cells originate outside of the bursa and migrate into it subsequently. Evidence of Ig (IgM) production can be found by day 14, and large numbers of lymphocytes are present within medullary follicles by 17 days' incubation. However, IgG production is not initiated until after hatching. The importance of the bursa to the *development of* **humoral immunity** can be seen in the consequences of bursectomy before hatching. Surgically removing the bursa at 17 days' incubation leads to agammaglobulinemia in a substantial number of cases. Moreover, bursectomy at 19 days' incubation, two days before hatching, can still reduce Ig production in chickens.

Spleen

The spleen arises from the dorsal mesentery and begins as a hemopoietic organ during the third month of gestation. Lymphocyte immigration does not begin until about 20 weeks' gestation, and lymphopoiesis can be demonstrated shortly thereafter. B and T cell regions are definable by 26 to 30 weeks. During the initial period, interdigitating reticulum cells appear to be present; however, by the thirtieth week of gestation both interdigitating and dendritic reticulum cells are present.

Among vertebrate species that lack a hemopoietic bone marrow, the spleen might serve as a "bursal equivalent." In amphibians, for example, splenectomy early in development is often associated with diminished Ab production. However, such a striking dependence upon the spleen for the development of humoral immunity does not occur among mammals.

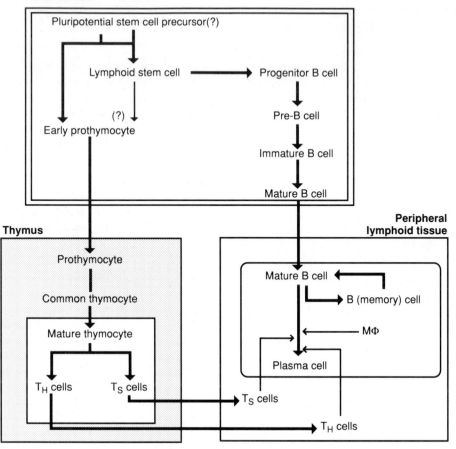

Bone marrow

Pluripotential stem cell precursor(?)

Lymphoid stem cell → Progenitor B cell

(?) ↓

Early prothymocyte

Pre-B cell

Immature B cell

Mature B cell

Thymus

Prothymocyte

Common thymocyte

Mature thymocyte

T$_H$ cells   T$_S$ cells

Peripheral lymphoid tissue

Mature B cell

B (memory) cell

MΦ

Plasma cell

T$_S$ cells

T$_H$ cells

FIGURE 20.3 Relationships and distributions of lymphocyte types during development. Lymphocytes at varying stages of differentiation are distributed among the bone marrow, thymus, and peripheral lymphoid tissues. Within the bone marrow, early commitments to T and B cell lineages occur. It is here that B cell differentiation takes place. In contrast, cells committed to the T cell lineage leave the bone marrow and migrate to the thymus, where further differentiation occurs. Cells competent for expression of humoral (B cell) or cellular (T cell) immunity enter the bloodstream and populate other lymphoid organs. The *question marks* denote that the pluripotential stem cell precursors might no longer be present beyond the earliest stages of lymphoid development, and that existing lymphoid stem cells might be incapable of producing T cell precursors once the original early prothymocytes have been produced.

Thymus

The thymus gland originates from outpocketings of the pharyngeal pouches. The precise level of origin and the subsequent developmental changes vary among diverse vertebrate groups. Most of the pharyngeal pouches (pouches two to six) participate in producing the thymus glands of the most ancient vertebrate classes, while fewer participate in more recently evolved vertebrate classes (e.g., pouches three and four in mammals). Furthermore, the thymic rudiments of more ancient classes of vertebrates do not coalesce into a single organ, as occurs in mammals, but remain apart forming bilateral thymus glands, as in amphibians and birds.

The thymus begins as a rather homogeneous population of basophilic cells surrounded by a loose collection of connective tissue cells. These events occur at approximately six weeks' gestation, in humans. Mitotic activity initially is very limited. Expansion of the thymus occurs in part by cellular immigration. In fact, in chickens, LeDouarin and associates have determined that the T cell pool of the thymus is derived

TABLE 20.3 Putative Thymic Hormones and Their Actions

Hormone	Molecular Weight	Functions Restored	Factors Stimulated
Thymosin	12 kD	Cellular immunity after thymectomy	Expression of Thy-1; cortisone resistance; lymphokine production; T_H, GVH, and MLC activity (mice); T cell number; PHA, and MLC activity (human)
Thymopoietins	7 kD		Expression of Thy-1; MLC reactivity; increase in T_S pool (mice)
Thymic factor	1 kD		Expression of Thy-1, mitogen responsiveness (mice)
Thymic humoral factor	Between 0.7 kD and 5 kD	Allograft and tumor rejection competence following thymectomy	MLC and GVH; lymphokine production; lymphopoiesis; B/T cell cooperation in production of Ab
Thymostimulin	<12 kD		Expression of Thy-1; cortisone resistance; IFN-γ production (mice)
Lymphocyte-stimulating hormone	15 kD and 60 kD		Production of Ab, number of plaque-forming cells (mice)

MLC = mixed lymphocyte culture; PHA = phytohemagglutinin; Thy-1 = mouse T lymphocyte differentiation Ag.
Sources: Hildemann, W. H. *Essentials of Immunology.* Elsevier, New York, 1984; Trainin, N., Pecht, M., and Handzel, Z. T. Thymic hormones: inducers and regulators of the T-cell system. In *T Lymphocytes Today.* Inglis, J. R. (ed.). Elsevier, New York, 1983.

from the second and third waves of lymphocyte precursors that populate the developing thymic rudiment. As development continues, two significant features emerge. First, at the cellular level, three populations of cells become readily recognizable. These are lymphocytes, lymphoblasts, and epithelial cells. The **epithelial cells** represent the *original thymic tissue* itself, while the **lymphocytes** and **lymphoblasts** represent *descendants of cells that migrated into the thymus.* The second feature is expressed at the tissue or organ level. Where the thymic parenchyma had formerly had a generally homogeneous appearance, it progressively segregates into two distinct regions, a central medulla and a peripheral cortex, surrounded by a capsule. By eight to nine weeks' gestation, interdigitating reticulum cells are discernible in the thymic perivascular spaces. Demarcation of a medulla occurs during weeks 12 to 14, at which time interdigitating reticulum cells are abundant. The normal architecture is achieved by 16 to 20 weeks' gestation, and the development of the thymus is complete by birth. After birth, the mass of the thymus remains fairly constant for several years but then progressively atrophies, by involution, after the onset of sexual maturity (puberty).

The thymus plays a *major role in the development of* **cellular immunity.** This is accomplished by providing the microenvironment in which T cell commitments occur. Moreover, the fetal thymus produces several important peptide hormones that influence the expression of numerous properties of T cells and cellular immune responses (table 20.3). In addition, the thymus also influences the expression of humoral immunity as fetal thymectomy leads to reduced Ab production as well as the loss of cell-mediated immunity, except for NK cytotoxicity.

Lymph Nodes, Peyer's Patches, and Related Sites

The first lymphatic cells are detectable at 12 to 14 weeks' gestation. They form in association with small lymphatic vessels and soon give rise to encapsulated organs. In humans, lymph nodes display myelopoietic activity at first. Typical T cell regions containing interdigitating reticulum cells are present by 16 to 20 weeks' gestation.

A variety of other lymphoid foci develop in association with the mucosa of the gastrointestinal and respiratory tracts. These **gut-associated lymphoid tissues** include the tonsils (pharyngeal and palatine), appendix, and Peyer's patches. These structures also begin to emerge at the time that the lymphatic system becomes anatomically defined. For example, Peyer's patches, which develop in association with the digestive tract (chiefly ileum, in humans), show distinct follicular architecture by the twentieth to twenty-fourth weeks of gestation.

In animals with extremely short gestation periods, the secondary lymphoid organs may not arise until rather late in development. For example, lymph nodes and Peyer's patches in mice (3-week gestation period) are very rudimentary structures at birth. They contain only a few lymphocytes and neutrophilic granulocytes within a reticular meshwork. This seems somewhat reminiscent of what is encountered in humans near the end of the fifth month of gestation.

DEVELOPMENT OF HUMORAL IMMUNITY
Acquisition of Humoral Immunity During Ontogeny

The *human fetus possesses a humoral defense* system. However, the Igs that constitute this defense during the six months preceding birth are supplied by the mother. These Igs, IgG, are delivered across the placenta through maternofetal circulation. This humoral defense, however, is soon augmented by Ab production by the fetus itself (fig. 20.4). By the twenty-fifth week of gestation, IgM can be detected in the fetal spleen and circulation. Initial levels are quite low, but they progressively rise. Production of other Igs, most notably IgG and IgA, are deferred until approximately 34 weeks' gestation for IgG and birth for IgA. At birth, maternal IgG levels fall sharply and are soon replaced by neonatal IgG, which rises sharply before assuming a more gradual, but sustained, rate of production thereafter. Ig levels of low birth weight, premature infants display a similar trend. It is curious that IgG levels at 10 months of age are only one-half that found in full-term, normal birth weight infants, whereas IgM and IgA levels are comparable.

Production of Igs shows *progressive increase throughout the first year* of life. This is undoubtedly a consequence of exposure of the infant to a broad range of foreign materials from the new environment. Thus, by the end of the first year of life, the child has acquired levels of IgM that are approximately 75% those of mature adults and levels of IgG and IgA that are approximately 60% and 20% of adult levels, respectively. These levels continue to rise, albeit at slower rates, as the child continues to mature. During this early period of new Ig synthesis, infants that are breast fed enjoy the benefit of supplementary humoral protection in the form of Igs, primarily secretory IgA (sIgA) (except cattle, which receive IgG), supplied in mother's milk.

Although Ig production, in humans, does not ordinarily begin until the thirtieth (IgM) to thirty-fourth (IgG) weeks of gestation, the capacity to produce Igs exists earlier, approximately 15 to 20 weeks of gestation. At this point in gestation, challenge by Ag can yield IgM, IgG, and IgA production. The magnitude of response differs among the three classes of Igs, however (fig. 20.5), and reflects the order in which these Igs would naturally develop.

B Cell Differentiation

Differentiation of B cells from **presumptive B cells** proceeds through three steps (table 20.4). These steps are (1) expression of cytoplasmic, but not surface, IgM; (2) expression of cytoplasmic and surface IgM; and (3) expression of a class-specific surface Ig (e.g., IgG, IgA, or IgD). In humans the first differentiation step begins near the end of the second month of gestation, while in mice this occurs around the twelfth day of gestation. Before this time, no cells can be detected that possess IgM, whereas at this time, *cells with cytoplasmic IgM* can be demonstrated. These cells, called **pre-B cells,** represent the earliest cells that can be truly identified as belonging to the humoral arm of the immune system. By 9.5 to 12.5 weeks' gestation, in humans, and day 17 of gestation, in mice, *cells with surface IgM* can be detected. These cells are **immature B cells.** These cells were found in fetal liver, but not in spleen or peripheral blood in humans, and in bone marrow, but not spleen or lymph nodes in mice. During this same period, *cells expressing surface IgG, IgA,* or *IgD also*

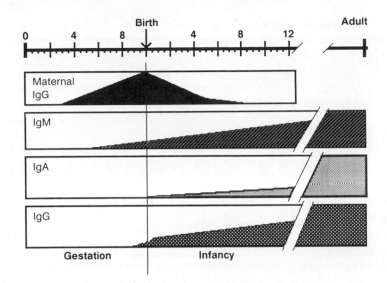

FIGURE 20.4 Relative Ig levels during gestation and infancy. Levels of various Igs that can be measured in fetal and neonatal serum are represented. Maternal IgG provides a significant contribution during pregnancy but later declines markedly. Fetal IgM and IgG levels rise slowly toward the end of pregnancy. IgA is not produced until birth. During the first year of life, all of these Ig levels rise. The relative height of the *shaded area* reflects the percent of adult level achieved by the end of the first year of life. The scale provided spans the entire period of pregnancy and the first year of neonatal life.

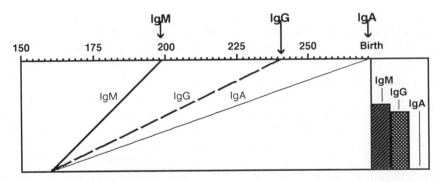

FIGURE 20.5 Premature stimulation of Ig expression during gestation. Although IgM (200 days), IgG (240 days), and IgA (birth) are expressed at varying times during gestation (*represented by arrows*), all can be induced from approximately 155 to 160 days' gestation (*represented by lines*). The consequences of early induction on the level of Ig detectable during gestation and at birth can be seen when compared against the level normally present at birth (*represented by bars on right*). Note that IgM is the predominant Ig and that IgA is **not** present ordinarily at birth

became detectable. These latter cells represent **mature B cells.** The order of appearance of surface Igs seemed to be IgM before IgG before IgA, with IgD appearing some time after IgM but not necessarily before IgG or IgA. (For a discussion of class switching in Ig expression, see chapter 4.)

These three steps in B cell differentiation are **Ag independent.** They occur *initially in the fetal liver,* in mammals. However, as fetal development progresses and a hemopoietically competent bone marrow arises, Ag-independent B cell differentiation is believed to *shift to the bone marrow.* These steps in B cell

TABLE 20.4 Differentiation of B Cells

Cell	Characteristics	Emergence*
Presumptive B cell	Lymphoid cell committed to B cell lineage but not expressing characteristics identifiable by existing techniques	4th–6th weeks (?) (by day 11)
Pre-B cell	Lymphoid cell possessing cytoplasmic IgM; first recognizable cellular element of humoral immunity	Approximately 7th week (12–13 days)
Immature B cell	Lymphoid cell possessing cytoplasmic IgM and expressing surface IgM	Approximately 9th–12th weeks (16–17 days)
Mature B cell	Lymphoid cell expressing surface IgM, IgG, IgA, or IgM/IgD	Approximately 9.5–12 weeks (after birth)
Ag-dependent Ig-secreting B cell	Mature B cell that has differentiated into plasma cell	Approximately 15th week

*Times of emergence of cells identified is given in weeks of gestation for humans and, in parentheses, in days of gestation for mice.

differentiation show a dependence upon a bursal environment since removal of this milieu profoundly affects B cell development. A tripeptide (gly-his-lys), designated bursin, has been found in the bursa of birds, which selectively stimulated B cell differentiation. However, neither the nature of comparable factor(s) produced by mammals nor the influence provided within the B cell–inducing microenvironment have yet been determined. Since the fetal liver and bone marrow of mammals cannot be removed as readily as the bursa, our understanding of this specific organ-dependent relationship is largely dependent upon work performed on chick embryos. In this system, removal of the bursa of Fabricius before the seventeenth day of incubation (four days before hatching) leads to a substantial reduction in the number of B cells found subsequently. Consequently, in the absence of the bursa, B cell differentiation either does not occur or is severely restricted. However, the results of at least one series of experiments suggest that differentiation of one class of IgM-bearing B lymphocytes can occur in the absence of the bursa, but switching to IgG expression remains severely depressed.

A further (fourth) maturational step can be identified. This is **Ag-dependent differentiation** of the mature B cells into Ig-secreting (plasma) cells and memory cells. In human fetuses, competence for this step cannot be demonstrated prior to the fifteenth week of gestation. However, at this early stage of develop-

ment, the magnitude of the response evoked is weak. This might simply reflect the relative immaturity of the existing T cell populations, since Ag-dependent B cell differentiation is dependent upon interactions with T cells. Animals that have undergone fetal thymectomy have normal numbers of B cells but reduced serum Ig levels, which is consistent with this dependence. This contrasts with the situation following bursectomy in which B cell numbers are reduced, but serum Ig levels can be normal or even elevated.

Furthermore, B cell differentiation is characterized by progressive acquisition of a variety of other surface markers. These include Ia (HLA-DR) Ag, Fc receptors (FcRs), complement receptors (CRs), and numerous other surface Ags and receptors. In mice, for example, Ia Ag is not expressed on immature B cells, but can be demonstrated on mature B cells. Human HLA-DR, in contrast, is expressed on both immature and mature B cells. In addition, FcRs are present on nearly all Ig$^+$ cells. Moreover, in mice, CRs can be found on most splenic B cells from adults but few splenic B cells from young (less than two weeks old) mice, while they are never found on B cells obtained from bone marrow. Thus, these maturational changes reflect idiosyncratic features of B cells, rather than mainstream B cell differentiation. Nevertheless, they still can be of value in identifying and studying B cell subtypes.

TABLE 20.5 Expression of T Cell Functions During Development

Function	Fetal Age	
	Human (38 weeks)	Rat/Mouse (3 weeks)
Participation in mixed lymphocyte culture (responder or stimulator)	7.5–10 weeks	19 days
Ag recognition/binding	10–13 weeks	–
Graft-versus-host reaction	13 weeks	birth
Response to mitogens	12–22 weeks	18 days
Lymphokine production	Midterm (?)	–
Cell-mediated cytolysis	7 months*	birth
Antigenic activation	Birth*	–
Ab-dependent cytotoxicity	Birth*	–
Suppressor function	–	14 days
Helper function	–	Birth (16 days [if primed with Con A])

Duration of gestation for humans (38 weeks) and rats/mice (3 weeks) is given in parentheses.

*Functions might be displayed at earlier age; however, this represents earliest age at which this function was studied.

Sources: Miller, M. E. *Host Defenses in the Human Neonate.* Grune & Stratton, Inc., New York, 1978; Waksman, B. H. (ed.). *Ontogeny of the Immune System.* Progress in Allergy Vol. 29. S. Karger, Basel, 1981.

DEVELOPMENT OF CELLULAR IMMUNITY
Acquisition of Cellular Immunity During Ontogeny

Lymphocytes bearing T cell surface Ags have been detected in human fetal liver as early as 5.5 weeks' gestation. However, lymphocytes do not begin to populate the developing thymus gland until approximately 9 weeks' gestation. By 10 weeks' gestation, T cell functions can be demonstrated (table 20.5). For example, rosetting of sheep erythrocytes is first observed at approximately 10 to 12 weeks' gestation, and by 18 weeks 50% to 96% of thymocytes display this ability. In addition, proliferative response of thymocytes to phytohemagglutinin is seen after the fourteenth week of gestation, but cannot be demonstrated earlier. Demonstration of these functions does not occur in the absence of the thymus, however. In contrast, effective participation of fetal lymphocytes in mixed lymphocyte reactions (MLRs) has been shown with cells from fetuses at 7.5 to 10 weeks' gestation. These cells can participate as either stimulators or responders. The age at which competence in MLRs occurred varied with the source of lymphocytes. For example, lymphocytes from fetal liver were effective by 10 weeks' gestation, while those from the thymus were not effective until 12 to 16 weeks, and lymphocytes from the spleen or blood failed to respond until 16 weeks' gestation.

Lymphokine production also appears to be expressed relatively late in ontogeny. For example, neonatal T cells produce only about 25% as much lymphotoxin as do adult lymphocytes. In addition, production of IFN-γ by T cells of newborn infants is limited, being less than 5% that of adults. The ability to produce IFN-γ rises sharply, however, reaching 50% of adult levels within the first year and 150% of adult levels between the ages of 2 and 10 years. The inability to generate IFN-γ does not appear to be a result of intrinsic T cell defects or deficiencies, but rather appears to be a consequence of inadequate stimulation by monocytes/Mϕs.

Thus, acquisition of competence in cellular immunity does not appear to progress in a linear fashion. That is, there is no clear progression from one property to the next that follows a hierarchical sequence. Expression of the potential for cellular immunity appears shortly after the emergence of the thymus, which exerts a profound influence on further acquisition and expression of cellular immunity. However, cellular immune responses have been demonstrated both before the thymus fully matures in normal mice and in athymic animals (e.g., nude mice). This indicates that thymus-independent differentiation of competent T lymphocytes is possible. Nonetheless, a pattern of progression does appear to exist. This general thread demonstrates the emergence of suppressor function before helper function. In fact, it is primarily this capacity that can be most easily demonstrated in fetal liver "T" cells and in T lymphocytes from nude mice. Acquisition of other characteristics of T cell function, such as mitogenic responsiveness, cytotoxicity, antigenic responsiveness, and helper functions all occur later in ontogeny. The majority of these developmental changes show a dependence upon the thymic environment for proper expression. In addition, full expression of cellular immune potential, *in vivo,* is affected by the maturation of auxiliary cells, like Mϕs.

T Cell Differentiation
Surface Antigenic Markers

In mice, four distinct T cell populations can be identified on the basis of surface markers. These are (1) *noncirculating thymocytes* that express TL and Thy-1 Ags; (2) a circulating population expresssing Ly-1 Ag, which is principally associated with a *helper* function; (3) a second circulating population expressing Ly-2 and Ly-3 Ags (Ly-2,3 cells), which is chiefly associated with *cytotoxic or suppressor* functions; and (4) a third circulating population that expresses all three Ly Ags (Ly-1,2,3), which can be induced to give rise to either Ly-1 or Ly-2,3 cells. (Ly-2 and Ly-3 Ags that are expressed on T cell surfaces are also designated as Lyt-2 and Lyt-3. This distinguishes them from their counterparts expressed on B cell surfaces, namely, Lyb-2 and Lyb-3, respectively.) The three circulating T cell subpopulations represent different portions of the circulating pool; Ly-1,2,3 = 50%, Ly-1 = 30%, and Ly-2,3 = 10%. Studies using fetal mice have demon-

strated that Ly-2,3 cells appear before either Ly-1 or Ly-1,2,3. However, in adult mice, Ly-1,2,3 cells appear to serve as precursors for Ly-1 and Ly-2,3 subsets.

The counterparts to these cells in humans also express distinguishing Ags (fig. 20.6). **Early thymocytes** expresses T9 and T10. When they differentiate into **prothymocytes,** T9 is replaced by CD1. However, expression of CD4 and CD8 also accompany this change. Consequently, prothymocytes have a T10$^+$,CD1$^+$,CD4$^+$,CD8$^+$ phenotype. Further differentiation into **common thymocytes** is associated with a replacement of CD1 by CD3, yielding an Ag profile of T10$^+$,CD3$^+$,CD4$^+$,CD8$^+$. (Immature T cells also exist that are double negative, [i.e., CD4$^-$,CD8$^-$]. However, their relationship to the immature T cells that are double positive [CD4$^+$,CD8$^+$] and to mature T cells remains controversial.) As the maturation process continues, T10 is lost and two major subpopulations are created through the segregation of CD4 and CD8. The population expressing CD3$^+$,CD4$^+$ displays **helper/inducer** (H/I) functions, while those expressing CD3$^+$,CD8$^+$ display **cytotoxic/ suppressor** (C/S) functions. The H/I population accounts for 55% to 70% of peripheral T lymphocytes, whereas the C/S population accounts for 25% to 40% of peripheral T cells. Each of these two populations, in turn, is divided into distinct functional subpopulations that can be distinguished by antigenic surface markers. For example, CD4$^+$,2H2$^+$,Leu8$^+$ cells are inducers of suppressor cells, while CD4$^+$,2H4$^-$,Leu8$^+$ cells are inducers of Ig synthesis by B cells. Similarly, CD8$^+$,Leu9.3$^+$ cells are predominantly cytotoxic, while CD8$^+$,Leu9.3$^-$ cells are predominantly suppressors.

In addition, during the course of differentiation within the thymic environment, the respective murine and human T cells become MHC restricted. Murine Ly-1$^+$ (or human CD4$^+$) cells recognize Ag primarily in conjunction with class II MHC Ags. On the other hand, Ly-2,3$^+$ (or CD8$^+$) cells recognize Ag when associated with class I Ags. Table 20.6 summarizes the principal changes in T cell surface Ags that reflect differentiation from presumptive thymocytes to fully mature T cell subsets that are the effectors of cellular immunity. T cells also express a constellation of other surface Ags; however, these do not appear to

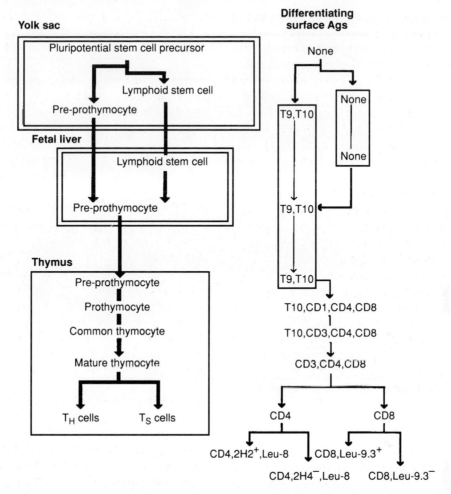

FIGURE 20.6 T cell differentiation and expression of antigenic markers. Lymphoid cells that participate in cellular immunity arise in the yolk sac and fetal liver before populating the fetal thymus. These prethymic cells first express primitive thymic-associated Ags before migrating to the thymus. Within the thymus, further differ-

entiation occurs. As differentiation takes place, the nature of surface antigenic markers changes. The identities of the lymphoid cells during T cell differentiation, and their locations during this process, are depicted *on the left.* The major surface markers associated with these stages of differentiation are aligned, in parallel, *on the right.*

provide specific diagnostic information about the subset identity or the stage of maturity of the T cell pool.

Maturation of T Cell Receptors

T cell activation in cell-mediated immune responses requires Ag recognition and subsequent clonal expansion. Ag recognition is accomplished by clonally expressed **T cell receptors (TCRs)**. (See chapter 9 for more detailed discussion.) TCRs are heterodimers that

recognize particular epitopes. TCRs undergo structural change during development that reflects differential use of loci within the germline gene sequence. For example, during mouse development, expression of TCR genes can be detected by day 14 of gestation. This coincides with early population of the thymus by lymphocytes. TCRs expressed at this time contain peptides encoded by the γ and δ TCR genes. Within three days, lymphocytes with TCRs containing peptides encoded by the α and β genes can be found. This

TABLE 20.6 Differentiation of T Cells

Cell	Characteristics	Distinguishing Antigens	
		Human*	**Mouse**
Early T cell	Lymphoid cell committed to T cell lineage; can be found in fetal liver *before* fetal thymus	T9$^+$,T10$^+$	Thy-1
Immature T cell (pro-T cell)	Noncirculating thymocyte; first stage to display evidence of thymic influence	T10$^+$,**CD1**$^+$,CD4$^+$, CD8$^+$	TL, Thy-1
Common T cell	"Immature" circulating T cell; serves as immediate precursor of T cell subsets	T10$^+$,**CD3**$^+$,CD4$^+$,CD8$^+$	Ly-1,2,3
Mature T cell	Cell displaying functional attributes for cellular immunity		
A. Helper/inducer	Class II, MHC restricted	(CD3$^+$,**CD4**$^+$,CD8$^-$)	
Helper	Stimulates B cells to Ig production	CD3$^+$,**CD4**$^+$,2H2$^+$,Leu-8$^+$	Ly-1
Inducer	Promotes expression of suppressor function by suppressor/cytotoxic cells	Cd3$^+$,**CD4**$^+$,2H4$^-$,Leu-8$^+$	Ly-1; Qa1
B. Cytotoxic/suppressor	Class I, MHC restricted	(CD3$^+$,**CD4**$^-$,**CD8**$^+$)	
Cytotoxic	Displays cytolytic properties when activated	CD3$^+$,**CD8**$^+$, Leu-9.3$^+$	Ly-2,3
Suppressor	Suppresses immunological expression (e.g., of Ig production by B cells)	CD3$^+$,**CD8**$^+$, Leu-9.3$^-$	Ly-2,3

*Specific differentiating Ags on human T cells are denoted in boldface.

reflects maturational change in TCR structure that occurs under thymic influence. In the absence of thymic influence (e.g., in nude mice), TCRs expressing the $\gamma\delta$ chain structure persist. Thus, one consequence of thymic influence on Ag-independent T cell development is a shift to α and β gene expression for Ag-specific TCRs.

Rearrangements of the germline TCR genes appear to be developmentally regulated and to proceed in sequential order. For example, in mice, some rearrangements of the δ chain are encountered before rearrangements of the γ chain. In addition, these rearrangements appear to precede rearrangements of the other peptide chains. In fact, one recent study describes three apparent stages in TCR maturation. The first wave of lymphocytes expresses TCRs containing $\gamma\delta$ chains. A second wave appears, also expressing $\gamma\delta$ chains; however, a new Vγ chain is used. The third maturational wave of lymphocytes expresses TCRs comprised of α and β peptide chains. Subsequent rear-

rangement within the selected genes determines the epitope specificity of the particular TCRs expressed.

Intracellular Enzymes

Changes in T cells during the course of their differentiation are not limited to the cell surface. Important intracellular changes take place as well. Among the changes that appear to reflect progressive differentiation are changes in the relative abundance and activity of enzymes involved in nucleotide metabolism. For example, prothymocytes have high levels of terminal deoxynucleotidyl transferase (TdT), which adds nucleotides to the ends of growing DNA chains, and adenosine deaminase (ADA), which degrades deoxyadenosine and adenosine; but low levels of purine nucleoside phosphorylase (PNP), which converts nucleosides to their corresponding bases, and 5'nucleotidase (5'NT), which converts nucleotide monophosphates to nucleosides. This pattern would appear to favor conservation of the nucleotide pool, which could be important to a proliferating population. With maturation, levels of ADA and TdT become reduced, and those of PNP and 5'NT are increased. Finally, in mature T lymphocytes, TdT is absent and ADA is much reduced while both PNP and 5'NT are abundant. This latter state would not favor maintenance of a large nucleotide pool, which is a condition that is acceptable to cells that are not engaged in proliferation.

Thymic Influence

The thymus influences differentiation of T cells and expression of cellular immune functions. One of the first manifestations of this influence occurs shortly after the thymus forms. This is expressed in two ways: (1) inducing the expression of Thy-1 Ag by presumptive thymocytes and (2) attracting T cell precursors to the developing thymus. How the thymus is able to draw precursor thymocytes to itself is not yet known with certainty. Nevertheless, experiments have shown that thymus rudiments can attract lymphocytes away from other lymphoid tissues (e.g., spleen) if placed in their vicinity. In addition, there exists a family of glycoprotein receptors on lymphocytes that can identify endothelial cells in an organ-specific manner. These might enable prethymic lymphocytes to recognize the location of the thymus. These "homing" receptors also play significant roles in general lymphocyte traffic throughout life (fig. 20.7). Evidence for this can be found in the relative distribution of lymphocyte types found in the bloodstream and lymphoid tissues. For example, the thymus contains 90% T cells, 5% B cells, and 5% null cells; while the bone marrow contains 90% B cells, 5% T cells, and 5% null cells. In contrast, lymph nodes and peripheral blood have 3:1 ratios of T/B cells, but the spleen has T and B cells present in equal proportions (45% each, with 10% null cells).

Once within the thymus, other interactions occur. The first of these is demonstrated in the form of *T cell differentiation* (outlined earlier). This influence on differentiation is displayed in the changing antigenic character of the T cells themselves and in modifications of their functional competence and

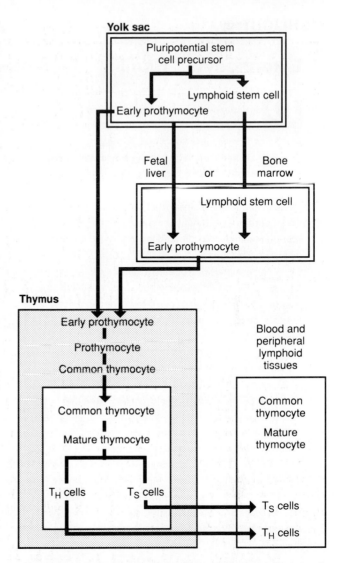

FIGURE 20.7 Distribution of T cell members during fetal development. Fetal T lymphocyte traffic leading to the seeding and populating of the lymphoid organs is outlined. All thymic precursors were derived from cells originally outside the thymus. Moreover, initial commitments to T cell lineage were probably made before migration to the thymus occurred. This figure shows that all T cells found in peripheral lymphoid organs had to pass through the thymus before reaching their final destinations.

Lymphocyte "Homing" Receptors: Immunological Zip Codes?

During embryonic and fetal development, lymphocytes migrate into and populate the various lymphoid organs. In addition, throughout life, T and B cells pass from these organs into the bloodstream and then back into the lymphoid organs. Similar receptors can be found on phagocytes, which seem to participate in directing migration to inflammatory sites. These journeys are not random. The cells that move about between the lymphoid organs and the bloodstream apparently do so in a directed manner. How do they know where they are going?

Lymphocytes possess *surface receptors* that belong to a family of glycoproteins, with a mass of approximately 90 kD, that seem to play an important role in this recognition. These receptors mediate interactions between lymphocytes and endothelial cells at points of entry into tissues. Although it is not known for certain, the nature of these interactions appear to be *organ specific*; that is, lymphocytes recognize one organ or class of organ and ignore others. For example, lymphocytes that recognize endothelium of peripheral lymph nodes do not interact with mucosal or synovial endothelium. However, recognition *does not appear to be species limited.* Lymphocytes with a given specificity from mice display this same specificity against human tissue, and vice versa.

These homing receptors change during the course of lymphocyte differentiation. Virgin B and T cells are believed to possess multiple homing receptors. Following stimulation, these cells pass through a nonmigratory period during which they undergo differentiation locally. Specific homing receptors might be selected for expression during this time, which affect where these cells then migrate. For example, *circulating T and B cells express high levels of an Ag called* **Hermes-1.** These cells *bind to lymph node, mucosal, and synovial endothelium.* Hermes-1 is only expressed at a low level by thymic cortical lymphocytes. Activation of B or T cells is accompanied by a period of downregulation of Hermes-1 Ag. In contrast, two other Ags, identified by MAbs, appear to be more specific. **Hermes-3** appears to be specific for cells that interact with *mucosal endothelium,* while **MEL-14** appears to be specific for cells interacting with *lymph node endothelium.*

Similar homing receptors seem to be expressed by other cell types as well. These seem to play important roles in the migration of phagocytes to sites of active inflammation, for example. In addition, transformed lymphoid cells display Hermes-1 Ag in relation to their ability to metastasize. Thus, the regulation of the expression of these receptors appears to be important both in health and in disease.

By extrapolation from studies using lymphocytes derived from adults, it might be supposed that similar, or the same, homing receptors play a role in the initial populating of the lymphoid organs. Thus, a particular homing signal might direct prethymic cells to the thymus, where further differentiation and maturation could occur. Other homing receptors might similarly direct presumptive B cells to the bursa of Fabricius in birds or the fetal liver and bone marrow in mammals. In this manner, precursors for cellular and humoral immunity could be directed preferentially to an environment appropriate to their further development into competent effectors of their respective arms of the immune response.

Jalkaren, S., Wu, N., Bargatze, R. F., et al. Human lymphocyte and lymphoma homing receptors. *Annual Review of Medicine* **38**:467, 1987.

expression. For example, the earliest thymocytes are corticosteroid sensitive and relatively incompetent, whereas later, presumably more mature, thymocytes are corticosteroid resistant and display progressively increased immunocompetence. This seems to be accomplished, in large measure, by a variety of hormonelike substances produced by the thymic stroma (table 20.7). These factors induce the expression of mitogenic responsiveness and lymphokine production. In addition, they can influence, either positively or negatively, the expression of helper or suppressor functions.

TABLE 20.7 Influences of Putative Thymic Hormones

Hormone	Actions
α-thymosins	*Induce differentiation and maturation of early and immature T-cells* Induce expression of Ly-1,2,3 Ags, E-receptors, TdT activity; induce mitogen responsiveness and production of MIF and LTX; augment expression of helper (α1) and suppressor (α7) function
β-thymosins	*Act on prethymic stem cells* Induce expression of Thy-1 and TdT activity
Thymopoietins	*Stimulate early T cell and inhibit early B cell differentiation* Induce expression of Thy-1, TL, and Ly-1,2,3 Ags; induce mitogenic responsiveness and augment T_S pool; increase cytotoxicity and response in MLC; stimulate NK cell activity (?)—inhibit tumor growth
Thymic factor	Induces expression of Thy-1 and mitogen responsiveness
Thymic humoral factor	*Promotes T cell differentiation* Induces expression of TL Ag and E-receptors; enhances mitogenic responsiveness and MLC reaction; enhances B/T cell cooperation in Ab production; augments expression of helper and suppression functions; induces production of IL-2 and LIF (mice); stimulates NK cell activity (?)—inhibits tumor growth; increases GM-CFU (human)
Thymostimulin	Induces expression of Thy-1 Ag and E-receptors; increases mitogen responsiveness and MLC reaction; stimulates helper function and IFN-γ production (mice)
Serum thymic factor	Induces expression of Ly-1,2,3; increases mitogen responsiveness and cytotoxicity

E-receptor = receptor for forming E-rosettes; GM-CFU = granulocyte-monocyte–colony-forming unit; IL-2 = interleukin 2; IFN-γ = interferon; LIF = lymphocyte-inhibiting factor; LTX = lymphotoxin; Ly-1,2,3 = mouse T cell differentiation Ags; MIF = migration-inhibiting factor; MLC = mixed lymphocyte culture; TdT = terminal deoxynucleotidyl transferase; TL = mouse T cell differentiation Ag; Thy-1 = mouse T lymphocyte differentiation Ag.
Sources: Hildemann, W. H. *Essentials of Immunology.* Elsevier, New York, 1984; Trainin, N., Pecht, M., and Handzel, Z. T. Thymic hormones: inducers and regulators of the T-cell system. In *T Lymphocytes Today.* Inglis, J. R. (ed.). Elsevier, New York, 1983.

In addition to inducing the expression of general T cell functional traits, the thymic environment provides another significant form of instruction. This leads to what is known as **MHC restriction.** (See chapter 9, Effectors of Specific Cellular Immunity, for additional discussion.) Associated with MHC restriction is instruction that leads to "self-tolerance," in a manner of speaking. During fetal development, cells of the thymic stroma express products of the MHC. In mice, this means K, D, and I Ags. These are expressed from very early stages of lymphoid development. Although certain of these gene products are also expressed early by other tissues, expression of I Ags (Ia) appears to be limited to thymic epithelium. Thus, it is only within the thymus that the developing thymocytes would be exposed to these Ags. The importance of Ia to acquisition of cytotoxic functions can be demonstrated in nude mice. This mutant mouse variant has severely restricted cellular immunity. The thymuses of these animals fail to develop properly and, in partic-

ular, have been shown not to express Ia. Consequently, a specific correlation exists between failure to express Ia in the fetal thymus and failure to properly express cellular immune response postnatally. Ultimately, as a result of undergoing primary differentiation within an environment that is enriched in the expression of MHC Ags, T cells learn to recognize Ag only when it is associated with either a class I (K or D) or a class II (Ia) self-MHC Ag.

It has been proposed that reaction against self does not occur to any appreciable degree because of "related instruction" that occurs within the thymus during this period. One popular model for explaining this lack of antiself reactivity is known as the clonal deletion model. According to this model, T_C cells that recognize (nonMHC) self-Ags in association with MHC class I Ags are deleted by some, as yet undefined, mechanism. Alternatively, these T_C cells might be suppressed, or induced to alter their specificity. However, regardless of the mechanism employed, T_C cells with antiself specificity are not expressed. The emergence, often later in life, of autoimmune phenomena would seem to argue against an absolute elimination of such T_C cells, but according to some investigators the possibility of somatic mutation producing a rogue clone of antiself T_C cells cannot be excluded. (See chapter 10 for further discussion of tolerance.)

An extrapolation of the *induction of self-tolerance* can be used to explain more general expression of tolerance to nonself Ags. For tolerance induction during the fetal and early neonatal periods, we might simply propose that exposure of differentiating T cells to any Ags (self or foreign) in conjunction with learning MHC restriction leads to identification of those Ags as self. Thus, Ags presented during this period of instruction will not be recognized as foreign upon reexposure. The result is tolerance of those Ags. For those cases, later in life, in which tolerance is demonstrated to novel Ags an alternative explanation is required. For these Ags, tolerance might occur because of similarities that exist between the new Ag, in association with self-MHC Ags, and self-Ag/MHC Ag complexes encountered during ontogeny. In this instance, tolerance arises because T_C cells that would have been expected to recognize these Ags have been excluded, or suppressed.

Development of Natural Killer Cell Activity

NK cell activity in rodents is nearly absent from fetal liver and spleen. However, it rises markedly approximately three weeks after birth. By six to eight weeks of age, NK activity reaches its peak, then falls. A similar age-related rise and fall in NK cell activity can be demonstrated in humans, although the progession is less impressive. NK cells have an innate capacity for killing tumor cells and certain bone marrow stem cells, at least in mice. Extrapolating from these features, we might consider that NK cells display a tendency to attack cells expressing embryonic, immature, or "primitive" Ags.

Several factors might account for the low level of NK cell activity seen in fetal and neonatal animals. One factor might be the existence of an extremely small population of NK cells at these early stages of development. Alternatively, low NK activity might be the result of direct regulation from other sources. For example, suppressor factors might be produced that either prevent the NK cell pool from expanding or from becoming activated. Evidence supporting this hypothesis can be found in the inverse relationship between NK cell density and availability of NK cell targets in adult tissues. Specifically, those organs that contain large numbers of NK cell targets, like the bone marrow, have the lowest concentrations of NK cells. Presumably, these organs produce factors that selectively exclude NK cells. On the other hand, the absence of stimulators might serve to keep NK cell activity in check. The most likely candidate for this role is IFN-γ, which is a potent modulator of NK cell expression. During fetal development, IFN production is extremely limited or absent. Consequently, this source of NK cell activation cannot be invoked. Other means of restricting NK cell activity might also exist. Nevertheless, the net effect is that NK cell numbers and functional expression are limited until after the majority of "early" fetal development has been concluded. This is a time when the expression of embryonic or fetal Ags is extremely restricted and when few endogenous targets for NK cells should be present.

Development of Monocyte/Macrophage Function

Mϕs are important participants in reactions of cellular immunity. Mϕs function as APCs and inducers of T cell proliferation. In adults, Mϕs are believed to arise from two sources: (1) blood monocytes and (2) other tissue Mϕs. Within this latter category are a variety of fixed tissue Mϕs, for example, Kuppfer cells (liver), alveolar Mϕs (lung), and microglia (nervous system). Excluding fixed Mϕs, most other Mϕs are perhaps derived from a common embryonic precursor. This precursor appears in the yolk sac and fetal liver. For example, in mice, Mϕs can be observed at 10 days' gestation in the yolk sac and at 12 days' gestation in the liver. Later in development, they take up residence in the bone marrow. The normal progression of differentiation for many, if not most, Mϕs is as follows: myelomonocytic stem cell $\rightarrow$ promonocyte $\rightarrow$ monocyte $\rightarrow$ Mϕ. The monocyte represents a transitional stage in the bloodstream before entry into tissues, where further differentiation into mature Mϕs occurs.

With progression through the maturational sequence, monocyte/Mϕs acquire a supply of proteolytic enzymes and the capacity for phagocytosis. In addition, Mϕs acquire the ability to process Ags in immune reactions. Fetal and neonatal Mϕs produce and use proteolytic enzymes, although not as efficiently as do Mϕs from adults. Moreover, fetal Mϕs appear to be ineffective in presenting Ag. Evidence is available suggesting that a subset of Mϕs expressing Ia is required for interactions with lymphocytes. These Mϕs are absent from fetal and early neonatal mice and do not emerge until three to four weeks after birth.

Development of Granulocyte Function

Granulocytes develop from the same precursor as the monocyte/Mϕ. However, the differentiation pathway differs: myelomonocytic stem cell $\rightarrow$ myeloblast $\rightarrow$ promyelocyte $\rightarrow$ myelocyte $\rightarrow$ metamyelocyte $\rightarrow$ granulocyte. In addition, three distinct classes of granulocytes can be produced: basophils, eosinophils, and neutrophils. These populations of leukocytes probably first appear toward the end of the first trimester of pregnancy. Basophils seem to function extensively in hypersensitivity reactions, while eosinophils are active in parasitic infestations. Neither population has been extensively explored during ontogeny. In contrast, neutrophils have been the object of greater investigation. These cells routinely participate in acute inflammatory reactions (see chapter 8) and in combating microbial infections (see chapter 12). Like the monocyte/Mϕ, there is progressive acquisition and expression of functional competence with differentiation and maturation.

Neutrophils from adults normally display active phagocytosis and microbicidal reactivity following appropriate stimulation. Activated neutrophils of older children and adults display a reserve capacity, demonstrated by a respiratory burst, that can be evoked under stress. In contrast, neutrophils from neonates show reduced levels of response in at least two areas: mobilization and microbial killing after phagocytosis.

Neutrophils from neonates generate a reduced intracellular reaction to receptor stimulation. Subsequently, motility and adherence were less than that observed with neutrophils from older children and adults. Decreased adherence seems to be associated with weaker upregulation of adhesive surface glycoproteins. For example, neonatal neutrophils display a diminished capacity (75% of adult) to express CR3 (a class of complement receptor, Mac-1), which is necessary for adherence and directed migration. Consequently, slow influx to inflammatory sites is observed. Moreover, neutrophils from "stressed" neonates display normal phagocytic capacity but decreased bactericidal capacity. This is paradoxical in light of a readily activated superoxide generating system that they possess. However, neonatal neutrophils produce relatively fewer hydroxyl radicals and possess less lactoferrin, which enhances the generation of hydroxyl radicals. Consequently, they are less efficient in expression of microbicidal activity than are adult granulocytes. The newborn infant possesses a granulocyte population that has not yet realized its full expressive potential. This, however, usually occurs during the first few weeks of life. The net effect is that the newborn infant is more susceptible to microbial infections.

DEVELOPMENT OF THE COMPLEMENT SYSTEM

The human fetus seems capable of producing complement. For example, C3 is detectable as early as 12 weeks of gestation and is present in measurable quantities in all fetuses by 15 weeks' gestation. C4 follows a parallel but slightly slower course, initially becoming detectable at 14 weeks and universally present by 18 weeks' gestation. In contrast, C1, C2, and C5 appear earlier, between 2 and 2.5 months' gestation. In addition, C1q, C3, and C4 can be produced by fetal tissues, at least in culture.

Although the human fetus undoubtedly produces several complement proteins, the concentrations (or activity) of these substances at birth is substantially less than that found in adults. For example, C1 through C7 are present at approximately one-half adult concentrations, whereas C8 and C9 are present at only 5% to 10% the adult concentrations. During the first four days of neonatal life, however, the serum levels of complement rise dramatically. The complement system matures more rapidly in other species. Full complement activity has been demonstrated in fetal sheep and goats, at 123 and 115 days' gestation, respectively. Moreover, in fetal calves and pigs, full complement activity has been achieved by the end of the first trimester, for example, 40 days in pigs whose gestation is 115 to 120 days.

S U M M A R Y

1. Fertility and reproduction can be influenced by immunological manipulation. For example, decreased fertility has been associated with naturally occurring immunity to sperm antigens, leading to decreased motility or survival of sperm. In addition, artificial manipulation of fertility is being sought through the development of vaccines against reproductive hormones, sperm, or oocytes. [pp. 512–513]

2. Interactions between the mother and fetus that involve the immune system occur almost from the time of conception. The first effects of the conceptus on maternal immune response are expressed as masking of trophoblast immunogenicity and suppression of maternal responsiveness. [p. 513]

3. Suppression of maternal immune response is achieved, in part, through soluble factors produced by the fetus and placenta and released into the maternal bloodstream and, in part, by other factors produced by the mother herself. Among the former are α-fetoprotein, β_1-glycoprotein, and soluble inhibitory factor, while α-macroglobulin is an example of the latter. [p. 513]

4. The mother contributes to the immune status of the fetus through immunoglobulins that she passes across the placenta. [p. 513]

5. Other interactions between the conceptus and mother can occur. Certain interactions lead to a syndrome of spontaneous abortions during the first trimester. Other interactions presumably involve a cytokine-mediated dialogue between the conceptus and maternal immune system. [pp. 513–515]

6. The fetus and neonate progress through three major stages of immunological competence: (a) relative incompetence during the first two to three months; (b) transitional competence during the middle trimester, when the immune system is being formed and maternal antibodies become increasingly abundant; and (c) progressive competence when differentiation of B and T cells is occurring and expression of independent immunological status is increasing. [pp. 516–517]

7. Maintenance of immune competence depends upon (a) an adequate number of cells; (b) their proper distribution into appropriate subsets; and (c) effective intrinsic functional competence. Although these are maintained throughout most of our lives, aging introduces defects that lead to a reduction in both cellular and humoral immune expression. [pp. 517–518]

8. The embryo and fetus go through three stages of hemopoiesis: (a) mesoblastic, in which blood formation occurs primarily in the yolk sac; (b) hepatic, when the liver is the predominant hemopoietic organ; and (c) myeloid, where hemopoiesis occurs in the bone marrow, which begins about midgestation and continues through adulthood. [pp. 518–519]

9. During embryonic and fetal development, several lymphoid organs emerge. These originate without lymphocytes, but are soon populated by lymphocytes that migrate from either the yolk sac, fetal liver, or bone marrow. Two of these organs play special roles as sites for B cell differentiation (bone marrow; bursa of Fabricius, in birds) and T cell differentiation (thymus). [pp. 519–520]

10. Expression of humoral immunity begins in the fetus at approximately 25 weeks' gestation with the production of IgM. Between that time and approximately one year after birth, there is progressive expression of IgG, IgD, and IgA which continues to increase until adult antibody levels are reached. [p. 522]

11. Competence to express humoral immunity is acquired with B cell differentiation and maturation. This involves a sequential progression through (a) expression of cytoplasmic IgM, (b) expression of surface immunoglobulin, (c) class switching, and (d) antigen-dependent immunoglobulin production. [pp. 522–524]

12. Expression of cellular immunity does not follow as clearly defined a pattern of progression and is dependent upon T cell differentiation. T cell differentiation begins outside of the thymus; however, it cannot be effectively completed in its absence. Prethymic cells "home" into the thymus, where they undergo further differentiation into one of several subsets of T cells. [pp. 525–526]

13. T cell differentiation is accompanied by changes in the nature of surface antigens expressed, modifications in the balance of intracellular enzymes, acquisition both of a variety of surface receptors, and a capacity to perform roles as either helper/inducer or cytotoxic/suppressor cells. [pp. 526–529]

14. Much of thymic influence is exerted through secretory products identified as thymic hormones. The thymus also provides instructions to diferentiating lymphocytes that lead to MHC restriction in antigen reactivity through the expression of K, D, and I antigens by thymic epithelial cells. [pp. 529–530]

15. Reaction against self might be prevented by deletion, or suppression, of cells that react against these antigens. A similar means of conditioning might be involved in the generation of tolerance, to self as well as nonself antigens. [pp. 531–532]

16. Expression of NK activity is low before birth, reaches a peak soon after birth, then declines to adult levels. These changes appear to be influenced, or regulated, by maturational changes in cellular immune expression. [p. 532]

17. Macrophages and granulocytes arise from a common precursor but follow divergent maturational pathways. Nevertheless, each displays progressive acquisition of functional potential with cellular maturation. In addition, each displays limitations in expression of full functional competence that requires further maturation of the individual to become apparent. In particular, at birth, macrophages are inefficient at processing antigen, while neutrophils lack full bactericidal competence. [pp. 532–533]

18. The complement system begins to develop before birth. Partial expression of the pathway is accomplished at birth and completed thereafter. Moreover, those complement proteins present at birth occur at only a fraction of the levels found in adults. [pp. 533–534]

READINGS

Abney, E. R., Cooper, M. D., Kearney, J. F., et al. Sequential expression of immunoglobulin on developing mouse B lymphocytes: a systematic survey that suggests a model for the generation of immunoglobulin isotype diversity. *Journal of Immunology* **120:**2041, 1978.

Audhya, T., Kroon, D., Hravner, G., et al. Tripeptide structure of bursin, a selective B-cell-differentiation hormone of the bursa of Fabricius. *Science* **231:**997, 1986.

Burgio, G. R., Ugazio, A. G., and Notarangelo, L. D. Immunology of the neonate. *Current Opinion in Immunology* **2:**770, 1990.

Cates, K. L., Goetz, C., Rosenberg, N., et al. Longitudinal development of specific and functional antibody in very low birth weight premature infants. *Pediatric Research* **23:**14, 1988.

CIBA Foundation Symposium. *Ontogeny of Acquired Immunity.* Elsevier/Excerpta Medica/North Holland, Amsterdam, 1972.

Cooper, E. L., Langlet, C., and Bierne, J. (eds.). *Developmental and Comparative Immunology.* Alan R. Liss, Inc., New York, 1987.

Hill, H. R. Biochemical, structural, and functional abnormalities of polymorphonuclear leukocytes in neonates. *Pediatric Research* **22:**375, 1987.

Isojima, S. Sperm and seminal plasma antigens relevant to contraceptive vaccine development. *Current Opinion in Immunology* **2:**752, 1990.

King, A., Kabra, P., and Loke, Y. W. Human trophoblast cell resistance to decidual NK lysis is due to lack of NK target structure. *Cellular Immunology* **127:**230, 1990.

Mitchison, N. A. Gonadotropin vaccines. *Current Opinion in Immunology* **2:**725, 1990.

Mowbray, J. F. Autoantibodies, alloantibodies, and reproductive success. *Current Opinion in Immunology* **2:**761, 1990.

Paterson, M., and Aitken, R. J. Development of vaccines targeting the zona pellucida. *Current Opinion in Immunology* **2:**743, 1990.

Royer, H. D., and Reinherz, E. L. T lymphocytes: ontogeny, function, and relevance to clinical disorders. *New England Journal of Medicine* **317:**1136, 1987.

van Eijk, W. T-cell differentiation is influenced by thymic microenvironments. *Annual Review of Immunology* **9:**591, 1991.

Waksman, B. H. (ed.). *Ontogeny of the Immune System.* Progress in Allergy Vol. 29. S. Karger, Basel, 1981.

Wegman, T. G. The cytoine basis for cross-talk between the maternal immune and reproductive systems. *Current Opinion in Immunology* **2:**765, 1990.

Wolf, R. L. Human placental cells that regulate lymphocyte function. *Pediatric Research* **23:**212, 1988.

Yabuhara, A., Kawai, H., and Komiyama, A. Development of natural killer cytotoxicity during childhood: marked increases in number of natural killer cells with adequate cytotoxic activity during infancy and early childhood. *Pediatric Research* **28:**316, 1990.

Young, M., and Geha, R. S. Human regulatory T-cell subsets. *Annual Review of Medicine* **37:**165, 1986.

CHAPTER 21

Comparative Immunobiology

OVERVIEW

The abilities of organisms at different phylogenetic levels to protect themselves against foreign agents are briefly reviewed. The cellular and humoral agents used for immunological defense by different species are examined. In addition, phylogenetic similarities and modifications in cellular and humoral immunity are related to the evolution of the mammalian immune system.

CONCEPTS

1. Elements of immunological defense exist at all phylogenetic levels, from protozoa to mammals; however, the defense mechanisms show considerable variability.

2. Significant advances in immunity during evolution are related to (a) the nature of the organs of the immune system, (b) the cells and mechanisms of cellular immunity, and (c) the agents that effect humoral defense.

3. Relationships have been found in the expression of cellular and humoral immunity between phylogenetically ancient organisms and phylogenetically more recent organisms that enable the tracing of progressive refinements in immunological strategies.

In the preceding chapter, the development of mammalian immunity was examined. This developmental sequence more or less recapitulates the progressive changes in immunological functions that have occurred through evolution. However, the organization and function of immune systems of nonmammalian organisms might be expected to differ from what was described for mammals. Comparative immunology focuses on the relationships, similarities, and differences in immune mechanisms among various animal groups and, thus, can provide insight into how the complex interrelationships in mammalian immunity evolved.

This chapter explores, in a general manner, the defense mechanisms and immunological capabilities of invertebrates and nonmammalian vertebrates. Bear in mind that the immune mechanisms of these animals might be less complex than those described in the earlier chapters; nevertheless, they are effective defense mechanisms for those animals that possess them. After all, many of these animal groups have been on earth millions of years longer than humans. The relationships between cellular and humoral immunity, as expressed in these organisms, will be compared with the progressive refinements in immunological strategies that culminate in the mammals.

■ ■ ■ ■ ■ ■ ■ ■ ■ ■ ■

DEFENSE MECHANISMS OF INVERTEBRATES

It has long been known that animals, no matter how simple, take steps to protect themselves against foreign invasion. Elie Metchnikoff, the father of cellular immunology, was the first to systematically explore the strategies used by invertebrates to counter assault from foreign materials. Some of his earliest observations document the aggressive role played by phagocytes in removing thorn slivers from sponges and embryos.

Since those early studies, we have learned considerably more about the defensive strategies and immune mechanisms used by members of the various animal phyla. We observe a progressive expansion of the defensive repertoire from an almost exclusively phagocytic system to one involving phagocytes, lymphocytes, and humoral agents (table 21.1). This section briefly surveys the strategies and mechanisms displayed by nonvertebrate groups.

Protozoa, Porifera, and Coelenterata

The ability to discriminate self from nonself exists even in single-celled organisms. This is supported by two kinds of experimental observation (fig. 21.1). If the nucleus is removed from an ameba and replaced with a nucleus from a "syngeneic" strain of ameba, the recipient ameba will survive (fig. 21.1a). However, if a nucleus from a "nonrelated" strain is used, it might not be accepted, resulting in the death of the recipient ameba. The more unrelated the amebas are, the more likely it is that the implanted nucleus will be incapable of rescuing the enucleated ameba from certain death.

In other instances, fragments of pseudopods from certain amebas (*Difflugia* and *Arcella*) will fuse with the cell from which they are derived (fig. 21.1b). The cell and pseudopod, separated by 500 μm or more, will migrate toward each other and fuse. This fusion will also occur with fragments from sister cells, but never with fragments from unrelated cells. This behavior is sharply contrasted with the behavior demonstrated by amebas encountering totally different species of protozoans, which are subsequently actively phagocytized.

These two modes of behavior reflect an ability of a single-celled organism to distinguish between itself (or closely related cells) and cells of a different type. Discrimination is mediated, in part, at the cell surface, as in the case of the fusion of pseudopodial fragments, and is associated, in part, with internal recognition (nuclear implantation). However, this form of recognition would appear to be more enzymatic than immunological.

It is among multicellular organisms, the Metazoa, that more forthright immunological strategies are encountered. This is related, in part, to the fact that with multicellularity particular roles are assigned to specific cell types. This is known as division of labor and has enabled organ systems to be established.

TABLE 21.1 Evolution of Mechanisms for Internal Defense

| Group | Phagocytic System (coarse discrimination between self/nonself) | Lymphoid System (finely tuned discrimination between self/nonself) | |
		Cell Mediated	Humoral
Invertebrates			
Protozoa	Absent (discrimination seems to be enzymatic, not immunological)	Absent	Absent
Metazoa	Well-established	Variable	Variable, no true Igs
Porifera/Coelenterata		Xenografts not tolerated	Absent
Protostomes		Xenografts not tolerated; allografts not tolerated by Annelids	Lysins and agglutinins
Deuterostomes		Allografts and xenografts not tolerated	Lysins and agglutinins
Vertebrates	Well-established	Established	Includes true Igs
Fish			Limited to IgM
Amphibians			IgM and IgG-like
Birds			IgA, IgG, and IgM
Mammals			IgA, IgE, IgG, IgM, IgD

Source: Modified and adapted from Manning, M. J., and Turner, R. J. *Comparative Immunobiology*. Halsted Press (John Wiley & Sons, Inc.), New York, 1976.

Among the Porifera (sponges) and Coelenterata, cells from another species are not accepted by the recipient organism. In both groups, cells that are recognized as nonself are not incorporated into the colonial organism. In the sponges, the foreign tissue is eliminated without damage or killing. In contrast, in the coelenterates, much tissue destruction is observed. In this latter instance, the destruction of the foreign tissue appears to be self-induced or suicidal, rather than caused by direct destruction by the host.

A class of freely wandering phagocytic cells, called **amebocytes,** are responsible for certain responses to foreign matter. In addition to phagocytosis, these cells provide defense by *encapsulation,* where foreign material too large to be engulfed is segregated from the organism by being walled-off from the remaining tissue. Although the amebocytes of the sponges and coelenterates can be viewed as immune cells of sorts, these cells are not organized into a recognizable coherent tissue.

Protostomes: Flatworms, Annelids, Molluscs, and Arthropods

Although no unequivocal documentation exists for graft rejection in flatworms, they do possess a population of phagocytes that eliminate foreign material. In contrast, their close relatives, the nemerteans, display transplantation reactions. Allografts are tolerated, but xenografts are rejected by apparently true immunological means. This is presumed because of the demonstration of accelerated second-set graft rejection, suggestive of immunological memory. Of further interest, the nemerteans are the most phylogenetically primitive organisms to possess a true circulatory system.

Rejection of allografts, as well as xenografts, occurs in annelids (fig. 21.2). Xenografts are destroyed in eight to 147 days at 15° C. Allografts are destroyed more slowly (15 to 255 days). Rejection rates are temperature sensitive, increasing with increasing temperature and decreasing with decreasing temperature. In addition, immunological memory is displayed. This

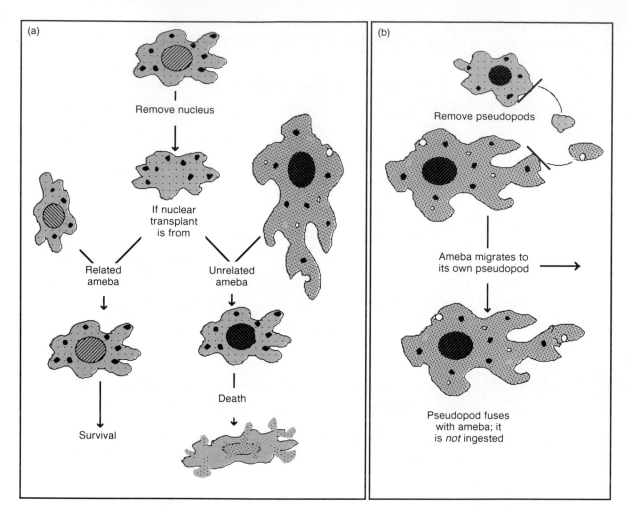

FIGURE 21.1 Features in protozoa that resemble, or mimic, a sense of self/nonself discrimination. (*a*) Transplanted nuclei into enucleated amebas are tolerated only if they are from a syngeneic ameba. Nuclei from amebas of other strains are rejected, leading to the eventual death of the host ameba. (*b*) If pieces of pseudopods are removed from amebas and placed nearby, migration toward these fragments can be observed. Movement is preferentially in the direction of the fragment that was originally a part of the ameba. Upon contact, the piece of pseudopod is incorporated as part of the ameba. This contrasts with the behavior displayed toward a piece of pseudopod derived from another ameba or toward another protozoan, namely, phagocytic ingestion and digestion.

memory can be either positive (accelerated rejection) or negative (delayed rejection). Expression of positive memory in annelids resembles sensitization to Ag, while negative memory seems to resemble induction of tolerance. Increasing temperature (from 15° C to 20° C) favors positive memory. Moreover, memory is specific, neither affecting nor being affected by third-party transplants.

Transplantation immunity in annelids resembles transplantation immunity displayed by vertebrates (table 21.2). Graft rejection in annelids seems to be accomplished by **coelomocytes.** These phagocytic cells (1) actively infiltrate the graft, (2) can transfer antixenograft immunity to nonimmune worms, and (3) appear in increased numbers in second-set grafts.

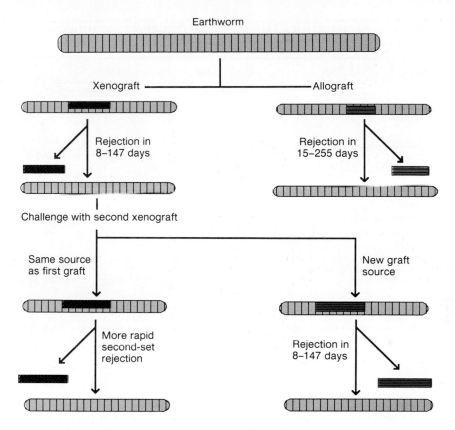

Earthworm

Xenograft ——————————————— Allograft

Rejection in
8–147 days

Rejection in
15–255 days

Challenge with second xenograft

Same source
as first graft

New graft
source

More rapid
second-set
rejection

Rejection in
8–147 days

FIGURE 21.2 Graft rejection in annelids. Earthworms reject xeno-grafts and allografts. Xenografts are rejected more rapidly than are allografts, although both are rejected chronically. Memory of the nature of the graft rejected is displayed in accelerated second-set rejection, whereas a third-party graft shows no enhancement in the rate of rejection.

Some manifestations of a **humoral immunelike capacity** exist in annelids. *No Igs* have been demonstrated. Nevertheless, the coelomic fluid of annelids possesses agents, called *lysins,* that are capable of causing cytolysis of foreign cells or tissues. These cytolytic factors are synthesized by free chloragocytes. However, it is somewhat presumptuous to refer to this as an actual counterpart to the humoral immune response of vertebrates.

Annelids are the first to display evidence of lymphoid tissues. Although rather primitive in organization, foci of tissue, hemal glands, from which red cells, phagocytes, and nonphagocytic granulocytes emerge are found adhering to blood vessels in the midgut region. In addition, ameboid cells regularly bud from "valves" in their dorsal blood vessel. Beyond these superficial features, no clear homologies have been described between these special aggregations and vertebrate lymphoid tissues.

Molluscs and arthropods appear to represent a step backward in terms of transplantation immunology. Studies of graft rejection in molluscs have not been decisive. They suggest that autografts, allografts, and xenografts can be distinguished. However, precise evaluation of specificity and memory is unavailable. In contrast, the experimental data seem to point to an inability of arthropods to recognize allografts and even xenografts. *Encapsulation* and elimination of foreign material by molluscan phagocytic **amebocytes** is well documented, however. Arthropods similarly display active phagocytosis and encapsulation as defensive strategies in dealing with foreign materials.

TABLE 21.2 Some Characteristics Displayed by Annelid Coelomocytes Participating in Transplantation Reactions

Cellular Response	Transplantation Reaction		Trait Seen in Vertebrates
	First Set	Second Set	
Proliferation of undifferentiated cells in response to graft	Yes	Yes	Yes
Assault on graft by responding cells	Yes	Yes	Yes
Migration of stimulated cells to other regions of host	Yes	Yes	Yes
Rapid response of sensitized cells to Ag	No	Yes	Yes
Accelerated rejection of second graft		Yes	Yes
Progenitors of cells involved in graft rejection respond to nonspecific mitogens	Yes	Yes	Yes
Stimulated cells can transfer antixenograft immunity to nonimmune recipient	Yes	Yes	Yes
Stimulated cells can produce reaction in mixed lymphocyte cultures	No	No	Yes

Source: Adapted from Manning, M. J., and Turner, R. J. *Comparative Immunobiology.* Halsted Press (John Wiley & Sons, Inc.), New York, 1976.

The basic strategies employed by all metazoa are expressed by molluscs and arthropods, although there is uncertainty as to the extent of their abilities to recognize the nature of transplants. It should be stressed that this latter deficiency results, in part, from limitations in available information. Transplantation immunity among these organisms has not received the same degree of attention as has been given to other phyla. Consequently, our knowledge remains incomplete and inconclusive.

In marked contrast, humoral factors of molluscs and arthropods that respond to foreign insult have been the object of considerable investigation. The hemolymph of members of both phyla contains a variety of hemagglutinins. These **agglutinins** can be highly specific. For example, the snail, *Helix,* possesses hemagglutinins capable of distinguishing Ags within the ABO and some MN blood group systems of human erythrocytes. (The ABO system represents the major human blood-grouping system, while the MN system represents a minor blood-grouping system. Ags within each system are surface glycoproteins.) In addition, the titers of these hemagglutinins vary as a function of Ag concentration and time after Ag challenge. The level of hemagglutinins rises sharply after challenge,

reaching a peak in about one to two days, and decines rapidly (fig. 21.3). This distinguishes it clearly from the Ig response of vertebrates that peaks after several days. Moreover, in arthropods, there is a definite correlation between hemagglutinin concentration and the number of hemocytes.

Both molluscs and arthropods also are capable of *opsonization.* The source and mechanisms of the factors involved in these reactions are not well understood. There is, nevertheless, some evidence that some opsonins are also hemagglutinins. In addition, Ags have been shown to be very rapidly and effectively cleared from the hemolymph of molluscs and arthropods. This Ag-clearing capacity appears to be associated with an immunological memory in that subsequent challenge by the same Ag leads to more rapid clearance. However, this memory appears to have a cellular, rather than a humoral, basis.

The organization of components of the "immune system" into specific tissues continues with the molluscs and arthropods. Among molluscs, there are discrete hemopoietic centers, and phagocytosis is often restricted to these specific sites. Among certain insects, an interesting and striking parallel with vertebrate systems occurs in these tissues. Immunization

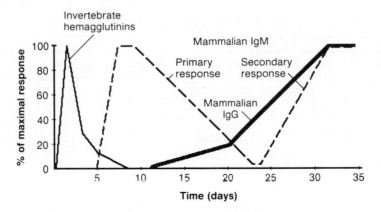

FIGURE 21.3 Comparison of humoral immune responses between invertebrates and vertebrates. Both invertebrates and vertebrates display humoral immune responses. Invertebrates release agglutinins (*light solid line*) that show no delay in rising, reach their peak quickly, then disappear. In contrast, vertebrates yield a biphasic response, the first portion of which is associated with a high molecular weight Ab (*dashed line*), while a low molecular weight Ab (*heavy solid line*) predominates, and far exceeds the concentration of low molecular weight Ab produced, during the second phase. This diagram does not show the relationship between concentrations of Abs produced during the humoral response of vertebrates but rather focuses on the temporal relationships of Ab release. Note that the time frame of the invertebrate response is so rapid that it has nearly run its course before the first phase of the vertebrate response would be initiated and has been totally extinguished before the major humoral response (second phase) would be inaugurated.

with live bacteria leads to two reactions in the hemopoietic tissues: (1) proliferation of cells with phagocytic and hemopoietic potential and release of young cells into the hemolymph and (2) differentiation of some reticular cells into secretory cells, which correlates with the appearance of antibacterial factors and antitoxins in the hemolymph. Injection of bacterial toxin alone produces only the second of these responses in these insects.

Deuterostomes: Echinoderms and Protochordates

Echinoderms and protochordates reject allografts effectively. In addition, *allograft rejection* mechanisms include *immunological memory*. Rejection of allografts by echinoderms occurs rather slowly; first-set allografts can persist for several months before elimination. Nevertheless, subsequent grafting of tissues from the same donor leads to progressively accelerated rejection. The cells of echinoderms and protochordates that reject foreign tissues resemble vertebrate **macrophages (Mφs)**, **lymphocytes,** and **granulocytes.**

Echinoderms possess several types of *coelomocytes*. These include (1) amebocytes, which resemble vertebrate Mφs; (2) red and colorless spherule cells, which are believed to produce collagenous material

used in tissue repair; and (3) vibratile cells, which release a mucoid substance that causes coelomic fluid to gel. Unlike the immunocytes of other invertebrates, lymphocytes from protochordates respond in mixed lymphocyte cultures.

The deuterostomes appear to possess humoral defense mechanisms. However, even the protochordates *lack any true Ig-like molecules.* Moreover, their immunocytes are produced in hemopoietic centers that resemble organized lymphoid tissues.

Recapitulation

Immunological defense mechanisms among invertebrates are designed, as in vertebrates, to preserve individual integrity, that is, maintain self intact. This seems to apply even to protozoans. However, for single-celled organisms, the mechanisms are more enzymatic and metabolic rather than immunological in nature. No specific immunocytes exist.

Among the Metazoa, where cellular specialization becomes possible, immunocytes can be found. The immunological defenses show a wide range of activities among the several invertebrate phyla (table 21.3). Common to all metazoan invertebrates are diverse sorts of manifestations of **cellular immunity.** *Phagocytosis and encapsulation* of foreign particles and

TABLE 21.3 Summary of Immunopotentialities of Invertebrates

Phylum or Subphylum	Immunocytes or Defensive Cells	Humoral Mechanisms	Allogeneic Cell-Surface Polymorphism	Specific Graft Rejection	Immunological Memory
Protozoans	None	None	Present	No	None
Porifera	Amebocytes	None	Present	Allografts and xenografts	Short-term only
Coelenterates	Amebocytes	None	Present	Allografts and xenografts	Short-term only
Platyhelminthes	Amebocytes	None	Present	Xenografts	Short-term (?)
Annelids	Coelomocytes	Lysins (produced by chloragocytes)	Present	Allografts and xenografts	Short-term only
Molluscs	Amebocytes	Hemagglutinins (produced by hemocytes)	Present	Allografts (?) and xenografts (?)	Uncertain
Arthropods	Amebocytes	Hemagglutinins (produced by hemocytes)	Present	Xenografts (?)	Uncertain
Echinoderms	Amebocytes, vibratile cells; red and colorless spherule cells*	Uncertain	Present	Allografts and xenografts	Short-term and long-term (?)
Protochordates	Lymphocytes; phagocytes†	Hemagglutinins	Present	Allografts and xenografts	Uncertain

(?) Denotes that there is evidence suggesting its possible occurrence; however, definite proof is lacking.

*Coelomocytes infiltrating grafts resemble vertebrate macrophages, eosinophilic granulocytes, and small lymphocytes.

†Lymphocytes and phagocytes present are morphologically similar to those of vertebrates.

Source: Adapted, modified, and expanded from Hildemann, W. H. *Essentials of Immunology.* Elsevier Publishing Co., Inc., New York, 1984.

infective agents (bacteria and viruses) occur throughout, while the *ability to recognize grafts,* whether allogeneic or xenogeneic, varies. In contrast, manifestation of **humoral immunity** is less universal. The most primitive colonial organisms (Porifera and Coelenterata) and flatworms lack such capability. The annelids, and more phylogenetically recent forms, possess humoral mechanisms for defense against foreign substances. These are typically in the form of *lysins and hemagglutinins.* Although they display some of the properties of Igs, they lack others. These humoral agents are proteins, are sometimes specific, and often possess opsonizing properties. In contrast to the Igs, however, few, if any, are inducible by the usual immunization procedures and their chemical structures are quite heterogeneous. Consequently, they are not related to the vertebrate Igs and are probably poor candidates as precursors to these molecules.

The various specific defense strategies among these groups provide effective defense for the organisms possessing them. Whatever cellular or humoral mechanisms exist at a particular phylogenetic level efficiently protect members of that phylum against the most common infectious agents.

IMMUNITY IN NONMAMMALIAN VERTEBRATES

There is great similarity in mediators and mechanisms of cellular and humoral immunity among vertebrates. Nevertheless, specific differences exist between classes (table 21.4). For example, all vertebrates reject allografts efficiently. However, the *rejection is chronic among most poikilothermic* (cold-blooded) vertebrates, but is *acute in homoiothermic* (warm-blooded) vertebrates. In addition, immunological *memory is displayed at all levels.*

TABLE 21.4 Characteristics of the Immune Systems of Nonmammalian Vertebrates

Group	Reaction to Allografts	Effector Cells	Thymus	Hemopoietic Bone Marrow	Immunoglobulins
Agnatha (hagfish and lampreys)	Moderate; chronic rejection	Lymphocytes, granulocytes, and Mφs	Absent	Absent	No Igs; molecule with some IgM-like properties present
Chondrichthyes (sharks and rays)	Moderate; chronic rejection	Lymphocytes, granulocytes, and Mφs	Present	Absent	IgM only
Osteichthyes (bony fish)	Moderate to strong; chronic rejection	Lymphocytes, granulocytes, and Mφs	Present	Present	IgM; some evidence for an IgG-like Ab called IgN
Amphibia (salamanders, newts, frogs)	Moderate to strong; acute and chronic rejection	Lymphocytes, granulocytes, and Mφs	Present	Absent (urodeles) Present (anurans)	IgM; some evidence for an IgG-like Ab
Reptilia (lizards, snakes, turtles)	Moderate; chronic rejection	Lymphocytes, granulocytes, and Mφs	Present	Present	IgM, IgG, IgN; some evidence for IgD (?)
Aves (birds)	Moderate to strong; acute rejection	Lymphocytes, granulocytes, and Mφs	Present	Present	IgM, IgY, IgA, IgD

Source: Adapted and modified from Hildemann, W. H. *Essentials of Immunology.* Elsevier Publishing Co., Inc., New York, 1984.

Humoral immunity among the most primitive vertebrates (hagfish) resembles that observed among invertebrates; namely, it is accomplished by hemagglutinins and lysins rather than by Igs. However, humoral agents with properties similar to IgM are also present. In contrast, all other vertebrate forms possess *Igs,* although their specific nature displays considerable variability. Moreover, among amphibians and birds clear evidence of immunological memory in humoral immunity can be found. In addition, an active cytolytic system, *complement,* exists in serum.

Unlike their invertebrate predecessors, *effector cells* of the immune system in vertebrates are the same in all classes: **lymphocytes,** assisted by **monocytes/Mφs,** and **granulocytes.** Another significant feature that distinguishes vertebrates from invertebrates is the presence of more *highly organized lymphoid tissues.* With the exception of the agnathans, these organs include the thymus and spleen. There is considerable heterogeneity in the architecture of these organs and in the presence of secondary lymphoid tissues as we progress up the evolutionary ladder. As a group, vertebrates possess a sophisticated immune system.

PHYLOGENY OF IMMUNOGLOBULINS AND RELATED MOLECULES

Invertebrates are able to respond to challenge by foreign Ags. For example, insects will respond to inoculation with heat-killed bacteria by producing bacteriolytic substances. The response is rapid and short-lived. However, the substances produced are apparently nonspecific—which differentiates them functionally from Igs. In addition, some bacteriolysins are not proteins, which contrasts structurally with Igs. On the other hand, naturally occurring hemagglutinins can be found in invertebrate blood that have electrophoretic mobilities similar to β- and γ-globulins. On this criterion, there is a resemblance to vertebrate Igs. More importantly, agglutinins might anticipate Igs functionally as a humoral means of defense in that they can entrap bacteria, thereby restricting their multiplication. This notwithstanding, no true Igs exist among invertebrate species.

Antibiotics Produced by Frog Skin

The natives of the Amazon River Basin have known for quite some time that amphibian skin possesses very powerful properties. They have taken ample advantage of this knowledge to prepare extracts from the skin of certain frogs in which to dip their darts. These extracts contain a very potent poison that we now know to be tetrodotoxin. This poison is used by the frogs as a protection against predators. Frog skin apparently also produces other substances for defense against predators of another nature. These substances are recently identified, naturally occurring antibiotics.

Between the summer of 1986 and the summer of 1987, Dr. Michael Zasloff, at the National Institute of Child Health and Human Development, pursued a course of investigation that led to the discovery of antibiotic peptides produced by the skin of *Xenopus laevis*. These peptides have been called **magainins.** Upon observing one of his frogs swimming in a murky aquarium only a few days after surgery, Zasloff was struck by the remarkable progress in wound healing that was occurring, *without infection.* Careful examination revealed that the wound was not heavily infiltrated by lymphocytes and phagocytes. Some other means of defense had to be operating.

Zasloff first demonstrated that fluid from the wound and from the frog's abdomen could arrest bacterial growth. The search was on! Over the next several months, Zasloff proceeded to isolate and characterize the active property in the frog's skin. This was accomplished by homogenizing frogs' skin and fractionating the extract. These fractions were tested to determine which contained the antibiotic property. By means of high-performance liquid chromatography, Zasloff isolated two peptides, which he designated as magainins I and II. With the assistance of two colleagues, Drs. Harry Chen and Brian Martin, the amino acid sequence of these peptides was determined.

The term "magainin," derived from Hebrew, means "shield." Magainins are peptides containing 23 amino acids. They are able to twist into long, spiral-shaped molecules with one hydrophobic (fat soluble) and one hydrophilic (water soluble) side. They are very similar to *cecropins*, which are defensive molecules produced by insects. They also are the proper length to span cellular membranes. But, more importantly, their chemical properties are suited for interactions with the surfaces of viruses, bacteria, and animal cells. Thus, they possess all of the characteristics required to be very effective antibiotic agents.

Two other important tests were also performed. One demonstrated that the magainins were actually produced by the frog's skin and were not merely an artifact created by the extraction procedures. Zasloff was able to isolate mRNA for the magainins and demonstrated that they are originally produced as a larger precursor in the cell, then processed before final release. The second demonstration required the preparation of synthetic magainins. These artificially produced peptides were shown to be functionally identical to those extracted from the frog's skin.

The dogged determination of one investigator converted a puzzling observation into an aggressive, systematic search that culminated in the discovery of a naturally occurring antibiotic from a vertebrate.

Zasloff, M. Magainins, a class of antimicrobial peptides from Xenopus skin: isolation, characterization of two active forms, and partial cDNA sequence of a precursor. *Proceedings of the National Academy of Sciences* (USA) **84**:5449, 1987.

Phylogenetic Distribution of Immunoglobulin Types

Igs, therefore, can be considered a *distinctive feature of vertebrate humoral immunity.* Igs can be found in all vertebrate classes, although the types of Igs present are not the same throughout. For example, mammals possess five classes of Igs (IgA, IgD, IgE, IgG, and IgM) while lampreys possess only one (an IgM-like species).

IgM appears to be the most primitive Ig type, since it occurs in the most phylogenetically ancient vertebrate groups. In lampreys, high (14S) and low (6.6S) molecular weight Abs occur. These Abs contain light (L) and μ heavy (H) chains, but lack disulfide bridges. In fish, similar Igs occur; however, they are slightly larger (with sedimentation coefficients of 17S to 19S and 7S) and contain disulfide bridges between H and L chains.

Among vertebrates, humoral immune response typically are biphasic (fig. 21.4). In agnathans and fish, the early phase of a humoral response to Ag challenge typically is associated with the high molecular weight Ab, while the late phase is associated with the low molecular weight Ab. In both instances, an IgM-like Ig is employed. In amphibians, at least anurans, a non-IgM Ig emerges during the later phase of a humoral response. This low molecular weight Ab has a γ type H chain and resembles mammalian IgG. This pattern is retained among reptiles and birds. Since the IgG-like molecules differ from mammalian IgG in physicochemical features, such as sedimentation coefficient (5.7S, 7.1S, or 7.5S) and molecular weight (35 kD to 38 kD or 64 kD to 68 kD), they have been designated as IgN and IgY. In addition, Igs resembling IgA have also been identified in birds.

Among mammals, IgM, IgG, and IgA are present, while IgN and IgY may also appear in some species. However, in addition, two new classes of Igs can be found. These are designated IgD and IgE. Thus, five distinct Ig classes can be identified: (1) IgM, the most ancient; (2) IgG and its relatives (IgN and IgY); (3) IgA, of intermediate ancestry; and (4) IgD and (5) IgE, which are phylogenetically recent additions to the Ig family.

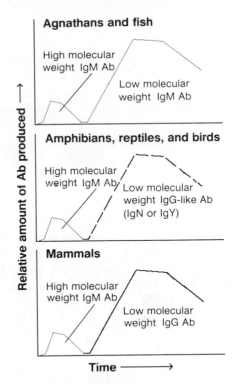

FIGURE 21.4 Comparison of Ab responses among vertebrates. Vertebrates display similar biphasic Ab responses. What distinguishes the specific responses at various phylogenetic levels is the identity of the low molecular weight Ab that appears during the second phase.

Phylogenetic Origins of Antibody Classes

Structural analysis of the diverse Ig classes reveals considerable similarity. All Igs are composed of two H chains and two L chains. In addition, these chains are composed of variable (V) and constant (C) domains, whose lengths are approximately 110 amino acids each. But more importantly, there is great similarity in the amino acid sequences among all vertebrate classes. This suggests that all Igs are derived from a common ancestor. One model proposes that gene duplication and diversification is responsible for the generation of the several Ig classes present today (fig. 21.5). According to this hypothesis, the ancestral gene was first duplicated giving rise to genes for future V and C domains. In turn, these V and C genes are duplicated.

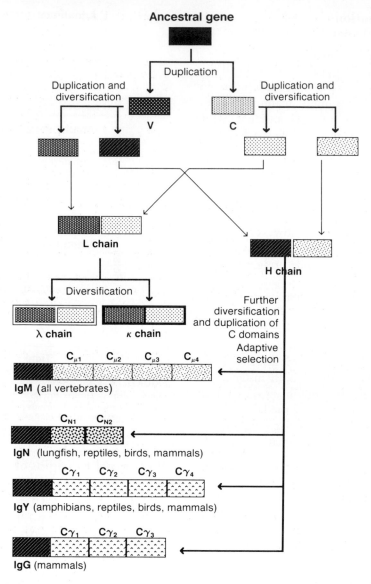

FIGURE 21.5 Model for the phylogenetic derivation of modern Igs. Modern Ig H and L chains are believed to have arisen from a common ancestral gene. Through the course of evolution, this gene has duplicated and diversified at several points, giving rise to genes for the C and V regions of L and H chains. Within the H chain family, considerably more duplication and diversification of the C region occurred, which enabled a variety of Ig classes to be produced in response to challenge by foreign Ag.

Through diversification, multiple V and C genes were produced within the genome. With further duplications of C genes, several contiguous genes for H chain C domains could be generated. Further diversification of C genes could later produce μ, N, and γ C gene classes. Adaptive selection and joining of V and C regions, following antigenic stimulation, could then give rise to Ab diversity.

From studies of the amino acid sequences of L chains, it appears that divergence from the L chain ancestral gene into κ and λ chains occurred approximately 460 million years ago. This corresponds roughly with the emergence of cartilaginous fish. In addition, representation of both types of L chains is highly variable among different vertebrate classes. For example, L chains are equally divided into κ and λ in turkeys and pigs. In guinea pigs and baboons, κ chains predominate by a 3:1 ratio. On the other hand, in cows, dogs, and horses λ chains represent over 90% of all L chains, whereas in rabbits and mice k chains account for over 90% of all L chains.

Similar analysis of H chain sequences is equally likely to provide information about differences between Ig classes and evolutionary relationships among Igs. Nevertheless, some insight into this latter question can be obtained by focusing attention on the V_H region, since it is this portion of the H chain that is involved in Ag-Ab reactions. Detailed analysis of amino acid residues of V_{H3} sequences of mammals and birds and of the antipolysaccharide Ab of sharks reveals considerable similarity. The amino acid sequences are 70% similar in the first 24 positions when comparing mammals and birds. The shark Ab displays 46% similarity compared with mammals and 33% similarity compared with birds in this same region.

Another means of seeking possible evolutionary relationships is to compare the binding characteristics of Abs from animals of different species. For example, these studies have shown that the Ag-combining site has remained well-conserved structurally, having an average depth of 11.5 Å in trout (IgM) and rabbits (IgG) and 12 Å in mouse IgA. In contrast, the binding affinities of different classes of Abs show marked variability. In comparing early Abs from fish

TABLE 21.5 Sequence Similarities Between Fc Regions of Human Immunoglobulins

C Gene Class	δ	α	ϵ	γ	μ
δ	100%	25.6%	23.8%	22.8%	22.5%
α	25.6%	100%	–	–	34.2%
ϵ	23.8%	–	100%	33.7%	27.5%
γ	22.8%	–	33.7%	100%	–
μ	22.5%	34.2%	27.5%	–	100%

Values of 100%, which appear running diagonally from upper left to lower right, are a reflection of H chain being compared with itself.

Dashes represent combinations for which no comparisons were made.

Boldface denotes percent sequence similarity between δ gene and other Ig genes.

Italics denotes percent sequence similarity between Ig genes other than δ.

Source: Lin, L.-C., and Putnam, F. W. Primary structure of the Fc region of human immunoglobulin D: implications for evolutionary origin and biological function. *Proceedings of the National Academy of Sciences* (USA) **78:**504, 1981.

(carp, IgM), reptiles (turtle, IgM and IgN) and mammals (rabbit, IgG), little difference was observed in binding affinities for the hapten DNP (dinitrophenyl). All binding affinities were low, 0.06 to 0.08 L/mol × 10^{-6} for IgMs and 0.20 L/mol × 10^{-6} for IgN and IgG. However, when comparing binding affinities of late Abs, a clear distinction emerged between IgM (16S and 19S) and IgG and IgN. The affinity of IgM for DNP remained low (0.5 to 0.15 L/mol × 10^{-6}), whereas affinities of IgN and IgG for DNP rose to 34 to 84 L/mol × 10^{-6}. This suggests that a distinct functional advantage was acquired when the newly evolved classes of Igs emerged.

Detailed study of the amino acid sequence of the Fc region of human IgD and a comparison of that sequence to the amino acid sequences of other Ig H chains provides an indication of the evolutionary relationships among the genes for the diverse H chain C domains. This analysis revealed less similarity between Fc$_\delta$ and other Fc classes (22.5% to 25.6% similarity) than between other pairings of Fc classes (27.5% to 34.2% similarity) (table 21.5). Two explanations could account for this phenomenon: (1) the δ chain gene arose

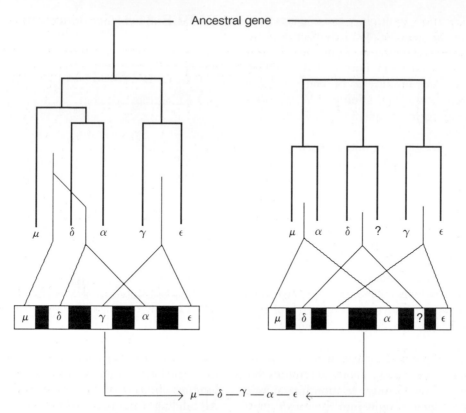

FIGURE 21.6 Phylogenetic relationships among H chain C genes. The several types of H chain C genes that exist today are believed to have arisen from a common ancestral gene. Their phylogenetic relatedness to each other and their order on the chromosome are believed to be the result of diversifications of existing gene elements at several points during evolution. Two models for this diversification are represented. (Modified from Lin, L.-C., and Putnam, F. W. Primary structure of the Fc region of human immunoglobulin D: implications for evolutionary origin and biological function. *Proceedings of the National Academy of Sciences* [USA] **78**:504, 1981.)

shortly after divergence between α and μ chain genes or (2) the δ chain gene has undergone mutation at a greater rate than other H chain genes since it originally arose. The available evidence provides support for both explanations. There appears to be a greater mutation rate in the δ chain gene than in other H chain genes. In addition, IgD has been demonstrated in primates, rodents, chickens, and possibly tortoises, which suggests that it might be as ancient as the α chain gene. Efforts to produce a phylogenetic tree to represent the emergence of the H chain genes generated two diagrams (fig. 21.6). According to one portrayal, the δ-chain gene arises shortly after the α and μ chain genes diverge; whereas in the other, the δ chain gene arises

from an independent branch. However, both models predict the same order for H chain genes, namely, μ–δ–γ–α–ϵ.

Immunoglobulin-Related Molecules

In addition to Igs, other proteins can be found in serum that have strong binding affinities for other molecules. Although these may not be related to Igs, as revealed from their physicochemical characteristics, they are functionally related to some extent. Examples of these serum-binding proteins include *lectins* of several invertebrate phyla, the *erythrocyte H(O)-binding protein* of lampreys and eels, the *fructosan-binding protein* of sharks, and *C-reactive protein* in humans.

TABLE 21.6 Conservatism of Amino Acid Composition Among Members of Immunoglobulin Superfamily

Molecule	Compared with	$S\Delta Q^*$
β_2-microglobulin	Ig chains	52–97
	α_1-acid glycoprotein	95
α_1-acid glycoproteins	Ig chains	54–106
MHC Ags	β_2-microglobulin	21
	α_1-acid glycoprotein	84
	Ig chains	63–79
L chain	γ and μ chains	24–26
γ chain	μ chain	29

*$S\Delta Q = \Sigma_j (X_{ij} - X_{kj})^2$, where i and k are proteins being compared, and X_j represents the content (per 100 residues) of a given amino acid of type j. $S\Delta Q$ for hemoglobins from 16 species of vertebrates = 80; for cytochrome c from 14 vertebrate species = 20; for Igs from 8 vertebrate species = 30.
Source: Marchalonis, J. J. *Immunity in Evolution*. Harvard University Press, Cambridge, Mass., 1977.

On the other hand, there are now several non-Ig proteins (or glycoproteins) that have been identified that possess strong similarities in amino acid sequences to those found in Igs. Many are believed to belong to the so-called Ig superfamily. This superfamily includes all currently known molecules involved in recognition of Ag by vertebrate B and T cells and several other cell-surface glycoproteins. Among the other molecules comprising the **Ig superfamily** are amyloid substance, β_2-microglobulin, α_1-acid glycoprotein, haptoglobin, class I and class II MHC Ags, T cell receptors (α, β, γ), and the Thy-1 Ag. In addition, there is some circumstantial evidence that C-reactive protein might also belong to this superfamily. However, the support for this relationship is not strong. There is a marked similarity in the amino acid composition between C-reactive protein and Igs, but analysis of the sequence similarities is lacking.

Using evaluation of $S\Delta Q$ (sum of squared differences), devised by Marchalonis and Weltman in 1971, to compare molecules that are considered part of the Ig superfamily, values less than 100 are often encountered (table 21.6). Such low values reflect possible relatedness between proteins. $S\Delta Q$ values for several members of this superfamily are comparable to that of hemoglobins ($S\Delta Q = 80$, comparing 16 vertebrate species). Further analysis enabled a diagram of probable phylogenetic relationship among these molecules to be constructed (fig. 21.7). Within this scheme, it is estimated that α_1-acid glycoprotein diverged from the Igs over 300 million years ago.

The striking sequence similarities among the molecules of the Ig superfamily provide evidence for their common ancestry. More importantly, they also raise questions about the origins of the immune system and about the interrelationships of its components. For example, the similarity between Thy-1 and Igs has raised the question of these two molecules serving as descendants of molecules comprising two separate arms of a primitive recognition system. According to this idea, the ancestral gene could have given rise to two related genes, one producing a receptor, or recognition molecule (Thy-1 precursor), and the other producing a triggering molecule (Ig precursor). These two molecules might have been used to communicate information about cellular specificity for various types of cell-to-cell interactions. Through the course of evolution, these components of this primitive communication system might have given rise to the Ab and histocompatibility systems that we recognize today.

PHYLOGENY OF COMPLEMENT

In mammals, two cytolytic systems are associated with serum. These are known as the classical and alternative complement pathways (see chapter 6). Although both

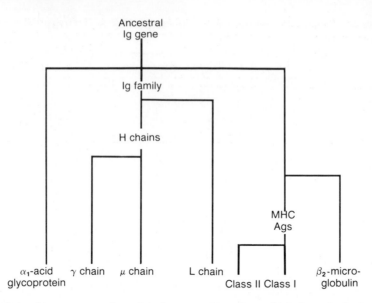

FIGURE 21.7 Phylogenetic relationship among members of the Ig superfamily. Members of the Ig superfamily have arisen from a common ancestral gene. The degree of apparent relatedness among the present-day members of the Ig superfamily are reflected in the positions from which they arise in the phylogenetic tree depicted. More closely related members are divergent branches from a common line. The relative positions of the branches reflect progressions through time.

systems employ the same components to achieve cytolysis, the C5–9 membrane attack complex, this point was arrived at through independent means. The classical pathway is Ab dependent, whereas the alternative pathway is Ab independent and makes use of accelerating cofactors such as properdin.

Most *metazoans possess cytolytic systems* in their hemolymph or serum. However, the nature of these systems is not the same. Using a hemolytic assay, invertebrates and agnathans do not show evidence of the classical complement pathway. However, hemolysis can be induced with the hemolymph or serum from these organisms if cobra venom factor (CoVF) is used. This suggests that components of the complement system associated with the lytic process, or closely related molecules, are present in these animals. In contrast, serum from other vertebrates will spontaneously induce hemolysis in this assay. This is indicative of the presence of the classical complement pathway. An interesting parallel emerges from this relationship: The *classical complement pathway appears to be present in all species in which true Igs exist.* Furthermore, it seems that the late-acting (lytic) components of the complement system emerged first, and only later in evolution did the components peculiar to the classical pathway (C1, C2, and C4) arise.

Although naturally occurring lytic systems appear in essentially all vertebrate species, the properties of these systems are not identical throughout (table 21.7). For example, differences in stability and temperature dependence exist. The cytolytic system of lampreys appears to be relatively stable to heating, while the lytic systems of other vertebrate classes are heat labile. In addition, the lytic systems of poikilotherms usually function most efficiently at 4° to 28° C, whereas the temperature optimum for homoiotherms is 37° C. But more importantly, incompatibilities can be demonstrated between complement components from different systems. Human C1 will not activate guinea pig C4 or C2, nor will guinea pig C1 activate human C4 or C2. In fact, mixing human C1 with guinea pig serum can inactivate C4 and C2. Thus, although analogous lytic systems can be found among vertebrate species, active complement components that are known to be serine esterases (e.g., C1, C4b2b, and C4b2b3b) appear to be highly species spe-

TABLE 21.7 Some Properties of Naturally Occurring Lytic Systems

Organism	Natural Hemolytic Activity	Antibody-Dependent Component	Optimal Temperature	Heat Lability
Invertebrates				
Arthropoda Echinodermata	None	No (Ig absent)	Probably 4° C–15° C	Uncertain
Vertebrates				
Agnatha	Yes	No	4° C	Relatively stable
Chondrichthyes	Yes	Yes	25° C–30° C	Yes
Osteichthyes	Yes	Yes	4° C–28° C	Yes
Amphibia	Yes	Yes	4° C–28° C	Yes
Reptilia	Yes	Yes	15° C–37° C	Yes
Aves	Yes	Yes	37° C	Yes
Mammalia	Yes	Yes	30° C–37° C	Yes

Sources: Gigli, I., and Austen, K. F. Phylogeny and function of the complement system. *Annual Reviews of Microbiology* **25:**309, 1971; Marchalonis, J. J. *Immunity in Evolution.* Harvard University Press, Cambridge, Mass., 1977.

cific with regard to the substrates on which they act. Moreover, this also suggests divergence, rather than conservatism, in the structures of several complement proteins through the course of evolution. It is especially interesting to observe that this apparent divergence applies more to the recently evolved components than to the more ancient components that form the attack complex itself.

PHYLOGENY OF LYMPHOID CELLS AND ORGANS

Invertebrates possess "circulating" defensive cells known as amebocytes, coelomocytes, hemocytes, and so forth. The majority of these display active phagocytic properties, although there is evidence of humoral activity among some coelomocytes and hemocytes. Nevertheless, **invertebrates lack lymphoid tissues.** It is only with the emergence of vertebrates, even the primitive agnathans, that lymphocytes and lymphoid tissues are encountered. Functionally, two major categories of lymphocytes can be anticipated, one associated with humoral immunity and the other with cellular immunity. All vertebrates possess lymphocytes

that display a similar morphology. In higher vertebrates (amphibians to mammals), a morphologically specific cell type, the plasma cell, represents the active Ab-producing cell. This particular cell type has not been identified in agnathans and primitive chondrichthyans, although they have populations of Ab-producing cells.

The distribution of lymphoid organs among vertebrates is more variable (table 21.8). In some instances, the organs are highly organized and numerous, whereas in other cases, they are represented by a few loosely associated clusters of lymphoid cells. Since the most primitive vertebrates possess circulating lymphocytes and rudimentary lymphoid tissues, these two characteristics most likely represent the minimal requirements for elaborating an immune response. In addition, their association with the gills and gut places them in locations where infectious, or foreign, agents are most frequently encountered.

In agnathans, aggregates of lymphoid tissue occur near the gills and in association with an invagination of the anterior gut. These aggregates might represent forerunners of the thymus and spleen, respectively. By the time jawed vertebrates diverged from

TABLE 21.8 Lymphoid Organs of Vertebrate Classes

Class	Thymus	Bursa	Spleen	Other
Agnatha	Diffuse (if present at all)	Absent	Present as diffuse precursor	Uncertain
Chondrichthyes	Present	Absent	Present	Gut-associated lymphoid accumulations; parenchyma of gonads and kidneys
Osteichthyes	Present	Absent	Present	Gut-associated lymphoid tissues; hemopoietic tissue near base of heart; pronephros
Amphibia	Present	Absent	Present	Gut-associated lymphoid accumulations; urodeles only—buccal and perihepatic regions; anurans only—bone marrow, lymph node precursors, kidneys
Reptilia	Present	Absent	Present	Gut-associated lymphoid tissues; kidney, lung, cloaca; lymphatic plexuses
Aves	Present	Present	Present	Gut-associated lymphoid tissues; lymphoid nodules
Mammalia	Present	Bursal equivalent present	Present	Gut-associated lymphoid tissues; lymph nodes

Source: Marchalonis, J. J. *Immunity in Evolution.* Harvard University Press, Cambridge, Mass., 1977.

the ancestral agnathans, approximately 400 million years ago, these ill-defined lymphoid accumulations had given rise to discrete organs, the thymus and spleen. The thymus develops embryologically from the pharyngeal pouches, which also give rise to the gills. Several other lymphoid organs are present. However, only the thymus exists as an exclusively lymphoid organ; since the other lymphoid organs are also hemopoietic tissues. In amphibians, an association between the thymus and cell-mediated immunity (allograft rejection) becomes frankly distinct. In contrast, no strict association emerges between the ability to effect a humoral immune response and any specific lymphoid organ. Nevertheless, in anurans, we can identify a separation into thymus-dependent and thymus-independent Ab responses. This suggests that a divergence of humoral responses along these two pathways occurred approximately 250 million years ago. Furthermore, with the advent of reptiles, the spleen's role in Ab production increases significantly. Two additional changes first appear in the anuran amphibians

and reptiles. These are (1) a displacement of certain hemopoietic activities from several of the secondary lymphoid organs to the bone marrow and (2) the appearance of primitive lymph nodules. However, it should be emphasized that these primitive lymph nodules are blood filters and not secondary lymphoid organs in these animals.

With the emergence of birds, further dissociation of humoral and cell-mediated arms of immunity occurred. A clear dependence upon the thymus for efficient cellular immunity originated with the amphibians. Now, there is an equally apparent association between efficient humoral immunity and the bursa of Fabricius. This uniquely avian organ is located near the cloaca and is necessary for proper B cell development and expression of humoral immunity. Nevertheless, the spleen retains an important position in Ab production, through the germinal centers for expansion of Ab-producing cell populations. However, its ability to execute this role is dependent upon prior action of the bursa. Although the essential features of cellular and humoral immunity first established in birds are also demonstrable in mammals, the site for B cell instruction and initial development remains unknown in this latter group. In the absence of a discrete bursa in mammals, the role played by this organ is now carried out by some other lymphoid organ, perhaps the bone marrow, gut-associated lymphoid tissue, or both. In mammals, the lymphoid nodules have been refined further into lymph nodes, where germinal centers play a more active role in immunity and are sites for Ag processing.

PHYLOGENY OF CELL-MEDIATED IMMUNITY
Cellular Immunity

In mammals, cellular immunity is carried out by T lymphocytes and their derivatives. Graft rejection is the form of immunological response most often called to mind. However, in considering cellular immunity more broadly, one must also consider collaborative cellular interactions, as can be demonstrated in mixed lymphocyte reactions (MLRs).

Graft Rejection

If liberal interpretation of cell-mediated defense is considered, manifestations can be found among all metazoans. However, this defense is not accomplished through the actions of lymphocytes in all cases. In fact, *lymphocytes are characteristically absent among invertebrates.* This function, therefore, is the province of amebocytes, coelomocytes, and hemocytes, depending upon the phylum. Moreover, defense is strongly dependent upon expression of phagocytic activity. This contrasts with the manifestations of cellular immunity in vertebrates, which is accomplished through the activities of T cells (see chapter 9, Effectors of Specific Cellular Immunity), although this might be accompanied by activities of phagocytes.

Refinements in the means of executing cellular immunity that have occurred in the course of evolution have not been restricted to a transfer of the primary role in this process from phagocytes to lymphocytes. The ability of an organism to recognize its own tissue as peculiar to itself and all others as foreign has changed over the ages. One way of visualizing this

progressive change is by surveying the types of grafts that members of the various metazoan phyla will reject or tolerate. At one end of the spectrum, we would expect that recognition would be so precise as to tolerate (accept) only our own tissues and reject all others (except perhaps an identical twin). At the other end, no recognition would occur and all grafts would be tolerated. Among existing metazoans, no case of complete tolerance seems to exist, but considerable variation exists in the extent to which nonself tissues are accepted or rejected.

Among the most primitive metazoans (Porifera, [sponges]) only xenografts are rejected consistently. Grafts of tissues from other members of the same species are often retained indefinitely. The capacity to recognize our own tissues as self and those of other members of the same species as foreign, manifested as allograft rejection, emerges with the Coelenterata. However, acquisition of a more refined sense of personal identity was not achieved as a discrete step. A loose sense of self also exists among members of the Platyhelminthes (flatworms) and Arthropoda, which will reject only xenografts. With the emergence of deuterostomes (echinoderms, protochordates, vertebrates) discrimination of self and related tissues has reached a point where xenografts and allografts are consistently rejected.

Two other features can be identified that display changes as a function of evolutionary progression. These are the nature and rate of allograft rejection and the occurrence of immunological memory. In this regard, rejection of allografts among invertebrates typically occurs slowly (chronic rejection). In addition, although there is evidence of immunological memory, it is short-term, that is, the rate of second-set graft rejection progressively increases as the time between graft challenges is increased. Among the more ancient vertebrate groups (Agnatha up through urodele amphibians), allograft rejection continues to be chronic but immunological memory becomes long-term. In contrast, the more recently evolved vertebrates (anuran amphibians through mammals) reject allografts acutely and possess long-term immunological memory.

Thus, the *phylogeny of graft rejection* is marked by three major advances, which did not occur simultaneously nor linearly over time. These advances were

(1) refinement in discrimination of self from nonself, leading to effective and consistent allograft rejection; (2) acceleration of the rate of allograft rejection from chronic (weeks) to acute (days); and (3) acquisition of long-term immunological memory that is reflected in persistence of more rapid second-set graft rejection.

Collaborative Cellular Interactions

Cooperative interactions among lymphocytes in expressing cell-mediated immune responses can be demonstrated *in vitro* by means of the MLR. Attempts to demonstrate MLR among nonmammalian vertebrates have yielded mixed results. Lymphocytes from vertebrates considered more primitive than anuran amphibians typically fail to produce positive responses in MLRs, while lymphocytes from animals considered more advanced produce positive responses. These responses are probably determined by minor lymphocyte stimulatory (Mls) Ags (see chapter 7). There are three factors that could account for the lack of response among more primitive species: (1) absence of Mls Ags on the lymphocytes used, (2) absence of a receptor for Mls Ags on the lymphocytes used, and (3) presence of suppressor cells. Which one, or combination, of these factors might account for the observed experimental findings has yet to be determined.

Collaboration can also be expressed as assistance, for example, in the cooperative interaction between T and B cells of mice to produce Abs against foreign erythrocytes. Attempts have been made to find evidence for "helper" cells in amphibians, birds, and agnathans (lampreys). In these investigations, hapten-carrier conjugates were used (fig. 21.8). Within this system, the hapten (e.g., DNP) is intended to interact with the Ab-producing cell, B (?) cell, and the carrier (e.g., sheep erythrocyte) will react with the helper cell, T (?) cell. The results of these experiments suggest that helper cell populations exist among amphibians and birds, but not agnathans. It is of particular interest, that helper cells seem to be present in urodele amphibians. Moreover, although agnathans did not appear to have a population of helper cells, their Ab-producing lymphocytes were able to respond to a small hapten.

From these observations, it might be inferred that assignment of particular roles to different subpopulations of T lymphocytes occurred progressively during vertebrate evolution. In addition, it is tempting to speculate that specific T cell subsets first emerged in the amphibians. However, considerable caution must be exercised in considering these possibilities. Moreover, there is only limited evidence presently available about collaborative interactions among lymphocytes in the lower vertebrates. On the other hand, a clear dissociation of lymphocytes into discrete B and T cell populations, as occurs in the chicken and mammals, has yet to be realized in these organisms.

Graft-versus-Host Reaction

In some vertebrates, another manifestation of cellular immunity has been demonstrated. This phenomenon is known as graft-versus-host (GVH) reaction. In contrast to traditional allograft rejection in which the host rejects the graft, in GVH it is the graft that reacts against the host. This phenomenon has not been studied in all vertebrate classes. It is known to occur in amphibians, reptiles, birds, and mammals. Consequently, its phylogenetic distribution is unknown, and possible evolutionary adaptations cannot be fully appreciated.

The Major Histocompatibility Complex

The major histocompatibility complex (MHC) is important in defining individual identity and in expression of cellular immunity (see chapter 7, Histocompatibility Systems). Mammalian MHCs give rise to proteins that are categorized as class I, class II, or class III. Some insight into the presence of similar products in more phylogenetically primitive vertebrates has been derived from comparisons of molecules believed to constitute the Ig superfamily (see above). Other efforts to explore this question are currently in progress using several very powerful techniques: (1) screening monoclonal Abs (MAbs) produced against nonmammalian blood cells, (2) seeking crosshybridization between cloned nonmammalian DNA and mammalian probes, (3) testing for crossreactivity with

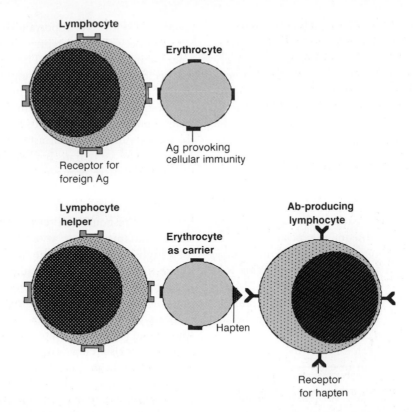

FIGURE 21.8 Model for cooperative cellular interactions in Ab production to hapten challenge. Lymphocytes responsible for cellular immunity (presumably T cells) recognize Ags on the surface of a foreign cell (e.g., an erythrocyte from another species) as nonself. If a hapten, which is too small to effectively provoke Ab production, is attached to one of these erythrocytes, the cell can act as a carrier. Its native Ags continue to present signals that can bind to appropriate lymphocyte receptors. If there is cooperation among cells of cellular and humoral immunity, this complex can be used to present the hapten to Ab-producing cells. Through this cooperation, hapten can effectively stimulate a humoral response. This approach has been used to demonstrate cooperative interactions among lymphocytes in amphibians.

xenoantisera. This last technique seeks crossreactivity, for instance, between Abs against isolated human MHC Ags and the unknown Ags being screened. Crossreactivity between the antiserum being used and the Ags being examined suggests similarities between these latter Ags and the Ag used to produce the antiserum.

Using crossreactivity to xenoantisera as a tool, evidence for class I Ags in axolotls (urodele amphibians) could not be found. This is in direct contrast to an earlier proposal that suggested that animals displaying poor allograft rejection lacked class II molecules. The results obtained with the xenoantisera argue for a reversal of the hypothesis. Thus, it seems that urodele amphibians (and perhaps other vertebrates that reject allografts chronically) possess class II Ags but lack class I Ags.

The sequence similarities among the molecules of the Ig superfamily, which includes the class I and II MHC Ags, provide evidence of their common ancestry. Thus, acquisition of the full spectrum of mammalian MHC Ags might have occurred progressively, paralleling the expansion of the number of elements in the Ig superfamily. According to this idea, an ancestral MHC gene could have duplicated and been modified to produce additional, but different, MHC genes and gene products. Although specific Ags that might represent predecessors of modern mammalian MHC Ags have not yet been identified among invertebrates or lower vertebrates, investigators are actively seeking them. One interesting candidate in these explorations is Thy-1, presumed by some to be a highly conserved descendant of an ancestral gene for the Ig superfamily and, by extension, of members of the MHC.

Memory and Tolerance

Memory

Immunological memory is expressed as a more rapid response to a second or subsequent exposure to a previously encountered foreign "signal." This might take the form of accelerated second-set graft rejection following exposure to appropriate allo-Ags (e.g., MHC Ags in mammals). Alternatively, in a humoral immune response, this would be expressed as more rapid elaboration of Abs to a second exposure to some provoking Ag. There is evidence of both forms of memory among metazoans. The distribution of each type of memory varies, however.

Immunological memory for cellular immunity is represented in essentially all metazoan phyla. Since members of each phylum are able to recognize xenografts, and in some instances allografts as well, responses to subsequent exposures to the same source of tissue can be examined. These studies have revealed that memory is essentially short-term among invertebrates and becomes long-term only among vertebrates. It is also interesting to observe that long-term immunological memory for cellular immunity occurs in animals that are capable of producing true Igs. However, there may not be any causal relationship between these two events.

The question of immunological memory for humoral immunity is somewhat more complex. Invertebrates do not produce Abs that are Igs. As a result, we cannot compare directly the responses in vertebrates and invertebrates. Nevertheless, we can ask if there are parallels in the memory characteristics of humoral factors used by invertebrates that are analogous to Igs. In general, the answer obtained is that there is *no memory for humoral immunity among invertebrates.* A possible explanation for this lack of memory might be

associated with two important distinguishing characteristics between invertebrate humoral agents of immunity and vertebrate Igs. These features are (1) a lack of specificity in the humoral responses and (2) the acute and monophasic nature of the humoral responses in invertebrates. For example, among invertebrates, the same humoral agents seem to be generated in response to a variety of Ags as contrasted with the Ag specificity displayed by vertebrate Igs. In addition, the invertebrate humoral response is initiated rapidly, achieves peak response within one to two days, then declines sharply. In contrast, vertebrates display a slower, more protracted response. Moreover, the response typically features an initial phase associated with the production of a high molecular weight Ab, followed by a second phase in which a low molecular weight Ab appears.

Among *vertebrates, immunological memory for humoral responses* is more universally demonstable. This appears to be related to the ability of vertebrate Ab-producing cells to generate *Abs specific for the provoking Ags.* This is also related to the retention of specific cells dedicated to the production of these particular Abs. The lack of specificity of the humoral response among invertebrates would make preservation of specific responder cells, or their descendants, unnecessary, since any other responder cell could apparently assume the same role. However, the inability to isolate a specific single product from these responder cells following stimulation by a particular Ag prevents absolute determination of the specificity of response by individual cells. That is, without the advantage of some unique product that can be recovered in quantity, like MAbs produced by individual plasma cells (particularly in myeloma), we cannot know for certain whether individual invertebrate responder cells elaborate and use only one or several humoral agents.

Although memory can be demonstrated among vertebrates, it is most definite among the more recently evolved classes. In particular, humoral immunological memory is most apparent in animals that display a biphasic response involving a switch in Ig class. That is, animals that display an initial response to Ag associated with an increase in IgM but followed by production and release of an IgG-like Ig (IgG, IgY, IgN) consistently display evidence of memory upon subsequent exposure to a given Ag. In contrast, members of those classes of vertebrates that display a second phase characterized by the presence of a low molecular weight IgM give weak, or no, evidence of immunological memory. A similar lack of memory seems to occur in amphibians and reptiles following challenge by Ags that do not produce a switch in Ig class. For example, a switch to an IgG-like molecule occurs when serum proteins or bacteriophage Ags are used, but only high molecular weight IgM is produced following exposure to bacterial Ags. Memory can be demonstrated to serum proteins and bacteriophage Ags but not to the bacterial Ags.

Thus, it appears that humoral immunological memory is influenced by, if not dependent on, two evolutionary acquisitions. The first is production of a humoral agent that is specific for a provoking foreign agent. This occurs with the emergence of vertebrates. The second is the ability to produce multiple classes of Igs and effect a transition to the more recently evolved class of Ig during the immune response. This acquisition occurs in anuran amphibians but seems lacking in urodele amphibians.

Tolerance

Tolerance can be viewed as a form of negative memory. As the result of previous exposure to some foreign signal, the host's immune system displays a reduced tendency to react upon subsequent exposure; in other words, the foreign signal is tolerated within what should be a hostile environment. This question has not been extensively explored among phylogenetically older vertebrates. It has not been explored among invertebrates, in which failure to reject a graft is principally an expression of an inability to recognize the graft as foreign.

Among amphibians, reptiles, and birds, it has been shown that prior exposure to foreign Ags can lead to a failure to mount a humoral response upon subsequent exposure to that same Ag. For example, the marine toad, *Bufo marinus,* can readily clear bovine serum albumin (BSA). However, by progressively increasing the dose of BSA used as a challenge, the rate of removal of BSA decreases. In fact, administration of

a large initial dose of BSA (250 mg) fails to induce Ab production. These toads are now tolerant to BSA. These animals will display a normal response to challenge with human IgG. Similar induction of tolerance can be demonstrated using human serum albumin (HSA) in chickens. However, in this case, an additional feature can be demonstrated. When suboptimal concentrations of HSA are used, tolerance results also. If, on the other hand, increasing concentrations of HSA are used within the optimal range, varying degrees of responsiveness are noted. At lower doses, there is a delayed onset in the appearance of Ab-producing cells. This is considered to represent the existence of populations of stimulated, but suppressed, cells or of unimpressed cells in the animals rendered tolerant.

In addition to tolerance in humoral immunity, animals of these same classes display tolerance in cellular immunity. Frogs can be made tolerant to tissues from a nonrelated frog during embryonic development. If tissues from one embryo (the donor) are transplanted to another embryo (the host), expressed surface Ags of the donor will become accepted when the host's immune system attains maturity. Thereafter, tissues from the donor can be presented to the host and the grafts will be tolerated. However, if similar transplants are performed in older embryos or tadpoles (when immunological competence is being acquired), it might be necessary to transplant a large quantity of donor tissue to the host in order to achieve tolerance. In these instances, small grafts might be recognized as foreign and be rejected, whereas the larger transplants might be capable of overwhelming the host's limited (immature) immune response. In cattle, tolerance can be induced in a somewhat similar manner when there is mixing of blood between two siblings *in utero.* In these instances, fetal calves that are not identical twins might become exposed to the Ags of their littermate if both share a common placenta. This allows blood from each of the developing calves to be exchanged. As development proceeds, and the immune systems mature, the Ags expressed on the exchanged cells come to be recognized as self and tolerance is established.

From these observations two notions emerge to account for the acquisition of tolerance. One interpretation suggests that tolerance is established because of a reduction in the availability of reactive lymphocytes. According to this notion, if the numbers of reactive lymphocytes are limited or depleted a state of tolerance will be achieved. Restoration of these reactive lymphocytes will break tolerance. Evidence supporting this hypothesis can be found in experiments using amphibians. Here, there is a mixture of blood cells in parabiosed frogs (these are frogs that were joined as embryos and have developed into conjoined, or Siamese, twins). The ratio of host-to-donor cells varies with age. Early in development, the ratio is close to 1; however, with further development, the number of donor cells decreases. Eventually, a point is reached at which sufficient host stem cells are produced that some now recognize the donor tissues as foreign. When this occurs, tolerance is broken and the graft is rejected. The second interpretation for tolerance relies upon the activity of suppressor cells. In this model, Ag stimulates certain cells that, when activated, prevent Ab formation against that Ag. Although there is evidence to support this mechanism in mammals, no experimental support for this mechanism has been generated in lower vertebrates. Tolerance, or at least the manner in which it is expressed, might reflect refinements and increased sophistication in the expression of immune responses among metazoan organisms, and vertebrates in particular.

S U M M A R Y

1. Comparative immunobiology explores the relationships in immune strategies among different groups of organisms. [p. 538]
2. The ability to discriminate between "self" and "nonself" exists even among protozoans, where it appears to be more enzymatic than immunological. [p. 538]
3. The Porifera and Coelenterata have populations of wandering defensive cells called amebocytes, but lack coherent immunological tissues. [p. 539]
4. Protostomes display evidence of both cellular and humoral immunity. Cellular immunity is slow and chiefly effective against xenografts, while humoral immunity is accomplished by lysins and agglutinins rather than by antibodies.

The first appearance of a closed circulatory system and of discrete hemopoietic organs occur among the protostomes. [pp. 539–543]

5. Deuterostomal invertebrates (a) display more effective cell-mediated immunity, rejecting allografts, and (b) have greater organization of hemopoietic centers. [p. 543]
6. Vertebrates have well-organized lymphoid tissues and display more advanced humoral and cellular immune responses. [pp. 544–545]
7. Humoral immunity among invertebrates is accomplished by lysins and agglutinins that are distinct from immunoglobulins, although some possess electrophoretic mobility similar to β- and γ-globulins. [p. 545]
8. Immunoglobulins, as agents of humoral immunity, first appear with the vertebrates. IgM is the most universally displayed immunoglobulin. Among fish and urodele amphibians, it can be expressed as both high and low molecular weight antibodies. IgG-like antibodies appear in anuran amphibians, while other classes of immunoglobulins (IgA, IgD, IgE) do not emerge until the advent of mammals. [p. 547]
9. All immunoglobulin classes are phylogenetically related. They appear to have arisen from a common ancestral gene through gene duplication and diversification. Numerous other molecules associated with immune function have strikingly comparable amino acid compositions or sequence similarities to the immunoglobulins. These molecules are believed to have also arisen from the same ancestral gene. Collectively these molecules comprise the immunoglobulin superfamily. [pp. 547–551]
10. Cytolytic systems exist in most metazoans, many with marked similarities to the mammalian complement system. Parallels to the alternative pathway are the most universal in these cases, suggesting that the lytic components (C5–C9) came first and the initial elements of the classical pathway (C1, C4, C2) appeared most recently during evolution. [pp. 551–553]

11. Lymphocytes do not occur in invertebrates, but are present in all vertebrates. Plasma cells, as morphologically distinct antibody-producing cells, exist in classes that have appeared since the time of the amphibians. [p. 553]

12. Beyond the agnathans, the thymus and spleen occur as discrete lymphoid organs. With progressive evolution, hemopoietic activities are shifted away from the spleen as they are assumed by other organs (e.g., bone marrow). In addition, other specialized secondary lymphoid tissues arise. [pp. 553–555]

13. The phylogeny of graft rejection mechanisms is marked by three significant features: (a) refinement in discrimination of self, (b) transition from chronic to acute rejection, and (c) acquisition of long-term memory. [pp. 555–556]

14. Cellular cooperation in the expression of immune responses occurs in amphibians and more phylogenetically recent vertebrates. This suggests a division of labor among lymphocytes in assigning specific roles during immune responses, both cellular and humoral immune responses. [p. 556]

15. Graft-versus-host reactions have been demonstrated in amphibians, reptiles, birds, and mammals, but its phylogenetic distribution is unknown since it has not been systematically sought in all vertebrate classes. [p. 556]

16. Histocompatibility systems have been documented in higher vertebrates. Evidence for similar systems has been provided for lower vertebrates and suggested for invertebrates. Studies of vertebrates suggest that class II antigens antedate class I antigens. Other evidence suggests that all histocompatibility systems might be related and descendant from an ancestral gene shared with the immunoglobulin superfamily. [pp. 556–558]

17. Immunological memory is associated with both cellular and humoral immunity at most phylogenetic levels. The quality of memory improves with progression up the phylogenetic ladder. [pp. 558–559]

18. Tolerance can be induced in amphibians, reptiles, birds, and mammals. Expressions of tolerance in humoral and cell-mediated immune responses show variations that parallel immunological refinement. [pp. 559–560]

READINGS

Bayne, C. J. Phagocytosis and non-self recognition in invertebrates. *BioScience* **40:**723, 1990.

Cohen, W. D. (ed.). *Blood Cells of Marine Invertebrates* (*MBL Lectures in Biology,* Vol. 6). Alan R. Liss, Inc., New York, 1985.

Cooper, E. L. Immune diversity throughout the animal kingdom. *BioScience* **40:**720, 1990.

Dieterlen-Lievre, F. Development of the compartments of the immune system in the avian embryo. *Developmental and Comparative Immunology* **13:**303, 1989.

Dunn, P. E. Humoral immunity in insects. *BioScience* **40:**738, 1990.

El Deeb, S. O., and Saad, A. H. M. Ontogenic maturation of the immune system in reptiles. *Developmental and Comparative Immunology* **14:**151, 1990.

Evans, D. L., and Cooper, E. L. Natural killer cells in ectothermic vertebrates. *BioScience* **40:**745, 1990.

Flajnik, M. F., and DuPasquier, L. The major histocompatibility complex of frogs. *Immunological Reviews* **113:**47, 1990.

Hadji-Azimi, I., Coosemans, V., and Canicatti, C. et al. Atlas of adult *Xenopus laevis laevis* hematology. *Developmental and Comparative Immunology* **11:**807, 1987.

Karp, R. D. Cell-mediated immunity in invertebrates. *BioScience* **40:**732, 1990.

Kaufman, J., Skjoedt, K., and Salomonson, J. The MHC molecules of nonmammalian vertebrates. *Immunological Reviews* **113:**83, 1990.

Klein, J., and Figueroa, F. The evolution of class I MHC genes. *Immunology Today* **7:**41, 1986.

Kokubu, F., Hinds, K., Litman, R., et al. Extensive families of constant region genes in a phylogenetically primitive vertebrate indicate an additional level of immunoglobulin complexity. *Proceedings of the National Academy of Sciences* (USA) **84:**5868, 1987.

Koppenheffer, T. L. Serum complement systems in ecothermic vertebrates. *Developmental and Comparative Immunology* **11:**279, 1988.

Kroemer, G., Bernot, A., Béhar, G., et al. Molecular genetics of the chicken MHC: current status and evolutionary aspects. *Immunological Reviews* **113:**119, 1990.

Lin, L.-C., and Putman, F. W. Primary structure of the Fc region of human immunoglobulin D: implications for evolutionary origin and biological function. *Proceedings of the National Academy of Sciences* (USA) **78:**504, 1981.

Litman, G. W., Amemiya, C. T., Haire, R. N., et al. Antibody and immunoglobulin diversity. *BioScience* **40:**751, 1990.

Manning, M. J., and Turner, R. J. *Comparative Immunobiology.* Halsted Press (John Wiley & Sons, Inc.), New York, 1976.

Mansour, M. H., Negm, H. I., and Cooper, E. I. Thy-1 evolution. *Developmental and Comparative Immunology* **11:**3, 1987.

Marchalonis, J. J. *Immunity in Evolution.* Harvard University Press, Cambridge, Mass., 1977.

Marchalonis, J. J., and Schluter, S. F. Origins of immunoglobulins and immune recognition molecules. *BioScience* **40:**758, 1990.

McCormack, W. T., Tjoelker, L. W., and Thompson, C. B. Avian B-cell development: generation of an immunoglobulin repertoire by gene conversion. *Annual Review of Immunology* **9:**219, 1991.

Sminia, T., and van der Knaap, W. P. W. Cells and molecules in molluscan immunology. *Developmental and Comparative Immunology* **11:**17, 1987.

Sun, S.-C., Lindström, I., Boman, H. G., et al. Hemolin: an insect-immune protein belonging to the immunoglobulin superfamily. *Science* **250:**1729, 1990.

Suzuki, T., and Mori, K. Hemolytic lectin of the pearl oyster *Pinetacla fucata martensii:* a possible non-self recognition system. *Developmental and Comparative Immunology* **14:**161, 1990.

Abbreviations and Acronyms

Å   angstrom unit

Ab   antibody

AC   adenylate cyclase

ACAID   anterior chamber–associated immune deficiency

ACh   acetylcholine

AChR   acetylcholine receptor

ACTH   adrenocorticotropic hormone

ADA   adenosine deaminase

ADCC   antibody-dependent cellular cytotoxicity

AFP   alpha-fetoprotein

Ag   antigen

AIDS   acquired immune deficiency syndrome

ALL   acute lymphocytic leukemia

ALS   antilymphocyte serum

APC   antigen-presenting cell

ARC   AIDS-related complex

A-T   ataxia telangiectasia

ATP   adenosine triphosphate

AZT   azidodeoxythymidine

Baso   basophil

BCDF   B cell differentiation factor

BCG   bacille Calmette-Guérin

BCGF   B cell growth factor

BFU-E   burst-forming unit–erythroid

BSA   bovine serum albumin

C   constant (domain or region)

C1–C9   complement component

CAM   cell adhesion molecule

cAMP   cyclic adenosine monophosphate

CD   cluster designation

CDC   Centers for Disease Control

cDNA   complementary DNA

CDR   complementarity-determining region

CEA   carcinoembryonic antigen

CFU-C   colony-forming unit–culture

CFU-E   colony-forming unit–erythroid

CFU-LM   colony-forming unit–lymphoid-myeloid

CFU-S   colony-forming unit–spleen

CFU-T   colony-forming unit–thromboid

CG   chorionic gonadotropin

cGMP   cyclic guanosine monophosphate

CH$_{-50}$ hemolytic unit of complement

CID   combined immunodeficiency disease

CLL   chronic lymphocytic leukemia

CMV   cytomegalovirus

CNS   central nervous system

Con A   concanavalin A

CoVF   cobra venom factor

CR   complement receptor

CRF   corticotropin-release factor

CRP   C-reactive protein

Cs   cyclosporine

CSF   colony-stimulating factor

CTF   chemotactic factor

Cy   cyclophosphamide

DAF   decay-accelerating factor

DAG   diacylglycerol

ddC   dideoxycytosine

ddI   dideoxyinosine

dL   deciliter

DNP   dinitrophenyl

DTH   delayed-type hypersensitivity

EAE experimental autoimmune encephalitis

EBV Epstein-Barr virus

ECF-A eosinophilic chemotactic factor of anaphylaxis

EGF epidermal growth factor

ELISA enzyme-linked immunosorbent assay

ELISpot enzyme-linked immunospot

EP endogenous pyrogen

F$_1$ first filial generation

Fab antigen-binding fraction

FACS fluorescence-activated cell sorter

FAF fibroblast-activating factor

Fc crystallizable fraction

FcE Fc domain of IgE

FcR Fc receptor

FGF fibroblast growth factor

FITC fluorescein isothiocyanate

FR framework residue

FSH follicle-stimulating hormone

G-6-PD glucose-6-phosphate dehydrogenase

GAF glucocorticoid-antagonizing factor

GALT gut-associated lymphoid tissue

GEF glycosylation-enhancing factor

GI gastrointestinal

GIF glycosylation-inhibiting factor

GM-CSF granulocyte-monocyte–colony–stimulating factor

GnRH gonadotropin-releasing hormone

gp glycoprotein

GTP guanosine triphosphate

GVH graft-versus-host

H heavy (chain)

H-2 murine histocompatibility complex

HAT hypoxanthine-aminopterin-thymidine

HbS hemoglobin S

HCG human chorionic gonadotropin

HEV high endothelial venule

HIM hemopoietic-inducing microenvironment

HIV human immunodeficiency virus

HLA human leukocyte associated

HPRT hypoxanthine phosphoribosyl transferase

HSA human serum albumin

HSP heat shock protein

HTLV human T lymphotropic virus

Ia mouse immune response gene antigen

ICAM intercellular adhesion molecule

ICSH interstitial cell-stimulating hormone

Id idiotope

IDDM insulin-dependent diabetes mellitus

IF immunofluorescence

IFN interferon

Ig immunoglobulin

IGF-I insulinlike growth factor-I

IL interleukin

IL-2R interleukin 2 receptor

Ir immune response (gene)

ITP inositol triphosphate

J joining (segment)

K$_a$ association constant

kD kilodalton

K$_d$ dissociation constant

L light (chain); also liter

LAK lymphokine-activated killer (cell)

LAV lymphadenopathy virus

LD lymphocyte defined

LE lupus erythematosus

Leu-CAM leukocyte CAM

LFA leukocyte function antigen

LGL large granular lymphocyte

LH leuteinizing hormone

LIF leukocyte-inhibiting factor

LMEF lymphocyte migration-enhancing factor

LMIF lymphocyte migration-inhibiting factor

LPS lipopolysaccharide

LTs leukotrienes

LTX lymphotoxin

M molar

MAb monoclonal antibody

MAC membrane attack complex

MAF macrophage-activating factor

mg milligram

mH minor histocompatibility (Ag)

MHC major histocompatibility complex

MIF migration-inhibiting factor

mIg membrane-bound or surface immunoglobulin

mL milliliter

MLC mixed lymphocyte culture

MLR mixed lymphocyte response

Mls minor lymphocyte stimulatory (gene)

mRNA messenger RNA

MS multiple sclerosis

MSF macrophage-stimulating factor

MSH melanocyte-stimulating hormone

MTD maximum tolerated dose

MW molecular weight

Mϕ macrophage

μg   microgram

μL   microliter

μm   micrometer

μM   micromolar

N   null (cell); also normal

NAD   nicotinamide adenine dinucleotide

NADP   nicotinamide adenine dinucleotide phosphate

NADPH   reduced NADP

NC   natural cytotoxic (cell)

NCF-A   neutrophil chemotactic factor of anaphylaxis

NGF   nerve growth factor

NK   natural killer (cell)

nm   nanometer

nM   nanomolar

NOD   nonobese diabetic

5NT   5′-nucleotidase

NZB   New Zealand black

NZW   New Zealand white

PAF   platelet-activating factor

PCA   passive cutaneous anaphylaxis

PCB   polychlorinated biphenyl

PCR   polymerase chain reaction

PDE   phosphodiesterase

PDGF   platelet-derived growth factor

PEG   polyethylene glycol

PG   prostaglandin

PHA   phytohemagglutinin

PK   protein kinase

P-K test   Prausnitz-Küstner test

pM   picomolar

PMN   polymorphonuclear neutrophil

PNI   psychoneuroimmunology

PNP   purine nucleoside phosphorylase

RA   rheumatoid arthritis

RAST   radioallergosorbent test

RB   retinoblastoma

RES   reticuloendothelial system

RF   rheumatoid factor

RIA   radioimmunoassay

RIST   radioimmunosorbent test

RLS   relative light scatter

S   Svedberg unit; also switch (sequence)

SAA   serum amyloid A

SAAI   serum amyloid A inducer

scid   severe combined immune deficient

SD   serologically defined

SIF   soluble inhibitory factor

sIgA   secretory immunoglobulin A

SIV   simian immunodeficiency virus

SLE   systemic lupus erythematosus

Slp   sex-linked protein

spp   species

SRBC   sheep red blood cells

SRS-A   slow-reacting substance of anaphylaxis

STLV-III   simian T lymphotropic virus, type III

S_w sedimentation coefficient

TAA   tumor-associated antigen

TAF   tumor angiogenesis factor

TAM   tumor-associated macrophage

T_C cytotoxic T (cell)

TCR   T cell receptor

T_D sensitized T (cell)

TdT   terminal deoxynucleotidyl transferase

T_{DTH} delayed-type hypersensitivity T (cell); another name for T_D cell

TGF   transforming growth factor

T_H helper T (cell)

$T_{H/I}$ T helper/inducer (cell)

TNF   tumor necrosis factor

TRF   T cell replacement factor

T_S suppressor T (cell)

TSH   thyroid-stimulating hormone

TSTA   tumor-specific transplantation antigen

V   variable (region or domain)

VLP   viruslike particle

xid   x-linked immune deficiency

XLR   x-linked lymphocyte regulatory (gene)

B Milestones in the History of Immunology

ontributions in several fields of the biomedical sciences (e.g., cell biology, medicine, microbiology, and pathology) that have been valuable to the advancement of our understanding of the immune system are identified. This list of contributors and their contributions is selective, not exhaustive. Other contributions can be identified that would be candidates for this list, but which we elected not to include. More importantly, this table lists those investigators that have played prominent roles in making these advances. As a result, other scientists who have participated in making these contributions are not identified.

Individuals awarded the Nobel Prize for their contributions to immunology are denoted in boldface type, with the year of the award indicated below.

Advances in the understanding of immunology that led to the award of a Nobel Prize are designated by *.

Dates	Investigator(s) or Contributor(s)	Contribution(s)
3000 B.C.–A.D. 200	Middle Eastern and Far Eastern cultures; Greek and Roman civilizations	Possessed awareness of transmission of infective diseases and acquired immunity; attempted induction of immunity by inoculation with virulent agents
9th/10th centuries	Rhazes	Advanced first recorded theory of acquired immunity
1546	Girolamo Fracastoro	Made first proposal of the transmission of "contagion" by infective agents; recognized different modes of infective transfer
1656	Athanasius Kircher	Was first to use microscope to study disease; reported association of "small worms" in plague victims
1798	Edward Jenner	Introduced vaccination with related, nonvirulent organism as means of inducing active immunity
1840s	M. J. Schleiden and Theodor Schwann	Formulated cell theory

Dates	Investigator(s) or Contributor(s)	Contribution(s)
1850s	Rudolf Virchow	Proposed continuity among cells; introduced cellular pathology
1860–1870s	Julius Cohnheim	Described cellular events of acute inflammation
1880–1890s	**Robert Koch** (1905)	Perfected methods for culturing pure strains of bacteria; proposed four criteria for identifying causative agents of infectious disease; discovered delayed (Type IV) hypersensitivity to tuberculin*
	Elie Metchnikoff (1908)	Defined role of phagocytes in immunity; developed first theory of cellular immunity*
	Louis Pasteur	Developed and applied attenuated vaccines for inducing active immunity
1888	Emile Roux and A. Yersin	Demonstrated that immunity to bacterial toxins (diphtheria toxin) was achieved by specific neutralizing substances, or antitoxins, in serum
1890s	**Emil von Behring** (1901) S. Kitasato	Discovered antibodies; developed antitoxins to diphtheria*
	Paul Ehrlich (1908)	Introduced methods for toxin and antitoxin standardization; proposed first selective theory of antibody formation*
	David Bruce and Ronald Ross	Demonstrated protozoa as causes of infectious diseases
	Max von Gruber, Herbert Durham, and Rudolf Kraus	Characterized agglutination and antibody-antigen precipitin reactions that made *in vitro* study of antibodies possible
1895–1910	J. Denys and J. Léclef; S. R. Douglas and Almroth Wright	Identified opsonization property of immune serum
	G. H. F. Nuttall	Exploited crossreactivity of antisera and demonstrated its usefulness as tool for diagnosis and exploration of taxonomic relationships
1900–1910	**Jules Bordet** (1919) R. Pfeiffer	Discovered roles of complement and antibody in cytolysis*; developed complement fixation test
	Charles Richet (1913)	Discovered and characterized nature of anaphylaxis*
	Theobald Smith	Discovered bacterial antigens; characterized role of maternal antibodies in passive immunization of newborn infants
	Maurice Arthus	Demonstrated local anaphylaxis
1900–1930	**Karl Landsteiner** (1930)	Described ABO blood groups; solidified chemical basis for antibody-antigen reactions*
1920s	Karl Prausnitz and Heinz Küstner	Identified reverse passive anaphylaxis; paved way for studies into mechanisms of anaphylaxis
	Clemens von Pirquet and Bela Schick	Described serum sickness

Dates	Investigator(s) or Contributor(s)	Contribution(s)
1930–1935	Michael Heidelberger	Advanced quantitive methodology for antibody determination; demonstrated that properties of antiserum are due to specific proteins
1940s	Albert H. Coons	Introduced use of fluorescently labeled antibodies for antigen localization
	Jules T. Freund	Developed means (adjuvants) of enhancing antibody response
	Karl Landsteiner and Merrill Chase	Demonstrated that delayed (Type IV) hypersensitivity could be transferred by using intact sensitized cells rather than circulating antibodies
	P. Levine and C. Stetson	Discovered that principal cause of erythroblastosis fetalis (hemolytic disease of the newborn) is Rh antibodies
	Orjan Ouchterlony	Introduced double diffusion method for evaluating similarities among antigens or antibodies
1945–1950	C. Hufnagel, D. Hume, E. Landsteiner, et al.	Refined methods for transplantation of cadaveric organs
1945–1955	Peter B. Medawar (1960)	Proved immunological basis for mammalian allograft rejection; contributed to elucidation of induced immunological tolerance*
1945–1980	George Snell (1980)	Characterized genetics of histoincompatibility reactions*
1950s	Jean Dausset (1980)	Described analogies between mouse and human histocompatibility systems*
	Pierre Grabar	Introduced immunoelectrophoresis
1950–1960s	C. Barnard, J. Hamburger, M. A. Hardy, R. Lillehei	Perfected techniques for successful transplantation of live organs*
	J. Murray (1990)	Performed first successful transplant of a living donor kidney to a host*
	E. D. Thomas (1990)	Pioneered procedures for chemical management of graft-versus-host disease in tissue organ transplantation*
	W. Dameshek and R. Schwartz	Discovered immunosuppressant property of 6-mercaptopurine
1950–1970s	G.B. Elion and G. H. Hitchins (1988)	Developed and exploited synthetic purine and pyrimidine antimetabolites*
	J. Borel	Discovered cyclosporin
1950–1980	Neils Jerne (1984)	Put forth biological selection theory of antibody formation similar to Ehrlich's but which also accounted for immunological tolerance; developed hemolytic plaque assay and demonstrated that individual antibody-producing cells made a single class of antibody; discovered idiotypes and characterized their role in immune regulation
	N. Kaliss and others	Showed regulation of immunological response by antibody produced against immunogen; categorized responses yielding immunoenhancement and specific immune suppression

Dates	Investigator(s) or Contributor(s)	Contribution(s)
1959	F. Macfarlane Burnet (1960)	Postulated clonal selection theory of antibody formation*
1960s	Gerald M. Edelman and Rodney R. Porter (1972)	Determined chemical structure of immunoglobulins*
	Rosalyn Yalow (1977)	Developed and refined radioimmunoassay*
1960–1970s	Baruj Benacerraf (1980) H. McDevitt	Identified immune response genes*
1969–1971	G. L. Ada, P. Byrt, M. C. Raff, M. Sternberg, and R. B. Taylor	Demonstrated that B cell receptor is immunoglobulin
1960–1980s	N. Cohen, E. Cooper, L. DuPasquier, W. Hildemann, J. Marchalonis, and others	Established field of comparative immunology
	E. Boyse, H. Cantor, R. Gershon, and others	Characterized T cell subtypes and their roles in cellular immunity
	H. Claman, M. Davis, J. F. A. P. Miller, G. F. Mitchell, and others	Described and characterized T and B cell cooperation in executing immune responses
1974	R. M. Zinkernagel and P. C. Doherty	Described phenomenon of MHC restriction in immune responses
1970–1980s	C. Milstein and G. Köhler (1984)	Developed hybridoma technology for production of monoclonal antibodies*
	S. Tonegawa (1987) L. Hood, E. Kabat, P. Leder, and others	Elucidated nature of antibody diversity in terms of recombination of C, V, and J genes*
	K. Haskins, J. Kappler, P. Marrack, and others	Characterized nature of T cell receptor
	J. M. Bishop and H. Varmus (1989)	Identified first cellular oncogenes and initiated studies characterizing their role in cellular function*

Sources

Bulloch, W. *The History of Bacteriology.* Dover Publications, Inc., New York, 1979.

Brock, T. (ed.). *Milestones in Microbiology.* Prentice-Hall, Inc., Englewood Cliffs, New Jersey, 1961.

Clark, W. R. *The Experimental Foundations of Modern Immunology.* John Wiley & Sons, Inc., New York, 1986.

Clendening, L. (ed.). *Source Book of Medical History.* Dover Publications, Inc., New York, 1960.

Gardner, E. J. *History of Biology.* Burgess Publishing Co., Minneapolis, 1972.

Hildeman, W. H. *Essentials of Immunology.* Elsevier Publishing Co., New York, 1984.

Lechevalier, H. A., and Solotorovsky, M. *Three Centuries of Microbiology.* Dover Publications, Inc., New York, 1974.

Long, E. R. *A History of Pathology.* Dover Publications, Inc., New York, 1965.

Paul, W. E. *Fundamental Immunology.* Raven Press, New York, 1984.

Characterization of Immune Status and Function

The immune system provides defense against insult, or invasion, by foreign agents. These insults can come in a variety of forms—infective microorganisms, parasites, microbial toxins, pollens, or other allergens. In addition, the immune system maintains active surveillance within the organism to ensure individual integrity, that is, preserving the identity of "self" intact. This is manifest in immunological defense against oncogenesis (tumor formation) and grafts of foreign tissues. In fulfilling these roles, the immune system is in constant flux, alternating between relative quiescence and active response (fig. A.1). For example, immunological defenses are set in motion in response to instigating signals but then abate once the source of the signal has been removed.

Therefore, the levels of activity of the components of the immune system vary over time (fig. A.2). Moreover, with the occurrence of various disease states, activities of the immune system, and its several subdivisions, display change. In most instances, we expect this change to appear as *increased* immunological activity, either humoral or cellular. However, circumstances might arise that lead to *reduced* expression of immunological activity. These changes can be viewed as shifts in the position of a balance—tipping in one direction when activities are reduced and in the opposite direction when they are increased.

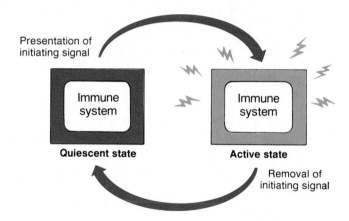

FIGURE A.1 Immune system activity.

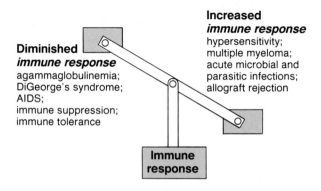

FIGURE A.2 Changes in immune response.

TABLE A.1 Alterations Affecting Expression of Humoral Immunity*

Diminished Activity	Increased Activity
Agammaglobulinemia: severely reduced γ-globulin levels *Bruton-type:* no circulating lymphocytes bearing surface Igs *Non-Bruton:* circulating B lymphocytes, but failure to differentiate into plasma cells and produce Igs	**Multiple myeloma:** unregulated production of single immunoglobulin class by affected cells; characterized by increased numbers of antibody-producing B cells (plasma cells)
Selective Ig deficiencies: production of single class of Ig does not occur—the class affected is usually IgG or IgA; may be accompanied by increased IgM	**Hypersensitivity** (Types I–III): increased levels of IgE in response to many allergens (Type I, e.g., allergies, anaphylaxis); increased IgG production binding to cells, eliciting cytolysis (Type II, e.g., transfusion reactions); increased IgG production with formation of immune complexes and inflammatory sequelae (Type III, e.g., serum sickness)
Tolerance: absence of B cell response due to absence of responsive clone (?) or inadequate signal input to induce B cell differentiation	**Autoimmunity:** Ig production against "self" Ags (e.g., experimental autoimmune thyroiditis)
Immune suppression: blocked expression of humoral immunity (e.g., through arrest of B cell proliferation by cyclophosphamide; or increased activity of T_S cells)	

*Sampling of states characterized by unresponsive or underresponsive B cell activity, on the one hand, and overresponsive B cell activity on the other hand. This does not represent a comprehensive listing of all possibilities of exaggerated or diminished B cell activity or expression.

Through the several chapters of this book, the composition, function, and integration of the immune system have been explored. We have described the nature and function of these elements in general terms (unit 1) and in more operational contexts (units 2 and 3). The various facets of immunological response have been characterized, and numerous means for evaluating these parameters have been defined and described. This appendix provides a summary of much of this information. We endeavor to provide, at a glance, an index of how humoral and cellular immunity are altered when immunological response (and responsiveness) are reduced or stimulated. This provides an indication of which participants in immunological reactions are more abundant or more active during states of heightened immunological activity and, alternatively, which are less abundant or less active during states of diminished activity (tables A.1 and A.2). In addition, methods (clinical and experimental) for visualizing and quantifying these changes are identified (table A.3). Details of these procedures are not presented. Rather, individuals who are interested in learning more about the performance of these tests, as well as the principles behind them and the interpretation of the results obtained, are referred to the brief descriptions provided within this text (see index for locations) or to books that are specifically dedicated to that objective (a few representative examples are provided at the end of this section).

TABLE A.2 Alterations Affecting Expression of Cellular Immunity*

Diminished Activity	Increased Activity
Thymic aplasia (DiGeorge syndrome): thymus fails to form, T cells absent	
Thymic hypoplasia/dysgenesis: (Nezelof's syndrome) abnormal thymus; greatly reduced T cell number; also abnormal Ig production	
Defective phagocytosis/killing: diminished response from NK, T_C cells, macrophages, or neutrophils (e.g., Chédiak-Higashi syndrome)	**Hypersensitivity** (Type IV): Ag-induced stimulation of T_C or T_D cell proliferation (e.g., poison ivy)
Acquired immune deficiency syndrome: destruction of T_H (CD4) cells	
Tolerance: absence of cellular immunity associated with failure to activate T_H cells	**Autoimmunity:** Ig produced against "self" Ags because of T_H stimulation (e.g., experimental allergic encephalitis)
Immune suppression: inhibition of cellular immunity (e.g., cyclosporine, inhibition of T cell proliferation, cytotoxicity, and lymphokine production)	

*Sampling of states characterized by unresponsive or underresponsive T cell activity, on the one hand, and overresponsive T cell activity on the other hand. Also included are alterations affecting other participants of cellular immunity (e.g., NK cells, null cells, and phagocytes). This does not represent a comprehensive listing of all possibilities of exaggerated, or diminished, cell-mediated activity or expression.

TABLE A.3 Evaluating the Status and Expression of Cellular and Humoral Immunity

Parameter	Immune Status Evaluated	Methods/Assays*
Lymphoid organs		
Morphology and cytology	Resting vs. active state of immune reactivity; immune competence	Immunohistochemistry, immunocytochemistry (e.g., immunoperoxidase)
Population sizes		
B cell	Competence for or level of humoral immunity	Assay B cell-specific surface markers; fluorescence-activated cell sorting; hemolytic plaque assay; mitogenic response to LPS, anti-IgA sera
T cell (general)	Competence for or level of cellular immunity	Assay T cell–specific surface markers; fluorescence-activated cell sorting; rosette formation with sheep erythrocytes; mitogenic response to Con A, PHA; level of IL-2 receptors in plasma or serum; lymphokine production
T cell subsets	T cell differentiation; quality of cellular immune response	Assay for differentiation Ags (e.g., CD4, CD8)

TABLE A.3 (cont.)

Parameter	Immune Status Evaluated	Methods/Assays*
Effective responses		
Antibody production	Level of humoral response	Serum electrophoresis; complement fixation; precipitin reactions; agglutination reactions; laser nephelometry
	Quality of humoral response Nature of Ab	Double diffusion assay (Ouchterlony gels)
	Thymus dependent vs. thymus independent	Evaluate Ig production with dependent and independent Ags
Complement activity	Classical pathway	Ab-dependent cytolysis
	Alternative (properdin) pathway	Ab-independent cytolysis (e.g., activated by CoVF)
Cellular immunity	Integrity of cell-mediated immunity	Allograft rejection; delayed hypersensitivity skin test (clinical); lymphocyte transfer; MLA
Lymphocyte subsets	Activated T_C cells	IL-2–stimulated proliferation and cytotoxicity
	T_H and T_D cells	Potentiation or augmentation of responses in MLA
	T_S cells	Reduction or suppression of responses in MLA
	N cells and NK cells	IL-2–independent, or spontaneous, cytotoxicity
Accessory cells		
Mononuclear phagocytes	Numbers available	Isolation by adherence to substrate or on Ficoll (or similar) gradient; fluorescence-activated cell sorting (cells recoverable from blood, bone marrow, peritoneal exudate, lung, or tumors)
	Activation or stimulation	Numbers of macrophages following challenge; assay IL-1, IFN, or TNF production using suitable responder cells
	Chemotactic responsiveness	Migration across filter of Boyden chamber in response to attractant
	Phagocytic responsiveness	Ingestion of radio-iron, latex particles, or microorganisms; NBT assay
	Cytotoxicity	Assay of nonspecific (NK) cytolysis using tumor cell lines; ADCC reaction
Neutrophils	Chemotactic responsiveness	Migration in Boyden chamber assay; induction of bipole shape following challenge by chemoattractant
	Phagocytic responsiveness	NBT assay
Eosinophils/basophils	Numbers available and status	Cell count and morphology

*Assays listed are not intended to be exhaustive, but they are representative of methods that can be used to assess aspect of immunity identified.

Ab, antibody; **ADCC,** antibody-dependent cellular cytotoxicity; **Ag,** antigen; **Con A,** concanavalin A; **CoVF,** cobra venom factor; **Ig,** immunoglobulin; **IFN,** interferon; **IL-1,** interleukin 1; **IL-2,** interleukin 2; **LPS,** lipopolysaccharide; **MLA,** mixed lymphocyte assay; **N,** null (cell); **NBT,** nitroblue tetrazolium; **NK**, natural killer; **PHA,** phytohemagglutinin; T_C, cytotoxic T (cell); T_D, sensitized (delayed hypersensitivity) type T (cell); T_H, helper T (cell); T_S, suppressor T (cell); **TNF,** tumor necrosis factor.

BACKGROUND SOURCES

Adams, D. O., Edelson, P. J., and Koren, H. S. (eds.). *Methods for Studying Mononuclear Phagocytes.* Academic Press, Inc., New York, 1981.

Coligan, J. E., Kruisbeek, D. H., Margulies, D. H., et al. (eds.). *Current Protocols in Immunology.* John Wiley & Sons, Inc., New York, 1991.

Colowick, S. P., and Kaplan, N. O. (series eds.). *Methods in Enzymology.* Academic Press, Inc., Orlando, Fla. (This series has published 11 volumes on immunological methods since 1980: Vols. 70 [1980], 73 and 74 [1981], 84 [1982], 92 and 93 [1983], 108 [1984], 116 [1985], 121 and 132 [1986], and 150 [1987].)

Greaves, M. F., Owen, J. J. T., and Raff, M. C. *T and B Lymphocytes: Origins, Properties, and Roles in Immune Responses.* Excerpta Medica, Amsterdam, 1974.

Mishell, B. B., and Shiigi, S. M. (eds.). *Selected Methods in Cellular Immunology.* W. H. Freeman & Co., Publishers, San Francisco, 1980.

Outteridge, P. M. *Veterinary Immunology.* Academic Press, Inc., Orlando, Fla., 1985.

Rose, N. R., Friedman, H., and Fahey, J. L. *Manual of Clinical Laboratory Immunology.* American Society of Microbiology, Washington, D.C., 1986.

Rowlands, D. T., Jr. Diagnostic Tests for Assessment of Immunity. In *Fundamentals of Immunology and Allergy.* Lockey, R. F., and Bukantz, S. C. (eds.). W. B. Saunders Co., Philadelphia, 1987.

Weir, D. M. (ed.). *Handbook of Experimental Immunology.* 4th ed. (Vols. 1–4). Blackwell Scientific Publications, Ltd., Oxford, 1986.

Human and Murine Cell–Surface Antigens

T he intensive scrutiny to which cells engaged in immunological expression have been subjected has led to the identification of a lengthy list of specific cell-surface markers or Ags. The number of surface markers that can be recognized have increased dramatically in recent years through the development of MAbs as diagnostic reagents. The surface Ags that have been recognized have enabled investigators to substantially extend our understanding of immunology in numerous areas.

Several means of identifying these diagnostic Ags have been employed through the years. Certain of these made use of designations used by individual laboratories to identify the specific MAb against the Ag in question. Other nomenclature has been adopted in an effort to provide more universal recognition of similar or identical Ags identified by different groups. These included schemes identifying major human T cell Ags with the letter "T" followed by a numeral and for identifying murine Ags by "Ly" followed by a numeral. More recently, a universal nomenclature has been adopted which considers each Ag as a cluster determinant and assigns each determinant a specific numerical identity. These Ags are known as cluster determination (CD) Ags. Ags expressed on human cells are used as the reference standard. Recognizable homologues expressed by cells from other mammals would have the same designation.

The following table lists most of the CD Ags recognized by the Fourth International CD Workshop (Vienna, 1989). CD Ags for which a murine homologue has been identified have the murine alternative listed in parentheses, while CD Ags for which no murine homologue is known are accompanied by a dash in parentheses. Provisional workshop designations are noted by "w" (e.g., CDw32). In addition, selected surface Ags with important roles in immunological function that are not CD Ags are also listed.

Chromosomal locations of each human and murine Ag listed are provided, if known; however, Ags for which no murine homologue is known are designated by – In addition, the cell types on which each Ag is expressed are identified. Furthermore, the molecular and functional characteristics of these Ags are summarized. These characteristics are based primarily on those of the human Ags. Last, for each Ag that is discussed in the text, relevant chapters are identified.

Antigen	Chromosome Location Human	Mouse	Cellular Expression	Characteristics Molecular	Functional	Chapter
CD Ags						
CD1 (–)	1q22–q23	–	Human thymocytes, dendritic cells, Langerhans cells, B cell subsets	Glycoproteins similar to MHC class I proteins; (three forms identified: CD1a, 49 kD; CD1b, 45 kD; CD1c, 43 kD)	Associates noncovalently with β_2-microglobulin	2, 20
CD2 (Ly-37)	1p13	3	Human T cells; murine thymocytes, T cells and B cells	50 kD single-chain transmembrane glycoprotein CAM (formerly called SRBC receptor)	Binds to LFA-3; stimulates or inhibits T cell activation (depending on conditions)	9
CD3	11q23	?	T cells (human and murine)	Consists of five peptides (γ, δ, ϵ, ζ, η)	Associates with TCR; mediates signal transduction during T cell activation	9
CD4 (Ly-4)	12	6	Human T cell subsets; murine thymocytes and T cell subsets	59 kD single-chain transmembrane glycoprotein	Participates in MHC-restricted (class II) Ag recognition; stimulates or inhibits $T_{H/I}$ or T_D cell activation (depending on conditions); is receptor for HIV	2, 3, 5, 7, 9, 12, 15, 20
CD5 (Ly-1)	11q12–13	19	Human and murine T and B cell subsets; murine thymocytes	67 kD single-chain transmembrane glycoprotein	Modulates CD3-mediated stimulation of T cell proliferation	—
CD6 (–)	?	–	Human T and B cell subsets	100 kD glycoprotein	Induces proliferation of accessory cell-dependent subsets	—
CD7 (–)	17q25	–	Human T cells	40 kD single-chain glycoprotein with V-like domain	Function is unclear	—
CD8 (Ly-2,3)	2p12	6	Murine thymocytes; human and murine T cell subsets	Glycoprotein dimer, either α,α or α,β	Binds MHC class I Ags; is responsible for MHC-restricted T_C and T_S cell activation	2, 5, 7, 9, 12, 15, 20
CD9 (–)	12	–	Human pre-B cells, monocytes, and platelets	24 kD single-chain protein	Role is unclear	2
CD10 (–)	3	–	Human lymphocyte progenitors, B cells (in germinal centers), and granulocytes	100 kD transmembrane glycoprotein (formerly called CALLA)	Expresses endopeptidase activity	—
CD11a	16p11–p13	7	Most human and murine leukocytes	180 kD glycoprotein (also known as LFA-1)	Complexes with CD18 to form CAM; recognizes CD54	8

Antigen	Chromosome Location Human	Mouse	Cellular Expression	Characteristics Molecular	Functional	Chapter
CD11b	16p11–p13	?	Human and murine monocytes; human granulocytes, and NK cells	165 kD glycoprotein (also known as CR3)	Complexes with CD18 to form CAM; has binding domains for complement, LPS, and fibrinogen	8
CD11c (–)	16p11–p13	–	Human monocytes, granulocytes, NK cells and B cell subsets	150 kD glycoprotein (also known as CR4)	Complexes with CD18 to form CAM; binds complement	8
CD12	Ag to be redefined (no identified murine homologue)					
CD13 (–)	15q25	–	Human monocytes and granulocytes	150 kD single-chain transmembrane glycoprotein	Displays aminopeptidase N activity; possibly modulates phagocytosis	—
CD14 (–)	5q23–q31	–	Human monocytes, and Langerhans cells	55 kD single-chain glycoprotein	Is receptor for LPS-LPS binding protein complexes	—
CD15 (–)	?	–	Human granulocytes	Trisaccharide, 3-fucosyl-N-acetyllactosamine, found in membrane proteins and lipids	Role is unclear, but might modulate phagocytosis	—
CD16 (–)	1	–	Human NK cells and granulocytes	50–65 kD single-chain glycoprotein (also known as FcγR III)	Is possibly involved in signal transduction during activation	—
CDw17 (–)	?	–	Human granulocytes, monocytes, and platelets	Specific membrane lipid chain, lactosyl ceramide	No function is yet described	—
CD18	21q22.3	?	All human and murine leukocytes	95 kD glycoprotein	Complexes with CD11 to form CAMs	8
CD19 (–)	all	–	Human B cells	90 kD transmembrane glycoprotein (part of Ig superfamily)	Might mediate activation of B cell proliferation; is FcR	2, 5
CD20 (–)	12a12–13	–	Human B cells	35 or 37 kD membrane phosphoprotein	Role in B cell activation is not clearly defined	—
CD21 (–)	1q 32	–	Human B subsets	140 kD single-chain transmembrane glycoprotein (also known as CR2)	Affects T cell–dependent B cell proliferation; binds Fc domains of Igs and complement; is receptor for EBV	5
CD22 (–)	?	–	Human B cell subsets	135 kD integral membrane glycoprotein	Binds Fc domains of Igs	5

Antigen	Chromosome Location Human	Location Mouse	Cellular Expression	Characteristics Molecular	Functional	Chapter
CD23	?	?	Murine B cells; human B cell subsets, activated monocytes, and eosinophils	45–50 kD integral membrane glycoprotein (also known as FcεR)	Binds Fc domain of IgE	5
CD24 (–)	?	–	Human B cells and granulocytes	38–41 kD single-chain sialoglycoprotein	Modulates B cell proliferation; modulates respiratory burst of granulocytes	—
CD25 (Ly-43)	10p14–15	?	Activated murine and human T and B cells; activated human monocytes	55 kD single-chain glycoprotein (α chain of IL-2R; also known as Tac-Ag)	Is low-affinity IL-2R; interacts with β chain of IL-2R to form high-affinity IL-2R	—
CD26 (–)	11	–	Human-activated T cells	120 kD single-chain transmembrane glycoprotein	Is a dipeptidyl peptidase; promotes expression by activated T cells	—
CD27 (–)	?	–	Human T and B cell subsets	Dimer of two identical 55 kD polypeptide chains with homology to NGFR and CD40	Modulates T and B cell proliferation	—
CD28 (–)	2q33–34	–	Human T cell subsets	Homodimer of two 44 kD polypeptide chains	Modulates T cell proliferation	—
CD29 (–)	10	–	Broadly distributed on human cells	130 kD glycoprotein	Mediates cell adhesion	—
CD30 (–)	?	–	Human-activated T and B cells	105 kD single-chain glycoprotein	Function is undefined	—
CD31 (–)	?	–	Human granulocytes, B cells, platelets, and monocytes	130 kD integral membrane protein with homology to FcγR and CAM	Function is not defined	—
CDw32 (Ly-17)	1	1	Human and murine monocytes and B cells; human granulocytes and eosinophils	39–48 kD proteins, related to FcγR II	Modulates monocyte and granulocyte activation	
CD33 (–)	19q13	–	Human progenitor cells and monocytes	67 kD single-chain transmembrane glycoprotein, related to CD22	Function is not defined	—
CD34 (–)	1	–	Human progenitor cells	105–120 kD single-chain transmembrane glycophosphoprotein	Function is not defined	—
CD35 (–)	1q32	–	Human granulocytes, B cells, and monocytes	Glycoprotein with four allelic forms (also known as CR1)	Can bind complement fragments C3b, iC3b, C3c, and C4b	8

| Antigen | Chromosome Location | | Cellular Expression | Characteristics | | Chapter |
	Human	Mouse		Molecular	Functional	
CD36 (–)	?	–	Human monocytes and platelets (possibly also B cells)	90 kD single-chain glycoprotein (also known as platelet glycoprotein IV)	Mediates platelet-platelet, platelet-monocyte, and platelet-tumor cell interactions; is receptor for *Plasmodium falciparum*–infected erythrocytes	—
CD37 (–)	?	–	Human B cells (possibly also T cells and monocytes)	40–52 kD single-chain transmembrane glycoprotein, related to CD53	Might participate with Ags binding to IgM and with BCGF in costimulating B cells	—
CD38 (–)	4	–	Human lymphocytes, progenitor cells, plasma cells, and activated T cells	45 kD single-chain transmembrane glycoprotein	Might be growth factor receptor for growth-related CAMs	—
CD39 (–)	?	–	Human B cell subsets (possibly also monocytes)	70–100 kD glycoprotein	No function is yet defined	—
CD40 (–)	?	–	Human B cells and carcinomas	45–50 kD integral membrane glycoprotein related to NGFR (some homology with CD27 and TNF receptor)	Modulates proliferation of activated B cells	—
CD41 (–)	?	–	Human platelets	135 kD heterodimeric transmembrane glycoprotein (called platelet glycoprotein GPIIb)	Participates with CD61 in forming receptor for fibrinogen, fibronectin, von Willebrandt's factor, and CAMs; plays role in ADP and collagen activation of platelet aggregation	—
CD42a (–)	?	–	Human platelets	23 kD single-chain glycoprotein	Interacts with CD42b to form receptor with possible role in platelet adhesion	—
CD42b (–)	?	–	Human platelets	170 kD heterodimeric protein (25 kD β chain, 135 kD α chain)	Interacts with CD42a to form receptor with possible role in platelet adhesion	—
CD43 (–)	16	–	Human T cells, monocytes, brain cells, and some B cells	95 kD integral membrane glycoprotein	Participates in T cell proliferation; has possible role on homotypic adhesion of T cells and monocytes	—

| Antigen | Chromosome Location | | Cellular Expression | Characteristics | | Chapter |
	Human	Mouse		Molecular	Functional	
CD44 (Ly-24)	11	2	Human leukocytes; murine thymocytes, B and T cells, and Mφs/monocytes	Synthesized as 37 kD polypeptide related to cartilage link protein family	Is receptor for hyaluronate; possibly modulates CD2-mediated functions	—
CD45 (Ly-5)	1q31–32	1	Human and murine leukocytes	180–220 kD single-chain transmembrane glycoprotein with four isoforms	Modulates signal transduction during activation; might modify function of other receptors	2
CD46 (–)	1q32	–	Human leukocytes	Glycoprotein doublet (56 and 66 kD)	Function is not clearly defined	—
CD47 (–)	?	–	Broadly expressed	47–52 kD glycoprotein	Has no defined function	—
CD48 (–)	?	–	Human leukocytes	41 kD glycoprotein (part of Ig superfamily)	Has no defined function	—
CDw49 (–)	?	–	Human platelets and possibly T cells	Glycoprotein complex (120 kD subunit plus 30 and 31 kD doublet) (part of the integrin superfamily)	Associates with CD29; acts as receptor for laminin	—
CDw49b (–)	?	–	Human platelets and cultured T cells	170 kD glycoprotein (part of integrin family)	Associates with CD29; acts as receptor for collagen or collagen/laminin	—
CDw49d	?	?	Human and murine B and T cells; human thymocytes, monocytes, and possibly Langerhans cells	150 kD glycoprotein (part of integrin family)	Associates with CD29; acts as receptor for fibronectin and vascular CAMs	—
CDw50 (–)	?	–	Human leukocytes	Structure is not defined	Function is not defined	—
CD51 (–)	?	–	Human platelets (weak expression)	140 kD glycoprotein dimer of disulfide-linked 125 and 25 kD subunits	Associates with CD61 to form vitronectin receptor	—
CDw52 (–)	?	–	Human leukocytes	21–28 kD glycoprotein	Function is not defined	—
CD53 (–)	?	–	Human leukocytes	35 kD transmembrane glycoprotein with homology to CD37	Is possibly involved in stimulating oxidative burst of monocytes	—
CD54	19	?	Murine B and T cells; numerous human cell types	90 kD integral membrane glycoprotein (also called ICAM-1)	Is adhesion ligand of CD11a; is rhinovirus receptor	—

Antigen	Chromosome Location Human	Location Mouse	Cellular Expression	Characteristics Molecular	Functional	Chapter
CD55 (–)	1q32	–	Broadly expressed	70 kD membrane glycoprotein (also called decay-accelerating factor)	Prevents formation of C42 and C3B; protects against complement-mediated injury	—
CD56 (–)	11q23	–	Human NK cells and T cell subsets	140 kD glycoprotein (isoform of N-CAM)	Mediates NK–target cell adhesion interactions	8
CD57 (–)	11	–	Human NK cells, T cells, B cell subsets, and brain cells	Carbohydrate, possibly attached to myelin-associated glycoprotein	Function is not defined	8
CD58 (–)	1	–	Human leukocytes and epithelium	45–66 kD glycoprotein (also called LFA-3)	Binds to CD2 on T cells with high affinity	—
CD59 (–)	11	–	Broadly expressed	18–20 kD glycoprotein	Mediates inhibition of MAC; modulates NK cell activation	—
CDw60 (–)	?	–	Human T cell subsets	Terminal carbohydrate on some gangliosides	Possibly mediates activation of T cells by costimulatory signals	—
CD61 (–)	?	–	Human platelets	33 kD glycoprotein	Forms complexes (e.g., Ca-dependent complex with CD41 vitronectin receptor with CD51)	—
CD62 (–)	1q21–24	–	Activated human platelets	140 kD glycoprotein	Promotes binding of monocytes and granulocytes to activated platelets; forms LEC-CAMs with other adhesion molecules	—
CD63 (–)	?	–	Activated human platelets and monocytes (weak on B and T cells granulocytes)	53 kD glycoprotein	Function is not yet known	—
CD64 (–)	?	–	Human monocytes (weakly expressed on activated granulocytes)	75 kD single-chain transmembrane glycoprotein (FcγR)	Binds Fc portion of IgG with high affinity	2
CDw65 (–)	?	–	Human granulocytes (weakly expressed on monocytes)	Fucoganglioside (also called ceramide dodecasaccharide)	Function is not defined	—
CD66 (–)	?	–	Human granulocytes	180–200 kD phosphoprotein	Function is not known, but reflects activation	—
CD67 (–)	?	–	Human granulocytes	100 kD PI-linked membrane protein	Function is not known, but correlates with activation	—

Antigen	Chromosome Location Human	Chromosome Location Mouse	Cellular Expression	Characteristics Molecular	Characteristics Functional	Chapter
CD68 (–)	?	–	Human Mφs	110 kD glycoprotein	Function is not defined, but is a Mφ-specific marker	2
CD69 (–)	?	–	Human-activated B cells and T cells	Dimeric glycoprotein (28 and 34 kD subunits)	Function unclear; expression is unregulated upon activation	—
CDw70 (–)	?	–	Human-activated B and T cells	Structure is not yet defined	Function is not yet known	—
CD71	3	?	Activated murine B and T cells; human Mφs and proliferating cells	Membrane glycoprotein homodimer, 95 kD subunits (also called transferrin receptor)	Mediates uptake of iron; modulates cell growth	—
CD72 (Lyb-2?)	?	?	Human B cells, murine B cells (?)	Glycoprotein dimer (43 and 39 kD subunits)	Function is unclear, but defines immature B cells	—
CD73 (–)	?	–	Human B and T cell subsets	69 kD PI-linked membrane glycoprotein	Has 5′-nucleotidase activity (reduced in immune deficiency)	—
CD74 (–)	5q32	–	Human B cells and monocytes	Tripeptide complex (known as MHC class II–associated invariant complex)	Function is not defined	—
CDw75 (–)	?	–	Human mature B cells (weakly expressed by T cell subsets)	Structurally identical to α-2,6-sialytransferase	Has sialytransferase activity	—
CD76 (–)	?	–	Human mature B cells and T cell subsets	Several gangliosides or possibly certain 67 and 87 kD glycoproteins	Function is not defined	—
CD77 (–)	?	–	Human resting B cells	Certain complex neutral glycosphingolipids	Function is not known	—
CDw78 (–)	?	–	Human B cells and possibly monocytes	Structure is not defined	Function is not defined	—

Other Ags

Antigen	Chromosome Location Human	Chromosome Location Mouse	Cellular Expression	Characteristics Molecular	Characteristics Functional	Chapter
(Ly-6)	–	15	Murine T and B cell subsets	12 kD PI-linked glycoprotein	Might mediate signal transduction during B and T cell activation	—
MHC Ags class I	6	17	Nucleated cells (human and murine)	40–45 kD polypeptide associated with β_2-microglobulin	Interacts with CD8 in MHC-restricted Ag presentation	2, 7, 9, 15, 20

Antigen	Chromosome Location		Cellular Expression	Characteristics		Chapter
	Human	Mouse		Molecular	Functional	
MHC Ags class II			B cells, activated T cells, Mφs/monocytes, myeloid stem cells, Langerhans cells, and spermatozoa (human)	Transmembrane glycoprotein heterodimer (28 and 34 kD)	Interacts with CD4 in MHC-restricted Ag presentation	2, 7, 9, 15, 20
mIg	Several	Several	B cell subsets (human and murine)	Membrane-associated glycoprotein (Ig type varies with cell maturity: IgD and IgM, immature; any Ig, mature)	Is Ag recognition receptor	3, 5, 20
TCR α chain β chain γ chain δ chain	Several 14 7 7 14	Several 14 6 6 14	T cell subsets (human and murine)	90 kD transmembrane protein heterodimer (each chain equals 45–55 kD; two forms identified: αβ, most T cells; γδ, minor T cell subsets and during development)	Is Ag recognition receptor; interacts with CD3 for signal transduction; interacts with CD4 or CD8 in MHC-restricted Ag recognition	2, 7, 8, 9, 20
(Thy-1)	–	9	Murine thymocytes and T cells (related molecule found on neurons)	Single-chain glycoprotein, (member of Ig superfamily)	Diagnostic of T lineage lymphocytes	2

Abbreviations: **ADP,** adenosine diphosphate; **Ag,** antigen; **BCGF,** B cell growth factor; **CALLA,** common acute lymphoblastic leukemia Ag; **CAM,** cell adhesion molecule; **CR,** complement receptor; **EBV,** Epstein-Barr virus; **FcR,** Fc receptor; **HIV,** human immunodeficiency virus; **ICAM,** intercellular CAM; Ig, immunoglobulin; **IL-2R,** interleukin 2 receptor; **LFA,** leukocyte function antigen; **LPS,** lipopolysaccharide; **MAC,** membrane attack complex; **MHC,** major histocompatibility complex; **mIg,** membrane-bound or surface immunoglobulin; **Mφ,** macrophage; **N-CAM,** neural CAM; **NGFR,** nerve growth factor receptor; **NK,** natural killer; **PI,** phosphoinositol; **SRBC,** sheep red blood cell; **TCR,** T cell receptor; **TNF,** tumor necrosis factor.

Source: Adapted from Coligan, J. E., Kruisbeek, A. M., Margulies, D. H., et al. (eds.). *Current Protocols in Immunology.* John Wiley & Sons, Inc., New York, 1991.

G L O S S A R Y

A

Ab Antibody.

ABO Blood Groups Family of major human blood group types. Depending upon the alleles present, yield blood types A (A/A or A/O), B (B/B or B/O), AB (A/B), or O (O/O).

ACAID Anterior chamber-associated immune deviation.

Accessory Cells Cells of macrophagic, lymphocytic, or epithelial lineage, possessing MHC markers, which present antigen and cooperate with T and B cells in the formation of antibody or T cell sensitization.

Acquired Immune Deficiency Syndrome Disease characterized by diminished immune responsiveness arising from impaired T_H function following infection by HIV.

Activated Lymphocytes Lymphocytes that have become functionally active following stimulation by antigen, cytokine, or mitogen.

Activated Macrophages Macrophages expressing elevated metabolic activity following stimulation by agents such as lymphokines.

Active (Acquired) Immunity Specific protection acquired after induction of an immune response following exposure to an antigen presented by immunization or infection.

Acute Lymphocytic Leukemia Cancer of the immune system characterized by a failure of lymphocyte maturation.

Acute-Phase Proteins Serum proteins that increase rapidly in the blood and remain prominent during early stages of infection and inflammation. They are nonimmunoglobulin factors, such as C-reactive protein, that are important in innate immunity.

Adaptive Immunity Antigen-specific protection against infectious agents, their products, or both that is acquired as a result of immunization or infection.

ADCC Antibody-dependent cellular cytotoxicity.

Adenoma Tumor affecting glandular tissues.

Adenosine Deaminase Deficiency Condition characterized by a deficiency in the enzyme adenosine deaminase. The direct consequence of this defect is an accumulation of adenosine within cells, leading to impairment of T_H cell function. Cellular and humoral immunity are depressed in individuals with this enzyme deficiency.

Adherent Cells Cells, such as monocytes and macrophages, that normally adhere readily to plastic or glass.

Adherins Substances produced and used by microbial pathogens to adhere to host tissues as a device to promote infection.

Adjuvant Substance capable of enhancing or potentiating an immune response to an antigen with which it is administered.

Adoptive Transfer Transfer of immunity from an immune individual to a nonimmune individual by the transplantation of immunocompetent cells.

Affinity Strength of attractive association between a ligand and its binding site. For antibodies, this refers to the attractive association between an antibody-combining site and an antigenic determinant.

AFP α-fetoprotein.

Ag Antigen.

Agammaglobulinemia Inherited immunological disorder characterized by a failure to produce γ-globulins.

Agglutination Aggregation of antigenic particles, or cells, by antibodies.

Agglutinin Polyvalent molecule that is capable of inducing agglutination, or crosslinking, of cells.

Agglutinogen Substance, often an antigen, that stimulates the production of an agglutinin.

Aggressins Substances produced and used by microbial pathogens to impair host immune responses.

Agretope Part of the antigen that combines with the desetope of an MHC molecule on an antigen-presenting cell.

AIDS Acquired immune deficiency syndrome.

AIDS-Related Complex Loosely defined group of conditions marked by the display of multiple systemic infections—but in the absence of clinically defined AIDS.

ALL Acute lymphocytic leukemia.

Allele Single form of a gene at a given locus that controls a particular characteristic.

Allelic Exclusion Phenotypic expression of only one of the two allelic forms of a gene present in heterozygous cells.

Allergen Environmental antigen that stimulates allergic reactions that are expressed as immediate (Type I) hypersensitivity responses mediated by IgE.

Allergy Hypersensitive state acquired through exposure to a particular allergen.

Allogeneic Genetic dissimilarity among members of the same species.

Allograft Graft of cells, tissues, or organs between allogeneic individuals. Also known as a homograft.

Allotypic Determinants Determinants found as allelic variants of antigens, such as immunoglobulin molecules, which may be found in some but not all members of a species.

α-Fetoprotein Antigen that is normally expressed by fetal tissues but abnormally occurs in association with certain forms of cancer. It is one of several substances, known as oncofetal antigens, that are used as tumor markers in adults.

α-Macroglobulin Serum protein of maternal origin that suppresses cell-mediated immune responsiveness against fetal antigens.

Alternative Complement Pathway Antibody-independent cytolytic pathway of serum proteins that includes complement components C3–C9 of the classical complement pathway and several other independent factors (Factors B, D, H, I, P). This pathway can be activated by microbial products. It is also known as the properdin pathway.

A$_m$ Marker Allotypic marker that appears in one of two forms on IgA light chains of some individuals.

Amebocyte Phagocytic immune effector cell of many invertebrate species. This represents an early (phylogenetically primitive?) nonspecific effector of cellular immunity.

Anamnestic Reaction Immune response involving immunological memory and heightened responsiveness upon exposure to a previously encountered antigen.

Anaphylatoxins C3a, C4a, C5a, which are released into blood following activation of complement. These can cause mast cell degranulation and histamine release capable of producing the symptoms of anaphylaxis.

Anaphylaxis Reaction characterized by vasodilation and smooth muscle contractions, possibly leading to hypotension, bronchoconstriction, and urticaria. It is an immediate (Type I) hypersensitivity reaction that follows exposure to an antigen in sensitized individuals that is induced by the release of mediators from IgE-coated mast cells.

Angiogenesis Process of blood vessel formation.

Anterior Chamber–Associated Immune Deviation Special case of selective suppression of delayed (Type IV) hypersensitivity reactions within the eye. Its occurrence can lead to adverse effects of infections on the visual system.

Antibody Serum protein formed in response to a single antigenic determinant, which is capable of binding specifically with the antigenic determinant or epitope that induced its formation.

Antibody-Dependent Cellular Cytotoxicity Form of cytotoxicity reaction in which target cells become coated with antibody and subsequently are lysed by leukocytes bearing Fc receptors.

Antigen Any foreign material that can be specifically bound by antibody or T cell receptors.

Antigen-Binding Site That part of an antibody molecule, or T cell receptor molecule, that binds to an antigenic determinant. It is also known as the paratope.

Antigen-Dependent Differentiation Differentiation of mature T or B cells into expressive elements of cellular or humoral immunity that is triggered by exposure to antigen.

Antigen-Independent Differentiation Differentiation of mature T and B cells from lymphocyte precursors. This process might begin in the fetal liver or adult bone marrow but continues in specific microenvironments where commitments are made to become mature, antigen-responsive T (thymus) or B cells (bursa or bone marrow).

Antigen-Presenting Cell Cell that processes and presents antigen, in association with MHC molecules, to lymphocytes such as T$_H$ cells.

Antigenic Determinant Single antigenic site, or epitope, on a molecule that reacts with antibody or T cell antigen receptor.

Antigenic Modulation Loss or change in expression of surface antigens displayed by infectious agents and cancer cells.

Antilymphocyte Serum Serum containing antibodies against lymphocytes that can be used to produce immune suppression.

Antinuclear Antibody Diagnostic feature of individuals afflicted with LE. Its presence is usually visualized by immunofluorescence microscopy.

Antioncogene A gene whose absence (or failure to be expressed normally) leads to cellular transformation or tumor expression. Also known as tumor suppressor gene.

Antiserum Serum from an immunized individual that contains antibodies against a particular antigen.

APC Antigen-presenting cell.

ARC AIDS-related complex.

Arthus Reaction Reaction appearing as a rash induced by deposition of immune complexes in cutaneous capillaries following repeated presentation of antigen.

Ataxia Telangiectasia Immune deficiency disorder characterized by uncoordinated muscular movement and vascular dilation. This developmental disorder occurs before hemopoietic stem cell maturation and leads to a progressive depression of cellular and humoral immunity and to defects in neural and endocrine function as well.

Atopy Genetically determined, IgE-mediated, immediate (Type I) hypersensitivity response to an allergen.

Autograft Tissue graft from one site to another in the same individual.

Autoimmune Hemolytic Anemia Reduction in erythrocyte mass (anemia) that is brought about by cytolysis of an individual's own red blood cells because of the presence of autoantibodies against erythrocyte antigens.

Autoimmunity Immune response to self-antigens, which can generate autoantibodies and autocytotoxic T cells.

Autosomal Pertaining to those chromosomes that are not "sex chromosomes." These include all chromosomes except X and Y.

Avidin A glycoprotein obtained from egg white which possesses a high affinity for biotin. Avidin is frequently used as a secondary reagent to amplify reactions in which binding of primary antibody to ligand might be difficult to visualize. As a secondary reagent, labeled avidin is allowed to bind to biotin-tagged (biotinylated) antibodies prior to being visualized by histochemical or enzymatic means.

Avidity Functional binding strength derived from the multiple affinities between a polyvalent antigen and its antibody.

B

B Cells Lymphocytes that have been conditioned in the bursal microenvironment and are precursors of plasma cells, which produce antibodies.

B Cell Antigen Receptors Membrane-bound, surface immunoglobulin (mIg) molecules displayed by B cells. These mIgs are expressed by the cell that produced them, and all possess a single antigenic specificity. The most prevalent mIgs are IgM and IgD.

B Complex Designation for the major histocompatibility complex in chickens.

Bacillus Calmette-Guérin Attenuated form of *Mycobacterium bovis* that can be used as an adjuvant or a vaccine.

Balanced Pathogenicity Situation in which a pathogen produces the least amount of damage to its host.

Basophil Infrequently encountered leukocyte (less than 1% of circulating leukocytes) containing prominent basophilic granules in stained blood smears. This cell participates in immediate hypersensitivity reactions releasing heparin, histamine, and other vasoactive amines contained in its granules. It possesses receptors for the Fc portion of IgE.

BCG Bacillus Calmette-Guérin.

Bence-Jones Protein Monoclonal immunoglobulin light chains present in the urine of patients with multiple myeloma.

Benign In reference to tumors, describes those that lack the ability to invade surrounding normal tissues.

β_2-Microglobulin Peptide member of the immunoglobulin superfamily that constitutes a portion of the MHC class I antigen.

Binary fission Means of reproduction employed by bacteria and fungi (e.g., yeast) in which a single organism subdivides into two offspring. This process is similar to mitosis used by most eukaryotic cells.

Biotin A small molecule that can be easily coupled to antibody without significantly reducing its biological activity. Biotin is frequently used to tag antibodies in assays coupled with labeled avidin as a secondary (amplification) reagent. Biotin-tagged (biotinylated) antibody that is bound to antigen can be visualized through the subsequent binding of labeled avidin. The resulting antibody-biotin-avidin-label complex is identified (or quantified) through histochemical or enzymatic reactions involving the label attached to avidin.

Blast Formation Generation of blast-stage cells. Usually, this refers to the emergence of lymphoblasts following activation of T or B cells (or both) induced by exposure to antigen or mitogen. This process is also called blastogenesis.

Blastocyst In mammalian development, this is the cystlike blastula that gives rise to the tissues and organs of the developing individual.

Blood Island Hemopoietic center in the embryonic yolk sac, where hemopoiesis first occurs during ontogeny.

Bradyzoite Stage of certain protozoal parasites that is formed within cysts. They are also known as cystozoites.

Burkitt's Lymphoma Lymphoproliferative disorder caused by the Epstein-Barr virus.

Bursa of Fabricius Site of antigen-independent development of B cells in birds; it is located near the cloaca.

Bursin A tripeptide product of the bursa of Fabricius which seems to stimulate B cell maturation and differentiation.

C1–C9 Designation for the serum components of the classical complement pathway.

C Receptor Cell membrane receptor for complement.

C Region (Constant Region) Carboxy-terminal portion of the heavy or light chain of immunoglobulins.

CAM Cell adhesion molecule.

Capping Regional aggregation of molecules on the lymphocyte cell surface following crosslinking between antigens and antibodies or mitogens and their receptors.

Carcinoembryonic Antigen Oncodevelopmental (oncofetal) antigen associated with certain tumors usually arising in the gut.

Carcinogen Cancer-causing substance or agent.

Carcinoma Tumor of epithelial origin.

Carrier Large immunogenic molecule to which an antigenic determinant is attached, rendering the determinant immunogenic.

CD Cluster designation. Defines a family of surface antigens that are used diagnostically to identify human leukocyte classes. For example, mature human T cells are CD1+3+, while T$_H$ cells also express CD4, and T$_S$ cells express CD8. Human B cells express CD19–22.

CD3 Surface antigen of T cells that is linked to the T cell antigen recognition receptor. This complex is composed of five peptides and is believed to be involved in signal transduction in T cell activation.

CD4 Diagnostic surface antigen of T$_H$ and T$_D$ cells. This antigen is associated with the T cell antigen recognition receptor and contributes to class II MHC restriction of these cells.

CD8 Diagnostic surface antigen of T_C and T_S cells. This antigen is associated with the T cell antigen recognition receptor and contributes to class I MHC restriction of these cells.

CEA Carcinoembryonic antigen.

Cell Adhesion Molecules Cell-surface glycoproteins that play important roles in ligand-specific cell-to-cell or cell-to-substrate interactions. These roles include lymphocyte homing and stabilizing interactions between cytotoxic cells and their targets.

Cell Cycle Representation of the stage of cellular proliferation, from one division to another. This cycle includes a period of DNA replication (S) and active division (M) separated by gap periods (G_1 and G_2). In addition, a designation for differentiation, lying outside the cycle, is often represented by G_0.

Cell (Cellular) Differentiation Developmental process whereby genetically identical cells become distinct one from another because of selective differences in the genes that they express.

Cell-Mediated (Cellular) Immunity Normally refers to specific acquired immunity, which is accomplished by effector T cells. This includes allograft rejection, delayed hypersensitivity, and cytotoxic reactions against intracellular parasites.

Cell (Cellular) Proliferation Process of increasing the numbers of cells in a population through cell reproduction. This is generally accomplished through mitotic division by existing cells.

Cercaria Free-swimming stage of trematodes that seeks out a new definitive host.

Cestodes Parasitic flatworms that include all tapeworms.

Chédiak-Higashi Syndrome Autosomal recessive disorder affecting phagocytes. Although displaying normal chemotaxis and microbial ingestion, neutrophils from individuals with Chédiak-Higashi syndrome have depressed killing times. This presumably reflects a defect in delivery of lysosomal enzymes involved in microbial killing to the phagosomes. Adaptive immunity appears normal, but NK cell killing is reduced in individuals

with this disorder. Also known as Chédiak-Higashi-Steinbrink syndrome.

Chemotaxis Movement of cells within a concentration gradient. Positive chemotaxis reflects movement toward the source of the gradient; negative chemotaxis is movement away from the source. In immune response, C5a, leukotrienes, and lymphokines are important positive chemotactic agents.

Chimera Organism or tissue composed of elements of two distinct genetic natures.

Chloragocyte Type of coelomocyte that is believed to produce lysins for nonspecific humoral defense against infection in annelids. They might represent an invertebrate precursor of vertebrate B cells.

Chorionic Gonadotropin Hormone produced by trophoblast cells that suppresses maternal immune response against the fetus.

Chronic Granulomatous Disease Disorder of phagocytes characterized by a failure to generate toxic forms of oxygen. Two forms of this disease are recognized: a sex-linked disorder affecting males and an autosomal recessive form expressed among females.

Chronic Lymphocytic Leukemia Form of cancer characterized by production of large numbers of functionally impaired mature lymphocytes.

CID Combined immunodeficiency disease.

Class I MHC Antigens Gene products encoded by HLA-A, HLA-B, and HLA-C loci, in humans, or H2-K and H2-D loci, in mice.

Class II MHC Antigens Gene products encoded by HLA-D locus, in humans, or the H2-I region, in mice.

Class III MHC Products Gene products encoded by genes located between the Ir region and the D locus, in mice, or between the HLA and D/DR loci, in humans, that are associated with the complement system.

Classical Complement Pathway Mechanism of antibody-dependent cytolysis that is accomplished by a family of serum proteins with autocatalytic properties. Activation of this pathway by antibody-antigen complexes on cell surfaces leads to

the formation of a membrane attack complex (MAC) and, ultimately, to cytolysis.

CLL Chronic lymphocytic leukemia.

Clonal Anergy One mechanism through which self-tolerance is believed to arise. Through this process, cells that are positively selected during development become nonresponsive to self-antigens.

Clonal Deletion Theory of tolerance induction, which proposes that cells possessing specificity for a given antigen are selectively deleted and, therefore, no longer available to respond upon subsequent exposure to that antigen.

Clonal Selection Theory Model that considers that the clones of effector B or T cells produced in immune responses arise from single cells specifically activated because of complementarity between their receptors and the instigating antigen.

Clone Population of cells arising from a single precursor (parental) cell.

Coelomocyte Any of the cells responsible for immune defense that are found in the coelomic fluid of several invertebrate groups from annelids through echinoderms.

Coisogenic Individuals that are genetically identical at all loci except one.

Combined Immune Deficiency Refers to a deficiency in immune expression that affects both cellular and humoral immunity.

Commensal Organism that lives in a symbiotic relationship with another organism from which it derives benefit but not at the host's expense.

Complement Family of serum proteins that generate a cytolytic complex when activated. Classically, complement is activated by immune complexes and mediates antibody-induced cytolysis.

Complement Fixation Binding, or fixing, of complement by antibody-antigen complexes. This is used as the basis for an assay of antibody-antigen content of serum.

Complement Receptor Member of the family of cell-surface receptors that specifically recognize one or another component of the complement system or products of their activation.

Complementarity-Determining Regions   Another name for the three hypervariable sequences in the variable regions within each of the immunoglobulin light and heavy chains.

Concanavalin A (Con A)   Lectin derived from the Jack bean that can stimulate the proliferation of T lymphocytes.

Concomitant Immunity   Resistance to infection or tumor establishment in individuals who are infected or have tumors.

Congenic   Strain of animals that differs from another strain within only one chromosomal segment.

Contact Sensitivity   Immediate (Type I) hypersensitivity reaction to chemicals coming into contact with the skin as, for example, with exposure to catechols released by poison ivy.

Contrasuppression   Immunoregulatory circuit that inhibits suppressor activity in a feedback loop.

Coomb's Test   Assay that can be used to identify the presence of antierythrocyte antibodies, particularly those directed against minor blood type antigens, such as the Rh antigen.

Cortex   Outer layer of an organ, as distinguished from its inner layer.

CR   Complement receptor.

Crossreactivity   Reaction of antibodies, or sensitized T cells, with more than one antigen because of shared, or similar, determinants.

Cryoglobulin   Serum globulin (protein) that spontaneously precipitates at low temperatures (below 37°C).

Cryptozoite   Stage in the life cycle of *Plasmodium* in which the parasite is within the host's tissues and is, therefore, inaccessible to the host's immunological defenses.

Cyclosporine   Immunosuppressive drug that is used to prolong survival of organ and tissue transplants (grafts).

Cysticercus   Stage of a cestode's life cycle that can embed within the intestinal wall of its definitive host.

Cystozoite   Another name for a bradyzoite.

Cytokine   Biologically active substance produced by cells that influences other cells. Cytokines are referred to as lymphokines if they are derived from lymphocytes and as monokines if they are derived from monocytes/macrophages.

Cytophilic Antibody   Antibody that binds to the surface of cells bearing appropriate Fc receptors, for example, IgE to mast cells in allergic conditions.

Cytotoxic T Cells (T$_C$ Cells)   Specifically sensitized T cells that recognize, attach to, and kill foreign cells.

D

Definitive Host   Host in which a parasite passes the adult or sexual phase of its life cycle.

Degranulation   Process whereby granulocytes discharge the contents of their cytoplasmic granules (lysosomes or specific granules). This occurs during the formation of phagolysosomes by neutrophils or in the discharge of specific granule content of basophils and mast cells.

Delayed (Type IV) Hypersensitivity   Hypersensitivity reaction mediated by sensitized T lymphocytes (T$_D$ cells). It is often associated with chronic inflammatory lesions in which lymphocytes and macrophages are prominent.

Dendritic Cell   Antigen-presenting cell found in lymph nodes and spleen that possesses long processes that interdigitate among lymphoid cells.

Desensitization   Loss of sensitization to an antigen, or induction of tolerance to an allergen.

Desetope   Part of the MHC molecule that associates, or binds, to the agretope of the antigen on the surface of an antigen-presenting cell.

Determinant   Portion of an antigen that is responsible for complementary interaction with the specific antibody or T cell receptor to which it binds.

Diabetes   Disorder characterized by an imbalance in the regulation of blood glucose levels. In *juvenile diabetes,* antibodies arise against the β cells of the pancreas and abolish the ability of the individual to produce insulin. In *maturity-onset diabetes,* antibodies are formed against the insulin receptors, blocking activation of target tissues.

Diapedesis   Passage of cells through intact walls of vessels into tissues.

Diethylamine   An agent frequently used to determine functional antibody affinity by ELISA because of its

ability to inhibit binding of low-affinity antibodies more strongly than binding of high-affinity antibodies.

DiGeorge Syndrome   Congenital disease characterized by near absence of cellular immune capacity resulting from a failure of the thymus to develop. Individuals with this disorder also lack parathyroid glands.

Disulfide Bonds   Chemical bonds between two sulfhydryl-containing amino acids, represented as —S—S—. These bonds are important in linking together immunoglobulin heavy and light chains or domains of immunoglobulin heavy and light chains.

Diversity Segment   One of several short sequences of DNA that may encode a part of the third hypervariable region of an immunoglobulin heavy chain, found on the 5′ of the J segments.

Domains   Segments of immunoglobulin heavy or light chains that are homologous. Each is approximately 110 amino acids long, folded three-dimensionally, and stabilized by internal —S—S— bonds.

Dysgammaglobulinemia   Condition in which the γ-globulin fraction is normal but in which the production of a single class of immunoglobulin is impaired.

Dysplasia   Refers to the display by tissues of characteristics that deviate from those normally associated with that tissue. This is frequently considered a sign of initial tumor formation.

E

E Rosette   Human T lymphocyte surrounded by a cluster, or rosette, of red blood cells. These rosettes are formed *in vitro* in assays using sheep erythrocytes.

EBV   Epstein-Barr virus.

ECF-A   Eosinophil chemotactic factor of anaphylaxis that is released from mast cells when bound IgE reacts with antigen.

Ectoparasite   Parasite that lives on the surface of its host.

Effector Cells   Cells capable of executing a function. For example, effector cells of cell-mediated immunity include cytotoxic T cells, suppressor T cells, and helper T cells.

Electroimmunodiffusion Technique in which antigen and antibody diffusion in a gel is accelerated by an electrical current.

Elementary Body Extracellular, infective form of mycoplasmas.

ELISA Enzyme-linked immunosorbent assay.

Encapsulation Means of elimination of foreign substances that is used by the Porifera and Coelenterata. This process leads to the segregation away from the organisms's tissues of foreign material that is too large to be phagocytized.

Endoparasite Parasite that lives within its host.

Endotoxins Lipopolysaccharides derived from the cell walls of gram-negative bacteria.

Enzyme-Linked Immunosorbent Assay Assay that identifies the presence of, and quantifies the concentration of, a ligand through the generation of a product from the reaction catalyzed by the enzyme linked to the antibody against that ligand.

Eosinophil Granulocyte present in low concentration (less than 5% peripheral leukocytes), with large specific cytoplasmic granules that are eosinophilic (i.e., stain pinkish-red). These granules contain cationic proteins that can modulate inflammatory reactions.

Eosinophil Chemotactic Factor of Anaphylaxis Product released from sensitized mast cells when bound IgE reacts with antigen. It attracts eosinophils to the site where antigen is located.

Epimastigote Transitional form in the life cycle of trypanosomal parasites. In this form, the parasite is somewhat rounded, and the undulating membrane is not fully developed.

Epitope Antigenic determinant.

Epitype Set of epitopes.

Epstein-Barr Virus Herpesvirus responsible for Burkitt's lymphoma.

Equilibrium Dialysis Technique used to measure the interaction (affinity) of a monovalent antigen (hapten) and its antibody.

Equivalence Ratio of antibody to antigen (optimal proportions) that yields maximal precipitation in liquids and gels.

Erythema Redness caused by capillary dilation that occurs during inflammation.

Erythroblastosis Fetalis Hemolytic disorder arising from the production of maternal antibodies against Rh antigens on the erythrocytes of the fetus. Also known as hemolytic disease of the newborn.

Erythrocyte Red blood cell.

Erythropoiesis Process of red blood cell production.

Exon Continuous sequence of DNA, bounded on either side by noncoding regions (introns), that encodes part of a gene product.

Exotoxin Toxic substances produced and released by some pathogenic microorganisms.

Extraembryonic Membranes Tissue membranes, such as the amnion and chorion, that are associated with the developing embryo but which lie outside of the embryo proper (the blastocyst).

Extravascular Occurring outside of blood vessels.

Exudate Accumulation of proteins, salts, fluids, and cells occurring extravascularly in an inflammatory site.

F

F$_1$ Hybrid First-generation heterozygote of a mating between genetically dissimilar parents, such as two different inbred strains of mice.

Fab Fragment Monovalent antigen-binding fragment of immunoglobulin molecules obtained by papain digestion.

F(ab')$_2$ Fragment Bivalent antigen-binding fragment of immunoglobulin molecules obtained by pepsin digestion.

Fc Fragment Crystallizable non-antigen-binding fragment obtained by papain digestion of immunoglobulin molecules.

Fc Receptor Cellular membrane receptor that binds the Fc fragment of different classes and subclasses of immunoglobulin. These receptors can be found on granulocytes, mast cells, monocytes/macrophages, B cells, certain T cells, and other accessory cells.

Factor B Component of the alternative complement pathway, also known as C3 proactivator, Factor B complexes with C3b and is cleaved by Factor D, yielding C3 convertase (C3bBb).

Factor D Serine esterase of the alternative complement pathway that, when activated, cleaves Factor B to form C3bBb (C3 convertase).

Factor H Serum glycoprotein that can impair binding of Factor B to C3b and facilitates inactivation of C3b by Factor I.

Factor I Serum glycoprotein that is a hydrolase which inactivates C3b.

Factor P Properdin, a serum protein of the alternative complement pathway, which stabilizes C3bBP (C3 convertase).

FcR Fc receptor.

Feedback Effect of a result, or product, of a series of actions on the component(s) of the system responsible for that result, or product. *Positive feedback* leads to an increase in the activity producing the result. *Negative feedback* leads to a reduction in the activity leading to the result.

Fibroblast Connective tissue cell that is spindle shaped and can be stimulated to produce extracellular matrix fibers.

Filaria Slender threadlike worm; a nematode.

First-Set Rejection Chronic, cell-mediated rejection by an individual of an initial histoincompatible graft.

Flagellum Long, whiplike filament used for locomotion by some organisms, such as flagellated protozoa.

Fluorescence Emission of light at one wavelength by a fluorochrome that was activated by light of a different wavelength.

Fluorescent Antibody Antibody conjugated to a fluorochrome that can be used to visualize, with a fluorescence microscope, the location of antigen on cells or microorganisms.

Framework Regions Sequences of amino acids located on either side of the three hypervariable sequences of variable regions of immunoglobulin heavy and light chains.

Freund's Adjuvant Water-in-oil emulsion that enhances immune responses. This adjuvant is "complete" when it contains mycobacteria and "incomplete" when it does not.

G

GALT   Gut-associated lymphoid tissue.

Gametocytes   Male and female sexual cells of protozoan parasites.

Gamma (γ) Globulins   Serum proteins (immunoglobulins) that show the lowest mobility to the positive electrode (anode) during electrophoresis. The γ_1 fraction contains a mixture of all five immunoglobulins and is faster than γ_2-globulin, which is mostly IgG.

Glomerulonephritis   Inflammation of the renal glomeruli, often brought about after the deposition of immune complexes.

Glomerulus   Capillary network within Bowman's capsules where filtration of blood occurs.

G_m Allotype   Allotypic antigenic determinant or marker that is present on IgG heavy chains of some individuals.

Goodpasture's Syndrome   Progressive glomerulonephritis arising from local deposition in the nephron of immune complexes produced by autoantibodies.

Graft-versus-Host Reaction   Reaction of a graft containing immunocompetent cells against the cells, or tissues, of a histoincompatible and immunodeficient recipient.

Granulation Tissue   Fibroblast-rich connective tissue associated with the repair phase of an inflammatory response.

Granulocyte   Member of the family of leukocytes characterized by the presence of cytoplasmic granules. This group is subdivided into three types, based on the nature of the granules present: (1) basophils, containing basophilic granules; (2) eosinophils, having eosinophilic granules; and (3) neutrophils, which lack any specific granules.

Granuloma   Tumorlike mass or nodule of modified macrophages (epithelioid cells), fibroblasts, lymphocytes, and giant multinuclear cells that may form in response to invasion by a foreign body.

Granulopoiesis   Production of mature granulocytes from their precursors.

Graves' Disease   Autoimmune disorder associated with excessive secretion of thyroid hormones. The hypersecretion by the thyroid gland arises because of stimulation caused by binding of antibodies to the thyroid-stimulating hormone receptor, which regulates the activity of the thyroid gland.

Gut-Associated Lymphoid Tissue   Lymphoid organs associated with the gastrointestinal tract. These include the palatine tonsils, the appendix, Peyer's patches, and lymphocytes in the submucosa.

H

H-2 Locus   Major histocompatibility complex of the mouse, which is located on chromosome number 17.

Haplotype   Set of genetic determinants, or closely linked genes, located on a single chromosome (half of a genotype).

Hapten   Incomplete antigen possessing a single epitope. A substance that can combine with antibody but cannot independently stimulate an immune response; it must be complexed to a carrier.

Hashimoto's Thyroiditis   Disease in which the thyroid gland is underactive because of autoimmune destruction of thyroid follicular cells.

Heat Shock Protein   One of several proteins found to be produced in response to heat shock and other forms of cellular stress. Several families of heat shock proteins have been identified. Certain of these are stress induced. However, others are routinely produced by nonstressed cells, where they appear to play a role in posttranslational processing of proteins.

Heavy Chain   Portion of an immunoglobulin molecule that is composed of one variable (V) region and three or four constant (C) regions. Together with another, similar, heavy chain and two light chains, it forms one immunoglobulin molecule.

Helminth   Worm.

Helper T Cells (T_H cells)   Subpopulation of T lymphocytes (CD4). When T_H cells become activated by antigen-presenting cells (APCs), they release lymphokines that help to promote the expression of cell-mediated and humoral immune responses. In addition, they can act as APCs in activating B cells during induction of antibody formation.

Hemagglutination   Aggregation, or agglutination, of red blood cells.

Hemal Glands   Primitive hemopoietic centers found in annelids.

Hemoblast   Earliest definable hemopoietic stem cell that appears in the mammalian embryo.

Hemolysis   Lysis or dissolution of red blood cells.

Hemopoiesis   Production of blood cells.

Hemopoietic Stem Cell   Precursor of mature blood cell types. These cells might be unipotent or multipotent.

Heterologous   Derived from a different species (synonymous with xenogeneic).

High Responder   This refers to the comparative capacity of an inbred strain of animal (e.g., mouse) to mount a strong response to a particular antigen. This capacity is related to the type of immune response (Ir) genes present.

Hinge Region   Amino acid sequence (proline rich), between the first and second constant regions of immunoglobulin heavy chains, which permits molecular flexibility. The angle between Fab regions can vary between 0° and 180°.

Histocompatible   Being matched in terms of major histocompatibility antigens.

Histotope   Part of MHC molecules that binds to the paratope of the T cell receptor during antigen presentation.

HIV   Human immunodeficiency virus.

Hives   Response of the skin, which can occur during an anaphylactic reaction. This reaction is mediated by histamine released from activated mast cells and can be accompanied by erythema and edema.

HLA   Human leukocyte-associated antigen. This designates the major histocompatibility complex in humans, which is located on chromosome number 6.

Hodgkin's Disease   Malignant lymphoma affecting spleen, lymph nodes, and occasionally the bone marrow.

Homeostasis   Actively maintained physiological steady-state conditions of an organism.

Homologous   Derived from the same source or the same species. When referring to amino acid sequences, denotes amino acid residues that are similar between molecules being compared.

Host Individual that receives a graft, implant, or transplant (transplantation) or is infected by a pathogenic organism (virus, bacterium, fungus, or animal parasite).

HSP Heat shock protein.

HTLV Human T lymphotrophic virus. Identifies a family of viruses that infects human T cells. This family of viruses formerly had been believed to include the agent responsible for AIDS.

Human Immunodeficiency Virus Family of retroviruses that is believed to be responsible for human acquired immune deficiency syndrome (AIDS).

Humoral Pertaining to plasma, lymph, and tissue fluids.

Humoral Immunity Active, specific, acquired immunity mediated by antibodies present in the plasma, lymph, and tissue fluids.

Hybridoma Transformed cell line formed by the fusion of two parental cell lines. A B cell hybridoma is formed by the fusion of a myeloma cell with a normal plasma cell, whereas a T cell hybridoma is formed by the fusion of a T lymphoma and a normal T lymphocyte.

Hyperplasia Display of increased cellular proliferation.

Hypersensitivity Reaction Allergic reaction accompanying a secondary immune response, which can produce tissue damage. These reactions can be mediated by antibodies (Types I, II, III) or T cells (Type IV).

Hypertrophy Increased cellular and tissue activity, often leading to an increase in tissue mass.

Hypervariable Region Amino acid residues within the variable (V) regions of immunoglobulin heavy and light chains, which show greater variability among V regions than do other sequences.

Hyphae Long, slender, stemlike portions of fungi.

Hypogammaglobulinemia Condition characterized by the underproduction of one or more classes of immunoglobulins.

Ia Antigen Class II histocompatibility molecules encoded in the I region of the MHC of mice.

Idiotope One of the epitopes or antigenic determinants making up the idiotype of immunoglobulin variable regions.

Idiotype Set of one or more unique idiotopes characteristic of the variable regions of specific immunoglobulin molecules.

Idiotype Network Series of idiotype-antiidiotype reactions postulated for the control of humoral and cell-mediated immune responses.

IgA Class of immunoglobulins that can be found in dimeric form in exocrine solutions such as intestinal fluids, saliva, and bronchial secretions, and in monomeric form in serum. IgA does not fix complement or cross the placenta.

IgD Prominent immunoglobulin class serving as antigen receptors on B lymphocytes and present in low concentrations in serum.

IgE Immunoglobulin class that binds to mast cells and basophils and is responsible for immediate (Type I) hypersensitivity reactions. IgE is present in external secretions and in serum at very low concentrations. Major sites for synthesis of IgE are the lymphoid tissues of the gut.

IgG Predominant serum immunoglobulin, which can be divided into four subclasses. This immunoglobulin crosses the placenta and can fix complement.

IgM Class of antibody normally produced first against antigens. This species of immunoglobulin can exist in monomeric form (usually on the surfaces of B cells) and as a pentameric molecule. Among immunoglobulins, it is most capable of fixing complement.

IgN Class of IgG-like immunoglobulin that occurs in some reptiles.

IgY Class of IgG-like immunoglobulins that can be found among birds.

Immediate (Type I) Hypersensitivity Allergic reaction that can occur in sensitized individuals within minutes of exposure to an allergen.

Immune Complex Macromolecular complex of antigen and antibody molecules bound together. Each antibody molecule within the complex is bound to a specific antigenic determinant.

Immune Response Genes Genes that control the ability of an individual to respond to thymus-dependent antigens. They are encoded in the major histocompatibility complex.

Immune Surveillance Postulated function of the immune system (humoral and cell mediated) that recognizes and destroys spontaneously transformed cells in the body.

Immunity Resistance to infectious disease or injury. Specific immunity is generally acquired as a result of previous exposure to an immunogen (antigen).

Immunization Process of creating a state of immunity to some foreign antigen. This can be accomplished actively through exposure to appropriate immunogens or passively by administration of specific antibodies derived from a sensitized individual or animal.

Immunoadsorption Removal of antibody molecules from a sample by reacting with an antigen, or removal of antigen by reacting with antibodies. This is generally accomplished by precipitation of antigen-antibody complexes or the use of a solid-phase system to which antibody or antigen is adsorbed.

Immunoblot Reaction of labeled antibodies with proteins absorbed (Western blot) to an insoluble matrix, such as nitrocellulose paper.

Immunocyte Any cell that participates in an integral manner in an immune response. This generally implies lymphocytes and antigen-presenting cells.

Immunoelectrophoresis Technique involving separation of protein antigens according to charge in an electrical field, followed by diffusion and precipitation in gels using antibodies against the separated antigens.

Immunofluorescence Microscopy Visualization of the location of antibodies, or antigens, in tissues through the use of antibodies labeled with a fluorescent tag. This approach makes use of a fluorescence microscope to actually see the location of the labeled probe.

Immunogen Antigen that is capable of inducing an immune response and reacting with the products of such a response.

Immunoglobulin Serum glycoprotein product of certain lymphocytes, composed of two heavy and two light chains, that displays specificity for a particular antigen.

Immunoglobulin Classes Groups of immunoglobulins based on significant differences in the amino acid sequence of heavy chains designated isotypic determinants. There are five class isotypes in mammals: IgA, IgD, IgE, IgG, and IgM.

Immunoglobulin Superfamily Sets of genes encoding immunoglobulins, T cell receptors, and MHC surface antigens. These genes are presumed to be related because of the high degree of conservatism in their nucleotide sequences.

Immunological Tolerance Refers to a state of specific immunological unresponsiveness to a particular antigen.

Immunologically Privileged Site Site displaying altered immunological intervention for one of several factors, which varies with the site, for example, differential entry of effectors of cellular immunity.

Indirect (Passive) Agglutination Agglutination of particles, or red blood cells, by antibodies generated against antigens that are chemically coupled to the particles or cell surfaces.

Inducer Cells Subpopulation of T lymphocytes (CD4) that cooperate with antigen-presenting cells and precursor T lymphocytes in cell-mediated immune responses.

Inflammation State existing when an inflammatory reaction is in progress. A condition characterized by the presence of four distinctive features: redness, swelling, pain, and heat.

Inflammatory Responses Reactions that occur during inflammation. Acute inflammatory responses are characteristically associated with neutrophils as primary effectors, while chronic inflammatory responses are mediated by macrophages and lymphocytes.

Innate Immunity Natural, nonspecific protection from infection and disease. This form of immunity is present from birth, is based on the constitution of the host, and does not require antigen-specific antibodies or T cells for expression.

Insulin Hormone produced by the β cells of the pancreas that acts on target tissues to lower blood glucose.

Interferons Proteinaceous cytokins originally recognized for their antiviral activity. Three types of interferons (α, β, and γ) are recognized. In addition to their antiviral activity, interferons can also modify immune responses.

Interleukins Family of cytokines that function principally as growth and differentiation factors. They are instrumental in propagating cellular or humoral immune responses (or both) once they are initiated.

Intermediate Host Host in which a transitional, or larval, stage is passed for parasites that infect more than one host.

Internal Image Idiotype of an antiidiotype antibody (Ab-2) that binds to the paratope of the antibody (Ab-1) formed against the foreign epitope. The internal image idiotope can be immunogenically substituted for the foreign epitope.

Interstitial Fluid Extracellular and extravascular fluid compartment of the body. This includes all fluids that bathe the tissues and organs.

Intron Structural gene segment that does not code for amino acid sequences in the gene product. The transcribed sequence is removed by splicing during the formation of mRNA.

Ir Genes Immune response genes.

Isograft Graft between genetically identical individuals.

Isotypic Determinants Antigenic determinants that define an immunoglobulin class or subclass (e.g., IgA1, IgA2; IgD; IgE; IgG1, IgG2, IgG3, IgG4; and IgM) and type of light chain (κ, λ). They are found on subsets of heavy and light chains in each human being.

J

J (Joining) Chain Polypeptide chain of about 15 kD, found in the polymeric forms of IgA and IgM, which links subunits.

J (Joining) Gene Short exon coding for part of the third hypervariable region (or complementarity region) of the immunoglobulin light or heavy chain. J segments translocate during differentiation to join V and C genes in light chains and D and C genes in heavy chains.

K

K (Killer) Cell Cell, lacking B and T cell differentiating antigens but possessing Fc receptors, that kills target cells by antibody dependent cellular cytotoxicity.

Kallikrein Plasma protein that enzymatically activates kinins (converts kinnogens to kinins).

Kaposi's Sarcoma Neoplastic lesion characterized by multiple, soft bluish nodules in the skin and hemorrhages. It is a common manifestation in individuals afflicted with AIDS.

Kappa (κ) Chains One of the two immunoglobulin light chain isotypes.

kD Kilodalton; represents 1,000 daltons and is a measure of molecular mass.

Kinins Inflammatory peptides that function as vasodilators by increasing vascular permeability and contraction of smooth muscle. Formed by the action of esterases on kininogens in plasma.

K_m Marker Allotypic determinant found on the κ light chain of immunoglobulins.

Kupffer Cells Fixed macrophages in the blood sinuses of the liver.

L

L3T4 A diagnostic surface marker for mouse $T_{H/I}$ cells.

LAK Cell Lymphokine-activated killer cell.

Lambda (λ) Chain One of the two immunoglobulin light chain isotypes.

Langerhans Cell Accessory, or antigen-presenting, cell found in the epidermis, which bears class II MHC antigens, Fc receptors, and complement receptors.

Large Granular Lymphocytes Lymphocytes with large cytoplasmic lysosomes that might serve as natural killer (NK) or killer (K) cells.

Latency The persistence of a virus within a host cell in an unexpressed (inactive) state. This is equivalent to lysogeny of bacterial viruses.

Latex Fixation Test Test in which polystyrene latex particles are used to adsorb antigen and which then can be agglutinated by the addition of specific antibody.

LAV Lymphadenopathy virus. Viruses that infect lymphoid cells and give rise to lymphomas. This group may be synonymous with HTLV.

LE Lupus erythematosus.

LE Cell Characteristic cell found in certain laboratory tests in individuals with LE. This cell is a neutrophil engorged by ingested nuclear material.

Lectins Proteins derived chiefly from plants that bind to sugars and oligosaccharides present in the glycoproteins of many cells. Certain lectins are especially mitogenic for lymphocytes, for example, concanavalin A and phytohemagglutinins.

Leukemia Form of cancer that affects leukocytes.

Leukocyte White blood cell.

Leukocytosis State characterized by an increased number of leukocytes in the blood.

Leukopenia State characterized by a reduced number of leukocytes in the blood.

Leukotrienes Biologically active agents, which are metabolic products of arachidonic acid generated by the action of lipoxygenases.

LFA Lymphocyte function antigen.

Ligand Molecule that binds to another substance.

Light (L) Chain Polypeptide chain, with a molecular weight of 22 kD, present in all immunoglobulin molecules. Each light chain has one constant (C) and one variable (V) domain. Two identical L chains are found in each immunoglobulin. These chains appear as either of two forms or isotypes, κ and λ.

Linkage Disequilibrium Occurrence of specific alleles to a greater extent than expected from random genetic distribution and recombination that arises because of apparent linkage between otherwise independent alleles.

Lipopolysaccharides Substances, produced principally by gram-negative bacteria, composed of lipid and polysaccharide that can have mitogenic (B lymphocytes), inflammatory, and pyrogenic effects.

LMEF Lymphocyte migration-enhancing factor.

LMIF Lymphocyte migration-inhibiting factor.

Locus Location of a gene on a chromosome.

LPS Lipopolysaccharides.

Lupus Erythematosus Complex of diseases associated with autoimmune reactions against a variety of self-components including DNA, RNA, and nuclear proteins. Vasculitis, red scaly skin patches, arthritis, and glomerulonephritis can develop.

Ly Antigens Surface markers of murine lymphocytes. Ly-1, Lyt-2, Lyt-3 are expressed by T cells, while Lyb-2 and Lyb-3 are expressed by B cells.

Lymph Fluid found in the lymphatic vessels.

Lymph Nodes Small lymphoid organs containing aggregates of lymphocytes, with macrophages and dendritic cells. Lymph nodes serve as filters through which foreign materials (antigens) pass and where activation of lymphocytes can occur.

Lymphocyte Mononuclear cell, approximately 7 to 12 μm in diameter, containing a large, round nucleus with densely packed chromatin and a small thin outer layer of cytoplasm. Several classes of lymphocytes are identified on the basis of surface antigens that they express and their roles in immune responses.

Lymphocyte Function Antigen Cell adhesion molecule that enhances efficiency of functional interaction between leukocytes and other cells. This antigen was first described through suppression of T cell cytotoxicity by monoclonal antibodies directed against it. They are expressed by T and B cells, granulocytes, and macrophages.

Lymphocyte Migration-Enhancing Factor A recently identified monokine that stimulates migration of lymphocytes into an area containing activated macrophages.

Lymphocyte Migration-Inhibiting Factor A recently identified monokine that suppresses migration of lymphocytes from an area containing activated macrophages.

Lymphoid Organs Organs of the body that contain large numbers of lymphocytes.

Lymphokine Cytokine produced by lymphocytes (chiefly T cells) and released following antigen or mitogen stimulation. Several lymphokines exist that act as intercellular mediators of the immune response.

Lymphokine-Activated Killer Cells Populations of K and NK cells that exhibit enhanced killing of target cells (e.g., tumor cells) following activation by interleukin 2.

Lymphoma Tumor of lymphoid tissues.

Lysogeny Process in which a bacterial virus remains unexpressed, or latent, within the bacterial host.

Lysosomes Cytoplasmic granules found in many cells, which contain hydrolytic enzymes that are normally inert until released. They play a critical role in the digestion of materials engulfed by phagocytes.

Lysozyme Low molecular weight cationic enzyme present in tears, saliva, and nasal secretions that digests mucopeptides in the cell walls of susceptible bacteria.

MAb Monoclonal antibody.

MAC Membrane attack complex.

Macrophage Large mononuclear phagocyte derived from bone marrow/blood monocytes. It can function as an antigen-presenting cell, a phagocyte, or a cytotoxic cell in ADCC reactions.

Macrophage-Activating Factor (MAF) Lymphokine that enhances the phagocytic (microbicidal) and cytotoxic (tumoricidal) capacity of macrophages.

Major Histocompatibility Complex Set of genes in close proximity on a chromosome (number 6 in humans; number 17 in mice), which encodes several products including histocompatibility antigens and factors influencing immune responses to antigens.

Malignant Referring to the property of a tumor to invade and displace surrounding healthy tissues.

Mantoux Test Intracutaneous test for evidence of exposure to tubercle bacilli (*Mycobacterium tuberculosis*).

Margination Attachment of leukocytes to the endothelium of blood vessels. This occurs to a limited extent normally and is enhanced during inflammation when it is a prelude to diapedesis.

Mast Cell Tissue granulocyte bearing FcE receptors. It resembles a peripheral blood basophil, having large cytoplasmic granules containing mediators of immediate (Type I) hypersensitivity.

Maximum Tolerated Dose The greatest dose of a carcinogen (or other test substance) that can be administered with little toxic effect (less than 1% mortality) on experimental animals.

Medulla Inner region of an organ, as opposed to its outer zone, or cortex.

Megakaryoctye Mature precursor within the bone marrow from which blood platelets are derived.

Membrane Attack Complex Complex formed by complement components C5b6789 that creates cytolytic pores in the membranes of cells in which it occurs.

Memory Cells Long-living progeny of B and T cells that were clonally expanded, following a primary response to antigen. These cells mediate specific immunological memory and rapid secondary immunological responses.

Merozoite Stage of *Plasmodium* parasites that can give rise to the male and female gametocytes.

Mesenchyme Loose embryonic connective tissue.

Metastasis Process of formation of secondary tumors that occurs when cells detach from a primary tumor and migrate by way of the bloodstream or lymphatic vessels to another site.

MHC Major histocompatibility complex.

MHC Restriction Limitation imposed upon activation of an immune response, unless antigen presentation occurs in association with either a class I or a class II MHC antigen.

Microfilaria Larval form of a roundworm.

mIg Membrane-bound or surface immunoglobulin; this is the B cell's antigen receptor.

Migration-Inhibiting Factor (MIF) Lymphokine produced by antigen-stimulated T lymphocytes that inhibits the movement of macrophages.

Minor Lymphocyte Stimulatory Gene One of several genes whose products act as superantigens. These genes appear to influence the expression of certain cytotoxic responses of lymphocytes to allogeneic lymphocytes in mixed lymphocyte cultures.

Miracidium Stage of schistosomes, and other trematodes, that infects the intermediate host.

Mitogen Any agent that induces DNA synthesis and proliferation of cells.

Mixed Leukocyte Reaction Reaction that occurs when leukocytes from two genetically distinct individuals are placed in culture. This is expressed as mutual stimulation of DNA synthesis, which is more pronounced in circumstances where the degree of histoincompatibility is great.

Mls Minor lymphocyte stimulatory (gene).

Monoclonal Antibody Homogeneous antibody produced by a clone of antibody-forming cells.

Monocyte Bone marrow–derived mononuclear phagocyte, which is large, amoeboid, and possesses an indented nucleus. It remains in the bloodstream for a short time before emigrating to tissues, where it develops into a macrophage.

Monokine Cytokine produced by activated macrophages/monocytes.

MTD Maximum tolerated dose.

Multiple Myeloma Neoplasm, or cancer, of antibody-forming cells (plasma cells).

Multiple Sclerosis Autoimmune neurological disorder characterized by progressive demyelination.

Multipotent Pertaining to stem cells, refers to the ability of the cell to give rise to progeny of more than one differentiated lineage.

Multivalent Capable of binding at more than one site; also called polyvalent.

Murine Pertaining to mice.

Myasthenia Gravis Autoimmune disorder in which normal neuromuscular interaction is blocked by antibodies against the acetylcholine receptor on skeletal muscle.

Mycology Study of fungi.

Mycoses Fungal infections.

Myeloperoxidase Enzyme that is present within granules of neutrophils that catalyzes the destruction of microorganisms mediated by hydrogen peroxide (H_2O_2).

Myxedema Autoimmune disorder of the thyroid gland that is characterized by the presence of antibodies against thyroglobulin and is associated with wasting of the thyroid gland.

N

Natural Antibody Antibody that is present in the serum of an individual who has never been immunized or clinically exposed to the antigen with which it reacts.

Natural Killer Cells Non-T, non-B lymphocytes that are present in nonimmunized individuals, which can be spontaneously cytotoxic to a variety of tumor cell lines without MHC restriction.

Nematodes Roundworms; comprise the largest group of helminthic parasites of humans.

Neoantigens Nonself antigens that might arise on cell surfaces during a disease state (such as cancer) and which are not derived from an exogenous source.

Neoplasia Generation of new growth; generally used to denote a tumor.

Network Theory Theory advanced by N. Jerne that proposes that idiotype-antiidiotype reactions involving antibodies (and T cell receptors) serve as immune regulators via physiological autoimmunity.

Neutrophil Most abundant leukocyte in the peripheral blood of healthy adults. It is a short-lived granulocyte with a multilobed nucleus and azurophilic granules. It is actively phagocytic and can perform in ADCC reactions since it possesses Fc receptors.

Nezelof's Syndrome Autosomal recessive immune deficiency disorder characterized by a marked reduction in T cells. Although B cell function is normal in individuals with this disorder, humoral immune responses are generally defective because of their dependence upon lymphokines from T_H cells.

NK Cell   Natural killer cell.

Nude Mouse   Inbred strain of hairless mice, which lacks a thymus and, consequently, is markedly deficient in T lymphocytes.

Null Cells   Lymphocytes that lack distinguishing phenotypic markers characteristic of T or B lymphocytes.

NZB Mouse   Inbred strain of mice produced originally in New Zealand that spontaneously develops autoantibodies and autoreactive T cells associated with autoimmune diseases. It serves as an animal model for lupus erythematosus.

Oncofetal Antigen   Antigen that is normally expressed during ontogeny but is inappropriate in its expression by adult tissues. Also referred to as an oncodevelopmental antigen.

Oncogene   Gene of either viral (viral-oncogene) or cellular origin (proto-oncogene) that can cause transformation of cells.

Oncogenesis   Process of tumor formation.

Oncosphere   Stage of cestode parasites that penetrates the intestinal wall to establish initial infection of the host.

Ontogeny   Development of an individual organism, from conception through maturation.

Opsonin   Substance, such as an antibody or complement, that can bind to the surface of a cell or particle, making it more readily phagocytized.

Ouchterlony Technique   Immunoprecipitation technique in which antigen and antibody, deposited in opposing wells within a gel, diffuse toward each other and form visible bands of precipitation in the gel in the region of equivalence.

Papain   Proteolytic enzyme, obtained from the papaw plant, used in hydrolysis of immunoglobulins to obtain Fab and Fc fragments.

Parasite   Organism that lives in association with another organism and derives benefit at the expense of its host.

Paratope   Antigenic determinant (epitope or idiotope) combining site found on an antibody or a T cell receptor.

Passive Cutaneous Anaphylaxis   Passive transfer technique for detecting, *in vivo,* the presence of allergen-specific cytophilic antibodies (IgE) responsible for immediate (Type I) hypersensitivity reactions.

Passive Immunity   Immunity conferred by the transfer of preformed immune products, such as antibodies or sensitized T cells, into a nonimmune host.

Pathogen   Disease-causing organism.

Pathogenicity   Potential, or ability, to produce disease.

PCR   Polymerase chain reaction.

Pepsin   Proteolytic gastric enzyme used to split polypeptide chains of immunoglobulins to form $F(ab')_2$ plus small peptide fragments from the remainder of the Fc fragment.

Perforin   Cytolytic molecules produced by T_C cells that create transmembrane channels in their target cells when activated by Ca^{2+}.

Peyer's Patches   Nodules of lymphoid tissue in the submucosa of the small intestines than contain follicles (germinal centers) and diffuse areas of abundant lymphocytes and plasma cells.

PHA   Phytohemagglutinin.

Phagocytes   Cells, such as monocytes/macrophages and granulocytes, that are capable of engulfing particulate matter.

Phagocytosis   Ingestion of cells or particles by phagocytes.

Phagolysosome   Membrane-limited vesicle that is the product of the fusion of a phagosome and a lysosome.

Phagosome   Intracellular vesicle, containing phagocytized material, that was formed by the invagination of the cell membrane.

Phenotype   Expressed cellular characteristics of an individual determined by the genotype and factors regulating gene expression.

Phylogeny   Development of a species through geological time.

Phytohemagglutinins   Lectins extracted from red kidney beans of *Phaseolus vulgaris.* In soluble form, they are T cell mitogens, while in insoluble form, they can serve as B cell mitogens.

Pili   Structural appendages of certain bacteria that are used for attaching to a prospective host.

Placenta   Tissue interface between the fetus and uterus of the mother, through which the fetus derives nutrients and other essentials during ontogeny. It consists of both fetal and maternal portions.

Plaque-Forming Cells   Antibody-forming cells that are visualized by the formation of hemolytic plaques. This occurs when B cells are induced to produce antibodies against erythrocytes, or antigens coating erythrocytes, and then plated with these erythrocytes in a semisolid medium containing complement. A hemolytic plaque forms as a result of antibody-dependent complement lysis of the red cells immediately surrounding the activated B cell.

Plasma   Fluid portion of the blood.

Plasma Cell   Differentiated, active antibody-producing cell derived by antigenic stimulation of a B cell.

Plasmacytoma   Plasma cell tumor or myeloma.

Plasmapheresis   Technique that passes blood through a machine in order to "purify" the plasma. In this process, cells are removed before "purification" (e.g., removal of immune complexes) and then returned to the plasma before being restored to the individual.

Plasmid   Extrachromosomal segment of DNA.

Platelets   Cytoplasmic fragments derived from megakaryocytes. They contain vasoactive substances and coagulation factors. Platelets are active in blood coagulation, inflammation, and allergic reactions.

Platyhelminthes   Flatworms; this taxon includes cestodes and trematodes.

Pokeweed Mitogen   Lectin derived from the pokeweed (*Phytolacca americana*), which can stimulate both B and T lymphocytes or only T lymphocytes, depending on the form used.

Polyclonal Activation   Stimulation of many different clones of lymphocytes, resulting in a heterogeneous immune response.

Polymerase Chain Reaction   A technique for producing large quantities of DNA (either isolated DNA segments or cDNA produced from isolated RNA). Through repeated cycles of DNA denaturation, primer annealing, and replication, multiple copies of isolated DNA or cDNA sequences are produced. This technique can be applied to define HLA polymorphism, characterize T cell receptor and immunoglobulin diversity, detect pathogens, and determine the expression of lymphokine genes.

Polymorphonuclear Granulocyte Neutrophil.

Pre-B Lymphocytes Immature B cells with diffuse cytoplasmic IgM but no membrane-bound immunoglobulin.

Precipitins Antibodies that react with antigens to form visible insoluble complexes or precipitates.

Primary Follicles Aggregates of small lymphocytes in the cortices of lymph nodes and the white pulp of the spleen after antigenic stimulation. They are the sites of germinal center development.

Primary Immune Response Initial immune response following exposure to an antigen, consisting chiefly of IgM antibodies and sensitized T cells.

Private Specificities Antigenic specificities of MHC-encoded proteins that are unique to particular haplotypes.

Proglottid Single segment of a tapeworm; it is a self-contained reproductive structure.

Properdin Factor P.

Properdin Pathway Alternative complement pathway.

Prostaglandins Biologically active lipids generated by the action of cyclo-oxygenases on arachidonic acid. Prostaglandins can inhibit platelet aggregation, increase vascular permeability, and promote smooth muscle contraction.

Protein A Protein derived from the Cowan strain of *Staphylococcus aureus* that binds to the Fc fragment of human IgG1, IgG2, and IgG4; murine IgG2a, and IgG2b; and rabbit IgG. It is frequently used for protein purification and immune-complex detection.

Protein C Surface protein of group C streptococci that can bind to the Fc fragment of all human IgG subclasses; murine IgG1, IgG2a, and IgG3; and rabbit IgG. It can be

substituted for protein A in immunoglobulin purification procedures.

Protein G Surface protein of group G streptococci that can bind to the Fc fragment of all human IgG subclasses; murine IgG1, IgG2a, and IgG3; and rabbit IgG. It can be substituted for protein A in immunoglobulin purification procedures.

Proto-oncogene Oncogene sequences that appear within the genomes of eukaryotic cells.

Protozoa Single-celled organisms possessing a distinct nucleus and cell membrane.

Prozone Effect Absence of agglutination or precipitation, or their suboptimal occurrence, when antibody is present in considerable excess over antigen.

Psychoneuroimmunology Study of interactions among the nervous, endocrine, and immune systems.

Public Specificities Antigenic specificities of MHC-encoded surface proteins that are common to the various allelic forms of a particular protein.

Pyrogens Substances that cause fever. They can be released by activated white blood cells.

Qa Antigens Class I murine histocompatibility antigens found on certain T lymphocytes. They are encoded by genes located between H2-D and T1.

Quiescent Not active; at rest.

R

Radioallergosorbent Test (RAST) Radioimmunoassay for the detection of specific IgE antibody in serum that has been allowed to react with specific insoluble allergens.

Radioimmunoassay Assay that enables the amount of a substance in a sample to be quantified by determining its competition for antibody binding against a known amount of radioactively labeled antigen.

Receptor Functional unit of a cell that can be located either on the cell surface (membrane receptor) or within the cytoplasm (cytoplasmic receptor) that leads to cellular activation when occupied by the specific ligand for which it possesses high affinity.

Recombinase Enzyme that mediates recombinatorial joining of immunoglobulin genes (or T cell receptor genes) during maturation and differentiation of B (or T) cells.

Reticular Dysgenesis Congenital immune deficiency disorder characterized by severe reduction, or absence, of lymphocytes and phagocytes.

Reticulate Body Form of mycoplasma found infecting a host cell.

Reticuloendothelial System (RES) Disperse mononuclear phagocyte system. Major concentrations of phagocytes of this system are located and operative in the liver, spleen, lymph nodes, and other lymphoid tissues.

Retrovirus RNA virus; upon infecting a host cell, this type of virus employs reverse transcriptase to produce a DNA copy of its genome for incorporation into the host cell genome.

Reverse Transcriptase Enzyme that makes use of an RNA template in order to produce a DNA transcript—essentially the reverse of what occurs in transcription.

Rh Factor Rhesus factor; a minor blood type antigen. Responsible for designation of blood type as positive (Rh^+) or negative (Rh^-).

Rheumatoid Arthritis (RA) Autoimmune disorder marked by severe inflammation of joints that results from antibodies (RF) against connective tissue antigens.

Rheumatoid Factor (RF) Antiimmunoglobulin antibody (autoantibody) mainly directed against IgG molecules. It is found in the sera of individuals afflicted with rheumatoid arthritis and other connective tissue diseases.

RIA Radioimmunoassay.

Ricin Toxin derived from the seed of the castor oil plant, which is capable of agglutinating red blood cells.

S

S Value Svedberg unit, which denotes the sedimentation coefficient of a protein. It can be obtained by analytical ultracentrifugation.

Sarcoma Tumor of mesodermally derived cells.

Schistosomule Stage of the schistosome's life cycle that occurs shortly after penetration into a definitive host. Also called a schistosomulum.

Schultz-Dale Reaction *In vitro* assay for immediate (Type I) hypersensitivity in which smooth muscle, passively sensitized with IgE antibody, contracts if exposed to allergen.

Scolex Head region of mature tapeworms that maintains physical attachment with the infected host.

SD Antigen Serologically defined antigen. This is a determinant found on an MHC gene product that is defined by its serological reactivity.

Second-Set Graft Rejection Rejection of a second allograft from the same source. This rejection is acute, occurring more rapidly than first-set rejection, since the histoincompatible host has developed immunity to the MHC antigens following primary exposure.

Secondary Immune Response More rapid and pronounced response that occurs in a previously primed individual following subsequent challenge with the priming antigen. This is due to the presence of memory lymphocytes.

Secretory IgA Dimer of IgA molecules linked to a secretory piece by the J chain, which may be found in exocrine secretions.

Secretory Piece Seventy kD molecule produced by epithelial cells, which may be associated with secretory immunoglobulins.

Sensitized Lymphocytes (T_D Cells) Cells that specifically respond and clonally expand following exposure to antigen.

Serology *In vitro* study of antibody-antigen reactions.

Serum Fluid portion of blood following clotting; this fluid lacks certain proteins normally encountered in plasma but consumed during clot formation.

Serum Sickness Adverse response following exposure to foreign antigens (e.g., serum) resulting in vasculitis, glomerulonephritis, and inflammation of joints due to intravascular immune-complex formation.

sIg Secretory immunoglobulin.

Simian Immunodeficiency Virus (SIV) Virus that produces an AIDS-like disease in rhesus (macaque) monkeys.

SLE Systemic lupus erythematosus; see lupus erythematosus.

Slow-Reacting Substance of Anaphylaxis Low molecular weight lipoprotein derived from arachidonic acid that is released by mast cells, which can promote smooth muscle contraction.

Splenocyte Mononuclear cell derived from the spleen.

Spores Propagation structures of bacteria, fungi, and certain invertebrates that are capable of withstanding adverse conditions. When conditions are favorable, spores are able to "hatch out" new offspring to continue the life cycle.

Sporozoa Group (phylum) of protozoan parasites that are responsible for toxoplasmosis (*Toxoplasma*) and malaria (*Plasmodium* spp.).

Sporozoite Stage of sporozoan parasites that is transmitted to and infects the definitive host.

TNF-β Lymphotoxin, a lymphokine produced by T_D and T_H cells, with properties similar to those of TNF-α.

Tolerance Active state of specific immunological unresponsiveness to one or more particular antigenic determinants.

Tolerogen Substance capable of inducing immunological tolerance.

Toxin Substance that is toxic to the host. In many instances, toxins are produced by infectious agents such as bacteria.

Toxoid Altered form of a toxin that retains its immunogenicity but has lost its toxicity.

Transfer Factor Dialyzable extract of sensitized lymphocytes that appears potentially capable of adoptively transferring delayed hypersensitivity to nonsensitized individuals.

Transformed Cell Cell that has undergone tumor transformation.

Transfusion Reaction Immunoprecipitation and hemolytic reaction that occurs following the administration of histoincompatible blood (wrong blood type) to an individual.

Transplantation Antigens Antigens, encoded by major and minor histocompatibility loci, that are expressed on cell surfaces. These antigens induce graft rejection, if the cells of the graft are not histocompatible with the host.

Transposon Transposable genetic element. This is a segment of DNA that can relocate to an alternative position(s) within the genome. These elements (which have been identified in fruit flies, yeast, and trypanosomes) provide tools for exploring the influence of the physical position of genes within the genome on their regulation and expression.

Transudate Protein-poor extracellular filtrate, can be found occasionally in an inflammatory site.

Trematodes Group of parasitic flatworms that includes schistosomes and flukes.

Trophoblast Extraembryonic peripheral cells of the mammalian blastocyst from which the placenta and extraembryonic membranes arise.

Trypanosome Flagellated protozoan of the subphylum Mastigophora. Trypanosomes are responsible for sleeping sickness and Chagas' disease.

Trypomastigote Mature, infective form of trypanosomes.

Tumor-Associated Antigens Cell-surface antigens found on transformed cells but not on normal cells.

Tumor-Associated Macrophage Macrophage found within a tumor. These macrophages appear to interact with tumor cells to promote angiogenesis and tumor growth.

Tumor Necrosis Factors Regulatory proteins produced by macrophages (TNF-α) and T lymphocytes (TNF-α and TNF-β) that contribute to the activation and proliferation of antigen-sensitive lymphocytes. They also can be cytostatic or cytocidal to transformed cells, stimulate bone resorption, and inhibit bone reformation.

Spreading Factors Products of certain microbial parasites that facilitate, or promote, their penetration of host tissues as an infection spreads.

Superantigen An antigen that can activate a large number of resting lymphocytes. For example, staphylococcal toxins and Mls gene products activate several-fold more resting lymphocytes than do most other antigens. These substances appear to induce activation through interaction with T cell receptors in a domain outside the antigen recognition site.

Suppressor Gene A gene whose absence (or failure to be expressed normally) leads to cellular transformation or tumor expression. Also known as an anti-oncogene.

Suppressor Lymphocyte (T_S Cell) Subclass of T cells that suppresses the expression of cellular or humoral immune responses to antigen exposure.

Switch Refers to a change in synthesis of heavy chain isotypes by a single cell, during differentiation, without affecting V region expression.

Syngeneic Refers to the relationship between genetically identical members of the same species.

T Cell Receptor Antigen recognition molecule of T lymphocytes. It is a member of the immunoglobulin superfamily and occurs in association with CD3 on mature T cells.

T_C Cell Cytotoxic T cell.

T_D Cell Sensitized T cell.

T_H Cell Helper T cell.

T_S Cell Suppressor T cell.

T Lymphocyte Bone marrow–derived lymphocyte that underwent antigen-independent differentiation in the thymus.

Tachyzoite Larval stage of certain sporozoan parasites (e.g., *Toxoplasma gondii*) that erupts from cysts in which they form and migrate to infect various organs of the host.

TAM Tumor-associated macrophage.

Theta (θ) Antigen (Thy) Alloantigen present on the surface of most thymocytes and peripheral T lymphocytes.

Thrombocyte Blood platelet.

Thymosin Thymic hormone of MW 12,000.

Thymocytes Lymphocytes in the thymus.

Thymus Central lymphoid organ, located in the thorax, that regulates the differentiation and maturation of T lymphocytes.

Thymus-Dependent Antigen Antigen that can induce an immune response only with the cooperation of T lymphocytes.

Thymus-Independent Antigen Antigen that can induce an immune response without direct cooperation from T cells.

TNF Tumor necrosis factor.

TNF-α Tumor necrosis factor or cachectin. A cytokine produced by macrophages, large granular lymphocytes, and T and B cells which can promote activation and proliferation of antigen-responsive lymphocytes. In addition, it can be cytostatic or cytocidal to transformed cells. Can stimulate bone resorption, and inhibit bone reformation.

Tumor Transformation Conversion process that a cell undergoes from normal expression to the expression of the traits of a tumor cell.

Unipotent Referrring to stem cells, designates a cell capable of producing offspring of a single differentiated lineage.

Urticaria Large wheal and flare reactions accompanied by edema that can be seen in immediate (Type I) hypersensitivity reactions.

V Region Variable sequences of N-terminal portions of immunoglobulin light and heavy chains.

Vaccination First relatively safe immunization procedure used to develop protection against smallpox by administering vaccinia virus to induce immunity. This term is now used frequently to indicate immunization against infectious disease agents.

Vaccine Preparation of antigenic material that is used to stimulate immunity against infectious agents.

Vascular Pertaining to blood vessels.

Vasculitis Inflammation of blood vessels.

Vasoactive Having an effect on blood vessels, usually inducing constriction or dilation.

Vector Organism that serves as a carrier, or transmitter, of an infectious agent.

Virulence Measure of infectivity of a pathogen.

Western Blot Detection of protein antigens following their transfer to an insoluble matrix, such as nitrocellulose, using labeled antibodies.

Wiskott-Aldrich Syndrome X-linked recessive combined immune deficiency disorder characterized by defects in T and B cell, and macrophage, function. IgM levels are usually depressed, although total immunoglobulin levels can be normal. Susceptibility to infections is extremely great.

Witebsky's Criteria A series of criteria, analogous to Koch's postulates, that are used to determine whether symptoms and expression of a particular disorder represent an autoimmune disease. These criteria specify that (1) a specific antibody must be found in association with the disease, (2) the antibody must be directed against a specific self-antigen of the affected tissue or organ, (3) the antibody must be capable of being induced by exposure to the antigen, and (4) symptoms of the disorder must be capable of being induced in an appropriate experimental model.

Xenogeneic Relationship between members of genetically distinct species.

Xenograft Cell, tissue, or organ graft between members of two different species.

Y

Yolk Sac In mammals, this highly vascularized extraembryonic membrane serves as the site for the earliest hemopoiesis during ontogeny. Unlike the yolk sac of phylogenetically older organisms (e.g., birds and reptiles), the mammalian yolk sac does not enclose a store of yolk.

antigen-dependent differentiation of, 63,
antigen-independent differentiation of, 63
B (bursal), 24
characteristics, 24t, 37–39, 37f, 38t
circulation of, 33–34
classes, 23–24, 24t, 38t
in deuterostomes, 543
distribution/migration during ontogeny, 520f
large granular, 41, 203, 247 (see also Natural killer (NK), cells)
non-B, non-T, 41–42, 203, 203t
null, 24, 41–42
surface receptors, 42–45, 43t, 44h
T (thymic), 24
tumor-infiltrating, 472h
Lymphoid organs, 28f, 29t
architecture, 28
embryonic/fetal, 519–22
phylogeny of, 553–55, 554t
primary, 29–32
secondary, 32–34
Lymphokine
in response to tumors, 461
in Type IV hypersensitivity, 351–53, 352t
Lymphokine-activated killer cell. See LAK cells
Lysozyme, 303

m

MAC. See Membrane attack complex
McDevitt, Hugh O., 180
Macroparasite, 272, 291–98. See also Arthropods Worms
eluding immune defense, by, 315–17, 316t
Macrophage, 24–25
as antigen-presenting cell, 46–47
derivation of, 46f
in deuterostomes, 543
development of function, 532–33
in graft rejection, 493, 495
as initiators of cell-mediated immunity, 205–9
in microbial infections, 303, 307, 308
migration, 205, 213–16, 215h
in parasitic infections, 312, 314
phagocytosis, 205–9, 206f
in response to tumors, 461, 463
roles, 46–47
secretions, 209
tumor associated, 467
in Type III hypersensitivity, 346
in Type IV hypersensitivity, 351–53
Macrophage activating factor (MAF), 241, 308, 352, 462

Macrophage chemotactic factor (MCF), 241, 308, 462
Magainins, 546h
Major histocompatibility antigens
Class I, 129, 182–84, 183f, 190, 232
Class II, 129, 185–86, 185f, 190–91, 232
Class III, 164, 186, 191
specificities, 181–82, 182f, 189–90
typing of, 182, 182f, 183f
Major histocompatibility complex, 22, 39
human (see HLA)
mouse (murine), 180–86, 181f (see also H-2 complex)
phylogeny of, 556–58
in relation to graft rejection, 191, 489–90, 490t
in tolerance induction, 256–58
Major histocompatibility genes, 180–81, 181f, 186–87, 187f
Mantoux test, 353, 354f
Mast cell, 49, 166, 210
degranulation in anaphylaxis, 330–35, 332f, 334h
Maximum tolerated dose, 430
Medawar, Peter B., 21
Megakaryocyte, 9
Membrane attack complex (C5b6789), 152, 156, 157f, 159, 161
Membrane-bound (surface) immunoglobulin, 38, 40, 120
Memory cell, 39, 118, 119, 126, 170, 229, 312
selective loss in AIDS, 390
Metaplasia, 432
Metastasis, 12, 434–36, 449–52
Metchnikoff, Elie, 20–21, 216
MHC. See Major histocompatibility complex
MHC restriction, 180, 184, 184f, 193, 193f, 231, 232–33, 307, 308, 462, 531
MHC self-education, 194–95, 194f
Microbe
life cycles, 273–76
modes of attachment to host cells, 278t
Microenvironments, inducing, 36–37
Microparasite, 272. See also Bacteria; Fungi; Protozoa; and Virus
entry in host, 277–79
evading/overcoming host defenses, 280t, 308–10, 309t
life cycles, 273–76
mechanisms of inducing damage to host, 280–83
spreading through host, 279–80
Migration inhibition factor (MIF), 205, 241, 262
assay for, 215f, 215h, 353
Milieu intérieur, 4
Milstein, C., 66, 137h

Mimetic, 324
Minor histocompatibility antigens, 195–96, 196f
Minor lymphocyte stimulatory genes, 195–96, 232, 263, 556
Mitogen, 44–45, 245, 353
Mitogen receptors, 44
Mixed lymphocyte reaction (culture), 182, 189, 491, 556
MLS genes. See Minor lymphocyte stimulatory genes
Molluscs, immunity in, 541–43
Monocyte, 46, 47f, 346, 532
Monokine, 245
Mononuclear cell, 9, 219. See also Lymphocyte; Monocyte
Montagu, Lady Mary, 17
Mucous membrane, as route of entry for infectious agents, 277–78
Multiple myeloma, 482
Multiple sclerosis, 414–15, 414f
Murray, Joseph, 496
Mutation, in carcinogenesis, 448
Myasthenia gravis, 415–16, 416f
Mycoses, 276
Myeloma, 64, 482
Myeloma protein, 64–65
Myxedema, 411–12

n

Natural cytotoxic (NC) cell, 42
Natural killer (NK)
activity, development of, 532
cells, 42, 170, 246
cytokines produced by, 204
role in graft rejection, 493, 495
role in infectious disease, 306, 314
role in innate cellular immunity, 203–5, 303, 312
role in nonspecific response to tumors, 461, 463
N cells. See Null cells
Nematodes, 296–97, 297f
Neoplasia, 12, 430–34. See also Cancer; Oncogenesis; Tumor
Neuroimmunoendocrinology, 368–72
Neutrophil (PMN), 47–49, 48f
chemotactic factor of anaphylaxis (NCF-A), 333
in innate cellular immunity, 209–10
in microbial infections, 303
in Type III hypersensitivity, 346–47, 348
Nezelof's syndrome, 365
Nitroblue tetrazolium assay (test), 366, 366f
NK cells. See Natural killer (NK), cells
Nude mouse, 32h, 365
Null cells, 42, 203

o

Oncofetal antigen, 465. *See also* α-fetal protein; Carcinoembryonic antigen
Oncogene, 14, 442–49
  cellular, 443, 445–46
  proto-, 443
  relationship between cellular and viral, 446, 446f
  theory/hypothesis, 443
  viral, 441–42
Oncogenesis. *See also* Cancer; Neoplasia; Tumor
  theories of, 437–49, 439t
Oncornavirus, 441–42. *See also* Retrovirus
Opsonin, 167
Opsonization, 167–68, 168f, 542
Ouchterlony, Orjan, 99
Ouchterlony technique, 99, 100f

p

Parasites, 272. *See also* Arthropods; Bacteria; Fungi; Macroparasite; Microparasite; Protozoa; Virus; Worms
  interaction with host, 276–77
  modes of entry to host, 276–79
Paratope, 56, 57f, 58, 124, 125f, 125t
Passive immunity, 17t, 19–20
Pasteur, Louis, 13h, 18
Paternity testing, 342–43, 343f
Pathogenesis, 11
Pathogenicity, 279
Pauling, Linus, 58, 62
Perforin, 204
Pernicious anemia, 407–8, 407f
pFc′ fragment, 70, 70f
Phagocyte, 9, 24t, 25. *See also* Granulocyte; Macrophage
  dysfunctions/disorders of, 366–68, 368t
Phagocytosis, 216
  disorders of, 224–25, 366–68
  microbicidal events of, 207–9, 208f
  stages of, 205–9, 206f
Plasma, 7
Plasma cell, 37f, 39, 40–41, 126
Plasma clotting factors, 216, 217f
Plasmagene theory, 443
Plasmid, 320f
Plasmin, 170
Plasmodium
  antigenic variation, 291h
  life cycle, 288–90, 289F
Platelet, 7, 49, 210
Platelet activating factor (PAF), 210, 333, 347, 348

PMN. *See* Neutrophil
Polymerase chain reaction, 396
Porifera, immunity in, 538–39, 539t
Porter, Rodney R., 22, 67, 71
Prausnitz-Küstner procedure, 335–36, 335f
Precipitin curve, 99, 99f
Precipitin reactions, 97–101, 98t
  in gels, 99–101
  in liquids, 98–99
Primary immune response
  cell-mediated, 229
  humoral, 117
Properdin, 162
Prostaglandins, 209, 212, 246, 333
Protostomes, immunity in, 539–43
Protozoa, 283–90, 285t
  immunity in, 538, 539t, 540f
  life cycles, 285–90, 286f, 287f, 289f
Provirus, 274

q

Qa region, 181f, 184. *See also* Histocompatibility, genes

r

Radioallergosorbent test, 336, 336f
Radioimmunoassay, 93–94, 104–5, 104f, 105h, 404, 405f
  solid phase, 93f
Radioimmunosorbent test, 336
Receptors
  antigen, 42
  assays for, 44h
  complement, 43
  Fc, 43
  surface, 42–45, 43t
Recombinase, 136
Recombinatorial germline theory, 134, *See also* Immunoglobulin genes
Red pulp. *See* Spleen
Repressor genes, 14. *See also* Suppressor gene
Reticular dysgenesis, 361
Retinoblastoma, 446, 450h, 451f
Retrovirus
  oncogene expression of, 441–42, 441f
  replication, 386f
Rheumatoid arthritis, 400, 406, 416–18, 417f
Rheumatoid factor, 102, 400, 406, 416, 418
Richet, Charles, 19–20
Rosette formation, 44f, 44h
Rous, Peyton, 440

s

Scatchard plot, 91–93, 92f
Schultz-Dale test, 336
scid. See Severe combined immune deficiency (*scid*)
Secondary immune response
  cell-mediated, 229
  humoral, 117–19
Serotonin, 212, 333
Serum electrophoresis, 63–64, 66f
Serum sickness, 347–48, 349t. *See also* Hypersensitivity, Type III
Severe combined immune deficiency (*scid*), 365–66
Signal sequences for V-J joining, 138
Simian immunodeficiency virus (SIV), 391
Skin, as site of entry for infectious agents, 277–78
SLE. *See* Systemic lupus erythematosus
Slow-reacting substance of anaphylaxis (SRS-A), 333, 338. *See also* Leukotrienes
Snell, George, 178
Soluble inhibitory factor, 513
Somatic mutation
  role in autoimmune disease, 401
  role in generation of antibody diversity, 146–47
Spacers, 138
Specificity
  antigen-antibody (*see* Antibody, specificity)
  private, 181, 182f
  public, 181, 182f
Spleen, 33–34, 33f, 519
Spleen colony assay, 36f
Splicing, gene, 142
Spontaneous generation, theory of, 13h
Steady state, 4. *See also* Homeostasis
Stem cells, 29, 30t
  disorders of, 361–63, 361t
  relation to derivatives, 35–37, 35f, 36f
Superantigen, 196, 232, 308
Suppressor factor, 127, 133, 244
Suppressor gene, 14. *See also* Antioncogene
Switch sequence, 145. *See also* Heavy (H) chain, class switching
Switch site, 145. *See also* Heavy (H) chain, class switching
Syphilis
  secondary, 351
  tertiary, 355–56
Systemic lupus erythematosus, 418–20
  characteristic cell, 419, 419f
  immunological activities of, 419–20, 420f